Reviewers

ELAINE ATKINS, RN
Louisiana Technical College–Huey P. Long Campus
Winnfield, Louisiana

JOYCE HARRIS, RN, MA Ed
Butler County Career and Technology Center
Hamilton, Ohio

MICHAEL JOHNSON, ADN, CEN, ACLS,
   PALS, ENPC, BTL
Tennessee Technology Center at Nashville
Nashville, Tennessee

LINDA KERBY, RNC, BSN, MA, BA
Educational Consultant
Leawood, Kansas

MARY A. DUESTERHAUS MINOR, MS, PT
Sanford-Brown College
Hazelwood, Missouri

VIRGINIA OSTING, BSN, MSN, RN
College of Health Sciences
Roanoke, Virginia

RON SCOTT, JD, LLM, MSBA, MSPT, OCS
Lebanon Valley College
Annville, Pennsylvania

GINA SIRACH, RN, BSN
Southeastern Illinois College
Harrisburg, Illinois

JULIE A. SLACK, RN, BS, ICCE
Dixie College
St. George, Utah

MARTHA E. SPRAY, RN, BSN, MS
Formerly, Mid East Ohio Vocational School
Zanesville, Ohio

GEORGETTA STREET, RN, ACLS, BLS
Tennessee Technology Center at Hohenwald
Hohenwald, Tennessee

ANN D. SUMNERS, BSN, MN, PhD
North Georgia College and State University
Dahlonega, Georgia

LYNNE TAYLOR, BSN, TNS, ACLS
Applied Technology Services
Chesterfield, Missouri

SANDRA WAKEFIELD, RN, BS Ed
Tennessee Technology Center at Nashville
Nashville, Tennessee

Foundations of
Mental Health Care

second edition

MICHELLE MORRISON VALFRE, RN, BSN, MHS, FNP

Health Care Educator/Consultant
Health and Educational Consultants, Inc.
Tucson, Arizona

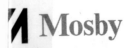

Mosby
Imprint of Elsevier Science
ndon Philadelphia Sydney Toronto

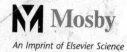
Mosby

An Imprint of Elsevier Science

Vice President and Publishing Director, Nursing: Sally Schrefer
Senior Editor: Terri Wood
Editor: Yvonne Alexopoulos
Developmental Editor: Kimberly Netterville
Associate Developmental Editor: Teena Ferroni
Project Manager: John Rogers
Project Specialist: Cheryl A. Abbott
Designer: Kathi Gosche

NOTICE

Pharmacology is an ever-changing field. Standard safety precautions must be followed, but as new research and clinical experience broaden our knowledge, changes in treatment and drug therapy may become necessary or appropriate. Readers are advised to check the most current product information provided by the manufacturer of each drug to be administered to verify the recommended dose, the method and duration of administration, and contraindications. It is the responsibility of the licensed prescriber, relying on experience and knowledge of the patient, to determine dosages and the best treatment for each individual patient. Neither the publisher nor the editor assumes any liability for any injury and/or damage to persons or property arising from this publication.

Mosby, Inc.
An Imprint of Elsevier Science
11830 Westline Industrial Drive
St. Louis, Missouri 63146

Printed in the United States of America

International Standard Book Number 0-323-01168-3

02 03 04 05 GW/KPT 9 8 7 6 5 4 3 2

Preface

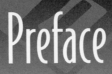

This book is intended for students and practitioners of the health care professions. Nursing students will find the information in this text useful and easy to apply in a variety of clinical settings. Students in fields such as social work, respiratory therapy, physical therapy, recreational therapy, occupational therapy, rehabilitation, and medical assistance will find concise explanations of effective and maladaptive human behaviors, as well as the most current therapeutic interventions and treatments. Practicing health care providers—anyone caring for clients in a therapeutic manner—will find this book a practical and useful guide in any health care setting.

The purpose of this book is threefold:

1. To help soften the social distinction between mental "health" and mental "illness," which is actually a matter of how effectively one is coping.
2. To assist nurses and other health care providers in working comfortably with clients who exhibit a wide range of maladaptive behaviors.
3. To apply the concepts of holistic care when assisting clients in developing more effective attitudes and behaviors.

CONTENTS

Unit One, **Mental Health Care: Past, Present, and Future,** provides a framework for mental health care. The evolution of care for persons with mental health problems from primitive to current times is described. Selected ethical, legal, social, and cultural issues relating to mental health care are explored. Community mental health care is explained, followed by chapters pertaining to theories of mental illness, therapeutic modalities, and psychotherapeutic drug therapy.

Unit Two, **The Caregiver's Therapeutic Skills,** focuses on the skills and conditions necessary for working with clients. Eight principles of mental health care are discussed and then applied to the therapeutic environment, the helping relationship, and effective communications. A chapter devoted to self-awareness encourages the reader to develop introspection—a necessary component for working with people who have behavioral difficulties. Characteristics of basic human needs, personality development, stress, anxiety, crisis, and coping behaviors help the reader explore behaviors common to us all. The section concludes with a description of the basic mental health assessment skills needed by every health care provider.

Unit Three, **Mental Health Problems Throughout the Life Cycle,** focuses on the growth of "normal" (adaptive) mental health behaviors during each developmental stage. The most common mental health disorders associated with children, adolescents, adults, and older adults listed in the *Diagnostic and Statistical Manual of Mental Disorders* (DSM-IV–TR) are discussed.

Unit Four, **Clients With Psychological Problems,** explores common behavioral responses and therapeutic interventions for illness, hospitalization, loss, grief, and depression. Maladaptive behaviors and mental health disorders are described in chapters on somatoform, anxiety, eating, sleeping, mood, sexual, and dissociative disorders.

The chapters in Unit Five, **Clients With Psychosocial Problems,** relate to the important social concerns of anger and its expressions, suicide, abuse and neglect, HIV/AIDS, and substance abuse. Sexual and personality disorders are also discussed. Chapters on schizophrenia and chronic mental illness focus on a multidisciplinary approach for treatment. A chapter titled "Challenges for the Future" concludes the section.

FEATURES

Throughout the text, cultural aspects of various mental health principles are explored. Because the majority of mental health care takes place outside the institution, the importance of using therapeutic mental health interventions during every client interaction is emphasized. Numerous **Case Studies** with thought-provoking questions encourage readers to consider the psychosocial aspects of providing therapeutic care in both community and hospital settings. Descriptions of each mental health disorder are drawn from DSM-IV–TR criteria. Nursing diagnoses are stated in terms approved by the North American Nursing Diagnosis Association (NANDA).

Each chapter begins with **Learning Objectives** and a list of **Key Terms**. The chapters conclude with a brief review of **Key Concepts, Suggestions for Further Reading** that encourage further exploration of the topics presented in that chapter, and, in some chapters, Internet site addresses.

Unique to this text are the **Review Worksheets** for each chapter, located in the back of the book. Because the worksheet sections are perforated, the sheets can be removed and submitted to the instructor, thus eliminating the need for a separate student workbook. Throughout the text, the liberal use of boxes, tables, and figures simplifies important concepts and stresses essential information. **Think About** and **Cultural Aspects** boxes stimulate critical thought and discussion. **Drug Alert** boxes identify important points relating to psychotherapeutic medications. New to this edition are multidisciplinary **Sample Client Care Plans,** which address how members of the health care team work together to meet client needs. Throughout the book, the holistic approach to care offers readers a view of the "whole person" context of health care.

Appendixes relating to the latest standards of mental health care, a list of DSM-IV–TR diagnoses, a tool for assessing the side effects of antipsychotic medication, and a mental status assessment tool are included. A **Glossary,** written in easy-to-understand terms, concludes the text.

INSTRUCTOR'S RESOURCE MANUAL

The *Instructor's Resource Manual* was developed to assist health care educators, from the novice to those with long-term teaching experience. Section I provides **Teaching Strategies.** Section II provides **Chapter Resources:** expanded **Learning Objectives** (which are referenced to the text by page numbers), **Lecture Outline, Guidelines for Discussion and Critical Thinking Case Study,** and **Clinical Enrichment Activities** for both hospital and community health care settings. A special feature called **Guidelines for Integration** helps instructors merge and blend the important principles of mental health care into all areas of client care. Section III provides the **Answers to Chapter Worksheets.** Section IV, a **Test Bank** with 500 NCLEX-style multiple-choice questions, completes the manual.

ACKNOWLEDGMENTS

No text is written alone. The continued support of my husband Adolph, friends, and colleagues has provided the energy to complete this project when my own was low. The guidance, expertise, and encouragement from Yvonne Alexopoulos, Editor; Kimberly Netterville, Developmental Editor; Terri Wood, Senior Editor; Teena Ferroni, Associate Developmental Editor; Catherine Ott, Editorial Assistant; and Cheryl Abbott, Project Specialist, is much appreciated. Finally, I would like to thank all the health care providers who so freely share their expertise with those who want to learn more about the dynamic and complex nature of human behavior.

Michelle Morrison Valfre

Brief Contents

Detailed Contents

Chapter 1

The History of Mental Health Care

Learning Objectives

1. Develop a working definition of mental health and mental illness.
2. List three major factors believed to influence the development of mental illness.
3. Describe the role of the Church in the care of the mentally ill during the Middle Ages.
4. Identify the contributions made by Philippe Pinel, Dorothea Dix, and Clifford Beers to the care of persons with mental disorders.
5. Discuss the impact of World Wars I and II on American attitudes toward the mentally ill.
6. State the major change in the care of the mentally ill resulting from the discovery of psychotherapeutic drugs.
7. Describe the development of community mental health care centers during the 1960s and 1970s.
8. Discuss the shift of mentally ill clients from institutional care to community-based care.
9. Explain how the Omnibus Budget Reconciliation Act of 1981 and the Omnibus Budget Reform Act (OBRA) has affected mental health care.

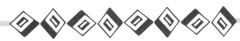

Key Terms

catchment area

deinstitutionalization

demonical exorcisms

electroconvulsive therapy

health-illness continuum

humoral theory of disease

lobotomy

lunacy

mental health

mental illness (disorder)

psychotherapeutic drugs

Mental or emotional health is interwoven with physical health. Behaviors relating to health exist over a broad spectrum, often referred to as the **health-illness continuum** (Figure 1-1). People who are exceptionally healthy are represented at the high-level wellness end of the continuum. Severely ill individuals fall at the continuum's opposite end. Most of us, however, function somewhere between these two extremes. As we meet with the stresses of life, our abilities to cope are repeatedly challenged and we strive to adjust in effective ways. When stress is physical, the body calls forth its defense systems and wards off physical illness. When the challenge is of an emotional or developmental nature, we respond by creating new (and hopefully effective) behaviors.

Mental health is the ability to "cope with and adjust to the recurrent stresses of living in an acceptable way" (Anderson, 1998). Mentally healthy people are able to successfully carry out the activities of daily living, solve problems, set goals, adapt to change, and enjoy life. They are self-aware, directed, and responsible for their actions. In short, mentally healthy people cope well.

Mental health is influenced by three factors: inherited characteristics, childhood nurturing, and life circum-

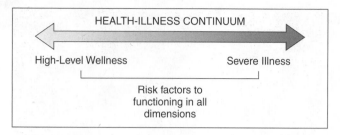

Figure 1-1 The health-illness continuum, ranging from high-level wellness to severe illness, provides a method of identifying a client's level of health.

stances. When a problem arises in any one area, the risk of developing ineffective coping behaviors increases. If behaviors interfere with daily activities, impair judgment, or alter reality, the person is said to be mentally ill. Simply put, a **mental illness (disorder)** is a disturbance in one's ability to cope effectively. History is rich with examples of changing attitudes toward people with mental health problems.

EARLY YEARS

Illness, injury, and insanity have concerned humanity throughout history. Illness and injury were easy to detect with the senses. Mental illness (insanity) was something different—something that could not be seen or felt—and therefore a condition to be feared.

Primitive Societies

Although the historical record is vague, it can be assumed that some care was given to the sick. Early societies believed that everything in nature was alive with spirits. Illness, both mental and physical, was thought to be caused by the wrath of evil spirits. People with mental illnesses were, therefore, possessed by demons or the forces of evil.

Treatments for mental illness focused on removing the evil spirits from the patient. Magical therapies made use of "frightening masks and noises, incantations, vile odors, charms, spells, sacrifices and fetishes" (Kelly, 1991). Physical treatments included bleeding, massage, blistering, inducing vomiting, and the practice of trephining—cutting holes in the skull to encourage the evil spirits to leave.

Mentally ill individuals were allowed to remain within society as long as their behaviors were not disruptive. Severely ill or violent members of the group were often driven into the wilderness to fend for themselves.

Greece and Rome

Superstitions and magical beliefs dominated thinking about illness until the Greeks introduced the idea that mental illness could be rationally explained through observation. Explanations about the cause and effect of illnesses gradually replaced most superstitions.

The Greeks incorporated many ideas about illness from other civilizations of the day. By the sixth century BC, medical schools were well established. The greatest physician in Greek medicine, Hippocrates, was born in 460 BC. He was the first physician to base treatment on the belief that nature has a strong healing force. He felt that the role of the physician was to assist in, rather than direct, the healing process. Proper diet, exercise, and personal hygiene were his mainstays of treatment. Hippocrates viewed mental illness as a result of an imbalance of humors—the fundamental elements of air, fire, water, and earth. Each basic element had a related humor or part in the body: blood, yellow bile, phlegm, and black bile. An overabundance or lack of one or more humors resulted in illness. This view (called the **humoral theory of disease**) persisted for centuries.

Plato (427-347 BC), a Greek philosopher, recognized life as a dynamic balance maintained by the soul. According to Plato, the soul was divided into a "rational soul," which resided in the head, and an "irrational soul," which was found in the heart and abdomen. He believed that if the rational soul was unable to control the undirected parts of the irrational soul, mental illness resulted. In theory Plato anticipated Sigmund Freud by almost 2000 years.

The principles and practices of Greek medicine became established in Rome around 100 BC, but most physicians still thought that demons caused mental illness. The practice of frightening away evil spirits to cure mental illness was reintroduced about this time and continued well into the Middle Ages.

The Romans showed little interest in learning about the body or mind. Most Roman physicians "wanted to make their patients comfortable by pleasant physical therapies" (Alexander and Selesnick, 1966), such as warm baths, massage, music, and peaceful surroundings. Reasons for the collapse of the Roman Empire remain unclear, but repeated invasions from barbaric tribes and plagues were two important elements in its downfall.

By AD 300 "six epidemics killed hundreds of thousands of people and desolated the land" (Alexander and Selesnick, 1966). Churches became sanctuaries for the sick, and soon hospitals were built to accommodate the sufferers. By AD 370 Saint Basil's Hospital in England offered services for the sick, orphaned, crippled, and mentally troubled.

Middle Ages

Dark Ages
From about AD 500 to 1100, care for the sick shifted from physicians to priests. The Church developed into a highly organized and powerful institution. Early Christians believed that "disease was either punishment for

sins, possession by the devil, or the result of witchcraft" (Ackerknecht, 1968). To cure mental illness priests performed **demonical exorcisms**—religious ceremonies in which the patients were physically punished to drive away the evil possessing spirit. However, these practices were tempered by the spirit of Christian charity as members of the community cared for the mentally ill with concern and sympathy.

As time passed, medieval society declined. Repeated attacks from barbaric tribes led to chaos and moral decay. Epidemics, natural disasters, and overwhelming taxes wiped out the middle class. Cities, industries, and commerce disappeared. "The population declined, crime waves occurred, poverty was abysmal, and torture and imprisonment became prominent as civilization seemed to slip back into semi-barbarianism" (Donahue, 1996). Only monasteries remained as the last refuge of knowledge.

Throughout the Middle Ages, medicine and religion were interwoven. However, by 1130, laws were passed forbidding monks to practice medicine because it was considered too disruptive to their way of life. As a result the responsibility for the care of the sick once again fell to the community.

In the late 1100s a strong Arabic influence was felt in Europe. Knowledge of the Greek legacy had been retained and improved on by the Arabs, who had an extensive knowledge of drugs, mathematics, astronomy, and chemistry, as well as an awareness of the relationship between emotions and disease. The Arabic influence resulted in the establishment of learning centers, called *universities*. Many were devoted to the study of medicine and surgery and the care of the sick.

Problems of the mind, however, received only spiritual attention. Church doctrine still stated that humans were the center of the universe and if a person was insane, it must be the result of some external force—a heavenly body such as the moon. Thus the term **lunacy** was coined and "literally means a disorder caused by a lunar body" (Alexander and Selesnick, 1966).

In time, large institutions were established, and the mentally ill were herded into these "lunatic asylums." Magic was still relied on to explain the torments of the mind. A few church scholars even suggested that witches might be the source of human distresses.

Superstitions, Witches, and Hunters

The Church's doctrine of imposed celibacy failed to curtail many of the clergy's sexual behaviors. The Church began an antierotic movement that focused on women as the cause of men's lust. According to the movement, women were carriers of the devil because they stirred men's passions. "Psychotic women with little control over voicing their sexual fantasies and sacrilegious feelings were the clearest examples of demoniacal possession" (Alexander and Selesnick, 1966). This campaign, in turn,

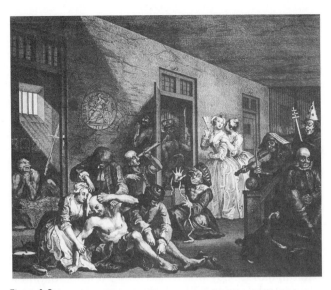

Figure 1-2 Bethlehem Royal Hospital in London. (William Hogarth, "The Rake in Bedlam," c. 1735. From the series entitled *The Rake's Progress*. Copyright The British Museum, London.)

flamed the public's mounting fear of mentally troubled people.

Witch hunting was officially launched in 1487 with the publication of the book *The Witches' Hammer*, a textbook of both pornography and psychopathology. Soon after its publication, Pope Innocent VIII and the University of Cologne voiced support for this "textbook of the Inquisition." As a result of this one publication, women, as well as children and the mentally ill, were tortured and burned at the stake by the thousands. There were few safe havens for individuals with mental illness during these troubled times.

Bethlehem Royal Hospital

The first English institution for the mentally ill was initially a hospice founded in 1247 by the sheriff of London. By 1330 Bethlehem had become a lunatic asylum that eventually became infamous for its brutal treatments. Violently ill patients were chained to walls in small cells. These patients provided "entertainment" for the public; the hospital would charge fees for their "tourist attractions" and conduct tours through the institution. Less violent patients were forced to wear identifying metal armbands and beg on the streets. The insane were harshly treated, but Bethlehem Hospital, commonly known as Bedlam (Figure 1-2), was preferable to burning at the stake.

By the middle of the fourteenth century the European continent had endured several devastating plagues and epidemics. One quarter of the Earth's population, more than 60 million people, perished from infectious diseases during this period in history. The feudal system lost power and declined. Cities began to flourish and house a growing middle class. "Luxury and misery, learning and ignorance existed side by side" (Donahue, 1996). Society was at last beginning to demand reforms. Yet, as the age of art, medicine, and science dawned, the hunting of "witches" became even more popular. It was a time of great contradictions.

The Renaissance

The Renaissance began about 1400 in Italy and spread throughout the European continent within a century. Upheavals in economics, politics, education, and commerce brought the real world into focus. The power of the Church to regulate people's activities slowly declined as an intense interest in material gain and worldly affairs began to develop. At the same time, the medieval view of a sinful, naked body was replaced by a celebration of the human form by such artists as da Vinci, Raphael, and Michelangelo. Thousand-year-old anatomy books were replaced by realistic anatomical drawings. Observation, rather than ancient theories, revolutionized many of the ideas of the day.

Sixteenth-century physicians, relying on observation, began to record what they saw. Mental illness was at last being recognized without bias. By the mid-1500s behaviors were accurately recorded for melancholia (depression), mania, and psychopathic personalities. Precise observations led to classifications for different abnormal behaviors. Mental problems were now thought to be caused by some sort of brain disorder—except in the case of sexual fantasies, which were still considered to be caused by God's punishment or possession by the devil. However, despite great advances the actual treatment of mentally troubled people remained inhumane.

The Reformation

Another movement that influenced the care of the sick—the Reformation—occurred in 1517. People were displeased with the conduct of the clergy and the widespread abuses occurring within the Catholic Church. Martin Luther (1483-1546), a dissatisfied monk, and his followers broke away from the Catholic Church and became known as Protestants. As a result of this separation, many hospitals operated by the Catholic Church began to close. Once again, the poor, sick, and insane were turned out into the streets.

Seventeenth Century

During the seventeenth and eighteenth centuries, developments in science, literature, philosophy, and the arts laid the foundations for the modern world. Reason was slowly beginning to replace magical thinking, but a strong belief in the influences of demons still persisted.

The 1600s produced many great thinkers. Knowledge of the secrets of nature brought a sense of self-reliance.

However, many people were uncomfortable so they, once again, moved toward the security of witch hunting as a means of protecting themselves from the unexplainable. It was during the seventeenth century that conditions for the mentally ill were at their worst. While physicians and theorists were making observations and speculations about insanity, the mentally troubled were bled, starved, beaten, and purged into submission. Treatments for these people remained in this unhappy state of affairs until the late 1700s.

Eighteenth Century

During the latter part of the eighteenth century, psychiatry developed as a separate branch of medicine. Inhumane treatment and vicious practices were now openly questioned. In 1792 Philippe Pinel (1745-1826), the director of two Paris hospitals, liberated the mentally ill from their chains "and advocated acceptance of the mentally ill as human beings in need of medical assistance, nursing care, and social services" (Donahue, 1996). During this period the Quakers, a religious order, established asylums of humane care in England.

In the American colonies the Philadelphia Almshouse was erected in 1731. It accepted sick, infirm, and insane patients, as well as prisoners and orphans. In 1794 Bellevue Hospital in New York City was opened as a pesthouse for the victims of yellow fever. By 1816 the hospital had enlarged to contain an almshouse for the poor, wards for the sick and insane, staff quarters, and even a penitentiary.

Unfortunately, the care and treatment of people with mental illness remained as harsh and indifferent in the United States as it was in Europe. The practice of allowing

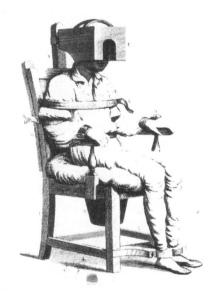

Figure 1-3 Tranquilizing chair. (Courtesy National Library of Medicine, Bethesda, Md.)

the poor to care for the mentally ill continued well into the late 1800s and was only slowly abandoned. Actual care of mentally ill persons in the United States did not begin to improve until the arrival of Alice Fisher, a Florence Nightingale–trained nurse, in 1884.

By the close of the eighteenth century, treatments for people with mental illness still included the medieval practices of bloodletting, purging, and confinement. Newer therapies included the tranquilizing chair, whirling devices, and circulation swings (Figure 1-3). The study of psychiatry was in its infancy, and those who actually cared for the insane still relied heavily on the methods of their ancestors.

NINETEENTH-CENTURY UNITED STATES

By the early 1800s the Revolutionary War had ended and the United States was a growing nation. Changes that occurred during this century had an enormous impact on the care of the mentally ill for years to come.

One of the most important figures in nineteenth-century psychiatry was Dr. Benjamin Rush, a crusader for the insane. Dr. Rush (1745-1813) graduated from Princeton University at age 15. By age 31 Rush had been a professor of chemistry and medicine, a chief surgeon in the Continental Army, and a signer of the Declaration of Independence. His book, titled *Diseases of the Mind,* was the first psychiatric text written in the United States. In his book he advocated clean conditions; good air, lighting, and food; and kindness. As a result of Rush's efforts the mentally troubled were no longer caged in the basements of general hospitals. However, only a few institutions for the insane were available in the United States at this time. Mildly affected people were commonly sold at slave auctions, whereas the more violent remained in asylums that were a combination of zoo and penitentiary.

During the 1830s, attitudes toward mental illness slowly began to change. The "once insane always insane" concept was being replaced by the notion that cure may be possible. A few mental hospitals were built, but the actual living conditions for most patients remained deplorable.

It was not until 1841 that a frail 40-year-old schoolteacher exposed the sins of the system. Dorothea Dix was contracted to teach Sunday school at a jail in Massachusetts. While there, she observed both criminals and mentally ill prisoners living in squalid conditions. For the next 20 years Dix surveyed asylums, jails, and almshouses throughout the United States, Canada, and Scotland. It was not uncommon for her to find mentally ill people "confined in cages, closets, cellars, stalls, and pens . . . chained, naked, beaten with rods and lashed into obedience" (Dolan, 1968).

Dorothea Dix's untiring crusade had results that shook the world. She presented her findings to anyone who would listen. The public became so aroused by Dix's efforts that millions of dollars were raised, more than 30 mental hospitals throughout the United States were constructed, and standards for the care of the insane were greatly improved.

By the late 1800s a two-class system of psychiatric care had emerged: private care for the wealthy and publicly provided care for the remainder of society. The newly constructed mental institutions quickly became filled, and soon chronic overcrowding began to strain the system. Cure rates fell dramatically. The public became disenchanted, and mental illness once again was viewed as incurable.

Only small, private facilities that catered to the wealthy had some degree of success, and those patients were well treated. State facilities evolved into large, remote institutions that became completely self-reliant and removed from society.

By the close of the nineteenth century, many of the gains in the care for the mentally ill had been lost. Overpopulated institutions could offer no more than minimal custodial care. Theories of the day gave no satisfactory explanations about the causes of mental problems, and current treatments were ineffective. It was a time of therapeutic despair for the mentally troubled and those who cared for them.

TWENTIETH CENTURY

The 1900s were ushered in by reform movements. Political, economic, and social changes were beginning. For the first time in history, disease prevention was emphasized. For the mentally ill, however, conditions remained intolerable until 1908, when a single individual began his crusade.

Clifford Beers was a young student at Yale University when he attempted suicide. Consequently, he spent 3 years as a patient in mental hospitals in Connecticut. On his release in 1908, Beers wrote a book that would set the wheels of the mental hygiene movement in motion. His book, *A Mind That Found Itself,* recounted the beatings, isolation, and confinement of a mentally ill person. As a direct result of Beers' work, the Committee for Mental Hygiene was formed in 1909. Along with prevention the group focused on removing the stigma attached to mental illness. Under Beers' energetic guidance, the movement grew nationwide. The social consciousness of a nation had finally been awakened.

Psychoanalysis

In the early 1900s a neurophysiologist named Sigmund Freud published the article that introduced the term *psychoanalysis* to the world's vocabulary. Freud believed that forces both within and outside the personality were responsible for mental illness. He developed elaborate theories around the central theme of repressed sexual energies (see Chapter 5). Freud was the first person who succeeded in "explaining human behavior in psychological terms and in demonstration that behavior can be changed under the proper circumstances" (Alexander and Selesnick, 1966). The first comprehensive theory of mental illness based on observation had emerged, and psychoanalysis began to gain a strong hold in the United States.

Influences of War

By 1917 the United States had entered World War I. Men were drafted into service as rapidly as they could be processed, but many were considered too "mentally deficient" to fight. As a result the federal government called on Beers' Committee for Mental Hygiene to develop a master plan for screening and treating mentally ill soldiers. The completed plan included methods for early identification of problems, removal of mentally troubled personnel from combat duty, and early treatment close to the fighting front. The committee also recommended that psychiatrists be assigned to station hospitals to treat soldiers who returned from combat with acute behavioral problems and to provide ongoing psychiatric care after soldiers returned to their homes.

Because of the war a renewed interest in mental hygiene evolved. During the 1930s new therapies for treating insanity were developed. Insulin therapy for schizophrenia induced 50-hour comas through the administration of massive doses of insulin. Passing electricity through the patient's head (**electroconvulsive therapy**) helped to improve severe depression, and **lobotomy** (a surgical procedure that severs the frontal lobes of the brain from the thalamus) almost eliminated violent behaviors. A new class of drugs that lifted the spirits of depressed people, *amphetamines,* was introduced. These therapies improved behaviors and made patients more receptive to Freud's psychotherapy. In 1937 the U.S. Congress passed the Hill-Burton Act, which funded the construction of psychiatric units throughout the country.

From 1941 to 1945 the United States was immersed in World War II. Many draftees were still rejected on enlistment because of mental health problems. A large number of soldiers received early discharges based on psychiatric disorders, and many active-duty personnel received treatment for psychiatric problems.

In 1946 Congress passed the National Mental Health Act, which provided funding for programs in research, training of mental health professionals, and expansion of state mental health facilities. By 1949 the National Institute of Mental Health was organized to provide research and training related to mental illness. New approaches to the care of the mentally ill (e.g., therapeutic community movement, family care, halfway houses) began to spark the public's enthusiasm.

The Korean War of the 1950s and the Vietnam War of the 1960s and 1970s contributed significant knowledge to the understanding of stress-related problems. *Posttraumatic stress disorders* became recognized among soldiers fighting wars. Today, stress disorders are now recognized as the basis of many emotional problems encountered by mental health care providers.

Introduction of Psychotherapeutic Drugs

Psychotherapeutic drugs are chemicals that effect the mind. These drugs alter emotions, perceptions, and consciousness in several ways and are used in combination with various therapies for treating mental illness. Psychotherapeutic drugs are also called psychopharmacologic agents, psychotropic drugs, and psychoactive drugs.

"By the 1950s, more than half the hospital beds in the United States were in psychiatric wards" (Taylor, 1994). Patients were usually treated kindly, but effective therapies were still limited. Treatments consisted of psychoanalysis, insulin therapy, electroconvulsive (shock) therapy, and water/ice therapy. More violent patients were physically restrained in straitjackets or underwent lobotomy. Drug therapy consisted of sedatives (chloral hydrate and paraldehyde), barbiturates (phenobarbital), and amphetamines, which quieted patients but did little to treat their illnesses.

In 1949 an Australian physician, John Cade, discovered that lithium carbonate was effective in controlling the severe mood swings seen in bipolar (manic-depressive) illness. With lithium therapy many chronically ill clients were again able to lead normal lives and were released from mental institutions.

Sparked by the apparent success of lithium, researchers began to explore the possibility of controlling mental illness with the use of various antipsychotic drugs. Chlorpromazine (Thorazine) was introduced in 1956 and proved to control many of the bizarre behaviors observed in schizophrenia and other psychoses (Keltner and Folks, 2001). The 1950s concluded with the introduction of imipramine, the first antidepressant. Soon other drugs, such as anxiety agents, became available for use in treatment.

As more patients were able to control their behaviors with drug therapy, the demand for hospitalization decreased. Many people with mental disorders could now live and function outside the institution. At this time the federal government began the movement called **deinstitutionalization,** the release of large numbers of mentally ill persons into the community. To illustrate, 560,000 patients were cared for in state hospitals in 1955. By 1994 the number of institutionalized patients had dropped to less than 120,000 people (Harrington, 1999). The introduction of psychotherapeutic drugs opened the doors of institutions and set the stage for a new delivery system—community mental health care.

FROM THE INSTITUTION TO THE COMMUNITY

The 1960s was a decade filled with social changes. With the introduction of psychotherapeutic drugs came the concept of the "least restrictive alternative." If patients could, with medication, control their behaviors and cooperate with treatment plans, then the restrictive environment of the institution was no longer necessary. It was believed that people with mental disorders could live within their communities and work with their therapists on an outpatient basis. In 1961 the Joint Commission on Mental Illness and Health published a 338-page report titled *Action for Mental Health*. The report motivated President John Kennedy to appoint a special committee to study the problem of mental illness and recommend specific actions. The recommendations from Kennedy's committee called for a bold new approach to mental health care, which included the development of an entirely new entity—the community mental health center.

Congressional Actions

As the population of people with mental illnesses shifted from the institution to the community, the demand for community mental health services expanded. To meet this demand, the federal government acted to establish a nationwide network of community mental health centers.

The Community Mental Health Centers Act was passed by Congress in October 1963. This act was designed to support the construction of mental health centers in communities throughout the United States. There, the needs of all people experiencing mental and emotional problems, as well as those of the acute and chronic mentally ill, would be met. Physicians (psychiatrists), nurses, and various therapists would develop therapeutic relationships with their clients and monitor their progress within the community setting. Each center was to provide comprehensive mental health services for all residents within a certain geographical region, called a **catchment area.**

It was believed that the community mental health centers would provide the link in helping mentally ill people make the transition from the institution to the community, thus meeting the goal of humane care delivered in the least restrictive way. Passage of the Medicare/Medicaid Bill of 1965, combined with the Community Mental Health Centers Act, led to the release of more than 75% of institutionalized mentally ill persons into the community (Morrissey and Goldman, 1984). Unfortunately, most chronically mentally ill people were "dumped" into their communities before realistic strategies, programs, and facilities were in place.

Community mental health centers expanded throughout the 1970s, but funding was inadequate and sporadic. Demands for services overwhelmed the system, and non–revenue-generating services (prevention and educa-

tion) were eliminated. Services for the general public dwindled and many centers began to close their doors. Finally, in 1975 Congress passed amendments to the Community Mental Health Centers Act that provided funding for community centers based on a complex set of guidelines.

The President's Commission on Mental Health was established in 1978 by President Jimmy Carter. Its task was to assess the mental health needs of the nation and recommend possible courses of action to strengthen and improve existing community mental health efforts. The commission's final report resulted in 117 specific recommendations grouped into four broad areas: coordination of services, high-risk populations, flexibility in planning services, and least restrictive care alternatives.

By 1980 Congress passed one of the most progressive mental health bills in history. *The Mental Health Systems Act* addressed community mental health care, clients' rights, and established priorities for research and training. However, before the recommendations could be nationally implemented, the country elected a new president, and mental health reform changed dramatically.

Just as legislation that comprehensively dealt with mental health issues was about to be enacted, the political climate changed. In 1981 Ronald Reagan's conservative administration drastically reduced federal funding for all mental health services (including research and training) through passage of the Omnibus Budget Reconciliation Act of 1981, which essentially repealed the Mental Health Systems Act. This resulted in *block grant funding* whereby each state received a "block" or designated amount of federal money. The state then determined where and how the money was spent. Unfortunately, many states proved less committed to mental health in the use of their block grant money. As a result many of the hospitalized mentally ill (especially the elderly) were transferred to less appropriate nursing homes or other community facilities.

To stem the practice of inappropriate placement for the chronic mentally ill, the Omnibus Budget Reform Act (OBRA) was passed in 1987. Because people with chronic mental problems could no longer be "warehoused" in nursing homes or other long-term facilities, many were discharged to the streets. As concern for a rapidly expanding federal budget deficit grew, funding for mental health care dwindled. By the late 1980s, funding was curtailed for most inpatient psychiatric care. Following the trend, most insurance companies withdrew their coverage for psychiatric care. At present, Congress is introducing bills that would require employers to provide *parity* (insurance for mental health care that is equal to that for physical care) for their employees.

Today, many of our population's most severely mentally ill wander the streets in abject poverty and homelessness as a result of federal and state funding cuts. Community mental health centers have closed their doors

Think About
- What are the most important priorities in a national health care plan?
- What priority would you give to care of people with mental illness?

or drastically reduced their services. Federal funding is limited to block grants (for all health care) to each state. The original goals of comprehensive care, education, rehabilitation, prevention, training, and research became lost in the efforts to curtail costs.

Currently, lawmakers in the United States are struggling to define a new national health policy. Models for delivering effective, cost-effective health care are being investigated. Other countries, such as Canada and the United Kingdom, are faced with similar mental health care issues. It is in all of our best interests that we accept the challenge to address and provide for our societies' mental and physical health care needs. The Think About box offers something to consider.

KEY CONCEPTS

- Mental health is the ability to cope with and adapt to the stresses of everyday life.
- Mentally healthy people are self-aware, directed, and responsible for their actions.
- Mental illness is an inability to cope, which results in impaired functioning.
- The history of mental illness and its treatment is based on superstition, magical beliefs, and demonic possession practices from primitive societies into the 1800s.
- Priests cared for the sick and exorcised demons, but the mentally troubled were treated with care by the Christian community during the Middle Ages.
- By the late Middle Ages large institutions (asylums) housed the insane and the belief that witches were the carriers of the devil led to the burning of thousands of women, children, and mentally ill people.
- By the 1500s psychotic behaviors were being accurately observed and recorded, but the Reformation movement returned many of the insane to the streets as church sanctuaries closed.

- During the 1800s Americans Dr. Benjamin Rush and Dorothea Dix crusaded for the humane care of the mentally ill.
- Standards for the care of the insane improved during the mid-1800s until huge waves of people overwhelmed the mental health care system, causing the conditions for patients to deteriorate.
- A book written by Clifford Beers about his 3-year experience as a mental patient set the mental hygiene movement of the early 1900s into motion.
- During the 1920s Sigmund Freud's psychoanalytical theories had become a popular method for treating emotional problems.
- The First and Second World Wars pointed out the need for comprehensive mental health care.
- With the introduction of psychotherapeutic drug treatment, many psychiatric institutions closed.
- Community mental health centers were built to accommodate the mentally ill during the 1970s, but a change in political climate left the project uncompleted.
- Today, many legislative changes again challenge us to develop comprehensive, cost-efficient care for society's mentally ill.

Suggestions for Further Reading

An excellent text about psychiatric practice through the ages is *The History of Psychiatry* by Franz Alexander and Sheldon Selesnick (New York, 1996, New American Library).

References

Ackerknecht EW: *A short history of medicine*, New York, 1968, Ronald Press.

Alexander FG, Selesnick ST: *The history of psychiatry*, New York, 1966, New American Library.

Anderson KN, editor: *Mosby's medical, nursing, & allied health dictionary*, ed 5, St. Louis, 1998, Mosby.

Dolan J: *History of nursing*, Philadelphia, 1968, WB Saunders.

Donahue MP: *Nursing: the finest art*, ed 2, St. Louis, 1996, Mosby.

Harrington SPM: New bedlam: jails—not psychiatric hospitals—now care for the mentally indigent, *The Humanist* 59(3):5, 1999.

Kelly LY: *Dimensions of professional nursing*, ed 6, New York, 1991, Pergamon Press.

Keltner NL, Folks DG: *Psychotropic drugs*, ed 3, St. Louis, 2001, Mosby.

Morrissey JP, Goldman HH: Cycles of reform in the care of the chronically mentally ill, *Hospital and Community Psychiatry* 35(89):785, 1984.

Taylor CM: *Essentials of psychiatric nursing*, ed 14, St. Louis, 1994, Mosby.

Chapter 2

Current Mental Health Care Systems

Learning Objectives

1. Describe the present system of mental health care delivery in Canada, the United Kingdom, Australia, and the United States.
2. State the differences between inpatient and outpatient psychiatric care.
3. Differentiate between voluntary and involuntary admission to mental health care facilities.
4. Explain the community support systems model of care, and list four settings for community mental health care delivery.
5. Identify five components of the case management method of mental health care.
6. Explain the purpose of the multidisciplinary mental health care team.
7. Name four high-risk populations served by community mental health centers.
8. List five community-based mental health services for people with HIV/AIDS.
9. Explain the concept of holistic care.

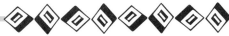

Key Terms

advocacy

case management

community mental health centers (CMHCs)

community support systems (CSS) model

consultation

crisis intervention

health maintenance organizations (HMOs)

holistic concept of care

homelessness

inpatient psychiatric care

involuntary admission

multidisciplinary mental health care team

outpatient mental health care

preferred provider organizations (PPOs)

psychosocial rehabilitation

recidivism

resource linkage

therapeutic environment

third-party payments

voluntary admission

The delivery of a population's health care varies with the culture. Because cultures, values, and beliefs differ, international comparisons of health care systems are difficult to make. The more developed nations have complex systems for providing health care for their citizens, and all societies are coping with the growing costs of high technology, drugs, and aging populations.

MENTAL HEALTH CARE IN CANADA

By the late 1960s Canada adopted a government-administered health insurance plan. Today, a "single-payer arrangement" is used in the Canadian health care system, which is based on five principles: universality, portability, accessibility, comprehensiveness, and public administration. Each guiding principle is explained in Box 2-1.

Each province or territory organizes, administers, and monitors the health care delivery system of its citizens. Benefits may vary, but all Canadian citizens are eligible for medical, hospital, convalescent, and mental health services. Medications for people over age 65, diagnostic procedures, and emergency and outpatient services are also provided. The official agency responsible for the health of Canadians is the Department of National Health and Welfare. It provides technical and financial support for each provincial health care program, enforces federal food and drug laws, promotes health, and administers social welfare programs.

Canada's health care system is divided into curative and preventive operations. As with the United States health care system, the major focus is on cure and treatment. Preventive services, including mental health, are delivered through public health departments. "Private psychotherapy, community mental health, other day programs, and hospital psychiatric services" (Kirkpatrick, 1999) are available to every Canadian based on need.

MENTAL HEALTH CARE IN NORWAY

Like other European countries, Norway has adopted a national insurance system. The National Insurance Act of 1967 provides access to health care for everyone living in Norway. Employees contribute a percentage of their wages and pay out-of-pocket fees for prescriptions and consultations until a payment ceiling (about $175) is reached. Thereafter, all services are covered except adult dental care.

Financing and delivery of health care services occur on three levels. "National authorities legislate health policy and monitor and supervise health service delivery" (Nylenna, 1995). Hospitals and specialized medical services are managed by Norway's 19 counties, and primary health care services are organized on the municipal level. Mental health care is available to all citizens of Norway.

MENTAL HEALTH CARE IN GREAT BRITAIN

All British citizens are provided health care through a government-managed national health care system. The Secretary for Social Services is responsible for setting fees for private physicians, budgets for hospitals, and salaries for hospital physicians. Parliament allocates funds for the health care system and regulates the rates at which general practitioners are paid. Tax revenues provide most of the financing for health care.

Mental health care is available for all British citizens as part of the standard benefit package. Physician services, emergency surgeries, hospital stays, and prescription drugs, along with preventive, home, and long-term care are all provided by the government. Eye care is not included and dental care is limited, but all other basic health care needs are provided. Private insurance is also available.

MENTAL HEALTH CARE IN AUSTRALIA

Australians are provided an interesting mix of health care plans. The government provides a public health plan that covers all public hospitals and physician services. Also available is a national private plan, which supplements the basic public plan. In addition, numerous private insurance plans are available for eye care, rehabilitative services, and psychiatric treatment.

National health care is financed by a tax on all citizens above a certain income. Policy and budget decisions are made at the federal level. Individual states are responsible for the administration and delivery of health care services, which are available through local government agencies, semivoluntary agencies, and profit-oriented organizations. Mental health care is not provided in Australia's basic health plan, so treatment for psychiatric disorders is more common for those with large incomes or private insurance plans.

MENTAL HEALTH CARE IN THE UNITED STATES

Health care in the United States is based on the private insurance model. Today, more than 75% of the population is covered by private insurance or public programs (Medicare and/or Medicaid). About 15.4% of U.S. citizens have no health care coverage at all (U.S. Bureau of Census, 1998).

Health Insurance

During the 1960s third-party payments became available. With **third-party payments,** medical costs were covered by a "third-party"—usually an insurance company or the state or federal government. By the late 1970s many employers provided insurance, which included some coverage for mental health care. Mental health care was available but expensive during the 1980s. Today, health care is delivered by independent practitioners, preferred provider organizations, and health maintenance organizations.

Preferred Provider Organizations

During the 1980s **preferred provider organizations (PPOs)** were established to help curtail the rapidly growing increases in health care costs. They consist of a network of physicians, hospitals, and clinics that agrees to provide care for different organizations at a discount. The client may see any health care provider within the network, and 80% to 100% of the costs to the client were covered.

Health Maintenance Organizations

Health maintenance organizations (HMOs) deliver health care to enrolled clients who pay a fixed, prenegotiated price. Health care costs are covered as long as clients receive care within the system. Physicians are salaried and clients may or may not have a choice of care providers. Costs are contained by monitoring the delivery of care and limiting access to specialists and/or expensive procedures.

Institutional Care

By the 1900s the U.S. government established a state hospital system specifically designed for treating the mentally ill. Once people were admitted to a state hospital, they usually stayed for months or years, regardless of their ability to function in the community.

Today, publicly financed mental health services are also available in community hospitals and clinics. Because the state hospital system is no longer in place, communities have been forced to provide increased emergency psychiatric services and short-term inpatient care for an expanding number of acutely ill psychiatric clients.

The distinction between public and private sector mental health care is beginning to blur. Federal funds (Medicare) and state funds (Medicaid) are being used to cover health care costs in both the private and public sectors. Medicare funds about 30% to 50% of all state mental health systems (Hogan, 1999).

CARE SETTINGS

Admission rates to psychiatric inpatient facilities were at an all time low by 1983. However, by 1988, hospitalizations for mental illness had again increased, as emergency rooms saw huge increases in clients with psychiatric problems.

Inpatient Care Settings

Individuals are admitted to **inpatient psychiatric services** on the basis of need. Several factors are considered when making the choice of an inpatient setting. The severity of the client's illness, the level of dysfunction, the suitability of the setting for treating the problem, the level of client cooperation, and the client's ability to pay for services all enter into the decision regarding inpatient psychiatric care. Clients who receive care in inpatient settings remain at the institution for 24 hours a day, where all aspects of the client's environment are focused on providing therapeutic assistance.

Inpatient psychiatric care settings provide clients with safe, stable, and therapeutic surroundings. This principle of the **therapeutic environment** is based on the concept that every interaction within the client's environment has therapeutic potential. Therefore the physical surroundings are pleasant but safe. Activities are structured, and clients are expected to participate in their treatment. Discharge from inpatient facilities occurs when client behavior has appropriately improved and treatment goals have been attained. Clients may be discharged into the community, to a group home or other structured setting, or to another institution for long-term psychiatric care.

The most important advantage of inpatient psychiatric care is that it provides clients with a safe and secure environment where they can focus on and work with the problems that brought them there.

Types of Psychiatric Admissions

The decision to seek psychiatric care, whether made by the client, family, or community, is difficult. Many misconceptions about mental illness still exist, and the majority of people are not accustomed to seeking help for emotional or mental health problems.

Voluntary Admission

When the client originates the request for mental health services, the admission is considered a **voluntary admission.** Because they are often aware of their problems, most voluntarily admitted clients are active participants in their treatments and therapies.

Normally healthy people may seek admission to work through specific problems or to obtain support during a crisis. Some clients seek to withdraw from addictive substances, and others feel the need for mental health educational services. Clients who seek voluntary admission to mental health services are usually able to function on a daily basis and have a low potential for violence.

Involuntary Admission

One of the characteristics of mental illness is a lack of insight into one's problems. When individuals engage in behavior that is harmful to themselves or others, the involuntary admission process is undertaken.

The 1953 Act Governing Hospitalization defines an **involuntary admission** as a process for institutionalization initiated by someone other than the client. When disturbed people become suicidal, violent, or acutely psychotic, they need to be protected from harming themselves or others. Involuntary psychiatric admissions provide a protected, therapeutic environment, which is usually necessary for the client's safety. Clients may stay for days to years.

Family members are often the first to notice abnormal responses. They usually admit a loved one through private physicians, local hospitals, or community agencies. Physicians, police, and representatives of a county administrator may commit an individual for emergency treatment without a warrant, but a court order is usually required for long-term stays. Procedures for psychiatric commitment in the United States vary from state to state. Each state has a mental health procedures act that governs involuntary admissions (see Figure 3-2, Chapter 3).

Clients may also be committed to psychiatric care by way of the criminal justice system. The legal aspects of involuntary commitment are discussed in Chapter 3. Society protects itself from its more dangerous members through the involuntary commitment process.

Outpatient Care Settings

As the emphasis shifts from institutional to community mental health care, the demand for outpatient psychiatric service grows. An **outpatient mental health care** setting is a facility that provides services to people with mental problems within their home environments. Outpatient psychiatric clients are able to remain within their communities, associating with the real world.

Mental health services are available through a variety of community agencies and support groups. Services offered in these settings focus on prevention, maintenance, treatment, and rehabilitation of mental health problems. Some agencies or groups limit their focus to one area (e.g., Alcoholics Anonymous focuses on treatment of alcohol addiction).

Unlike the controlled, limited environment of inpatient treatment facilities, community-based mental health therapy occurs within a dynamic society. Supervision is limited, and the responsibility for controlling behavior lies squarely with the individual. Clients are assessed in relation to their environment, and therapies are designed to assist them to function appropriately within their communities. Unfortunately, the number of outpatient psychiatric care facilities in the United States is being rapidly outpaced by the mental health needs of a nation undergoing many changes.

COMMUNITY MENTAL HEALTH CARE

Federal funding for mental health care has shifted from state psychiatric hospitals to general hospitals. It was not until 1998 that "state mental health programs had moved strongly in the direction of implementing a community support" (Hogan, 1999) system of care delivery.

Mentally ill people make use of community services only sporadically. Many wait until major problems occur before seeking treatment. When services are used, a "Band-Aid" approach that treats only the presenting complaint is often used. Consequently, many of the mentally ill in need of inpatient psychiatric care end up in the emergency rooms of general hospitals or county jails. Today, it is estimated that "between 600,000 and one million jail admissions annually are mentally ill" (Harrington, 1999).

Unable to cope in the community setting, people with chronic psychiatric problems often return to institutions or use community services on a revolving door basis. This behavior pattern is known as **recidivism** and means a relapse of a symptom, disease, or behavior. Recidivism is a major problem in mental health care. It is associated with increased frustration for staff, negative treatment outcomes, and inappropriate use of services. Lower rates of recidivism are seen in communities where coordination and cooperation among community agencies and mental hospitals exist.

Psychiatry and mental health care policies are based on the medical treatment model: identify and treat the symptoms. This point of view worked well for institutionalized psychiatric clients, but it became inadequate after clients were released into the community. A broader, community-oriented, more flexible outlook was needed.

Community Support Systems Model

For mentally ill people to function well within their communities, a wide range of support services is necessary. The **community support systems (CSS) model** views clients holistically—as individuals with basic human needs, ambitions, and rights. The goal of the CSS model is to create a support system that fosters individual growth and movement toward independence through the use of coordinated social, medical, and psychiatric services. Effective community support systems are consumer oriented, culturally appropriate, flexible enough to meet individual needs, accountable, and coordinated. A typical program may include such services as health care, housing, food, income support, rehabilitation, advocacy, and crisis response (Figure 2-1).

The most successful community mental health centers have forged strong links with available community agencies, services, and government. Other centers have developed slowly, but the CSS model of mental health care

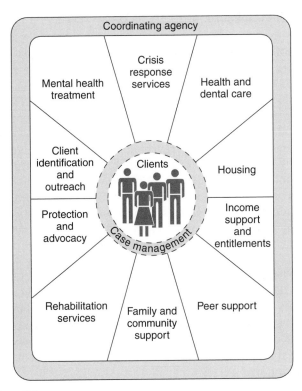

Figure 2-1 Community support system. (Redrawn from Stroul BA: *Psychosocial Rehabilitation Journal* 12:14, 1989.)

is proving to be one of the most comprehensive and workable concepts for the future.

DELIVERY OF COMMUNITY MENTAL HEALTH SERVICES

Mental health services and support systems are available through several community and civic organizations. Individuals, families, and the community itself benefit from the activities of various groups. Box 2-2 lists several examples of commonly available community services.

Mental Health Care Settings

Community mental health services are based on the identified needs of specific populations. Also, mentally ill people must be treated in the least restrictive manner. Therefore a wide range of services is offered in various settings throughout the community.

Emergency Care

This is available through emergency psychiatric clinics in large cities and general emergency rooms at local community hospitals. The primary focus is to stabilize the client, assist with the crisis, and locate appropriate resources in the community for referral. Staff members include nurses, psychologists, counselors, therapists, and social workers. Many of the chronically mentally ill use

---

Box 2-2 Examples of Community Services

Serving Individuals

Rape crisis center
Churches and synagogues
Employment and job training agencies
Recreational clubs
Adult education programs
Literacy programs
Mediation groups
Meals-on-Wheels
Colleges and universities
Mental health agencies

Serving Families

Women, Infants, and Children (WIC)
Nutritional services
Community "Welcome Wagon"
Family planning agencies
Recreation centers
Children's groups (e.g., Camp Fire Girls)
Church groups
Day care centers for the young, disabled, and elderly
Family recreation centers and groups
Shelters for victims of domestic violence

Serving the Community

Environmental groups
Education groups (e.g., American Lung Association and March of Dimes)
Utility companies
Community emergency shelters
Government agencies
Police and fire departments
Fair housing bureau or agency
Prisons
Performing arts centers
Public forests and parks

From Haber J and others: *Comprehensive psychiatric nursing*, ed 5, St. Louis, 1997, Mosby.

psychiatric emergency settings as an entry into the mental health services network.

Residential Programs

These programs offer the chronically mentally ill a protected, supervised environment within the larger community. Services provided include the provision of food, shelter, clothing, supervision of personal care, and counseling. Vocational training is frequently provided. Opportunities for leisure and socialization activities are included in most programs. Types of residential programs range from group homes to single-room occupancies, but all provide direct therapeutic support and treatment for the chronically mentally ill.

Psychiatric Home Care

These services deliver mental health assistance to individuals and families in their homes. With short institutional stays and the release of people with chronic mental illness into the community, the need for home psychiatric care providers to fill the gap between institution and community is rapidly growing. Psychiatric clinical nurse specialists (CNSs) ease the transition from hospital to home for clients and their families and assist clients in gaining entry into the mental health care system. They also provide psychosocial crisis interventions and collaborate with clients, families, and other professionals to deliver the most appropriate, effective, and cost-accountable psychiatric care. The case history presented in the box below illustrates the role of the mental health CNS in the home care setting.

 Case Study

Joanne is a 59-year-old woman with severe depression, anorexia, and suicidal ideation. The psychiatric home care referral was an effort by her husband to prevent nursing home placement. Joanne presented with a 30-yearhistory of scleroderma (a disfiguring skin condition), numerous surgeries and hospitalizations, and a 10-year psychiatric history with numerous suicide attempts. She has severe anxiety and agoraphobia (fear of crowds and open spaces). Her anorexia was severe, with her weight at 77 pounds. Medical and psychiatric problems were interwoven, and she needed comprehensive intervention. The certified nurse specialist (CNS) served as case manager.

Because Joanne could not leave home and needed medication management, a psychiatrist made home visits. Companion services were supplied while the husband was at work. The husband was actively involved in the decision making regarding his wife's care, but he needed supportive interventions.

Over a 4-month period, Joanne progressed from a severely withdrawn, suicidal person to someone who was dealing with her panic attacks, agoraphobia, and scleroderma. Her weight had increased to 90 pounds. Although she would continue to cope with a chronic illness, her hopelessness was gone, and her ability to function in her daily life had markedly improved. She was able to continue living in her home and community with the help of community mental health services.

♦ What follow-up care would you plan for Joanne?
♦ What activities would help Joanne meet her social needs?

Modified from Mellon SK: *Issues in mental health nursing* 15:229, 1994.

Partial Hospitalization

Day treatment programs provide more structure and intensive therapy than outpatient or clinic services for clients who are not dysfunctional enough for full-time hospitalization but too ill to be independent within the community. Usually partial hospitalization or day treatment programs last from 30 to 90 days and require attendance for 6 to 8 hours a day for 5 days a week. Programs are staffed by psychologists, nurses, therapists, and counselors. Multidisciplinary assessments help to formulate individualized care plans, which are reviewed by the staff at weekly intervals. Treatment methods include various therapies, education, and vocational training. Clients are gradually reintroduced into the community after support systems are in place and coping behaviors are appropriate.

Clients enrolled in these programs become more adept with work and social situations, have fewer psychiatric symptoms and return hospitalizations, and are able to function within the community. With the current emphasis on cost containment and limited health care resources, partial hospitalization programs are effective methods for working with the mentally ill.

Community Mental Health Centers

These centers assist individuals and families in coping with life's problems and provide services for persons with severe mental illness. Services offered by most **community mental health centers (CMHC)** include crisis intervention, individual and family counseling, and mental health education. Clients with chronic mental illness also receive regular medication reviews, medical care, and vocational and social skills training. CMHCs are staffed by mental health professionals (psychologists, nurses, social workers, and therapists and their assistants).

Those CMHCs with firm funding also focus on prevention, education, and interventions aimed at reducing mental disorders. Unfortunately, financing for many community mental health programs has been sporadic, resulting in fragmented services. As the country's policy makers struggle to define a national health policy, consumers and mental health professionals continue to grapple with the everyday problems of mental illness within their communities. The future holds many changes for mental health care in the United States as social, political, and economic forces shape health care policies.

Case Management Systems

Defined as a holistic system of interventions, **case management** is designed to support the transition of mentally ill clients into the community. The major components of case management include psychosocial rehabilitation, consultation, resource linkage (referral), advocacy, therapy, and crisis intervention. Clients are involved with the assessment, planning, and evaluation of their care. Goals are stated as client outcomes. Success is measured in terms of client satisfaction, improved coping behaviors, and appropriate use of services. The overall goal of case management is a successfully functioning client who is able (with support) to avoid relapse and achieve productive patterns of living. A look at each component of case management may help clarify the process.

Psychosocial Rehabilitation

Use of multidisciplinary services to help clients learn the skills needed to carry out the activities of daily living as actively and independently as possible best describes **psychosocial rehabilitation.** Clients are first assessed for physical, social, emotional, and intellectual levels of functioning. Then specific plans for teaching needed skills are developed. If clients are capable of work, vocational rehabilitation is offered.

The psychosocial rehabilitation (also called *psychiatric rehabilitation*) model of care encourages decision making, thus empowering clients. This empowerment fosters a sense of self-esteem and mastery, which results in improved coping abilities. As clients feel the success of making their decisions, they are encouraged to take control over other areas of their lives. Education is also a strong component of psychosocial rehabilitation because mastering daily living skills motivates clients to more productive and independent levels of functioning.

Consultation

In mental health care, **consultation** is defined as a process in which the assistance of a specialist is sought to help to identify ways in which to cope effectively with client problems. The case management system relies on the expertise of psychiatrists, nurses, psychologists, social workers, counselors, and various therapists. Their objective is to find ways for clients to receive the services and support that helps them achieve their goals. For example, a nurse might work with a client on personal grooming skills while a social worker is locating supported housing and the vocational counselor seeks out an appropriate work setting. By covering all the bases, care providers hope to maintain clients in the least restrictive setting (the community) and assist them with their needs.

Resource Linkage

The process of matching clients' needs with the most appropriate community services best describes **resource linkage.** Health care providers have traditionally referred clients to other services, but resource linkage adds the component of periodic monitoring. The advantages of coordinating and linking services are several: clients can be more easily moved into different programs because background information moves with clients; duplication of services is avoided; and as the clients' level of functioning improves, services can be tailored to support the new, more effective behaviors. With resource linkage, the focus for treatment of clients with chronic mental illness is on care instead of the more traditional emphasis on psychiatric symptoms and illness (see Think About box).

Advocacy

A critical concept of case management, **advocacy,** is providing the client with the information to make certain decisions, but advocacy for the mentally ill involves more. Advocates work to protect clients' rights, help to clarify expectations, provide support, and act on behalf of clients' best interests. Every person involved in mental health care can act as an advocate by supporting community efforts and policies that encourage healthy living practices.

Therapy

Therapy is provided for each client based on assessed needs, client cooperation, and available services. Medications may be included as part of the overall plan of treatment. Therapies may include the use of counseling, support groups, vocational rehabilitation programs, and techniques to assist clients with problem-solving and adaptive behaviors.

Crisis Intervention

This component of case management is crucial to the success of the client. People with chronic mental dysfunction have great difficulty in coping with stress. What may be bothersome or inconvenient to us could provoke a crisis in someone with mental illness. When problems, frustration, anxiety, or even loneliness become too intense, a crisis erupts; the client becomes unable to cope and retreats into the safety of his or her illness. **Crisis intervention** describes a short-term, active therapy that focuses on solving the immediate problem and restoring the client's previous level of functioning. Crisis services help stabilize the client, prevent further deterioration, and support the client's readjustment process. The use of crisis services also results in better distribution of

Think About
You are a health care provider who has recently moved to this area. As a staff member in a CMHC, you are responsible for helping refer clients to appropriate agencies.
◆ How would you go about locating the agencies in the community that provide services for the mentally ill?

resources. Emergency room visits decrease, rehospital-ization is prevented, and law enforcement resources are better focused on those who break the law instead of apprehending mentally ill individuals. For clients with severe, treatment-resistant mental illness, a new approach, known as *continuous intensive case management,* is being used.

A new, highly flexible model of care, known as *Assertive Community Treatment (ACT),* provides "medical, psychosocial, and rehabilitation services by a community-based team that operates 7 days a week, 24 hours a day" (Salkever and others, 1999). The team usually consists of a social worker, psychiatrist, addictions counselor, and four clinicians (two social workers and two registered nurses). Clients are seen individually and in supportive therapy groups. They attend day treatment programs or pursue vocational training. Many clients live in supervised housing arrangements. Table 2-1 provides a summary of the continuous care team's treatment activi-

ties. In short, the continuous care team directs the client's treatment during all encounters with the mental health care system.

Intensive case management programs and ACTs have demonstrated that clients with chronic and severe mental illness can be effectively stabilized within the community with appropriate support systems. As the pressures of increased demand for services and cost restrictions force the system into trying new approaches, mental health care professionals must not lose sight of the most important element in the equation—"the client."

CLIENT POPULATIONS

Community mental health care was originally designed to provide prevention, education, and treatment services for all members of a community. Community mental health services for the general public include crisis interventions, working with businesses to decrease the costs of mental health programs while improving their effectiveness, and providing aid for individuals and families to adjust to life difficulties.

However, there are groups of people who are at a high risk for developing mental health problems in every community, large or small. They include the more obvious populations, such as the homeless, and more subtle high-risk groups, such as children, families, adolescents, the aged, and people who are HIV-positive. Clients living in rural areas present a challenge because of distances between services.

Many community mental health services offer assistance for homeless people. Currently, short-term strategies for working with the homeless include temporary shelters, assisted housing programs, and volunteer efforts such as Habitat for Humanity.

Clients with HIV infection or AIDS are using community mental health services in ever-growing numbers. To illustrate, in1984, 7354 cases of AIDS were reported in the United States. By 1996 those figures had exploded to almost 67,000 AIDS cases with 39,200 deaths (U.S. Bureau of Census, 1998). With statistics like these, it becomes easy to understand that AIDS is likely to become a major mental health problem.

People with AIDS face overwhelming physical, emotional, and social consequences. Mental health problems associated with HIV disease include organic problems, such as impairments in memory, judgment, or concentration progressing to dementia. Psychosocial problems include anxiety, depression, adjustment disorders, increased substance abuse, panic disorders, and suicidal thoughts. In addition, many researchers believe that stress directly affects the immune system. Fear of AIDS may hasten the onset of complications in HIV-positive persons. AIDS-related anxiety can increase everyday apprehensions in the lives of many people.

Table 2-1 Continuous Care Team Treatment Strategies	
Setting	**Mental health care team interventions**
Community	Meets with clients 2-4 times a week
	Accompanies client to appointments and other community activities
	Helps with daily living/social skill needs
	Monitors medications
	Nurtures relationships with persons interested in client's well-being
	Encourages client to call team instead of using ER
Emergency room	Prearranges for ER staff to notify clinician on arrival of continuous care client
	Conducts assessment of client and planning of care jointly with ER physician
	Avoids unnecessary hospitalizations
Hospital	Care team psychiatrist and primary therapist remain in charge of the client's case
	Helps with decisions regarding admission, treatment, and discharge
	Coordinates treatment with inpatient staff

Modified from Arana JD, Hastings B, Herron E: *Hospital and Community Psychiatry* 42(5):503, 1991.
©American Psychiatric Association, Reprinted by permission.
ER, Emergency room.

Comprehensive community mental health services for people with HIV/AIDS are not yet available in all communities. CMHCs that offer comprehensive services focus on three groups: persons with AIDS, their families and friends, and the general public. Clinicians at CMHCs accept referrals from other agencies, provide mental status and suicide risk assessments, offer crisis intervention services, and provide individual or group therapies for clients with HIV/AIDS. Family members and significant others are encouraged to join support groups. Some CMHCs train family members in techniques for keeping clients oriented or on task. Respite care (time off for the caregiver) services are sometimes coordinated through the CMHC. At the community level, CMHCs work with other interested groups to provide prevention strategies and education about AIDS for all citizens of the community.

Clients living in rural areas present a special challenge for community mental health care providers. Small villages, settlements, and farms dot the country landscape of the United States and Canada. In the United States, rural residents define and relate to health differently than people in cities. Children and adolescents living in rural areas have less access to mental health services. Mental health care providers (e.g., nurses, therapists) who work in rural areas cope with clients of all ages and with all types of problems. They are also expected to provide and coordinate comprehensive mental health care with few resources.

Other populations such as families, the elderly, children, and adolescents are vulnerable to mental health problems. Community mental health services are a vital link to the well-being of a population. Social and economic changes will continue to influence community mental health care, but as the system matures, the goal of individualized, holistic mental health care for all people should not be forgotten.

MULTIDISCIPLINARY MENTAL HEALTH CARE TEAM

Professionals working within the mental health system have various educational backgrounds. In the past, each would work with clients from their particular point of view or specialty. This approach resulted in disjointed, fragmented client care. In some cases, care providers worked at cross-purposes, leaving clients unsure and confused. The need for coordinated assessment and treatment was filled by the **multidisciplinary mental health care team** concept.

The main purpose of the team approach to treating mental illness is to provide effective client care. The mental health care team "provides a forum where psychiatrists, social workers, psychologists, nurses, and others can democratically share their professional exper-

tise and develop comprehensive therapeutic plans for clients" (Haber and others, 1997). The team approach can also be cost-effective by preventing duplication of services and fragmentation of care. Clients and their significant others contribute to the plan of care and remain actively involved throughout the course of treatment.

Multidisciplinary mental health care teams exist in both inpatient and outpatient settings. The number of team members may vary, but the "core" of the team is usually composed of a psychiatrist, psychologist, nurse, and social worker. Other team members, known as adjunct therapists, join the team as needed.

Each team member holds a degree or certificate in a specialized area of mental health. This approach allows for clients to be assessed and treated from various points of view. As data are compiled, a broad, hopefully holistic picture of the client emerges and individualized therapeutic plans are developed. Table 2-2 identifies team members, their educational preparation, and their function.

Client and Family

No discussion of the mental health team is complete without including the client. As the consumers of services and the focus of therapeutic interventions, clients contribute important information that may make the difference between the success or failure of therapeutic plans. Including clients and their families in the treatment process "reflects a fundamental change in attitude toward those who have a mental illness and their families" (Taylor, 1994). Mental illness today is considered to be a manageable, even treatable, complex of disorders.

TRENDS TOWARD HOLISTIC CARE

Most current mental health care delivery systems are diagnosis and treatment oriented. Traditionally, most people received mental health care only after the onset of behavioral signs and symptoms. This resulted in more acute conditions that were more difficult and expensive to treat. Emphasis was rarely on prevention or early diagnosis.

During the 1970s and 1980s, researchers found that emotions caused chemical changes within the body that in turn affected the physical state. As health care models were developed to recognize the interrelatedness of mind, body, and environment, a new movement (known as holism) began to emerge. The word *holism* is derived from the Greek word holos, meaning "whole." Holism today is a philosophical concept in which a person is viewed as more than just the sum of his or her parts.

The concept of holism helps to blend many aspects of mental health care. The primary goal of nurses and other mental health care providers is to "help clients develop strategies to achieve harmony within themselves and with others, nature, and the world" (Rawlins, Williams, and

Table 2-2 Mental Health Team Members

Team member	Educational preparation	Responsibilities and functions
Psychiatrist	MD with residency in psychiatry	Physician; leader of the team; responsible for administration and planning; diagnostic and medical functions are main tasks
Clinical psychologist	PhD in clinical psychology	Specializes in study of mental processes and treatment of mental disorders; performs diagnostic testing; treats clients
Psychiatric social worker	Master's degree in social work (MSW)	Evaluates families; studies environmental and social causes of illness; conducts family therapy; admits new clients
Psychiatric nurse	Master's degree; advanced level preparation; baccalaureate degree; diploma nurse; associate degree nurse; licensed practical nurse	Responsible for client's activities of daily living/ environment management and individual, family, and group psychotherapy; coordinates care team activities; supervises technicians and psychiatric assistants; active in various community roles
Psychiatric assistant or technician	High school education; special on-job training in setting of employment	Supervised by professional nurse; assists in providing basic needs of clients; carries out nursing functions; maintains the therapeutic environment; supervises leisure-time activity; assists with individual/group therapy
Occupational therapist	Advanced degree in occupational therapy (OT)	Assesses potential for rehabilitation; provides socialization therapy and vocational retraining
Expressive therapist	Advanced degree and specialized training in art therapy	Helps make use of spontaneous creative work of the client; works with groups; encourages members to analyze artwork; adjunct to care team in diagnosis and treatment of children
Recreational therapist	Advanced degree and specialized training in recreational therapy	Provides leisure-time activities for clients; teaches hospitalized clients useful pastimes; uses pet therapy, psychodrama, poetry, and music therapy
Dietitian	Advanced degree and special training in dietetics (RD)	Provides attractive, nourishing meals; helps treat food-related illnesses
Auxiliary personnel (housekeepers, volunteers, clerks, secretaries)	Various backgrounds and on-job training	Assists clients with activities of daily living and other practical jobs; can be invaluable in helping clients
Chaplain	Seminary pastoral counselor or rabbinical education	Attends to the spiritual needs of clients and families; pastoral, marital counseling

Modified from Haber J and others: *Comprehensive psychiatric nursing*, ed 5, St. Louis, 1997, Mosby.

Beck, 1993). This statement reflects the **holistic concept of care.** We are no longer content to treat the illness. We are learning to treat the whole person.

IMPACT OF MENTAL ILLNESS

Mental illness affects everyone directly or indirectly. Many people know of someone with behavioral problems. Indirectly, mental illness costs taxpayers millions of dollars as the costs of care escalate. Today, health care reform is part of an overall strategy to distribute scarce resources and control expenses.

Incidence of Mental Illness

Although exact statistics are unavailable, it is estimated that at any given time "at least 19% of adults in the United States . . . (and) 7.5 million children" (National Mental Health Association, 1999) suffer from mental-emotional disorders. Chronic severe mental disorders, such as schizophrenia and depression, have emerged as major challenges to treatment. Substance abuse has become a national problem. Two million divorces each year place families in crisis situations (U.S. Bureau of Census, 1998). The incidence of Alzheimer's disease and other dementias is currently estimated at more than three million; that number is expected to increase threefold over the next 15 years. Social problems such as AIDS, homelessness, violence, and abuse may be related to mental problems. It is easy to see why there is a growing number of mentally troubled people in today's society.

Economic Issues

The nationwide movement to treat people with mental illness in the least restrictive environment is part of a plan to reduce mental health care costs while still providing ongoing care. Unfortunately, funding has not kept pace with the need for services. Because insurers have "capped" or limited the amount of money they will pay for psychiatric care, strict limits have been set on mental health care. Some gains have been made. By mid 1999, 19 states required *parity* for mental health treatment. This means that insurance plans had to provide coverage for mental health care equal to that for physical care.

Inpatient stays for acute problems in those states without parity are usually funded for a maximum of 14 days. Clients who require longer periods of treatment can be funded for up to 60 days. Long-term stays are less common as clients are discharged rapidly into the community.

To control costs, Congress established the Health Care Financing Administration (1983) who developed a cost-containment method where health care providers are paid at predetermined rates. A group of more than 400 diagnostic-related groups (DRGs) classifies each illness. Medicare, the funded health plan for the elderly and disabled, adopted these groups. Payment guidelines, based on clients' average lengths of inpatient stay, determine each DRG. If clients are not discharged from hospitals within the specified time, funding is stopped and the facility or client becomes responsible for payment.

Today, about 5400 mental health facilities provide services for more than 30 million mentally troubled people in the United States. Present levels of service cost taxpayers more than $33 million in 1994 (U.S. Bureau of Census, 1998).

Mental illness also influences economics in less direct ways. Unemployed, homeless, and troubled families cost society in many ways more than dollars. Loss of productivity and unfulfilled potential are difficult to appraise financially. Clearly, economic issues have and will continue to play a major role in the availability and delivery of mental health care.

Social Issues

Many social problems are related to mental illness. Changing lifestyles, work patterns, family structures, and health are a few of the many changes that are influencing society. The mentally ill, however, are likely to be coping with more basic issues such as poverty, homelessness, and substance abuse.

By 1996 nearly 14% of U.S. citizens lived below the poverty line and another 18% lived close to it (U.S. Bureau of Census, 1998). Of those, a significant number are incapable of making a living as a result of mental problems. They exist along the fringes of society, attempting to meet the most basic needs of food, shelter, and clothing. Within this environment of poverty, hopelessness grows, and it becomes easier to retreat into one's mental illness than face the grim reality of poverty.

After a time, homelessness becomes poverty's companion. The National Academy of Sciences defines **homelessness** as the lack of a regular and adequate nighttime dwelling. Millions of our nation's citizens are homeless on any given day. About 10% of the homeless are older than 60. Many are families, and as many as 85% of the homeless suffer from addictions or mental disturbances (Walker, 1998).

Homelessness is a national problem that continues to grow. The actual number of homeless people is difficult to count because with no regular housing they tend to melt into society and disappear into the world of soup kitchens and temporary shelters. In the past, most homeless people were single men, usually with alcohol problems. However, today's statistics present a different picture. Women, children, and families now account for as many as one third of the homeless.

Several factors contribute to homelessness. Social conditions such as a lack of low-income housing, public assistance eligibility requirements, and the movement of chronically mentally ill people into communities that lack adequate support systems have all had an adverse impact on homelessness. Community factors relating to available housing, steady employment, and welfare services affect homeless people. Family dysfunction, poverty, and health status all relate to the homeless problem.

Many families live "from paycheck to paycheck," with just enough money to scrape by until the next check. Even a small event can trigger a crisis. An increase in the rent, for example, may force a family out of their home.

Society's use of mind-altering chemicals has resulted in many of the mentally ill becoming addicted to "recreational drugs" such as crack, cocaine, LSD, and heroin. When used in combination with prescribed psychotherapeutic drugs, overdoses, permanent psychotic states, and death occur. Street drugs also cost money. It is not uncommon for people with mental problems to spend money on drugs before they buy food. Addicted people with mental disorders suffer from two separate disorders, with each compounding the severity of the other. Illicit drugs and mental illness become a vicious circle.

The current mental health care system in the United States is undergoing major changes as budgets decline, social issues emerge, and needs for treatment grow. Organization and technology may address some of the system's problems, but the provider-client contact is and will remain the core of mental health treatment.

KEY CONCEPTS

◆ The health care systems of many developed countries are undergoing financial strains as the result of the increasing cost of high technology, drugs, and aging of the populations.

◆ Canada's health care system is administered by each province under the guidance of the Department of National Health and Welfare and includes coverage for most medical, hospital, convalescent, and mental health services.

◆ All British citizens are provided health care through a government-managed national health care system.

◆ Norway's health care is delivered on national, county and municipal levels.

◆ Australians are provided a mix of health care plans. These include a public health plan, which covers all public hospitals and physician services; a supplemental national private plan; and private insurance plans for eye care, rehabilitative services, and psychiatric treatment.

◆ Funds for health care in the United States are provided through federal (Medicare) and state (Medicaid) programs, private insurance coverage, and direct client payments.

◆ Admissions to inpatient mental health care settings are usually on a voluntary basis, but people with acute illness can be admitted involuntarily if they pose a threat to themselves or others.

◆ The community support systems (CSS) model for mental health care is defined as an organized network of people committed to assisting people with mental illness to develop their potential without isolation from the community.

◆ Community mental health care settings include psychiatric clinics, general hospitals, residential care programs, day treatment facilities, and psychiatric home care.

◆ Case management is a holistic system of interventions designed to support the integration of mentally ill clients into the community.

◆ Psychosocial rehabilitation is the use of multidisciplinary services to help clients learn or reestablish the skills and supports needed to carry out the activities of daily living as actively and independently as possible.

◆ Psychosocial rehabilitation, consultation, resource linkage, advocacy, crisis intervention, and therapy are the basic components of the case management system.

◆ Intensive case management may use continuous care or Assertive Community Treatment teams who assume responsibility for the client in and out of the hospital.

◆ Community mental health services serve high-risk (or vulnerable) populations such as children, people in crisis situations, the homeless, clients with HIV/AIDS, clients living in rural areas, and the elderly.

◆ Mental health services are commonly delivered by the multidisciplinary care team—a group of physicians, nurses, psychologists, therapists and their assistants who each contribute to the client's plan of care and treatment.

◆ Holistic health care focuses on assisting clients work for harmony and balance within their lives.

◆ Social and economic issues must be considered when discussing mentally troubled persons.

Suggestions for Further Reading

Your daily newspaper offers discussions about our current health policies, proposed changes to the health care delivery system, proposed and adopted mental health care legislation, and events that shape attitudes toward the mentally and emotionally troubled.

References

Edelman CL, Mandle CL: *Health promotion throughout the lifespan*, ed 4, St. Louis, 1998, Mosby.

Haber J and others: *Comprehensive psychiatric nursing*, ed 5, St. Louis, 1997, Mosby.

Hamdy RC and others: *Alzheimer's disease: a handbook for caregivers*, ed 3, St. Louis, 1998, Mosby.

Harrington SPM: New bedlam: jails—not psychiatric hospitals—now care for indigent mentally ill, *The Humanist* 59(3):9, 1999.

Hogan MF: Medicaid and mental health: can this relationship thrive? *Policy and Practice of Public Human Services* 57(1):41, 1999.

Kirkpatrick DC: Mental health care above and below the 49th parallel, *Harvard Mental Health Letter* 15(11):1, 1999.

Mellon SK: Mental health clinical nurse specialist in home care for the 90s, *Issues in Mental Health Nursing*, (15):229, 1996.

National Mental Health Association: *National prevention coalition position statement* (9):1, 1999.

Nylenna M: Norway's decentralized single-payer health system faces great challenges, *Journal of the American Medical Society* 274(2):120, 1995.

Rawlins RP, Williams SR, Beck CK: *Mental health-psychiatric nursing: a holistic life-cycle approach*, ed 3, St. Louis, 1993, Mosby.

Salkever D and others: Assertive community treatment for people with severe mental illness, *Health Services Research* 34(2):577, 1999.

Taylor CB: *Essentials of psychiatric nursing*, St. Louis, 1994, Mosby.

U.S. Bureau of Census: *Statistical abstract of the U.S.: 1998*, ed 118, Washington, DC, 1998.

Walker C: Homeless people and mental health, *American Journal of Nursing* 98(11), 1998.

Chapter 3

Ethical and Legal Issues

Learning Objectives

1. State the differences between values, rights, and ethics.
2. Explain the purpose of Patient's Bill of Rights.
3. List the five steps for making ethical decisions.
4. Identify the legal importance of practice acts.
5. Describe the process of involuntary psychiatric commitment.
6. Name four areas of potential legal liability for mental health care providers.
7. Know the difference between the legal terms *negligence* and *malpractice*.
8. Explain three legal responsibilities that relate to nursing and health care providers.

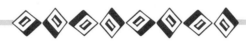

Key Terms

assault
attitudes
autonomy
battery
belief
beneficence
civil law
codes of ethics
confidentiality
contract law
controlled substances
criminal law
defamation

duty to warn
elopement
ethical dilemma
ethics
false imprisonment
felonies
fraud
informed consent
invasion of privacy
involuntary commitments
laws
libel
malpractice

misdemeanors
morals
negligence
nonmaleficence
Patient's Bill of Rights
professional (nurse) practice act
reasonable and prudent care provider
right
slander
standards of practice
tort law
value
values clarification

Health care professions are defined by certain beliefs, rights, and principles that serve as the basis for ethical and legal concepts. A framework for delivering effective therapeutic interventions is rooted in these concepts.

Attitudes, beliefs, values, and morals influence who we are. To be effective with mentally ill clients, we must first understand these concepts within ourselves and then as they apply to our clients and their support persons.

VALUES

Attitudes are ideas that help make up our points of view. The term can also describe one's outlook, such as "He has a cheerful attitude."

A **belief** is a conviction that is intellectually accepted as true, whether it is based in fact. A **value** is something that is held dear, a feeling about the worth of an item, idea, or behavior. Values are formed in childhood.

They shape our reactions, influence our behaviors, reflect the society in which we live, and are often used as a basis for making decisions. Values are individual and may change.

Morals reflect one's attitudes, beliefs, and values and define right or wrong behavior. Once established, morals become deeply ingrained and are not easily changed.

Acquiring Values

As children grow, they observe and adopt the reactions of others in their environment. These adopted reactions become our earliest attitudes. Preschool children learn the difference between "right" and "wrong" behavior and adopt the family's beliefs and traditions. As attitudes and beliefs develop, values begin to form.

Children are exposed to a variety of values at school. They develop work habits, learn to solve problems, and make decisions. Parental values are still modeled as the family remains the major source of values until adulthood.

During the teen years, adolescents begin to identify their own significant values. By early adulthood, an individual value system is established. Adults may feel secure with their values or discard them for new ones. Older adults may feel threatened by the changing social values, but they tend to hold onto their value systems.

Culture, society, personality, and experiences all shape our values. How values are shared largely depends on the sociocultural environment. Most societies use a combination of modeling, moralizing, laissez faire, reward/punishment, and responsible choice to transmit values (Potter and Perry, 2001) (Table 3-1).

People who choose to work in the health care profession usually arrive with a strong set of personal values. Human values that enhance the giving of care include a concern for the welfare of others (altruism), respect for the uniqueness and worth of people (human dignity), equality, justice, truth, freedom, and acceptance. Caring is the foundation of health care, for if we are unable to care for clients, we will be unable to effectively treat, teach, or work with them.

Values Clarification

Every society has a value system. Habits, customs, and traditions are important to more traditional societies. Modern societies are rapidly changing, and we are not always aware of our values and do not think about them until something goes wrong. When we are experiencing difficulties, we become more aware of our values.

Values clarification is a step-by-step process that encourages one to identify significant values. The process helps care providers become aware of how their values affect interactions with clients. Value clarification involves three steps: choose, prize, and act (Table 3-2).

Table 3-1	How Values Are Transmitted
Mode of transmission	**Definition**
Modeling	Copying an example—One person behaves in the ideal or preferred manner, while the other copies the behavior.
Moralizing	Sets standards for right and wrong—Choice is not allowed.
Laissez-faire	Unrestricted choices—No direction is given. One is free to explore and learn from experiences. This mode of transmission may result in confusion or frustration.
Reward/punishment	Rewards valued behaviors and punishes undesirable acts; authoritarian—Children learn that strength is right. This mode of transmission may send the message that violence is acceptable.
Responsible choice	A balance of freedom and restriction—One may choose among stated options. New behaviors and consequences are explored.

Modified from Potter PA, Perry AG: *Fundamentals of nursing*, ed 5, St. Louis, 2001, Mosby.

To illustrate the process, let us assume that you worked at the local clinic. A large, scruffy man who has not bathed in weeks presents himself for care. There is a wild look in his eye, and he is arguing with himself as he approaches you. What you really want to do is run, but you must cope with this client. How does the value of caring apply here?

First, you have freely chosen to care about people; otherwise you would have selected another line of work. Second, you prize the value of caring, because your clients see you as compassionate and concerned for their welfare. Third, you act on your values by accepting the unkempt, scruffy man as a person worthy of care. You ask him what you can do to help. He begins to cry and tells you that since the death of his wife and children in a house fire, no one has cared if he lives or dies. By acting on your value (caring), you have touched this person and paved the way for him to improve his situation. You have chosen to care. You cherish the value of caring enough to act, even when that value is threatened. Be clear about *your* values. Be aware of your client's values because they are the guidelines for one's lifestyle, conduct, and interpersonal relationships.

Table 3-2	Values Clarification Process
Step	**Process**
Choosing	Consider all possible alternatives.
	Consider all possible consequences.
	Choose freely without pressure or coercion from others.
Prizing	Cherish or prize the choice.
	Share choice with others.
	Reaffirm importance of value.
Acting	Make value a part of behaviors (internalize value).
	Generalize value to all situations.
	Repeatedly act with consistent behavioral pattern.

RIGHTS

A **right** is described as a power, privilege, or existence to which one has a just claim. Rights have several roles in society; they can be used as expressions of power, to justify actions, and to settle disputes. Rights help define social interactions because they contain the principle of justice; they equally and fairly apply to all citizens. For example, we all have the right to be respected as human beings and treated with dignity. Rights also have obligations. You may have the right to drive down the road, but inherent in this right is the obligation to obey traffic laws.

Client Rights

The 1972 **Patient's Bill of Rights** states that all clients have the rights to respectful care, privacy, confidentiality, continuity of care, and relevant information. It also addresses clients' rights to examine their bills, refuse treatment, and participate in research. In addition, it serves as a model for the development of specific bills of rights for many health care organizations. Statements of rights now exist for the old, young, disabled, pregnant, dying, developmentally disabled, and mentally ill—the most vulnerable people in society.

People with mental illness tend to lose their rights in two ways. First, the problems with which they are coping require energy. Sometimes reality eludes them. Many mental health clients are not able to recognize their rights, much less exercise them. Second, the mental health delivery system can impose limits on clients' abilities to exercise their rights. To protect their rights, the Mental Health Systems Act Bill of Rights was passed by the U.S. Congress in 1980. This bill served as a pattern from which state bills of rights for the mentally ill were developed (Box 3-1).

Box 3-1	Mental Health Bill of Rights

1. The right to be informed about one's benefits, including the design, usage, contractual limitations, appeals or grievances, and services of the plan.
2. The right to professional expertise, including choice of services and providers and information about treatment and explanations of its objectives, potential adverse effects, and alternatives.
3. The right to refuse treatment, except in an emergency or as provided by law.
4. The right to confidentiality of mental health care records.
5. The right to freedom from restraint or seclusion, except in an emergency or when prescribed as a part of treatment.
6. The right to a humane treatment environment.
7. The right to access own mental health care records, except to that information provided by third parties and information deemed by a mental health professional to be detrimental to the client's health.
8. The right to convenient and reasonable access to the telephone and mails, and to see visitors, except when denied access to a particular visitor as part of the written treatment plan.
9. The right to referral to other providers of mental health services on discharge.
10. The right to exercise these rights without reprisal or denial of appropriate, available treatment.

From American Nurses Association: *ANA fact sheet: mental health bill of rights,* Kansas City, Mo, 1999, The Association.

It must be remembered that the basis for the development of these statements was a basic dissatisfaction with the treatment of health care clients. Nurses and other care providers must ensure that each person's rights are protected and advocated.

Care Provider Rights

The rights of nurses and other care providers relate to respect, safety, and competent assistance. Care providers have the right to *respect* as individuals. Nurses have the right to full and equal participation as members of the health care team. All health care providers have the right to set standards for quality and develop policies that affect client care.

Every health care provider has the right to function within a *safe* environment. This right applies to both the physical environment (e.g., properly maintained equipment) and the affective or feeling environment. Nurses, technicians, and other care providers who work to minimize the physical and emotional stresses of the working environment are exercising their right to function safely.

The right to *competent assistance* includes the right to receive assistance with nursing care by people who are capable of performing at the stated level. For example, the CNA who is assigned to work with a nurse is able to function adequately and safely as a nursing assistant. Health care providers need to exercise their rights. It is through the exercising of rights that we remind the system of the therapeutic values inherent in the caregiver-client relationship.

ETHICS

Ethics is a set of rules or values that govern right behavior. Ethics reflect values, codes of morality, and principles of right and wrong. The purpose of ethical behavior is to protect the rights of people. Health care ethics focus on the moral aspects of health care availability, delivery, and policy. They are also called *biomedical ethics, bioethics,* or *medical ethics*.

Ethical Principles

Ethical principles are the general concepts that form the basis for professional codes of ethics (Edelman CL and Mandle CL, 1998). They are the behaviors that define what is good or right conduct. Ethical codes serve two purposes: (1) they act as guidelines for standards of practice and (2) they let the public know what behaviors can be expected from their health care providers.

The concepts of autonomy, beneficence, nonmaleficence, and justice are the main ethical principles on which codes of ethics are established. Remember these principles because they will serve you well as you encounter the many ethical situations inherent in health care.

Autonomy refers to the right of people to act for themselves and make personal choices, including refusal of treatment. Caregivers who practice the principle of autonomy encourage clients to participate in informed decision making. The procedure known as **informed consent** promotes client autonomy by providing relevant information and choice for the client.

Beneficence means to actively do good. Actions that promote client health are beneficent. Choosing the action that is the most therapeutic for the client is an example of beneficence.

The principle of **nonmaleficence** can be stated in three words: do no harm. Perhaps it is the most important

Table 3-3 Codes of Ethics for Nurses	
Registered nurse	**Practical/Vocational nurse**
Participates in activities that contribute to ongoing development of profession's body of knowledge	Knows scope of maximum utilization of the LPN/LVN and functions within that scope
Participates in profession's efforts to implement and improve standards of nursing	Recognizes and appreciates cultural backgrounds and spiritual needs
Participates in profession's efforts to establish and maintain conditions of employment that encourage high-quality care	Respects religious beliefs of individual patients
Participates in profession's effort to protect the public from misinformation and to maintain integrity of nursing	Safeguards confidential information acquired from any source about clients
Collaborates with health professionals and other citizens in promoting community and national efforts to meet health needs of public	Refuses to give endorsement to sales and promotions of commercial products or services
Provides services with respect for human dignity and uniqueness of the client unrestricted by considerations of social or economic status, personal attributes, or nature of health problems	Upholds high standards of personal appearance, language, dress, and demeanor
Safeguards client's right to privacy by judiciously protecting confidential information	Accepts responsibility for membership in NFLPN and participates in its efforts to maintain established standards of nursing practice and employment policies that encourage quality client care
Acts to safeguard client and public when health care and safety are affected by the incompetent, unethical, or illegal practice of any person	Safeguards client's right to privacy by judiciously protecting confidential information
Maintains competence in nursing	Safeguards client and public when health care and safety are affected by incompetent, unethical, or illegal practice of any person
Exercises informed judgment and uses individual competence and qualifications as criteria in accepting responsibilities, delegating nursing activities, and seeking consultation	Maintains competence in nursing
	Exercises informed judgment and uses individual competence and qualifications as criteria in accepting responsibilities and seeking guidance

From American Nurses Association: *Codes for nurses with interpretive statements,* Kansas City, Mo, 1985, The Association; and The National Federation of Licensed Practical Nurses: *Code for licensed practical/vocational nurses,* Garner, NC, 1979, The Federation.
NFLPN, National Federation of Licensed Practical Nurses.

ethical principle of the caregiving professions. Although nurses must sometimes carry out procedures that result in pain, the procedure is considered in light of the benefits gained. Therapeutic interventions are delivered only after client safety and comfort are considered. Nonmaleficence ensures that clients will not be harmed during care.

Justice implies that all clients are treated equally, fairly, and respectfully. Because health care resources are limited, the application of justice can be difficult. However, all clients deserve respect and a share of the available resources.

The concepts of confidentiality, fidelity, and veracity are other important ethical principles. The client's rights to privacy, truth, and duty are protected by these ethical principles. **Confidentiality** is the duty to respect private information. It is a legal and ethical duty of health care providers to keep all information about clients limited to only those directly involved with client care. Sharing private information is not only unethical but also may be grounds for legal action.

Fidelity is the obligation to keep your word. Telling the client that you will return in 10 minutes is a promise. Keep that appointment because your client relies on you, and your credibility grows or diminishes depending on how well you keep your promises. Do what you say or do not say it.

The final principle, *veracity,* is the duty to tell the truth. Be careful here. Answer clients' questions honestly, but remember to stay within your standards and limitations of practice. It is not within your realm, for example, to discuss the disease prognosis or lead a client toward a certain decision.

Codes of Ethics

Codes of ethics for practical (vocational) and registered nurses have been developed by the International Council of Nurses, the American Nurses Association, the National Federation of Licensed Practical Nurses, and the Canadian Nurses Association (Table 3-3). Codes of ethics have been developed for other health care professions and may differ slightly, but all codes of ethics are based on the same ethical principles. Provide information to clients, be truthful, and support your clients, but consult your supervisor if there is any question of appropriateness. It is important to practice your profession with ethical principles in mind.

Ethical Conflict

In today's world of advanced technologies and complex situations, no clear-cut answers exist for complicated questions that arise. **Ethical dilemmas** (conflicts) exist when there is uncertainty or disagreement about the moral principles that endorse different courses of action.

In the health care profession, ethical dilemmas arise when problems cannot easily be solved by decision making, logic, or use of scientific data. Answers to ethical dilemmas usually have a broad impact. Because of this, many health care institutions have established bioethics committees to study, educate, and assist staff members in coping with ethical dilemmas.

Most of the time no clear-cut solutions exist for ethical dilemmas. Although each ethical dilemma is unique, the method for making ethical decisions can be applied to all situations. Guidelines for dealing with such dilemmas are seen in Box 3-2. "Making ethical decisions in an orderly systematic manner increases one's ability to deal with the dynamic and sometimes complex issues relating to ethics. The quality of one's care depends on the skills and ethical integrity of the practitioner" (Morrison, 1993).

LAWS AND THE LEGAL SYSTEM

Every health care provider must be familiar with the basic concepts of the legal system. **Laws** are the controls by which a society governs itself. They are derived from rules, regulations, and moral and ethical principles, and they include all members of society.

General Concepts

Laws exist at every level of government. In the United States, federal law "defines or establishes the very organization of the government" (Creighton, 1986). Federal law is based on the U.S. Constitution. Laws at the

---

Box 3-2 Guidelines for Making Ethical Decisions

1. *Identify all elements* of the situation. Gather data. Identify each person involved in the decision-making process.
2. *Assume good will.* All care providers want a satisfactory resolution to the problem. When working with emotionally charged issues, remember that there is no need for competition.
3. *Gather relevant information.* Thoroughly assess lifestyle, preferences, wishes, and support systems. Try to form an "ideal picture" of the resolution for the dilemma.
4. *List and order values.* Using the ethical principles, decide which principles are most important in the situation. List them in order of importance, then determine a plan or course of action.
5. *Take action.* Implement the plan. Monitor any changes.
6. *Evaluate* the effectiveness of the plan.

Modified from Potter PA, Perry AG: *Fundamentals of nursing,* ed 5, St. Louis, 2001, Mosby.

state level are derived from the state's constitution and apply to citizens living within its boundaries. Local and city laws evolve from state law.

Laws change as society changes, but they are all based on four fundamental principles: justice (fairness), change, standards, and individual rights and responsibilities. Laws have several functions in our society. They define relationships, describe which behaviors are or are not acceptable, and explain what kind of force is applied to maintain rules. Laws help provide solutions for many social and legal problems and serve to protect the rights of people, while defining the limits of acceptable behaviors.

There are two types of law: public law and private law. *Public law* focuses on the relationship between the government and its citizens. The division of public law that is of importance to caregivers is known as **criminal law.** Its main function is to protect the members of society. Serious crimes, known as **felonies,** are punishable by death or imprisonment. Less serious crimes are called **misdemeanors,** with punishments ranging from fines to prison terms of less than 1 year.

Private law is commonly called **civil law.** Its function is to deal with relationships between individuals. Two important types of civil law for caregivers are contract law and tort law. **Contract law** deals with agreements between individuals or institutions. These agreements or contracts may be written or implied. To illustrate, on employment, health care providers enter into contracts with the employing institution.

"A tort is a legal wrong that is committed against the person or the property of another individual" (Morrison, 1993). **Tort law** relates to individuals' rights and includes the need to compensate a person for a wrong. Tort law is of special importance to caregivers because many potential legal problems exist in all health care settings. Figure 3-1 lists the areas of law that are most significant for care providers.

Legal Concepts in Health Care

Each health care profession is governed by rules and standards. Nursing, for example, is regulated by state boards of nursing that define the practice of nursing through nurse practice acts and regulate the profession through licensing procedures and disciplinary actions. Each state's board of nursing defines the limits and scope of nursing practice through a series of regulations known as that state's *nurse practice act.* Nurses need to be familiar with their state's nurse practice act because it is the legal framework for practice in that state. Other health care providers are responsible for knowing their state's governing regulations. Nurses are legally responsible for their actions. They are expected to know what is contained within their **professional (nurse) practice act**s.

Institutional policies also help to define health care practices. *Policies* are statements that define a course of

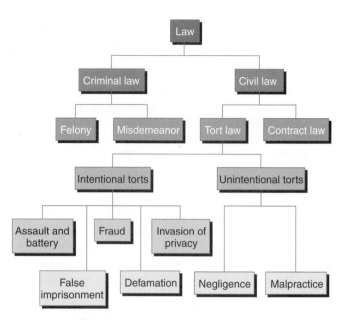

Figure 3-1 Laws important for nurses.

action. "What" is to be done is stated in policies. "How" a task or skill is to be performed is defined in the institution's procedure manual. *Job descriptions* define the job, its functions, its qualifications, and to whom the caregiver reports. Guidelines for sound health care practice can be found in each state's practice act, professional standards, and the employing institution's policies.

A *standard* is a measurement for comparison by which one evaluates an action. Every health care provider practices with certain standards, called **standards of practice.** They are usually developed by each specific discipline. Standards of nursing practice, for example, are a set of guidelines that provide measurable criteria for nurses, clients, and others to evaluate the quality and effectiveness of nursing care. Psychiatric mental health standards for nursing practice can be found in Appendix A.

LAW AND MENTAL HEALTH CARE

Historically, people with mental illnesses were afforded few legal rights. Only recently have mental health clients been able to exercise their claims to fair and adequate treatment in settings helpful to their care. Nurses and their colleagues need to be aware of their clients' legal rights to freedom, privacy, and choice. Laws relating to mental health issues "attempt to balance the basic rights of the individual against society's interest in being protected from persons who, because of mental disorder, present a threat of harm" (Keltner, Schwecke, and Bostrom, 1998).

Client-Caregiver Relationship

An awareness of the obligations relating to the client-caregiver relationship ensures safe, legal practice. From a legal point of view, the caregiver and client enter into an implied contract on acceptance of service. The caregiver provides services that are accepted by the client. This idea of contractual obligations is one legal aspect of the caregiver-client relationship. Two other important aspects that relate to nursing are liability and standards of care.

The concept of liability states that nurses are legally responsible for their professional obligations and behaviors. This concept includes the obligation to remain competent, maintain a current knowledge base, practice at a level appropriate to one's education, and practice unimpaired by drugs, disability, or illness.

Standards of care (practice) are defined by practice acts and professional organizations. They help to define legal limits by stating how a "reasonable and prudent care provider" would behave. These concepts will assist you in providing the respectful mental health care so needed by clients.

Clients still retain their legal rights when they enter the mental health care system. The 1980 Mental Health Systems Act states that the mentally ill have rights to obtain information and treatment within a supportive, humane environment. The Patient Self-Determination Act of 1991 gives clients the right to make decisions about their care, especially if or when their ability to make decisions has been lost (Loewy, 1998). Individuals who are admitted to psychiatric facilities retain the right to vote, to buy and sell property, and to possess a driver's license.

People with mental illness may be unaware of their legal rights or unable to exercise them. Clients' judgments may be limited as the result of their illness. It is important to recognize and safeguard clients' legal rights. Behind every mental disorder lives a real person.

Adult Psychiatric Admissions

Admission to an inpatient mental health facility is usually voluntary. Clients seek out treatment and agree to receive treatment and abide by the rules. Voluntarily admitted clients may legally discharge themselves at any time.

Admissions that occur against a client's will are known as involuntary admissions or **involuntary commitments.** Each state establishes its standards for commitment, but most laws allow involuntary commitment only if the person is dangerous to self or others or cannot function in a reasonable manner. Most states have similar procedures for involuntary admissions.

The commitment process begins when a formal petition is filed. The client is then assessed by one or two physicians and a determination is made to either release or hospitalize the person. (Stuart GW and Laraia MT, 1998). If the client is hospitalized, the length of stay may be on an emergency, temporary, or indefinite basis. Clients who are indefinitely hospitalized must be gravely disabled and unable to provide for themselves as a result of mental

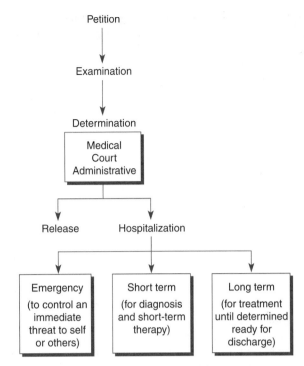

Figure 3-2 The involuntary commitment process. (Redrawn from Stuart GW, Laraia MT: *Principles and practice of psychiatric nursing,* ed 7, St. Louis, 2001, Mosby.)

illness. Indefinite commitments are most often an action of the courts, which usually provide a guardian or conservator to protect the client's rights. They are subject to yearly review and clients retain the right to consult a lawyer and petition the court for discharge. Figure 3-2 illustrates the process of involuntary commitment.

Areas of Potential Liability

Mental health care providers are placed in the unique position of balancing their clients' rights with the need to protect society. Many legal issues relate to the care of the mentally ill and an awareness of the potential liabilities helps safeguard caregivers', as well as clients' rights.

The most common crimes in the health care settings are homicide, controlled substance violations, and theft. Legally, *homicide* is the killing of a human being, whereas *murder* is killing with intent. For example, a nurse who unknowingly gives a client the wrong drug that causes death may have committed homicide. However, a nurse who knowingly administers a lethal drug may be guilty of murder.

The Controlled Substances Act of 1970 was passed by Congress to regulate the supply and distribution of certain powerful drugs. **Controlled substances** currently include narcotics, stimulants, depressants, hallucinogens, and some tranquilizers (Table 3-4). As agents of the physician, nurses administer controlled drugs. They are responsible

Table 3-4	Controlled Substances
Classification	**Drugs**
Schedule I	No accepted medical use in the United States
Schedule II	Narcotics, amphetamines, amobarbital, pentobarbital, secobarbital
Schedule III	Nonnarcotic depressants, short-acting barbiturates
Schedule IV	Long-acting barbiturates, tranquilizers, depressants
Schedule V	Exempt narcotics (e.g., cough syrups that contain codeine)

Think About

You overhear two psychiatric aides discussing Mrs. Samson while making the bed in Mrs. Jones' room.
◆ How would you handle this situation?
◆ Are there any ethical principles being violated by the aides' behaviors?

for adhering to their institution's policies and procedures regarding storage, distribution, and documentation of controlled substances.

Robbery, theft, and *larceny* all describe the taking of another person's personal property. Clients who lose valuable items can hold the agency liable for theft. Ensuring that a valuables disposition list is completed for every client is an important protection against theft.

Fraud is the giving of false information with the knowledge that action will be taken based on the information. For example, a technician documents that a treatment was given when it was not. The physician then bases a decision on the client's lack of response. The technician is guilty of fraud. Practicing with the utmost honesty is the best protection against fraud.

Defamation is defined as a false communication that results in harm. It is subdivided into two categories: written defamation, or **libel,** and verbal defamation, referred to as **slander.** Psychiatric care providers should base their communications on objective data and clinical observations, not judgments or opinions.

Assault is any act that threatens a client. No physical contact need occur, just a threatening action. Telling a client that he or she will be physically forced to do something if one does not cooperate is an example of assault. **Battery** is when touching occurs without the client's permission. The best prevention against assault or battery is clear communication. Make sure clients understand what you intend to do before you begin.

An important area of potential liability relates to **invasion of privacy.** "The right to privacy includes privacy related to the body, confidential information, and the right to be left alone" (Morrison, 1993). An invasion of privacy occurs when a client's space, body, or belongings are violated. Although caregivers must be continually vigilant to protect a client's privacy, those rights may occasionally be outweighed by the need to ensure the client's safety. For example, a client who behaves suicidally may have his or her belongings searched for potentially dangerous objects.

The client's right to privacy also includes confidentiality, which is the sharing of information about the client only with those people who are directly involved in care. Discussing any client with noninvolved people constitutes a breach of confidentiality (see Think About box).

All mental health care providers can protect the client's privacy by treating each person with dignity and respect. Caregivers who work in inpatient settings need to orient clients to their environment and inform them of their privacy rights, as well as how those rights may be restricted. Clients trust their care providers to maintain, nurture, and safeguard that trust.

Detaining a competent person against his or her will constitutes **false imprisonment.** Any time a client's freedom of movement is restrained the potential for liability exists. See Box 3-3. Both physical force and verbal intimidation are included in the concept of false imprisonment. For example, threatening a client with confinement constitutes grounds for false imprisonment.

Involuntarily committed clients may make false imprisonment claims in some states, but usually the public's right to safety takes precedence over a client's claim of false imprisonment. Health care providers can confine mentally ill people only to protect safety and prevent injury; medical or legal authority must be obtained as soon as possible.

The application of *protective devices* and *restraints* may constitute false imprisonment. Restraints must be used only to protect the client, not for the staff's convenience. The least restrictive measures should first be attempted and documented. A written medical order for restraints must be on file in the client's chart. Once restraints have been applied, the caregivers have an increased obligation to observe, assess, and monitor the client every 15 minutes. The restraints must be removed, one limb at a time, and exercised every 2 hours. All observations and actions must be documented. Restraints should be removed as soon as the client's behavior is under control.

The concepts of both negligence and malpractice are rooted in the "reasonable and prudent person" theory. **Negligence** is defined as the omission (or commission) of

Box 3-3 Criteria for False Imprisonment

1. Client is aware of the confinement.
2. Intent to confine exists.
3. Confinement takes place against the client's will.

an act that a reasonable and prudent person would (or would not) do. For example, a public swimming pool owner who did not repair a slide that then caused a child's injury could be guilty of negligence.

The concept of **malpractice** usually applies to professionals and is defined as a failure to exercise an accepted degree of professional skill that results in injury, loss, or damage. To be considered negligent, professional misconduct must meet four requirements:

1. The care provider owed a duty to the patient.
2. The care provider did not carry out the duty (breach).
3. The patient was injured as a result of the care provider's action or inaction (proximate cause).
4. Actual loss or damage resulted from the actions.

To illustrate, a suicidal client is to be continuously observed (duty). The staff goes to lunch, leaving the client alone (breach of duty). During this time, the client commits suicide (proximate cause) and dies (damage). The staff is guilty of malpractice because no reasonable and prudent caregiver in a similar situation would leave a client unattended.

CARE PROVIDERS' RESPONSIBILITIES

The main responsibility of mental health care providers is to help clients cope with their mental and emotional problems. Dignified, humane treatment includes the protection of rights as human beings, citizens, and clients. Mental health clients have specific rights to treatment, refusal of treatment, informed consent, examination by the physician of their choice, confidentiality, and freedom from restraints. Other legal issues that relate to psychiatric care include elopement and the duty to warn.

Informed consent is an agreement between the client and providers of care that documents knowledge of and agreement to treatment. The client must be aware, informed, and capable of consenting. Mental health clients are presumed competent and able to consent to treatment. Obtaining consent for treatment is the physician's responsibility.

A special situation, known as **elopement,** sometimes arises during hospitalization when clients run away or elope from the institution. Caregivers who fail to prevent client elopement may be held liable if the client is injured as a result of the elopement. Keeping clients under supervision, plus accurate documentation of client behav-

iors and therapeutic actions, can prevent elopement from occurring.

All caregivers have the **duty to warn.** In situations where serious harm or death may occur, mental health professionals have a duty to protect potential victims from possible harm by a client. For example, if your client states that he intends to kill his barber, you have a duty to warn the barber. Contact the client's physician and your supervisor, and document the situation.

In some states, nurses and their colleagues have a duty to report certain information. Examples of reportable data include suspected incidents of abuse, gunshot wounds, and certain communicable diseases. The rights of the client must sometimes be balanced by the right of the public to be protected.

Documentation in client records is used in court to prove or disprove a claim. All client records should be completed in ink, dated and timed, and be legible and complete. Data should be objective, with client statements in quotation marks. Documentation should reflect the nursing process, standards of care, and client responses. Accurate, objective documentation is an excellent defense against potential legal problems.

The Reasonable and Prudent Caregiver Principle

The law judges professional actions by asking, "What would a **reasonable and prudent care provider** do under similar circumstances in a similar situation?" Then a comparison between behaviors is made. Practice "reasonable and prudent" care by following standards of practice and the employing agency's policies, procedures, job descriptions, and contracts. Safe practice is based on your knowledge of the limits that define caregiving in your practice setting.

Health care providers have the overall responsibility to practice in a competent, safe manner. This involves an active pursuit of new knowledge, as well as a willingness to conduct oneself according to ethical and legal standards. Even so, areas of potential liability exist in many situations. Awareness of your actions, as well as any possible problems, will help you practice safely and effectively.

KEY CONCEPTS

- ◆ Many aspects of society are defined by common values, morals, and rights that serve as foundations for making decisions.
- ◆ Values clarification is a three-step process to identify one's significant values.
- ◆ Rights are described as powers or privileges to which one has a just claim.
- ◆ Clients' rights are addressed by each state in its Patient's Bill of Rights and the federal Mental Health Systems Act Bill of Rights.

◆ Health care providers have the right to practice their professions in safety and with competent assistance and respect.

◆ Ethics are a shared set of codes, rules, or laws that govern right behavior.

◆ Ethical principles for nurses have been organized into codes of ethics by several nurses' organizations based on primary and secondary ethical principles.

◆ A five-step process assists health care providers in resolving ethical dilemmas.

◆ Laws are the controls by which a society governs itself. They function to define relationships, describe acceptable behaviors, maintain rules, and protect the public.

◆ Legal concepts that govern health care providers are found in state practice acts; standards of practice for the specific profession; and institutional policies, procedures, and job descriptions.

◆ Health caregivers are obligated to protect their clients' rights and provide competent care at the appropriate level of education and according to standards of care (practice).

◆ Because detaining a person against his or her wishes violates rights, most states have a formal commitment process that limits and monitors inpatient stays in psychiatric facilities.

◆ Care providers who care for people with mental illnesses need to be aware of the potential liabilities inherent in many client care situations.

Suggestions for Further Reading

Seven Common Legal Pitfalls in Nursing, by Tina Rae Eskreis in *The American Journal of Nursing,* (98[4]:34) describes common reasons for legal actions. All caregivers will find this an interesting article.

References

American Nurses Association: *ANA fact sheet: mental health bill of rights,* 1999, Kansas City, Mo, The Association.

Creighton H: *Law every nurse should know,* ed 5, Philadelphia, 1986, WB Saunders.

Edelman CL, Mandle CL: *Health promotion throughout the lifespan,* ed 4, St. Louis, 1998, Mosby.

Keltner NL, Schwecke LH, Bostrom CE: *Psychiatric nursing,* ed 3, St. Louis, 1998, Mosby.

Loewy EH: Ethical considerations in executing and implementing advanced directives, *Archives of Internal Medicine,* 58(4):32, 1998.

Morrison MW: *Professional skills for leadership: foundations of a successful career,* St. Louis, 1993, Mosby.

Potter PA, Perry AG: *Fundamentals of nursing,* ed 5, St. Louis, 2001, Mosby.

Stuart GW, Laraia MT: *Stuart and Sundeen's Pocket guide to psychiatric nursing,* ed 4, St. Louis, 1998, Mosby.

Chapter 4

Sociocultural Issues

Learning Objectives

1. Compare the concepts of culture, ethnicity, and religion.
2. Describe the consequences of stereotyping mental health clients.
3. List seven characteristics of culture.
4. Identify three ways in which culture influences health and illness behaviors.
5. List six components of cultural assessment.
6. Explain the importance of recognizing clients' spiritual or religious practices.
7. Identify four topics to be included in the assessment of a client who is a refugee.
8. Integrate cultural factors into a holistic plan of therapeutic care.

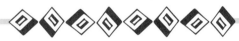

Key Terms

cultural competence	gender roles	refugee
culture	illness	religion
disease	norms	role
environmental control	nuclear family	spirituality
ethnicity	prejudice	stereotype
extended family	race	territoriality

Culture has a profound influence on mental illness and its treatment. Mental illness is defined within a cultural context. What may be appropriate behavior in one culture might be considered insanity in another. This is an important point because awareness of each client's cultural background will help us understand the client as a whole person, thus improving our therapeutic effectiveness.

NATURE OF CULTURE

Concepts are ideas that, when grouped together, form a "picture" of something. The "picture" of a person is incomplete without consideration of the cultural, ethnic, and religious concepts that define and guide an individual's life.

Simply put, **culture** is a total way of life. It is the learned pattern of behavior that shapes our thinking and serves as the basis for social, religious, and family structure. Culture is a shared system of values that provides the framework for who we are. **Race** is a biological term that describes a group of individuals who share physical characteristics that are distinct, such as skin color, facial features, and hair texture.

Ethnicity is a social term associated with the socialization patterns, customs, and cultural habits of a particular (ethnic) group. Ethnic groups function as a subsociety within a larger society and play important roles in preserving cultures. The values, traditions, expectations, and customs of a society are passed from one generation to another within ethnic groups. Because ethnic groups function as focal points for evaluating the value systems of other groups, ethnicity contributes to one's point of view.

Spirituality and religion play important roles in the concept of culture. The term **spirituality** refers to a belief in a power greater than any human being. **Religion** relates to a defined, organized, and practiced system of worship. Religious groups may have values that range from allowing for individual variation to requiring a commitment to place the religion before family, work, and friends. Often mental health clients have religious components to their illnesses. "Delusions of religiosity" may be ingrained in the illness. "The challenge to the nurse is to balance pathological behavior with appropriate cultural expression of religion" (Taylor, 1994).

Characteristics of Culture

Culture is an abstract concept, composed of the values, beliefs, roles, and norms of a group. Large multicultural societies such as our own have many cultural variations and subgroups. Health caregivers have varied cultural backgrounds themselves. Knowing how one's culture relates to clients' cultural backgrounds is a key to establishing effective care.

Cultural values strongly influence the thinking and actions of a culture's members. Because people of different cultures respond in various ways to time, activity, relationships, the supernatural, and nature, learning about the client's cultural values is important if health care providers are to be effective (Lester, 1998).

A culture's *belief system* develops over generations, formed by the feelings and convictions that are believed to be true within the society. Belief systems can be found in a culture's political, social, and religious practices. Conflicts in cultural value systems can lead to mental illness. People may also express one value and then act out another. Observing behaviors, rather than merely listening, allows caregivers to gain a more accurate picture of the client's values.

Beliefs about mental health have a strong impact on the outcome of treatment. When people believe in the treatment and in their care providers, successful outcomes are much more frequent. Know and respect the client's beliefs. Some things that you find strange may be of great cultural importance to the client.

Values and beliefs help define norms, which are a culture's behavioral standards. **Norms** are the established rules of conduct that define which behaviors are encouraged, accepted, tolerated, and forbidden within the culture. Simply put, norms are the rules for behavior.

A **role** is an expected pattern of behaviors associated with a certain position, status, or gender. Cultures commonly describe roles based on age, sex, marital status, and occupation. Individuals within the culture are expected to fulfill their roles and conform their behaviors to meet the expectations defined by the role. Some cultures have clearly defined role expectations, whereas others may be vague and ambiguous.

Case Study

Hauni is a 22-year-old woman who recently arrived from Sumatra. She has been ill for 3 days and arrives at the clinic with a friend. Although Hauni speaks English, the nurse who is obtaining her history must frequently repeat her questions. With patience, Hauni responds to the questions, but she immediately freezes when Dr. Dankin enters the examination room. Although she feels very ill, she refuses to be examined. Sensing the client's uneasiness, the nurse confers with Dr. Dankin, who recommends that the case be turned over to Dr. Linda Smith. Hauni responds immediately to Dr. Smith, even to the point where she becomes talkative.

- What difference did the recognition of the client's cultural background make in her care?
- What do you think would have happened if the client's culture was not considered?

"A **stereotype** is an oversimplified mental picture of a cultural group" (Haber and others, 1997). Some beliefs about certain groups are passed on through generations and tend to color the perceptions and influence the behaviors of people who hold them. Stereotyping may take negative, positive, or traditional forms. The extreme form of negative stereotyping is called **prejudice**. Traditional stereotyping occurs when one assumes that all members of a culture behave in the traditional manner.

Stereotypes develop unconsciously in many people, especially those who have had little exposure to culturally diverse groups Health care providers need to know and understand their own racial, ethnic, religious, and social stereotypes. Clients, especially those with mental problems, are very sensitive to discrimination. If they sense such treatment, they will resist receiving care. By removing stereotypes, you allow each person to be treated as an individual, with the respect and dignity that is his or her right.

Caregivers who assess the behaviors of culturally different clients without personal biases are better able to distinguish adaptive behaviors from dysfunctional ones (see Case Study box).

Cultures vary greatly in values, beliefs, and behaviors, but they all share several characteristics Table 4-1 presents a brief description of the main characteristics of culture.

Culture is a social phenomenon. First, culture is *learned* through life experiences as a part of the society. Second, culture is *transmitted* or passed from one generation to another through language, symbols, and practices. Third, culture is *shared*. Values, beliefs, and standards of behavior that are known to all members

Table 4-1 Characteristics of Culture

Characteristics	Description	Example
Culture is learned.	Culture is a learned set of shared values, beliefs, and behaviors and is not genetically inherited.	Cuban family members learn that humor is a way of making fun of people, situations, or things called *chateo*. Humor also includes modifying situations through exaggeration, jokes, and satirical expressions or gestures.
Culture is transmitted.	Culture is passed from one generation to another.	In the Asian culture the concept of family extends both backward and forward. The individual is seen as a product of all generations of the family from the beginning of time. This concept is reinforced by rituals, such as ancestor worship and family record books. Personal actions reflect on not only the individual but also all generations.
Culture is shared.	Culture is a shared set of assumptions, values, beliefs, attitudes, and behaviors of a group. Members predict one another's actions and react accordingly.	In the Arab culture a woman will not make eye contact with a man other than her husband. All decisions are made by her husband. Because a woman may not be touched by another man, health care may be provided only by another woman.
Culture is integrated.	Universal aspects of culture include religion, politics, economics, art, kinship, diet, health, and patterns of communication. All categories of culture are interrelated.	In Ireland and the United States, the primary cultural force and national unifier of Irish culture has been the Catholic Church. The parish, rather than the neighborhood, has traditionally defined the family's social context.
Culture contains ideal and real components.	Ideal cultural patterns are called norms, which prescribe what people ought to do and may be legally or socially reinforced. Real behavior may diverge from ideal behavior and still be acceptable.	The American mainstream culture condemns the drinking of alcohol on a daily basis. However, those who do so but "hold their liquor well" are regarded with only minimal disapproval.
Culture is dynamic and continuously evolving.	Cultural change is an ongoing process. All aspects do not change at the same time. Cultural habits and newer behaviors are easier to alter than deep-rooted values and beliefs.	Although Italian-Americans have become an integral part of American society, values regarding the family roles of men and women are often more traditional than values regarding the roles of men and women in the workplace.
Individual behavior is not necessarily representative of the culture.	Although culture defines the dominant patterns of values, beliefs, and behaviors, it does not determine all the behaviors in any group. Variation from the major pattern of behavior is called *eccentric behavior*. The meaning of this behavior within the culture will determine whether it is regarded as normal, eccentric, or deviant.	Male and female roles are strictly defined in traditional Greek culture. Women are secondary; the man is the head of the family. Men work and provide for their families; it is a dishonor if the wife works outside the home. Within this cultural context, a Greek woman who is a proponent of the feminist movement might be viewed as eccentric or deviant.

Modified from Haber J and others: *Comprehensive psychiatric nursing,* ed 5, St. Louis, 1997, Mosby.

allow children to learn right from wrong and adjust their behaviors according to the cultural norms. Fourth, culture is *integrated* into an interwoven framework of political, social, religious, and health practices. Fifth, because a culture reflects its members, it is *dynamic,* changing, and adaptive. Sixth, cultural habits are also *satisfying.* They fill a need within the society and result in gratification. Seventh, an individual's behavior may or may not represent the culture. Individual behaviors may differ from the major behavioral patterns and still be tolerated, but only to a certain extent. When a person's actions go beyond a culturally acceptable point, they are considered eccentric, maladaptive, or deviant. Each of these seven characteristics helps to explain the framework of a culture. To deliver holistic, effective mental health care, all care providers must assess the impact and meaning that each cultural characteristic has for the client.

INFLUENCES OF CULTURE

People base many health decisions on both scientific and cultural values. As a result, many individuals seek health care from folk healers, as well as medical practitioners.

Health and Illness Beliefs

The practice of Western medicine is based on scientifically proven treatment methods and tends to disregard that which cannot be explained by scientific research. Providers of health care are specifically licensed and trained in one area of expertise. Health care is offered in institutions and is often delivered in an impersonal, assembly-line manner.

Folk medicine, "on the other hand, embodies the beliefs, values and treatment approaches of a particular cultural group" (Edelman and Mandle, 1998). Its foundation is based on empirical knowledge—observation and experience without an understanding of cause or effect. Folk practitioners explain disease culturally as an imbalance of energies. Caregivers may receive training through an experienced practitioner, religious groups, or self-study. Care is provided in the home or community in a personal, individualized manner (Table 4-2). Providers of health care within the Western system of medicine need to know about clients' folk medical practices, because many people seek out professional care only after folk healing proves inadequate.

Traditional health beliefs involve explanations of the causes of health and disease. For example, Navajo and traditional black cultures view health as a state of harmony with nature. The mind and body are one and function in harmony with the earth and the supernatural. Disease is a state of disharmony.

Chinese cultures consider health to be a balance of positive and negative energy forces (yin and yang). An imbalance of yin or yang results in disease. Hispanics feel that good health is a gift from God, sprinkled with good luck. Illness is an imbalance of the hot and cold body properties and is considered God's punishment (Geissler, 1998). Low-income families define health as the ability to work. Illness is seen as unpreventable. Throughout the years, millions of people have sought health care from alternative (folk) sources. Understanding and respecting the client's cultural health beliefs and practices promote effective treatment for those who seek the Western system of health care.

Illness Behaviors

Disease is a condition in which a physical dysfunction exists, whereas **illness** is a state of social, emotional, intellectual (as well as physical) dysfunction. Culture has no impact on disease, but illness, and its attendant behaviors, are strongly influenced by culture.

When the signs and symptoms of illness appear, an individual may choose one of four courses of action: (1) do something to relieve the symptoms, (2) do nothing, (3) vacillate without taking any real action, or (4) deny the existence of the problem. Several studies have compared the illness behaviors of men from various cultural backgrounds. Results revealed that Italian-Americans sought medical help when social or personal relationships were affected by the illness. Irish-Americans sought help for their symptoms only after receiving approval of

Table 4-2 Comparison Between Folk and Western Health Care Systems		
Criteria	**Western**	**Folk**
Philosophy of care	Curative	Curative
Approach to care	Fragmented specialization Often impersonal	Personalized
Setting for services	Institutions	Homes, community, other social places
Treatments	Technology Approved pharmacological agents	Herbs, charms, amulets, massage, meditation
Providers	Licensed professionals	Healers, shamans, spiritualists, priests, other lay unlicensed therapists
Support for care	Other ancillary personnel and agencies	Family, relatives, friends
Payment for services	Third-party insurers Personal funds	Negotiable
Philosophy of health	Influenced by the professional's definition and dealt with in terms of illness and treatment	Reflected as a quest for harmony with nature
Definition of disease	Result of cause-effect phenomena; cure is achieved by scientifically proven methods	Imbalance between person and physical, social, and spiritual worlds

From Edelman CL, Mandle CL: *Health promotion throughout the lifespan,* ed 4, St. Louis, 1998, Mosby.

others. Americans of Anglo-Saxon origin required medical assistance only when their symptoms interfered with specific activities.

Illness behaviors are also affected by ideological beliefs (e.g., Christian Scientists do not seek medical help for illness) and culture. For example, if headaches are considered a sign of weakness, to seek treatment would be to act counter to the cultural heritage. To be effective, health care providers must assess each client's attitudes and behaviors relating to illness.

On Mental Illness

Clients and their care providers may have very different belief systems about mental disorders. Members within a culture may define normal and abnormal behaviors differently than those outside the culture. To illustrate, in several cultures the practice of altered states of consciousness or trances is considered acceptable. Nurses must ascertain their clients' cultural definitions of mental health and illness.

Cultural descriptions of mental dysfunction are classified as naturalistic illness or personalistic illness. According to Haber and others (1997), "naturalistic illnesses are caused by impersonal factors without regard for the individual." Forces that exist outside the individual cause mental illness. Illnesses that are categorized as personalistic illnesses are seen as aggression or punishment directed toward a specific person. Examples include voodoo, witchcraft, and the evil eye.

Beliefs in witchcraft are widespread in Haitian, Puerto Rican, and African-American cultures. Spells, hexes, and incantations are used to cause a person injury, illness, or even death. Mental illness is considered the result of witchcraft, magic, or evil spells.

The practice of voodoo calls forth the spirits of the dead back to the world of the living to bless or curse specific people. People with mental disorders are thought to be cursed by spirits. Although the causative forces exist outside the body, the chosen individual "takes on" or internalizes the behaviors associated with the hex.

Stress and Coping

All cultures classify their members by sex and age. Age and sex roles contain certain norms, status, and expectations. Some cultures, for example, value the elderly and respect their acquired wisdom, whereas others consider their elders as nonproductive burdens. Clearly the role of elders in the latter example is associated with more stress.

Adolescence in many cultures can be a stressful time. Societies that clearly define adolescence and its roles tend to be less stress inducing than cultures who lack a clear definition of adolescence.

Women are often placed in stressful roles as a result of their culture. Traditional Greek culture, for example, sees the man as the breadwinner for the family. A Greek wife who works brings embarrassment to the entire family group. A great deal of stress would result for a working woman in this culture.

Stress is associated with various culturally defined roles. Ways of coping with role-induced stress are also culturally determined. Crying, screaming, and other displays of emotion are viewed as healthy outlets in one culture, whereas others expect quiet, unemotional responses to stress. Caregivers who are aware of clients' cultural stresses and their associated behaviors are better able to assist them in developing effective coping skills.

CULTURAL ASSESSMENT

Cultural competence is the process of continually learning about the cultures with which we work and developing cross-cultural therapeutic health care skills. "Rather than impose personal cultural values on others, the professional nurse is an active listener and analyst who develops appropriate care plans based on the insights, knowledge, and beliefs of other cultures" (Deloughery, 1998). Transcultural nursing is the application of culturally sensitive therapeutic interventions (Lipson and others, 1996). All care providers must guard against the tendency to transfer their own cultural expectations onto clients or make generalizations about clients based on their own cultural attitudes. Each client is uniquely molded by his or her culture.

It is the responsibility of all care providers to learn how clients perceive and cope within their worlds. Cultural assessments are the tools that allow us to do that. Several tools have been developed, but all have in common six areas of assessment: communication, environmental control, space and territory, time, social orientation, and biological factors (Figure 4-1) (Giger and Davidhizar, 1999).

Communication

People of all cultures communicate with one another. The process of communication, however, involves more than just the use of language. Communication is a complex, interwoven tapestry of voice, gesture, and touch. Both verbal and nonverbal components of communication have cultural meaning (Table 4-3).

Clients communicate their emotional states based on their cultural backgrounds. In some cultures, verbal expressions of emotion are approved, whereas members of other cultures value communicating indirectly and may resent the frankness of mental health care providers. Clients require sensitivity if we are to be therapeutically effective. We all communicate; some of us are just louder than others.

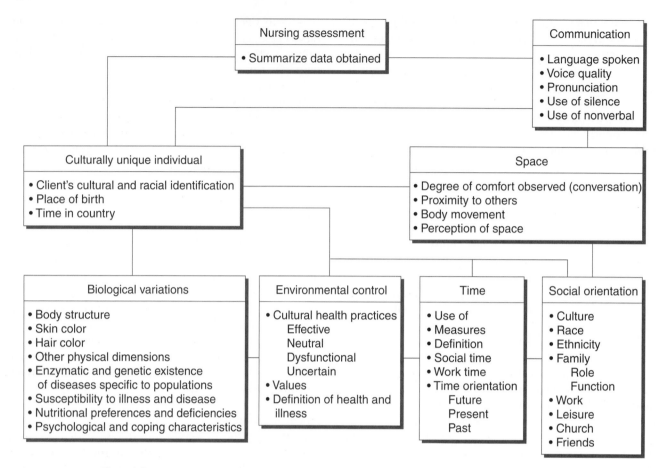

Figure 4-1 Cultural assessment. (Redrawn from Giger JN, Davidhizar RE: *Transcultural nursing: assessment and intervention,* ed 3, St. Louis, 1999, Mosby.)

Table 4-3	Cultural Communication Assessment

Verbal communications	Nonverbal communications
Language 　Dialect 　Pronunciation 　Voice quality 　Rate of speech 　Style of speech 　Volume of speech 　Use of small talk, laughter Music Written language 　Formal usage 　Regional usage Communicates emotions verbally More verbally oriented	Touch 　Use of touch 　How touch is perceived and received Space 　Interpersonal distance Use of silence, eye contact, facial gestures (e.g., smiles, frowns) Communicates emotions nonverbally More behaviorally oriented

Cultural traditions, practices, and kinship systems all communicate. A society's religious practices communicate its basic beliefs. Attitudes toward children, family health care, and dying are all communicated through cultural customs. It is wise to learn the important customs of a culture if one is caring for many of its members (see Cultural Aspects box).

Environmental Control

Environmental control focuses on the individual's ability to perceive and control the environment. Does the client feel that the power to effect change lies within, or is everything the result of fate, chance, or luck? What are the client's values relating to the nature of man, the supernatural, health, and illness? How are the causes and treatments for mental illnesses viewed?

Environmental control includes an assessment of clients' cultural health practices. Have any alternative practitioners been consulted? What were the treatments? Were they effective? What is their definition of "good health," and what is done to maintain health? When alternative (folk) practices are assessed, both clients and their care providers increase the potential for success.

Space, Territory, and Time

Also included in the cultural assessment are the concepts of space and territory. *Space* is the area that surrounds the client—an invisible "bubble" that travels with the person. The physical distance that a person maintains between himself or herself and others is influenced by one's culture. People consciously maintain a "comfortable" distance from each other. Mental health clients often have additional perceptions about space. For example, some clients feel the need to be *closer* to people for feelings of safety and security. Space comfort areas are divided into four distances: public, social, personal, and intimate (Figure 4-2). Observe and respect your client's degree of comfort at each distance, and their use of surrounding space.

Some clients have a need to establish territory. **Territoriality** is the need to gain control over an area of space and claim it for oneself. For many people a territory helps to provide a sense of identity, security, autonomy, and control over the environment. People will protect their territory (even if it is the size of a hospital bed), and health care providers can be casually careless about invading these precious spaces. Caregivers, especially nurses, need to know and respect the client's territorial space if culturally appropriate holistic care is to be given.

The concept of *time* is rooted in a culture's basic orientation. Cultures oriented to the past (e.g., Chinese, Amish) strive to maintain the customs and traditions of previous generations. Present-oriented cultures focus on current daily events but may not follow a schedule. Many Native Americans are present oriented but not to time. Cultures with future time orientations use today as a tool for meeting future goals. Schedules are established and people are oriented to the time of day. An example of a future-oriented culture is the middle class of the United States and Canada. Western society's concept of time is linear. For some cultures the linear concept of time is difficult to understand.

Clients with mental dysfunctions frequently have misperceptions about time. An inability to tell the difference between day and night can exist, and difficulty following schedules is commonplace. Problems with time may be based in the client's cultural orientation or psychiatric illness. Until the caregiver can discover the difference, the delivery of effective care is difficult.

Social Orientation

To assess a client's social orientation, caregivers must consider the family unit within the culture. The family unit and its importance in the society are culturally defined. The family unit imparts the culture's important traditions, beliefs, values, and customs. Social orientation also includes the meaning of work, gender roles, friends, and religion to the client.

Although the functions of the family (e.g., caring for the young, providing identity, security) remain similar among most cultures, the size and composition differ.

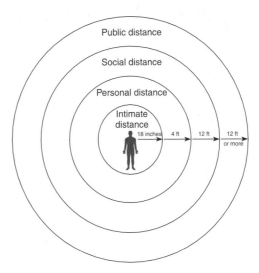

Figure 4-2 Space and distance zones.

Middle-class Americans live within a **nuclear family** unit consisting of a father, mother, and one or more children. In many cultures, aunts, uncles, grandparents, cousins, and/or godparents are also included in the family. This family unit is called an **extended family,** and its importance to the client may be significant. Many groups—such as traditional Chinese, Mexicans, and Puerto Ricans—believe the family to be the supreme social organization. Family causes take priority over personal or national causes in these cultures. When care providers fail to consider the whole family, culturally sensitive care goals cannot be achieved.

Gender roles are expected behavioral patterns based on sex. The traditional roles for men and women in one society may collide with the expectations of another. Women who have learned to fill a serving, passive gender role may have great difficulty assuming the assertive and outspoken role of the modern Western woman. Be sensitive to this area of assessment. Few women will identify themselves as having a culturally based gender role conflict. Mental health problems more frequently seen in women include eating disorders, phobias, and depression. Men, on the other hand, tend to demonstrate more violent and abusive behaviors. Cultural norms that identify gender roles often encourage the expression of conflict in different ways.

Assessment of social orientation also includes the client's religious beliefs and practices. Religious beliefs and practices serve many functions in a culture. They bind people together in a common belief system. Religion helps to explain the unexplainable, such as unexpected deaths or natural catastrophes, and it helps to provide meaning and guidance for living.

Religious beliefs and practices vary widely. Attitudes toward health, illness, death, burials, procreation, food, and stress all have religious components. Although it is impossible to discover the inner workings of every religion, it is necessary to be aware of the religious practices of those clients with whom you frequently interact.

Biological Factors

The final area of cultural assessment focuses on the biological or physical differences that exist among different cultural groups. When assessing the client's cultural group for biological factors, consider the following: physical variations, enzymatic and genetic variations; susceptibility to disease; and psychological characteristics.

Physical variations include differences in body structure, eyes, ears, noses, teeth, muscle mass, and skin color. People of some races are taller than others. For example, African-Americans are usually taller than Asian-Americans. The shape of the eyelids and nose vary from one racial group to another. Teeth may also vary in size and shape: "Australian aborigines have the largest teeth in the world, as well as four extra molars" (Giger and

Davidhizar, 1999). In contrast, white Americans tend to have small teeth. Certain muscles of the wrist and foot are absent in some racial groups. Differences in skin color range from pale white to black. Mongolian spots, for example, are bluish discolorations of the skin that may be found in black, Asian, Mexican, and Native American newborns. In this case, knowing the client's cultural background may prevent possible misdiagnosis because Mongolian spots can be mistaken for bruises resulting from child abuse.

A person's *genetic makeup* is largely determined by racial group. Physical appearance, metabolic activities, enzyme functions, and susceptibility to disease are all influenced by racial factors. To illustrate, sickle cell anemia is commonly found in the African-Americans but rarely in white Americans. Lactose (milk) intolerance is very common in black, Native American, and Asian groups yet is rare in northern European whites. Tuberculosis is common in Native Americans, whereas diabetes is rare in Eskimos. Relationships between race and physical health have been well documented, but the relationship between race and mental health remains hazier.

Certain *psychological characteristics* may be related to different cultural groups. The low socioeconomic status of some groups can affect mental health when housing, education, and health care are substandard. Feelings of insecurity can result when a client's views of health care are threatened. The Hmong people of Laos, for example, believe that "losing blood saps strength and may result in the soul leaving the body, causing death" (Rairdan and Higgs, 1992). Therefore great anxiety is produced in a Hmong client when blood is drawn. Cultural factors do affect mental health. Nurses and their colleagues must become aware of group differences if they are to consistently deliver culturally appropriate mental health care.

CULTURE AND MENTAL HEALTH CARE

No society is immune to mental disorders, but research is needed to study mental illness from a worldwide perspective. The definition and treatments of mental illness vary among cultures. To understand and treat clients from diverse backgrounds, the concept of **cultural competence** has evolved. As the name implies, cultural competence seeks to deliver appropriate client care based on a knowledge of the client's culture.

It is important here to understand the unique status of refugees. By definition, a **refugee** is a person who, because of war or persecution, flees from his or her home or country and seeks refuge elsewhere. Many refugees have seen or experienced imprisonment, torture, and harrowing escapes. Some have lost family members, and all must learn to cope within a new reality.

When assessing a person who is a refugee, be extra sensitive to the possibility of stress-related problems. In addition to the routine cultural assessment, tactfully obtain the following information: immigration history, time in the new country, a history of the flight and arrival in the new country, and who or what was lost (Lipson, 1993). Because of a usually traumatic history, higher incidences of depression, anxiety, and stress disorders occur in refugee groups. Nurses who work with the whole person are sensitive to the special circumstances of refugees.

Clients from other cultures may evaluate their health care differently. Haitian-Americans, for example, may feel that improvement in health was not the result of good care but the mystical healing power of the tree leaves kept close to the body. There exist many such customs and beliefs (see Think About box). If culturally sensitive health care providers are able to consistently view clients as unique, dynamically functioning individuals, then effective, appropriate health care will be one step closer to becoming a reality.

KEY CONCEPTS

◆ Culture is a learned pattern of behaviors, values, beliefs, and customs shared by a group of people.
◆ Stereotyping is basing one's behavior on an oversimplified mental picture of a cultural group.
◆ Culture is learned, transmitted, shared, integrated, dynamic, and satisfying.
◆ Culture influences people's health beliefs and practices.

◆ Because illness behaviors are influenced by one's perceptions and cultural outlook, each client's definition of health and illness must be assessed.
◆ Cultural assessments focus on six areas: communication, environmental control, space and territory, time, social orientation, and biological factors.
◆ Working with refugees requires added assessments and great tact because of their frequently traumatic experiences and losses.
◆ Because no universal descriptions of mental health and illness exist, the definition and treatment of mental illness vary among cultures.
◆ Culturally competent health care seeks to deliver the diverse therapeutic actions necessary for appropriate, effective client care.
◆ When caregivers are able to consistently view each client as a unique dynamic individual functioning within a sociocultural context, then culturally appropriate health care will become a reality.

Suggestions for Further Reading

Transcultural nursing: assessment and intervention, ed 3, by J.N. Giger and R.E. Davidhizar (St. Louis, 1999, Mosby) is interesting reading and an excellent source of information for several cultural groups. It is highly recommended for all health care providers.

References

Deloughery GL: *Issues and trends in nursing*, ed 3, St. Louis, 1998, Mosby.

Edelman CL, Mandle CL: *Health promotion throughout the lifespan*, ed 4, St. Louis, 1998, Mosby.

Geissler EM: *Pocket guide to cultural assessment*, ed 2, St. Louis, 1998, Mosby.

Giger JN, Davidhizar RE: *Transcultural nursing: assessment and intervention*, ed 3, St. Louis, 1999, Mosby.

Haber J and others: *Comprehensive psychiatric nursing*, ed 5, St. Louis, 1997, Mosby.

Lester MA: Cultural competence, *American Journal of Nursing* 98(8):26, 1998.

Lipson JG: Afghan refugees in California: mental health issues, *Issues in Mental Health Nursing*, 14:411, 1993.

Lipson JG and others: *Culture and nursing care: a pocket guide*, San Francisco, 1996, UCSF Press.

Rairdan B, Higgs ZR: When your patient is a Hmong refugee, *American Journal of Nursing* 92(3):52, 1992.

Taylor CM: *Essentials of psychiatric nursing*, ed 14, St. Louis, 1994, Mosby.

Chapter 5

Early Theories and Therapies

Learning Objectives

1. Explain how theories can be applied to mental health care.
2. Identify the theory of human behavior that was popular from 350 BC to AD 1400.
3. Describe how Darwin's theory of evolution changed attitudes toward mental illness.
4. List three parts of Freud's psychoanalytic theory of human behavior.
5. Name four therapeutic techniques used in psychotherapy.
6. Identify how humanistic and behavioral theories differ in their viewpoints.
7. Discuss how Maslow's human needs theory can be used in the care of people with emotional problems.
8. Explain why it is important for health care providers to be familiar with different theories of human behavior and their explanations of mental illness.

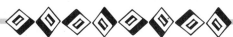

Key Terms

affective	inferiority	psychoanalysis
anxiety	libidinal energy	psychotherapy
cognitive	model	soma
defense mechanisms	natural selection	superego
ego	personifications	theory
id	psyche	unconscious

Human beings exist within an orderly but changing universe. As our ancestors evolved, they began to observe the world about them and develop ideas to explain nature and its cycles. Eventually their ideas became related to each other. When related ideas were combined, they provided a framework or point of view that helped provide possible explanations for the workings of their world.

Today, a **theory** is defined as a statement that predicts, explains, or describes a relationship among events, concepts, or ideas. Modern theories are developed through observation and research. Earlier theories evolved through observations and deductions. Later,

theorists used models to help explain their ideas more simply. A **model** is an example or pattern that helps explain a theory. For example, a model of an airplane can be used to explain the theory of flight.

Models and theories about human behavior help explain the complicated creature known as the human being—the physical, psychological, social, and cultural aspects of people. Theories are also used to help describe the psychodynamics of people: the basic needs, drives, conflicts, perceptions, values, attitudes, belief systems, and cultural influences that shape every individual. Nurses, physicians, therapists, and others in the helping professions use theories as frameworks for describing the relationships between people and various aspects of their environments.

HISTORICAL THEORIES

Some of the earliest questions about human nature began with the observations of a Greek physician, Hippocrates (460-377 BC) (see Chapter 1). His *humoral theory* of disease and mental illness linked personality types (temperaments) to each basic element or humor of the body. The humoral theory influenced the fields of medicine and philosophy for almost 15 centuries.

Symbolic and magical thinking was used to explain how the world worked in medieval times. "For the Middle Ages there was a perfect spiritual world just beyond the imperfect world of physical suffering and decay; one could attempt contact with the perfect reality through visions, religious ecstasy, or sorcery, and by deciphering the spiritual meaning behind everyday events" (Corsini, 1994).

Paracelsus (1493-1541) revolutionized the study of mental health and illness by distinguishing between natural (physical) illnesses and spiritual (psychological) illnesses. He is credited with being the first to recognize the role of unconscious forces in illness.

Darwin's Theory

Charles Darwin (1809-1882) was a naturalist, but his theory of evolution was to have a lasting impact on the emerging field of psychiatry. Basically, Darwin's theory explained why some animal species became extinct while others flourished. His theory stated that only the fittest organisms would adapt and survive and that, through the process of **natural selection,** increasingly superior creatures evolved. In this way, nature culls the weak and preserves the strong.

During the latter half of the nineteenth century, Darwin's theory led to the persistent belief that people who were impaired or unsuccessful in life were, by nature, lower on the evolutionary scale. Poverty, disease, alcoholism, and mental illness were all claimed to be the product of an inferior genetic makeup. High incidences of tuberculosis, rickets, infant mortality, and low adult life expectancies all indicated that Nature was at work. This popular theory may have continued for many years had not the work of new theorists challenged the commonly held beliefs of the time.

Functional Psychology

William James (1842-1910), was educated in Europe, England, and the United States. He taught the first psychology course in an American university (Harvard) in 1875 and published the first textbook on psychology in 1890. However, he is best remembered for his view of the human mind as "functional, adaptive mental processes" (Corsini, 1994).

James built on Darwin's theory of natural selection by viewing behaviors as adjustments to the environment. His theory stated that the general causes of emotions were internal, physical, and nervous processes, not just psychological events. This innovative approach laid the groundwork for a new system of thinking in psychology known as *functionalism.* Followers of functionalism thought that psychology should have practical applications and deal with commonsense issues. They believed that mental functions were part of a whole complex world that included both physical and mental adaptive processes. Although functionalism no longer exists as a separate theory, it contributed to our understanding by including studies relating to adaptation, experience, intelligence testing, learning, child behavior, and abnormal behavior. Many of the principles of functionalism have been incorporated into the mainstream of American psychology.

Psychoanalytical Theories

By the middle of the nineteenth century, various theories of mental health and illness had circulated throughout the scientific world. Physicians everywhere were exploring new curative treatments for mental illness. Dr. Joseph Breuer (1842-1905) employed the technique of hypnosis along with a new method of "talking out" symptoms. A brilliant young neurosurgeon, Sigmund Freud, heard of this "talking cure" and sought to work with the distinguished physician. By 1895 Breuer and Freud had published *Studies in Hysteria,* a collection of successful case histories in which the therapeutic use of hypnosis and the "talking cure" were used. Freud's association with Breuer faded as disagreements over the use of hypnosis therapy grew, and Freud alone delved further into the use of talking as a therapy.

After years of observation and documentation, Freud came to believe that unconscious thoughts and emotions have a strong impact on mental functioning and behavior. By 1902 Freud had become convinced of the talking cure's value. He called his approach to therapy **psychoanalysis,** which means to explore the unconscious. Weekly discussions about psychoanalysis, attended by a number of Freud's colleagues (e.g., Alfred Adler, Otto Rank, and Carl Jung), later provided the framework for various new and different theoretical beliefs.

The nucleus of Freud's theories focused on behaviors of which the patient was unaware. His study of the unconscious processes of the mind evolved into theories about the development, structure, and dynamics of the personality. These ideas, together with Freud's ability to apply his concepts to such varied topics as dream content, hysterical paralysis, and the biological nature of people, made psychoanalysis the most influential set of theories in the early twentieth century.

For the next 30 years Freud worked to develop and test his theories. By the 1920s the one definition of psychoanalysis had broadened into three: Freud's theories of personality, a therapy for certain emotional disorders, and a method for investigating the workings of the mind. Today, the term **psychotherapy** is used to describe any therapy relating to mental illness. Freud's theories that are of importance to health care providers relate to the development, dynamics, and defenses of the personality.

Freud's Theories of Personality

Freud believed that the human mind was made up of three interacting structures, which he labeled id, ego, and superego. The **id** is the storage site for all the basic drives and early childhood experiences. It contains the instinctual drives for self-preservation, reproduction, and association with others. For example, drives arising from hunger, cold, physical discomfort, and isolation are centered in the id. The demand, "I want what I want *now*," is characteristic of id behavior. Freud stated that the id is governed by the "pleasure principle." It seeks out immediate pleasure or avoidance of pain for all impulses without regard to the outcome. Because infants disregard all other parts of their environment as they demand immediate attention, they are often described as "bundles of id."

The word **ego** is derived from the Latin word meaning "I" and is the part of the mind in active awareness. In other words, the ego is the conscious mind. When people discuss one's personality, character, or intellect, they are referring to the ego. The ego develops when the child becomes aware of "self," usually around 2 years of age. During growth the reality-based ego gradually gains control over the more primitive id and develops into the personality that copes with the external world.

The **superego** is the last to develop. All the attitudes, values, role expectations, taboos, rules, ideals, and standards to which the child is exposed help form the superego. There are two parts to the superego: the conscience, which punishes the individual through guilt and anxiety when behaviors move away from its strict, rigid standards, and the ego ideal, which rewards with feelings of satisfaction and well-being for behaviors that are in keeping with the superego's expectations. The superego does not base rewards or punishments on reality. It uses internal standards of right and wrong that were learned early in life. These standards, according to Freud, are primarily stored in the **unconscious,** where they remain unavailable to awareness but still influence the ego. The superego is the controller of the id as a result of its strict and rigid, moralistic rules. The statement, "I want what I know is the right thing," is characteristic of the superego.

According to Freud, id and superego demands go straight to the ego, unhampered by values or external world rules. Therefore the ego must maintain the delicate balancing act of meeting id and superego needs within the limitations of the real world.

People with strong egos are considered to have a great degree of control. Behavior that is ruled by the superego can result in repressed, guilt-ridden, inhibited individuals. Id-dominated behavior may result in antisocial, lawless people with little control. The mentally healthy adult is said to be one who has achieved a dynamic balance among all the elements of the personality.

Freud's theory of personality development has the central theme of sexual instinct growth through four stages from newborn to adult. He believed that the most powerful primitive motivation was the drive to reproduce. He described this drive, known as **libidinal energy,** as the need to seek sexual pleasure. Freud's stages of personality development became known as the *psychosexual theory* of development.

Freud placed great emphasis on early childhood experiences and their impact on personality development. He believed that what happens to the child during each particular stage becomes part of the adult character. He then characterized each stage with a primary erogenous zone (an area of the body that serves as a focus for excitation and pleasure) and named them the oral stage, anal stage, phallic stage, latency stage, and genital stage. Freud believed that mental health results when an individual successfully moves through each stage and, as an adult, can maintain a mature sexual relationship. On the other hand, mental difficulties arise when an individual becomes fixated or stuck in a particular stage. To illustrate, followers of Freud consider activities such as smoking or overeating to be the remnants of unresolved oral stage demands.

According to Freud, emotional disturbances and behavioral dysfunctions arise from five sources: (1) instinctual-biological drives, (2) early childhood experiences, (3) deeply buried unconscious experiences and attitudes, (4) fixations arising from earlier psychosexual stages of development, and (5) defensive maneuvers that help prevent the person from changing. Freud believed that all individuals have some conflict embedded within themselves and thus use psychological tools to help to lessen negative feelings. He called these psychological tools **defense mechanisms** and defined them as "psychological strategies by which persons reduce or avoid negative states such as conflict, frustration, anxiety, and stress" (Corsini, 1994) (Table 5-1). Defense mechanisms are used to avoid negative emotional states, but individuals are not consciously aware when they are being used. Furthermore, most defense mechanisms contain some inaccurate pictures of reality. No matter which mechanism is used, the goal remains the same—to reduce uncomfortable negative emotions.

Table 5-1 Common Defense Mechanisms

Mechanism	Definition	Example
Compensation	Attempt to overcome feelings of inferiority or make up for deficiency	A girl who thinks she cannot sing studies to become an expert pianist.
Conversion	Channeling of unbearable anxieties into body signs and symptoms	A boy who injured an animal by kicking it develops a painful limp.
Denial	Refusal to acknowledge conflict and thus escapes reality of situation	A child covered with chocolate refuses to admit eating candy.
Displacement	Redirecting of energies to another person or object	A husband shouts at his wife, the wife then berates her child, who then scolds the dog.
Dissociation	Separation of emotions from situation; isolation of painful anxieties	A soldier casually describes the battle in which he lost his legs.
Fantasy	Distortion of unacceptable wishes, behaviors	A teenager doing poorly in school daydreams about owning a private jet airplane.
Identification	Taking on of personal characteristics of admired person to conceal own feelings of inadequacy	Teen-aged adolescents dress and behave like the members of a popular singing group.
Intellectualization	Focusing of attention on technical or logical aspects of threatening situation	A wife describes the details of nurses' unsuccessful attempts to prevent the death of her husband.
Isolation	Separation of feelings from content to cope unemotionally with topics that would normally be overwhelming	A soldier humorously describes how he was seriously wounded in combat.
Projection	Putting of one's own unacceptable thoughts, wishes, emotions onto others	A woman is afraid to leave her house because she knows people will ridicule her.
Rationalization	Use of a "good" (but not real) reason to explain behavior to make unacceptable motivation more acceptable	A student justifies failing an examination by saying that there was too much material to cover.
Reaction formation	Prevention of expression of threatening material by engaging in behaviors that are directly opposite to repressed material	A young man with homosexual feelings, which he finds to be threatening, engages in excessive heterosexual activities.
Regression	Coping with present conflict, stress by returning to earlier, more secure stage of life	A 4-year-old boy whose parents are going through a divorce starts to suck his thumb and wet his pants.
Restitution	Giving back to resolve guilt feelings	A man argues with his wife and then buys her roses.
Sublimation	Unconscious channeling of unacceptable behaviors into constructive, more socially approved areas	A hostile young man who enjoys fighting becomes a football player.
Substitution	Disguising of motivations by replacing inappropriate behavior with one that is more acceptable	A man who is attracted to pornography campaigns to ban adult book stores in his community.
Suppression	Removal of conflict by removing anxiety from consciousness	A woman with a family history of breast cancer "forgets" her appointment for a mammogram.
Symbolization	Use of an unrelated object to represent hidden idea	A girl who feels insignificant draws a picture of her family in which she is the smallest character.
Undoing	Inappropriate behavior that is followed by acts to take away or reverse action and decrease guilt and anxiety	A man physically abuses his wife and then cleans her wounds and nurses her back to health.

Psychoanalytical Therapies

Early therapies based on Freud's work were designed to assist the patient in discovering the causes of unconscious, repressed conflicts and working through fixations (anxieties) that resulted from those conflicts. Freud used *dream analysis* to delve into the origins of the patient's symptoms. He believed that, during sleep, the individual's censor (superego) is less active; therefore the unconscious (id) could express itself in dreams. Therapy centered around interpreting the dream's symbols to discover the unconscious wishes that were causing the conflicts.

The technique of *free association* soon followed. With free association, the patient was presented with a series of words or phrases and then asked to state the first words that came to mind. The therapist would then "interpret" each response and give the patient the "real" meaning behind each association. This process, Freud thought, would eventually lead to the discovery of the patient's problems.

Psychoanalysis was the main form of therapy for Freud and many of his followers. Because behavioral problems were considered to arise from several different factors, the process of psychoanalysis lasted for many sessions, sometimes for years. The therapist and the patient would develop and work through an intense transference relationship, in which the patient remembered past experiences, then actually transferred emotions associated with significant people in the past to the therapist. Reliving the original maladaptive responses allowed the patient to use adult strengths to solve emotional difficulties that were overwhelming as a child. To achieve a cure in psychoanalysis, the patient must first recall past events and then develop insight into the meaning of each event.

Many of Freud's theories are challenged today. Psychoanalysis is a long and expensive form of therapy. There has been frequent criticism for his strong focus on sexual drives as the primary motivation for all behavior, and it appears that Freud himself suffered from some of the very anxieties he described. However, his contributions have influenced the fields of psychiatry, psychology, the humanities, education, history, and the social sciences. Sigmund Freud's revolutionary theories "brought about a new level of awareness and, for better or worse, a permanently altered image of humankind" (Corsini, 1994).

NEW THEORIES EMERGE

The early 1900s was a time for several new, but related, theories about the nature of man. By this time it was generally agreed that people were more than just physical bodies. The term **psyche** was borrowed from Plato and used to define the mental or spiritual part of the person (as compared with the term **soma,** which relates to the body). Interest in this new area of study attracted such people as Carl Jung, a noted German physician; Alfred Adler, a Viennese ophthalmologist and neurologist; and other visionaries. Here we consider a few of the more important contributions to the understanding of human nature.

Analytical Psychotherapy

Carl Jung, the founder of analytical psychotherapy, was a physician and university lecturer whose theories differed from Freud's in two basic respects: (1) the energy that

Freud labeled sexually-based libido was, according to Jung, actually a more generalized life energy, and (2) Freud stated that personality is determined in childhood, whereas Jung believed that personality could be changed during adulthood and is actually influenced by future plans, goals, and dreams (Jung, 1968).

Jung built on Freud's theory of personality by dividing the psyche (mind/spirit) into three levels: the conscious ego, the personal unconscious, and the deeper collective unconscious, which stores all the experiences of man's ancestral past. The components, or parts, of the collective unconscious he called *archetypes*. He also coined the terms *extroversion* and *introversion* to describe outward-going and inward-focused personalities.

Jung's concept of the self focuses on the importance of balance and wholeness. His theory goes beyond Freud's by recognizing the spiritual realm and creative power of the individual, as well as the potential for psychological growth in every person.

Jung's ideas became known as the analytical theory or school of thought. Although Jung used traditional psychoanalytical techniques, he believed that the primary effort in life was to gain more awareness. He helped patients understand their problems and conflicts by uncovering the symbolic meanings of their disorders. Jung and his followers also encouraged patients to experience rather than just intellectually understand something. Patients were encouraged to contact and value their inner worlds.

The analytical view of psychotherapy did not survive as a separate discipline, but many of its concepts remain in the mainstream of psychological thought. Jung himself wrote many books and articles, but translations of his works did not reach the United States until the 1950s. He died in 1961 while working on the draft for his twenty-ninth book titled *Man and His Symbols*.

Individual Psychotherapy

Alfred Adler graduated from the Vienna School of Medicine as an ophthalmologist in 1895. As a result of his interests in public health issues, Adler was invited to attend Freud's weekly discussion sessions on psychoanalysis. By 1918 he had developed his theory of personality and a new way of thinking that became known as individual psychology (also called Adlerian psychology).

Adler's personality theory states that the human infant, because of dependency and helplessness, starts out in this world in a position of **inferiority** (of being inadequate or less than others). The child must learn to master his or her world by assessing the environment and then making certain conclusions. Each person wants to belong, to be considered as significant, and to be treated as an individual. Thus as children grow, they find where they fit within the family. Adler believed the perception of children's positions within the family helped to create their evaluations of self and other people. These evaluations, in turn, become incorporated into adult lifestyle and influenced people's movements throughout life.

Adler theorized that the general goal of life is to gain mastery over the environment. To do this the adult must cope with three tasks. First is work, which includes schooling, vocational choices, use of leisure time, satisfaction with work, and retirement. Second is the social task, subdivided into the tasks of belonging and social interactions. Third is the task of coping with members of the other sex. (Adler disliked the term "the opposite sex" and thought it encouraged conflict between the sexes.) Later analysis of Adler's writings uncovered two additional life tasks, those of self and spirit. The task of self states that people must define themselves and find meaning in their lives. Tasks of the spirit include considerations of religious, philosophical, and spiritual questions.

Adlerian or individual therapy uses the fundamental techniques of psychoanalysis but adds several of basic assumptions. For one, the human being is viewed as a total organism, functioning within the environment. Because all behavior is goal directed, people are capable of perceiving and assessing events to arrive at conclusions. However, each individual perceives the world subjectively from an individual, unique point of view. To understand a person the therapist "must be able to see with his eyes and listen with his ears" (Adler, 1964). Adlerians believed that people have the ability to make choices and are responsible for their behavior.

Behavior is best understood within a social context. Therefore behavior becomes meaningful only when viewed within the social setting. As a result, Adlerian psychology is often called *social psychology*.

The concept of a value system was introduced by Adler. The highest value is the value for people (social interest). The concepts of choice, individual responsibility, and finding the meaning in life evolved and later became the foundation for the humanistic school of psychology.

Adlerian psychologists dislike the use of labels and do not categorize people into groups. People with mental dysfunctions are not considered psychopathic or mentally ill. They are referred to as "discouraged." Therapy is designed to encourage them to assume responsibility for

directing their lives in more positive ways. To summarize, the Adlerians see people as creative, evolving, responsible individuals who are moving toward goals within a social world—the first holistic point of view.

Other Therapies

Other therapists during the early twentieth century also broke with the Freudian tradition. Karen Horney (1855-1952), an early follower of Freud, stressed the importance of social and environmental conditions on personality development. Her concept of basic anxiety stated that a child's isolation is not inherited, but results from culture and social upbringing.

Erich Fromm (1900-1980) stressed human loneliness as the motivation for social interaction (Fromm and Xirau, 1968). His general theme of productive love is seen in many of his writings. Fromm also developed several personality or character types (Table 5-2).

Interpersonal Psychology

Harry Stack Sullivan's (1892-1949) comprehensive theory of interpersonal relationships emphasizes the social nature of people and the critical role of anxiety in the formation of the personality (Sullivan, 1968). He viewed the personality as a pattern of interpersonal relationships, where social interactions serve as the process for the development and treatment of mental disturbances. Mental health problems were considered to be the result of the patient's distorted images of certain relationships. Sullivan called these distorted images **personifications** and believed that these images and behavioral patterns arising from one relationship spill over or transfer into other relationships. Therapy thus becomes a matter of assisting the patient in discovering which personifications are unhealthy and substituting more effective behavioral patterns.

A central theme of Sullivan's theory is the concept of **anxiety,** which he defined as a vague feeling of uneasiness felt in response to stress. Threats to one's security bring anxiety. To decrease anxiety the infant discovers which behaviors are most desired by other people. Behaviors bringing approval are strengthened, and conversely, behaviors bringing disapproval are inhibited. If the infant fails to have its needs consistently met, it experiences

Table 5-2 Fromm's Personality Types	
Personality type	**Description**
Exploitative character	Satisfies needs through use of behaviors such as force and cunning
Hoarding character	Sees outside world as threat; keeps all he or she has to self and does not share
Marketing character	Considers self as commodity that can be bought, sold, or traded
Receptive character	Demands all that he or she can get; willing to take, but resists giving
Productive character	The most desirable; realizes own potentials; devotes self to welfare and well-being of all people

Table 5-3	Sullivan's Stages of Interpersonal Development	
Developmental stage	**Age**	**Description**
Infancy	Birth–18 mo	Uses crying to communicate; needs human contact; organizes patterns of sensation and emotional responses
		Task: to develop security by learning to rely on others to meet needs
Childhood	19 mo-6 yr	Identifies self; masters space, objects, language; needs interaction with peers and adults; shows anxiety, guilt, shame, and anger
		Task: to learn to accept outside control and interference with own wishes
Juvenile	7-9 yr	Uses competition, cooperation, compromise to cope; needs to be accepted; develops self-esteem
		Task: to develop satisfying relationships with peers
Preadolescence	10-12 yr	Uses cooperation, group agreement as tools; needs a chum, friend or loved one; develops compassion and capacity to love
		Task: to learn to relate to same-sexed friend
Early adolescence	13-14 yr	Needs intimacy; experiences lust and anxiety; develops capacity for love and empathy
		Task: to develop satisfactory relationships with members of opposite sex and become independent
Late adolescence	15-21 yr	Masters social conventions; develops capacity for happiness
		Task: to become interdependent and establish intimate and durable sexual relationships

much anxiety. As a result, avoiding anxiety becomes a central goal in later years. Sullivan described six stages of psychological interpersonal development, beginning with infancy and ending with late adolescence (Table 5-3). One of Sullivan's greatest contributions was his great sensitivity to the isolation and anxiety experienced by disturbed people. Many forms of therapy have benefited from his theories.

Psychoanalytical therapies have expanded to include several different techniques, but the foundation of treatment still lies in the use of "talking therapies." Psychoanalytical theories and therapies have had an enormous impact on the treatment of mental disorders. As new information about the complexities of human functioning arises, many old ideas will be challenged. Psychotherapeutic techniques will evolve as well, but the striving for a deeper understanding of ourselves never changes.

DEVELOPMENTAL THEORIES AND THERAPIES

Using Freud's theory of personality as a foundation, many theorists offered their views of human psychological development. Jean Piaget and Erik Erikson attempted to understand the relationships among the body, mind, and society throughout the life cycle. One of the most commonly used theories in health care is Erikson's eight stages of psychosocial development, which represents the first attempt to explain human behavior throughout the entire life cycle.

 Case Study

Susan is an attractive 42-year-old housewife and mother of four teenage children. She has been married to Jeff, a long-haul truck driver and her high school sweetheart, for 22 years. The family is well respected in the community, and Susan frequently volunteers for charitable projects. The children are considered well behaved and polite. In all respects, Susan is a model wife, mother, and community member. Last week, however, Susan announced her unhappiness, left everything behind, and ran away with a 25-year-old traveling salesman.

◆ How would Erikson's theory of psychosocial development explain Susan's behavior?

Psychosocial Development

Erik Erikson (1902-) described the human life cycle as composed of eight stages (Table 5-4). According to Erikson, each stage is marked by a developmental or core task—a normal crisis that must be confronted and resolved. As each crisis is resolved, it leaves an impression on the developing person that contributes to one's total personality. The uniting of the personality occurs as each developmental psychosocial task is mastered. Erikson believed that success with the crises of one developmental stage prepares individuals to move into the next stage.

Table 5-4 Erikson's Stages of Psychosocial Development

Developmental stage	Age	Core task and associated quality	Description
Oral-sensory (infancy)	Birth–1 yr	Trust/mistrust Associated quality: hope	Dominated by biological drives and needs; learns to trust that needs will or will not be met; learns to trust or mistrust others and world in general
Anal-muscular (early childhood)	1-3 yr	Autonomy/shame and doubt Associated quality: will (to do the expected)	Demands for self-control influence feelings of self-confidence vs. shame and doubt in own abilities; ego is developing; parallel play
Genital-locomotor (preschool years)	3-6 yr	Initiative/guilt Associated quality: purpose	Actively explores environment; activities are directed with purpose; conscience develops; cooperative play; uses fantasy; imitates adults; beginning to evaluate own behavior
Latency (school age)	6-12 yr	Industry/inferiority Associated quality: competence (learning skills of adult)	Site of learning moves from home to school; masters skills and tasks valued by teachers and society; learns to behave according to rules; develops confidence and perseverance; practices self-restriction
Puberty (adolescence)	12-18 yr	Identity/diffusion Associated quality: fidelity (commitment to value system)	Combines experiences to form sense of personal identity; forms sexual relationships; plans for future; feels confused and indecisive; if successful with prior crises, will develop strong sense of identity; peer groups important
Young adulthood	18-25 yr	Intimacy/isolation Associated quality: love	If has strong sense of identity, is willing and able to unite own identity with another; develops devotion; commits to relationships, career If weak sense of identity, has impersonal, short-term relationships; shows prejudice; becomes socially isolated
Middle adulthood	25-65 yr	Generativity/stagnation Associated quality: caring	Strives to actualize identity that was formed in earlier stages; generates or produces children, ideas, products, services; is creative, productive, concerned for others; demonstrates caring through parenting, teaching, guiding others; adults who do not care become stagnant, self-indulgent, absorbed in themselves
Maturity	65 yr–death	Integrity/despair Associated quality: wisdom (to accept one's life and value contribution that one has made)	Adjusts to changes; senses flow of time, past, present, and future; accepts worth and uniqueness of own life as it was and is; finds order and meaning in own life; despairs when life is viewed as waste; adults who focus on what "might have been" blame others, feel a sense of loss and contempt for others

Poorly resolved developmental (core) tasks continue to haunt the person throughout successive stages until they are mastered. The Case Study presents a person with an inadequately resolved developmental task. Erikson's theory is commonly used by caregivers as a framework for assessing and planning individualized client care.

Cognitive Development

Jean Piaget (1896-1980) devised a theory of intellectual (**cognitive**) development. He theorized that personality is the result of interrelated intellectual (cognitive) and emotional (**affective**) functions (Piaget and Inhelder, 1969). Growth is an increasing intellectual ability to organize and integrate (combine) experiences. Piaget observed that certain behaviors occurred in steps at certain age groups, so he divided these patterns into four main stages of intellectual growth (Table 5-5).

Piaget believed that children struggle to find a balance between themselves and their environments through assimilation and accommodation. *Assimilation* is the process of developing abilities to handle new situations using existing coping mechanisms. The process of *accom-*

Table 5-5	Piaget's Stages of Intellectual (Cognitive) Development			
Developmental stage	**Age**	**Developmental task**	**Description**	
Sensorimotor	Birth–2 yr	To recognize permanence of objects	Unable to do things or distinguish self from environment; reflexes evolve into repeated actions that become coordinated movements; learns that objects in environment are still present even when they are not seen, touched, tasted; begins goal-directed and imitative behavior	
Preoperational	2-7 yr	To develop symbolic mental abilities	Thinking limited; centered on self; learns to use language as tool; establishes routines; thought is focused on only one part of situation; cannot understand more than one dimension of object; justifies own behavior at all costs	
Concrete operations	8-11 yr	To develop logical, objective thinking	Understands numbers, length, mass, area, weight, time, and volume; can see interrelations; able to reflect and discover relationships in environment	
Formal operations	12-15 yr	To learn to think abstractly	Able to consider all possibilities of situation; can think in terms of probability and proportions; uses problem-solving approach to conflicts	

modation occurs when children must handle new situations or experiences that go beyond their previous coping abilities. The *equilibration process* (as Piaget called it) is the weaving of new knowledge into one's existing structure. Although no specific therapies are based on Piaget's work, his theories have become essential in the understanding of intellectual growth and development.

Theories of psychological and personality development are important for health care providers. By understanding where clients are in their development, we are better able to provide effective health care and individually tailored emotional support. Time spent in supporting clients through their developmental phases may help move them toward success.

BEHAVIORAL THEORIES AND THERAPIES

The foundation for the behavioral theories and their therapies lies in the assumption that all behavior is learned. The behavioral school of thought stated that human behavior is the outcome of past learning, current motivation, and biological differences (Corsini and Wedding, 1989). Learning is a behavioral change that results when individual actions repeatedly prove successful and are reinforced. Dysfunctional behaviors are the result of learned maladaptive behaviors. Behavioral theories take a mechanical approach to human behavior by focusing only on objective, observable, and measurable behaviors. The influence of the environment on both human and animal subjects is stressed, but all behaviors are seen as responses to stimuli. Four important figures were instrumental in

establishing the behavioral movement: Pavlov, Watson, Skinner, and Wolpe.

Ivan Pavlov (1849-1936) became the director of the physiology department at the Institute of Experimental Medicine in Saint Petersburg, Russia. There he pioneered his experiments and devised his theories on conditioning for which he was awarded the Nobel Prize in 1904 (Pavlov, 1941).

Pavlov's precise and objective research methods allowed him to evaluate the responses of dogs to various stimuli. By studying animal behaviors, Pavlov discovered that a given behavior was the response to a given stimulus. His famous experiment of conditioning dogs to salivate when they heard a bell demonstrated the mechanical aspects of behavior. Pavlov then went on to discover that behaviors were more likely to be repeated when they were rewarded or reinforced and faded or became extinct when ignored or not rewarded. Successful behaviors became generalized over time and were applied to current situations. Pavlov's work on conditioning laid the foundation for the development of the American behavioral movement.

The behavioral school of thought was established in the United States during the 1920s by John B. Watson (1878-1958). He developed the basic viewpoint for behaviorism: psychology is an objective science—the science of behavior. He published two books on behaviorism and, when he died in 1958, his views on behaviorism were a strong force in American psychology.

B.F. Skinner

Burhus Fredrick Skinner (1904-1990) was one of the most influential minds of the twentieth century. As a crusader for objective psychology, Skinner stated that only observed behaviors in current situations were open to analysis. He pursued this idea by developing the concepts of operant conditioning, positive and negative reinforcement, and shaping (Skinner, 1963).

Skinner's first research efforts were focused on developing a set of learning principles. White rats and pigeons were taught to press a certain lever in their cages to receive a pellet of food, which Skinner labeled a *reinforcer*. Positive reinforcers served as rewards for specific behaviors, as demonstrated by the results of his experiments with animals. He also found that negative reinforcers produced anxiety when the animal engaged in specific unacceptable behaviors. (Punishment is an example of a negative reinforcer.) Skinner believed that all organisms moved toward pleasure and away from pain. His theory proposed that the continual rewards of positive conditioning strongly enforce the desired behaviors, whereas negative reinforcements weaken and fade out undesirable behaviors. The process of guiding the individual to replace unacceptable responses with more desirable behaviors was called *shaping*, and the overall approach to changing observable behavior became known as *operant conditioning*.

By 1953 Skinner was applying his theories of behavior and learning to human subjects. His results were published in his book titled *Science and Human Behavior*. Throughout the 1960s Skinner crusaded for improvements in the educational system in the United States. He developed the concept of *programmed learning*, a process whereby new knowledge is broken down to small bits of information and presented at the learner's pace. Today, programmed learning techniques are commonly used in business and industrial training courses.

Other Behavioral Therapies

During the 1960s Joseph Wolpe explained neuroses and anxiety as conditioned responses. Concurrently, researchers Dollard and Miller developed their *stimulus-response theory*, which emphasized reward as the most important element in forming new behavioral responses. Today's behavioral therapists believe that emotional problems stem from poor learning, conditioning, dysfunctional self-thinking, lack of skills, avoiding anxious situations, and misconceptions about reality. Therapeutic techniques focus on understanding the client's current behavior. The "past" is important only to the extent to which it affects present actions.

Behavioral therapists teach clients to change dysfunctional thought and behavioral patterns by using *behavior modification therapies*. These therapies are then used to replace undesirable behaviors with more appropriate actions. They also provide social skills training and assist clients in learning to control the stimuli that cause them problems. *Assertiveness training* teaches clients to express themselves in constructive, nonaggressive ways. The behavioral school of thought also promotes continual research as a tool for the refinement and improvement of treatment strategies.

HUMANISTIC THEORIES AND THERAPIES

By the middle of the 1950s, the two main schools of thought in the study of human behavior were the psychoanalytical and the behavioral. One school stressed the powers of the unconscious, whereas the other defined behavior in terms of stimulus and response. Much of the data was collected through experimental research, and most of the work was conducted within the academic setting. Critics, however, believed that something was missing in the theories of the day, and several of them began to look at human nature from a different point of view. As a new humanistic outlook was considered and adopted, a "third force" in American psychology evolved into the field of humanistic psychology.

Humanistic theories are an important part of many of today's therapies. The humanists view a person as a whole and emphasize the totality of an individual. All realms of the human condition are therefore considered important. The physical, emotional, spiritual, intellectual, and social aspects of one's life influence the journey toward reaching one's greatest potential. Humanists also believe in the innate goodness of human nature and focus on the positive aspects of humanity. In short, humanistic psychology views people as holistic and multidimensional (many-sided) individuals—adapting to stress within a changing environment. These ideas serve as the foundation for the concept of holism and the model of comprehensive health care delivery.

Perls and Gestalt Therapy

The first contribution to the humanistic movement was made by Fredrick Perls (1893-1970), a German-born physician who worked with brain-injured soldiers after World War I. Although he studied psychoanalysis, it was his years of work with his injured patients that sparked the idea of the gestalt, which means "whole." From this concept, Perls developed his psychotherapy, which he termed *Gestalt therapy*.

Perl's therapy accepted the notion of unresolved conflicts in the past, but he also stressed the present, freedom, responsibility, and attempts to become whole (or "actualized," as it was later called). Clients were encouraged to "act out" their emotions, frustrations, and conflicts to work through their difficulties. The therapist assumed an authoritarian role, which emphasized frank emotional expression. Critics considered this approach to be too strict to foster personal growth, but the contributions of Perls' Gestalt therapy paved the way for further exploration into human nature.

Maslow's Influence

Abraham Maslow (1908-1970) and his theories had a strong impact on the practice of nursing and health care. His background was in Gestalt therapy, which fueled his ideas about holistic psychology. He published extensively on the subjects of personality, motivation, self-actualization, and human nature. Maslow died in 1970, leaving behind a rich legacy of the more positive aspects of humanity.

The core concept of Maslow's theories is that human nature is essentially good and contains the inherent potential for self-fulfillment (Maslow, 1968, 1971); Maslow explored how people cope with and adapt to their situations. His investigations of people who function at highly successful levels led to his theory of motivation that has become widely adopted throughout the health care professions.

Maslow grouped human needs into a hierarchy or ranking (Figure 5-1). The lower order needs include the physical and social requirements of the human organism. Without the fulfillment of these fundamental needs, the individual will perish. The physical (physiological) needs for air, water, food, elimination, and reproduction take first priority. For example, when the relief worker asked the starving child who he was, he replied "I am hungry." The child's need for self-respect was not as great as his need for food.

Second-priority needs relate to safety, security, and protection. Intellectual and social growth are difficult when a person must be constantly vigilant or protective. Love and belonging needs come next. Everyone needs to feel accepted as part of a group or family. People who are lonely or isolated have unfulfilled belonging needs. Last are the needs for esteem and respect, which include the needs for self-respect and the respect of others.

The higher order needs for optimal functioning include aesthetic and self-actualization needs. Aesthetic needs relate to the values of beauty, goodness, order, justice, and simplicity, whereas self-actualization needs encourage individuals to develop to their highest potential—to be the best one can be. Maslow believed that when these needs go unmet, the individual can develop illnesses. For example, unmet needs for truth may result in suspiciousness and a distrust of others, whereas the lack of beauty can result in a vulgar, negative outlook. To understand the nature of self-actualized people, Maslow studied individuals who were highly successful. He found they had several similar characteristics (Box 5-1).

Today, Maslow's hierarchy of needs serves as a basis for planning client care. His theories also serve nurses as a method for prioritizing care. For example, maintaining a client's airway (a physical need) takes priority over his or her need for belonging. Many clients encountered in today's health care environments are suffering from unmet basic needs. To deliver effective health care, providers must be able to accurately assess and plan therapeutic interventions according to the client's most critical unmet needs. Teaching a client to correctly self-administer insulin, for example, will be ineffective if the client has no home or way of obtaining regular meals. Maslow was instrumental in the development of humanism, but he also gave health care providers the tools for designing effective health care.

Rogers' Client-Centered Therapy

Carl Rogers (1902-1987) developed a new approach to psychotherapy. Rogers studied Freud's teachings and worked as a child guidance therapist. He became

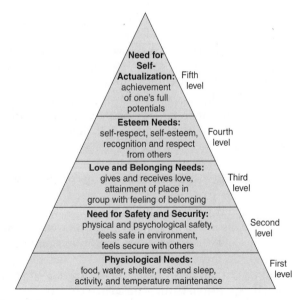

Figure 5-1 Maslow's hierachy of needs. (Data from Maslow A: *Motivation and personality*, ed 2, New York, 1970, Harper & Row.)

Box 5-1 Characteristics of Highly Self-Actualized People

Comfortable with reality
Expresses self spontaneously
Independent, self-directing
Has emotional depth
Has a high social interest
Expresses creativity
Shows democratic values
Accepts self and others
Able to solve problems
Needs privacy and detachment
Identifies with humanity
Appreciates life
Has gentle sense of humor

influenced by the theories of Otto Rank, a psychoanalyst who stated that people have a self-directing ability that emerges during therapy. Rank broke from the traditional, mechanical techniques of therapy by stating that the client should direct the therapeutic relationship using the therapist as a guide to self-understanding. Inspired by Rank's ideas, Rogers moved to Ohio State University and began work on a new system of psychotherapy.

Rogers also built on Maslow's work by stressing the goal of self-actualization (Rogers, 1961). He believed that the goal of therapy is to assist clients in becoming increasingly more aware of their experiences and emotions. Rogers felt that the therapeutic relationship should foster an open and trusting climate in which clients can safely and freely express themselves. He believed that the therapist's task is to reflect clients' feelings and support their work toward healthy functioning and self-actualization.

Rogers continued to refine his theories and spent the last 15 years of his life applying his methods to areas outside psychology (Rogers, 1980). His efforts have benefited the disciplines of nursing, pastoral counseling, and education. He also worked with many leaders, policy makers, and groups experiencing conflict, but his greatest legacy was his focus on the positive, achieving side of man's nature, which gave many people permission to accept themselves.

Current Humanistic Therapies

Many humanistic theories are with us today. The concept of holism has led to the development of a holistic health care model in which every client is viewed as a unique person functioning within a changing environment. The concept of basic needs is used to plan and prioritize health care, to allocate scarce resources, and to assist clients achieve their best.

Mental illness, from the humanistic point of view, results when individuals refuse to risk living fully, are unwilling to control their lives, overconform, or refuse to experiment with their desires and emotions. Therapy is designed to promote change by helping clients to find a sense of inner truth, release emotions, and take charge of their lives.

Several new therapies have evolved from the humanistic movement. Everett Shostrom developed a system of

therapy based on the goal of self-actualization rather than cure. His actualizing therapy assists clients in learning to trust their inner or "core" selves despite life's negative influences.

Viktor Frankl's psychotherapy is based on a person's need to search for meaning and values in life. He called his system of treatment *logotherapy,* based on the Greek word *logos,* which is defined as "meaning." His ideas of human worth and dignity grew out of his 3-year experience in a concentration camp (after having lost his entire family) during World War II.

Even the psychoanalytical school of Freud was influenced by humanism. I.H. Paul blended traditional analysis with Roger's client-centered therapy and developed nondirective psychoanalysis, a 2- to 4-year system of therapy that involves reflection and a willingness to look into oneself. Newer therapies will continue to evolve, but each will be grounded in the basic premise of humanism: people are dynamic and multidimensional beings who strive for personal fulfillment.

Early theories about human nature sparked inquiries that encouraged investigations and experiments of new thoughts, as well as refinements of old ideas. Because of these efforts, our ideas of human behavior are much different from those of Freud's time. Our understanding of human nature will continue to expand and encourage us to explore the most complex of all worlds, the one inside the self.

KEY CONCEPTS

◆ Theories and models help to explain human development and behavior.

◆ The humoral theory began with Hippocrates around 400 BC and remained popular until the 1400s.

◆ Charles Darwin's theories led to the belief that mental illness was the result of inferior genetic makeup and a lower place on the evolutionary scale.

◆ Sigmund Freud's study of the unconscious processes of the mind evolved into theories about the development, structure, defenses, and dynamics of the personality.

◆ Analytical psychology was founded by Carl Jung, who built on Freud's theories and recognized the spiritual and creative powers of people, as well as their potential for growth.

◆ Alfred Adler's individual therapy focuses on the ideas of choice, individual responsibility, and finding the meaning in life.

◆ Harry Stack Sullivan described six stages of interpersonal (social) development and believed that the therapist's role was to sensitively assist clients in understanding how distorted images contribute to the anxiety and isolation in their lives.

Think About

The client, a 22-year-old female, has been admitted with anxiety, an inability to retain food or fluids, and shortness of breath. She has no health insurance and has lived alone since her recent divorce.

◆ Using Maslow's hierarchy, list the client's problems (unmet needs) in order of priority.

◆ Erik Erikson's theory of the stages of psychosocial development states that as each developmental (core) task is mastered, the individual builds and unites his or her personality.

◆ Jean Piaget's theory of cognitive development describes four stages of intellectual and emotional growth.

◆ The foundation for behavioral theories and their therapies lies in the assumption that all behavior is learned and is seen as responses to stimuli.

◆ Ivan Pavlov developed the concept of conditioning.

◆ John B. Watson stated that psychology was the objective science of behavior and began the movement known as behaviorism.

◆ B.F. Skinner's experiments found that positive reinforcement enforced behaviors, whereas negative reinforcement weakened behaviors.

◆ Behavioral therapies today assist clients in learning how to change their dysfunctional thoughts and behavioral patterns. Examples include behavior modification techniques, assertiveness training, and training in the social skills.

◆ Humanistic theories view the individual as a multidimensional person who adapts to stress within a dynamic environment while striving for self-fulfillment.

◆ The concept of gestalt led Fredrick Perls to develop a system of therapy that stressed the present, personal freedom, and attempts to become a whole person.

◆ Maslow's hierarchy of needs theory categorizes physical and psychological requirements for optimal functioning and describes the characteristics of successful, highly self-actualized people.

◆ Carl Rogers built on Maslow's work by stressing the goals of self-actualization and awareness.

◆ Current humanistic theories have led to the ideas of holistic health care, planning based on priorities of human needs, and therapies designed to assist clients in taking charge of their lives.

Suggestions for Further Reading

Toward a psychology of being by Abraham Maslow (New York, 1968, vanNostrand Reinhold) presents an interesting discussion of the potential we all are capable of achieving.

References

Adler A: *The individual psychology of Alfred Adler: a systematic presentation in selections from his writings,* ed 2, New York, 1964, Harper & Row.

Corsini RJ, editor: *Encyclopedia of psychology,* ed 2, New York, 1994, John Wiley.

Corsini RJ, Wedding D, editors: Current psychotherapies, Itasca, Ill, 1989, FE Peacock.

Fromm E, Xirau R: *The nature of man,* New York, 1968, Macmillian.

Jung CG: *Analytical psychology: its theory and practice,* New York, 1968, Random House.

Maslow AH: *Toward a psychology of being,* ed 2, New York, 1968, vanNostrand Reinhold.

Maslow AH: *The farthest reaches of human nature,* New York, 1971, Viking Press.

Pavlov IP: *Conditioned reflexes and psychiatry,* New York, 1941, International Publishers.

Piaget J, Inhelder B: *The psychology of the child,* New York, 1969, Basic Books.

Rogers CR: *On becoming a person,* Boston, 1961, Houghton Mifflin.

Rogers CR: *A way of being,* Boston, 1980, Houghton Mifflin.

Skinner BF: Behaviorism at fifty, *Science* 140:951, 1963.

Sullivan HS: *The interpersonal theory of psychiatry,* ed 2, New York, 1968, Norton.

Chapter 6

Contemporary Theories and Therapies

Learning Objectives

1. Explain the main concept underlying systems theories.
2. Discuss how Glasser's reality therapy differs from Ellis' rational-emotive-behavioral therapy.
3. Describe the concept of homeostasis.
4. Explain how Selye's theories of stress and adaptation influence the delivery of health care.
5. List five physical responses to stress.
6. State the primary purpose of crisis intervention.
7. Discuss why psychobiology is being called a revolution in mental health care.
8. Describe three kinds of psychotherapy used in the treatment of mental disorders.
9. List three somatic therapies for treating mental illness.

Key Terms

acupuncture

biofeedback

closed system

cognition

coping mechanisms

covert modeling

crisis

crisis intervention

equilibrium

homeostasis

life space

neuropeptides

neurotransmitters

open system

phototherapy

psychobiology

psychoneuroimmunology (PNI)

psychotherapy

somatic therapies

stressor

By the 1950s four schools of thought (psychoanalytical, behavioral, Gestalt, and humanistic) existed in American psychiatry. Behaviorism was popular until the 1960s when the "cognitive revolution" emerged as an attempt to expand its narrow "stimulus-response" viewpoint of pure behaviorism. Since then, theories about human systems, communications, sociocultural natures, and biobehavioral responses have been developed. Separate fields of study have combined their efforts and developed into multidisciplinary sciences as explorations of human nature spilled over into the disciplines of anthropology, sociology, medicine, nursing and health care, and economics.

SYSTEMS THEORIES

Systems theorists view humans as functioning within a set of related units (called *systems*). Historically, the origins of systems theories lie in Gestalt psychology. Royce and Powell (1983) built on earlier theorists' work by developing the "open and closed systems" concept. They defined an **open system** as having boundaries that are permeable, passable, and accessible. Energy and information pass easily among open systems; thus the organism grows and flourishes. A **closed system,** however, has rigid, impermeable boundaries that shut out information and energy. If the system remains closed, the organism no longer grows and eventually will die.

Kurt Lewin (1890-1947), who was trained in Gestalt psychology, developed his "field theory," which proposed that to understand behavior, it must be considered within the total situation. Lewin rejected any notions of past, future, or cause and effect and focused only on the immediate situation. He thought of people as systems, who interact with other systems across boundaries. His concept of **equilibrium** states that each system attempts to maintain a balance or steady state within itself and among other systems.

Lewin also developed the concept of **life space**—the psychological field or space in which one moves. Life space includes oneself, other people, and objects. Behavior is thus viewed as a function of life space. Lewin also posed the concept of *psychological tension*, which results from the interaction of opposing forces or systems. Although his work is complex, Lewin's theories influenced the development of several therapies.

The idea of systems with mechanisms that influence behavior sparked further studies of the body's self-regulating systems. Maxwell Maltz published a popular book in 1960 titled *Psycho-cybernetics*, which explained how "positive thinking" works by programming one's behavior to achieve the self-image that has been adopted. Maltz defined *psychocybernetics* as the study of the automatic control system formed by the brain and nervous systems. He believed that thoughts influence this system, so positive thoughts and images would encourage the system to replace unwanted behaviors with new actions (Maltz, 1960).

Systems theory psychology has provided a point of view that differs from other approaches. Systems theorists believe that behavior does not occur in response to an external stimulus but originates *within* the organism. All living creatures are open systems with input, output, and regulating feedback mechanisms. People are open systems in a state of continual exchange, interacting with other people, their environment, and within themselves. The systems theorists developed the concept of *people as dynamic and evolving*.

COGNITIVE THEORIES AND THERAPIES

The word **cognition** is a general term that means "to know." It includes the mental activities of attention, language, imagery, memory, perception, and problem solving. The development of modern cognitive psychology began in the 1890s with the work of Paul DuBois, a Swiss psychologist who believed that mental illness resulted from incorrect ideas. His *rational psychotherapy* changed the incorrect ideas through the use of reason and logic. Alfred Adler's individual therapy and Jean Piaget's work contributed to cognitive psychology by demonstrating the importance of intellectual factors in human development.

Albert Bandura's *social learning theory* established a relationship between cognition and behavior. His work focused on the importance of learning through imitation, the use of symbols, and one's capacity for self-regulation through reflection and control. People learn by observing the outcomes of various situations (Bandura, 1986). These observations then develop into expectations and emotions. As a result people compare themselves with others and make judgments based on their expectations and emotions. Thus our decisions act to determine our behaviors.

Today's cognitive therapies differ from traditional psychotherapies. The importance of intellect is stressed more than emotion and behavior. The understanding of an event triggers emotions and thus causes behavior. The main goal of all cognitive therapies is to replace dysfunctional beliefs and thoughts to cause a change in personal, private viewpoints. Clients develop successful self-control strategies by attacking dysfunctional behaviors and then learning specific coping skills. Current cognitive therapeutic techniques are grouped into three categories: cognitive restructuring, coping skills, and problem-solving skills.

Cognitive Restructuring Therapies

The best examples can be seen in theories developed by Ellis, Beck, and Meichenbaum. The first two approaches focus on changing or restructuring faulty beliefs and assumptions, whereas the third approach focuses on changing one's self-talk.

During the 1950s Alfred Ellis developed a theory, called *rational-emotive-behavioral therapy* (REBT), and treatment based on the irrational beliefs and unrealistic expectations people hold of themselves. He saw emotions as arising from the understanding of an event. It is not the event but the "value" placed on the event that determines behavior.

The goals of REBT are to help clients (1) gain insight into the irrational beliefs that cause their disturbed behaviors, (2) cease actively reinforcing the disturbed behaviors, (3) monitor the effects of their thoughts, and (4) adopt more appropriate outlooks by practicing more effective thoughts. Beck's *cognitive therapy* helps clients recognize their self-defeating tendencies and replace them with more adaptive thinking.

Donald Meichenbaum's *self-instructional training* takes a different approach to therapy. He believes that undesirable behaviors are the result of faulty instructions given in childhood (Meichenbaum, 1989). Therapy consists of learning a pattern of new self-instructions. The techniques of imagery, modeling, and anxiety control are used to help clients adopt new self-talk patterns.

Coping Skills Therapies

Several models have been introduced to teach clients how to develop more successful daily living skills. During the 1970s Joseph Cautela described the process of **covert modeling**—the act of mentally rehearsing a difficult performance or event before actually doing the activity. This mental practice has been used by sport psychologists to improve the performance of their players.

Coping skills training is similar to covert modeling except that anxiety is first induced and then the client is trained to "relax the images away." Coping skills taught by cognitive therapists include training in anxiety management, assertiveness, progressive relaxation, and techniques to reduce physical responses to stress.

Problem-Solving Therapies

Some cognitive therapists believe that the cause of dysfunctional emotions is an inability to successfully solve problems. (Matheny and Kern, 1994). *Problem-solving therapy* teaches clients to solve their problems in more constructive and satisfying ways. Box 6-1 lists the steps in the problem-solving process. Note the similarities between this and the nursing (therapeutic) process.

Reality Therapy

William Glasser M.D. (1925-) founded the Institute for Reality Therapy to educate people about his therapeutic techniques. Glasser's theory, like Maslow's, states that people are born with certain basic needs. The most important needs are to be loved and belong, followed by needs to gain self-worth, respect, and recognition.

Unlike Freud, Glasser believed that the problems of mental illness are rooted in the failure in the social realms (areas) of human functioning. His "three Rs" of therapy encourage clients to do what is "realistic, responsible, and right" (Glasser, 1965).

Reality therapists help clients to examine and evaluate the effectiveness of their behaviors, face their situations, and then develop more effective ways to satisfy their

needs. Therapists and clients plan the behavioral changes that will best fulfill the clients' most basic needs first. Contracts are made and both agree to abide by them. The use of contracts builds rapport, trust, and commitment between client and caregivers. It has become a valuable tool in treating chemical dependency problems.

Glasser defines *responsibility* as the ability to satisfy one's needs in a way "that does not deprive others of the ability to fulfill their needs" (Glasser, 1965). He described people with mental illness as irresponsible and believed that values, ethics, and morals provide the basis for right behaviors. Glasser's methods have been taught to thousands of educators who follow the principles of his book, *Schools Without Failure*.

SOCIOCULTURAL THEORIES

Theories that focus on human social nature were introduced in the early twentieth century with the inquiries of George Mead. He believed that the social setting is extremely important in the concept of self that is developed through interactions with significant others. Mead believed that as children learn the rules and norms of their society, they take on the behaviors associated with those controls. Breaking the rules results in social rejection and labeling if behaviors do not fall within acceptable social limits. Mead's concepts encouraged theorists to consider the social aspects of behavior.

Mental Illness as Myth

Thomas Szasz was a psychiatrist who, in the 1950s, began to publish a series of books and articles attacking the concepts of mental illness. His main argument was that deviant (different) behavior was culturally defined. Szasz stated that all societies have individuals whose behaviors are considered abnormal. He believed that societies must have a way of controlling their more undesirable members. Many do this by labeling these people as "mentally ill" and removing them to institutions where they are taught to conform to society's approved behaviors (Szasz, 1974).

According to Szasz, people are responsible for their behavior. Even those labeled mentally ill have the choice to take part in the labeling process by allowing it to occur. He also strongly objected to describing maladaptive behaviors as illnesses. Mental illness is not an illness but a socially defined condition. Szasz believed that the purpose of institutionalization is to remove the labeled individual from the community and exert some control over the person's behaviors.

Szasz felt that clients should be able to choose their therapist and treatment based on the premise that clients can be helped only if they ask for it. Clients initiated therapy, defined the problems they wanted to solve, and worked with the therapist to change. The role of the

---

Box 6-1 Problem-Solving Process

1. State the problem.
2. Collect information about the problem.
3. Identify the causes or patterns of the problem.
4. Examine all possible options.
5. Choose the best option and apply it to the problem.
6. Examine the outcomes of the option's application.
7. Evaluate and revise actions based on outcomes.

therapist was to make suggestions, point out possible ways to change, and act as the client's advocate, but it was never direct or pushed the client. Therapy was completed when the client felt satisfied with the behavioral changes. Szasz's perspective has sparked a reexamination of the moral, legal, and political aspects of modern psychiatry.

The field of *community psychology* has evolved to focus on promoting changes in society at the community level. Community therapists work with local groups and organizations to improve social conditions such as hunger, homelessness, teen pregnancies, and social conflict.

BIOBEHAVIORAL THEORIES

Biobehavioral theories follow the medical model, which states that mental and physical illness is the result of abnormalities in the structure, function, or chemistry of the body. Mental health practitioners using the medical model focus on the biological aspects of the problem. A medical history and physical examination are performed. Next, tests, imaging techniques, and electroencephalograms (brain wave recordings) are used to assist in diagnosis. The problem-solving approach is then applied to the data, and treatment plans are developed. Therapy is considered effective when the cause of the problem has been eliminated. Today, the fields of *behavioral medicine* and *psychobiology* are dedicated to uncovering new knowledge about the inner chemical and biological workings of the body.

Homeostasis

Walter Cannon, in the 1920s, was the first theorist to consider the physical or biological aspects of mental illness. His research on the changes in the body's

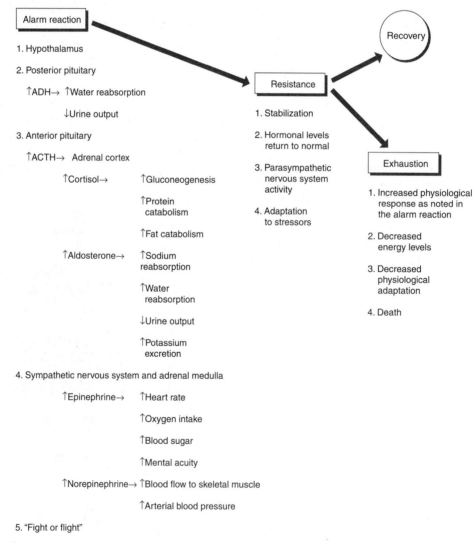

Figure 6-1 General adaptation system. *ADH,* Antidiuretic hormone; *ACTH,* adrencortico-tropic hormone. (Redrawn from Potter PA, Perry, AG: *Basic nursing: a critical thinking approach,* ed 4, St. Louis, 1999, Mosby.)

physiology during emotion led to the observation that the body always attempts to stabilize itself. Cannon believed that an emotion is a reaction that causes the body to use its resources. He described an *emergency syndrome,* which consists of a total body response that results in fright, fight, or flight behaviors when the individual is challenged or threatened. He also identified the roles of the hypothalamus and adrenal glands in the stress response. These and other discoveries about the autonomic nervous system led Cannon to formulate the concept of **homeostasis,** which he defined as the tendency of the body to achieve and maintain a steady internal state. Disease, in his view, was the fight to maintain the body's homeostasis (balance) within an open system. Cannon's concepts served as the foundation for many later developments. The concept of homeostasis has also been applied to family systems, holistic health, and world ecology.

Stress Adaptation Theory

Hans Selye (1907-1982) was educated in France, Italy, Germany, and Canada. During his many years of study, he repeatedly observed students who were "just feeling sick." This undefinable syndrome led him to study Cannon's emergency syndrome, which launched Selye toward years of research into the physical and biochemical changes associated with stress. The results of his studies led Selye to believe that many physical problems (e.g., hypertension, arthritis, coronary artery disease) are related to an individual's inability to control stress (Selye, 1976).

Selye described the physical response of the body to stress. He defined a **stressor** as a nonspecific response of the body to any demand placed on it. Selye thought that every person coped with many stressors on a daily basis. This daily dose of stressors created what Selye called the "wear and tear" on the body. His objective measurements demonstrated that people respond to stress in the same physical manner regardless of the stressor.

Selye's stress adaptation theory (also called the *general adaptation syndrome*) describes the body's physical responses to stress and the process by which people adapt. The general adaptation syndrome states that the body reacts to stress through three stages of adaptation: alarm, resistance, and exhaustion (Figure 6-1).

When stress is first perceived, Selye noted that the brain triggers an alarm reaction that releases hormones (epinephrine, norepinephrine) and prepares the body to stand and defend itself or run away from the threat, the fight-or-flight response (Figure 6-2). If the individual successfully adapts by coping with the stress, the body's heightened level of functioning returns to its usual state. However, if the stress cannot be resolved, the body continues to function at a high metabolic rate and progresses toward the next stage of adaptation.

The stage of resistance is the body's optimal attempt to cope with the stress. All the individual's coping skills and defense mechanisms are mobilized. Hormone levels and other physical measurements may return to normal, but problem solving becomes difficult. The individual becomes more susceptible to other, unrelated stresses. During the stage of resistance, one either adapts to the stress or progresses to the body's final attempt at homeostasis, the stage of exhaustion.

When stressors are overwhelming or lasting too long, the individual's resources become depleted (used up) and the organism begins to exhaust itself. Body processes begin to break down as glands fail to produce the elevated levels of hormones required to meet the threat. Thinking becomes illogical and distorted. Problem solving and sometimes communication are ineffective. Unless the stress is removed or adapted to, the individual continues to use all physical and emotional resources until death from exhaustion results. Chilling examples of Selye's general adaptation syndrome can be observed in the accounts of prisoners of war and concentration camp survivors of the World War II. Selye's work reminds us that effective health care can neither be given nor received if stress levels are ignored.

Crisis Intervention

When experiencing stress, people use their resources to decrease their discomfort. These efforts are known as **coping mechanisms,** and they are defined as any thought or action aimed at reducing stress. We all use coping mechanisms. They are the tools that help us work through

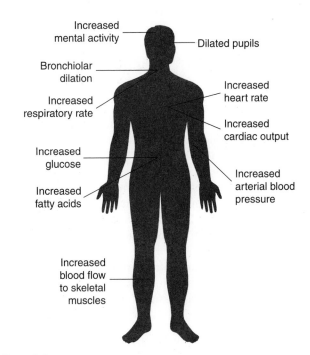

Figure 6-2 Physical assessment findings of fight-or-flight response. (Redrawn from Potter PA, Perry, AG: *Basic nursing: a critical thinking approach*, ed 4, St. Louis, 1999, Mosby.)

Increased mental activity
Dilated pupils
Bronchiolar dilation
Increased respiratory rate
Increased heart rate
Increased cardiac output
Increased glucose
Increased fatty acids
Increased arterial blood pressure
Increased blood flow to skeletal muscles

Table 6-1	Types of Coping Behaviors	
Mechanism	**Description**	**Example**
Psychomotor (physical)	Efforts to cope directly with problem	Confrontation, fighting, running away, negotiating
Cognitive (intellectual)	Efforts to neutralize threat by changing meaning of problem	Making comparisons, substituting rewards, ignoring, changing values, using problem-solving methods
Affective (emotional)	Actions taken to reduce emotional distress; no efforts are made to solve problem	Ego defense mechanisms such as denial and suppression; see Chapter 5 for other ego defense mechanisms

the ups and downs of daily living. A **crisis** is an upset in the homeostasis (steady state) of an individual.

All aspects of the personality are involved with coping mechanisms. They are divided into three main types: psychomotor (physical), cognitive (intellectual), and affective (emotional) (Table 6-1). When coping mechanisms are successfully used, an individual is able to solve problems and reduce stress. These are considered adaptive or constructive coping mechanisms. However, when efforts to decrease stress are used without resolving the conflict, then the coping mechanism is labeled as maladaptive or destructive. Table 6-1 describes each type of coping mechanism.

A crisis has several characteristics that separate it from other stressful situations. First, the definition of crisis is an individual matter that depends on the perception of the event, the severity of the threat, and the available coping strategies and resources. The crisis can be viewed as a threat to basic needs, a loss, or a challenge. If the crisis is viewed as a challenge, a mobilization of energy and purposeful problem-solving activities are more likely to occur.

Second, a crisis occurs when an individual's usual coping mechanisms are ineffective. The crisis demands a new solution outside of the person's previous life experiences. The individual must now strive to develop new coping strategies.

Third, crisis is self-limiting. Because human organisms cannot endure high levels of continued stress, crises are usually resolved within a short time. The solution may result in a return to the precrisis state, a higher level of functioning, or maladaptive behaviors and a lower level of functioning.

Fourth, a crisis usually affects more than one person. Every significant other within the person's social support system is affected by the crisis. No therapeutic intervention is successful until clients are assessed within the context of their total situation and appropriate social systems are considered.

As people experience a crisis, they travel through similar stages: perception, crisis, denial, disorganization, recovery, and reorganization (Figure 6-3). Once an event

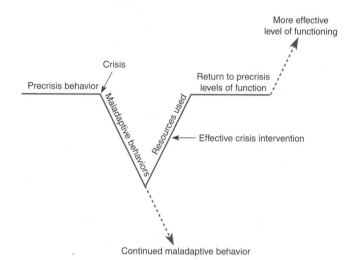

Figure 6-3 Stages of crisis.

is perceived as a crisis, an overwhelming feeling of denial is experienced. This emotion serves to protect the individual from a sudden, intense stress. An increase in tension is felt as attempts are made to eliminate the problem. All efforts to cope are ineffective, and the individual or family enters the stage of crisis in which everything seems to "fall apart."

During the disorganization phase, activities of daily living are no longer continued as individuals become preoccupied with the crisis situation. Past experiences may be symbolically linked to the present situation, and the individual becomes "flooded" with anxiety. Attempts are made to reorganize or escape. Individuals may blame others or consciously pretend the situation does not exist, but neither behavior defuses the crisis. This is the stage at which most people seek help. Once all attempts to deny, solve, escape, or ignore the problem have failed, the individual slowly moves toward the recovery.

Recovery begins when attempts to cope with the problem result in success. One success provides the encouragement to try something else. Soon one success builds on another and the stage of reorganization is entered. Normal activities are resumed. When a crisis is

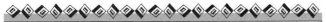

successfully resolved, the individual functions at a higher level than before the crisis. Growth has taken place, and the individual becomes stronger and more capable.

Crises can also result in unsuccessful resolutions or pseudoresolutions (Taylor, 1994). Unresolved crises result when maladaptive behaviors are used to hide the problem. An example is the husband who sends his wife to counseling for depression while he continues to abuse her when he drinks. Crises with unsuccessful resolutions usually result in a return to homeostasis but at a lower level of functioning.

Pseudoresolution occurs when nothing is learned from the crisis. As a result there is no change in the level of functioning because the opportunity for growth was missed. However, the appearance of any new stressors may trigger the buried conflicts of the unresolved crisis. The inability to solve future crises may be compounded by these old conflicts (see Think About box).

The main goal of **crisis intervention** is to help individuals and families manage their crisis situations by offering immediate emotional support. People are then assisted in developing effective coping mechanisms, which allows time to reorganize resources and support systems.

Victims of crisis are treated in such settings as emergency rooms, clinics, jails, places of worship, homes, and even over the telephone. Crisis hotlines are 24-hour telephone lines that are staffed by volunteers trained in crisis intervention techniques. Emotional support and referral to various community resources are offered to any caller.

Guidelines relating to crisis intervention have been developed and refined by the National Institute for Training in Crisis Intervention and other organizations. These guidelines have been taught to health care providers, educators, police officers, attorneys, ministers, and volunteers. Because crisis situations are high-stress encounters for all parties, the following guidelines can assist in providing safe effective crisis interventions:

First, *care is needed immediately.* As soon as the client is encountered, actions must be taken to reduce anxiety levels. Sometimes this may require only reassurance. In other instances, actions must be taken to ensure safety and prevent harm.

Second is *the issue of control.* People experiencing a crisis are often unable to exercise control over themselves or their situation. Safety for both client and care providers must be considered. The therapist or caregiver must quickly assume control but only until the client is able to recover self-control. Again, the level of control is determined by the individual situation. Some people are relieved that someone else is in control, whereas others resort to physical aggression during a crisis. Control is important in a crisis because without it, the client cannot be helped to work with the problems that triggered the crisis.

Third is *assessment.* Although assessment usually is the first step in the care process, the issues of immediacy, safety, and control must be considered first in crisis. During this phase, the situation is assessed thoroughly. Ask direct questions such as "What happened?" Have the client explain the crisis situation and review the events of the past 2 weeks. A quick and accurate assessment of the total situation helps to determine the best therapeutic interventions.

Fourth, the client's *disposition* is determined. A treatment plan is developed that assists the client with working on the problems triggering the crisis. The plan encourages clients to work things out themselves. The focus of crisis intervention therapy is not to resolve clients' problems but to help them manage their problems more effectively.

Fifth is *referral,* an often overlooked part of crisis intervention. Once emotionally stabilized and in control, clients may be referred to professional, community, or support group resources. The most successful referrals are the result of matching the client's needs with the most appropriate service. Know which resources are available within your community before interacting with the client. Avoid looking through the Yellow Pages during a crisis because this generates lack of confidence and invites problems.

Sixth is *follow-up,* the last guideline of crisis intervention. Care providers must see if the referrals were actually contacted. A follow-up telephone call to a person seen in a crisis will often reveal new problems that prevent the client from receiving needed care.

All people experience crisis. When new coping mechanisms are needed but are unavailable because of immaturity, an individual experiences a developmental or maturational crisis. Severe stresses within one's environment may cause a situational crisis. Assisting people in crisis to mobilize their resources is an important goal for all providers of health care (see Chapter 22).

PSYCHOBIOLOGY

"**Psychobiology** is the study of the biochemical foundations of thought, mood, emotion, and behavior" (Wilson, 1994). By applying the latest developments in imaging technology and biochemistry, researchers are exploring human mental experiences and emotional states. Techniques such as positron emission tomography (PET) and magnetic resonance imaging (MRI) are linked to powerful computers that are now able to "see" thought processes. The techniques "show how specific regions of the brain 'light up' when activities such as reading are performed and how neurons and their elaborate cast of supporting cells organize and coordinate their tasks" (Raichle, 1994). Researchers are using these technologies to learn about mood disorders, schizophrenia, language problems, and other conditions. Biochemists are exploring the role of neurotransmitters and other messenger systems in behavior, while immunologists are attempting to unravel the secrets of the body's defense systems, especially when exposed to stress.

Research is spawning new theories, fields of study, and therapies. Psychobiological theories about the causes of mental illness relate to genetics, neurotransmitter activity, viruses, fetal development, and immune system dysfunction. The field of *neuropsychology* is devoted to the study and treatment of behaviors related to brain functioning. The interdisciplinary field of *cognitive psychophysiology* blends the disciplines of psychology and physiology to study mental processes by monitoring selective body systems, and the new science of *neurobehavioral toxicology* is exploring behavioral changes that result from exposure to toxins in the environment.

Psychoneuroimmunology

The division of man into parts was made by Plato. The viewpoint that one set of laws governed physical events, whereas a separate set of laws governed mental events dominated for centuries. Recently, however, researchers are favoring models that unite mind and body into one wholly functional unit.

In the early 1960s, Jonas Salk developed a model of disease that encompassed the genetic, neurological, immune, and behavioral systems (Salk, 1961). Ader (1981) later built on this model. His studies on the effects of stress on the immune system led him to coin the term *psychoneuroimmunology (PNI)*. **Psychoneuroimmunology (PNI)** is the study of interactions between the body's central nervous system, its immune system, and aspects of the personality.

Ader's studies demonstrated that anxiety and depression can decrease immune system functions. Other researchers found that opiate (pain-relieving) mechanisms in the brain could be activated by the body's neuropeptides (endorphins) (Wickramasekera, 1988). Pain control by activating the opiate pathways of the brain has been seen in athletes, yogis, and women during labor. Some nurses are using this knowledge to help their clients cope with severe pain by teaching them to turn on the body's pain-relieving mechanisms.

Research into **neurotransmitters** (the body's chemical messenger system) uncovered the existence of **neuropeptides,** a neurotransmitter composed of amino acid strings. Further research found that amino acid strings of neuropeptides actually connect the endocrine, immune, and nervous systems. It is believed this neurobiochemical system provides the pathway for emotional reactions. As research continues to expand our knowledge, there is mounting evidence that emotions, stress, and attitudes have an impact on the body's immune response.

New studies are beginning to demonstrate that various interventions can have a positive impact on the immune system. Research found that relaxation exercises increased the production of antibodies. Positive emotional states, humor, and laughter, have been shown to increase an immune component in saliva (Dillon, Minchoff, and Baker, 1986). As the results of new research become known, our concepts of mental health and illness will change during the upcoming psychobiological revolution. Current mental health therapies are grouped into two basic categories: psychotherapy and somatic therapy.

PSYCHOTHERAPIES

Psychotherapy is defined as the treating of mental and emotional disorders by psychological, rather than physical, means. Psychotherapies began with Freud's psychoanalysis and now include behavior therapies, cognitive therapies, crisis intervention, and hypnosis. Psychotherapeutic sessions take place on an individual basis or in a group setting.

Individual Therapies

Clients who work on a one-to-one basis with a therapist are involved in individual therapy. *Psychoanalysis* is a type of individual therapy where clients analyze the meaning of certain behaviors and symbols and learn to cope with their problems by understanding the meaning or significance of their behaviors.

Client-centered psychotherapy is based on the premise that "every person has within themselves the resources for constructive change" (Smoyak, 1993). In client-centered therapy, the therapist expresses empathy to encourage growth and healthy change. Mobilizing the client's inner resources through the therapeutic relationship is the goal of client-centered therapy.

Cognitive therapy helps clients intellectually identify and correct their distorted thinking and dysfunctional beliefs. The therapist's role is focused on solving the problem within a limited time. Recently, a form of this type of therapy, called *brief-term therapy,* has been introduced in the United States. Studies have demonstrated that six to twelve sessions of therapy can be as effective as long-term psychotherapy. The focus of brief-term therapy is on the problem that faces the client at the moment.

Brief-term therapy has been effective for managing depression, marriage and family problems, and stress (Cade and O'Hanlon, 1993). Further research is needed to determine the impact on clients with more severe problems.

Behavioral therapy is a type of individual therapy that is tailored to each person's needs, behavior, and environment. Behavior modification techniques are used by therapists and clients to define positive behaviors and develop programs with specific reinforcements to change behaviors. This type of therapy has proven effective with developmentally disabled persons and those with severe forms of mental illness.

Hypnosis and *meditation,* although not distinct therapies, are often used in combination with individual psychotherapies. The traditional definition of hypnosis is the induction of a relaxed, trance-like state in which the individual is receptive to appropriate suggestions. However, Bierman (a full-time emergency room physician) focuses on the concepts of human patterns and consciousness. He believes that no special training, relationship, or process is required. Hypnosis is just ideas and responses. His work with acutely traumatized clients demonstrates the power of the health care providers' words and actions. (Bierman, 1995). The Case Study illustrates the use of Bierman's response-evoking hypnosis.

Meditation has been used as a part of Eastern religions for more than 2500 years. It has recently gained popularity in the West as a tool for combating stress. Many therapists who recommend meditation for their clients practice meditation daily themselves. Although there are many techniques for meditation, each has four common elements: concentration, retraining the attention to one item while excluding all other thoughts, mindfulness, and an altered state of consciousness. The physical effects of twice daily meditation sessions include "slower

heart rate, decreased blood pressure, lower oxygen consumption, and increased alpha brain wave production" (Moore, 1994). Meditation techniques have been used successfully in the fields of education, business, medicine, and mental health care.

Group Therapies

The use of groups to help people in distress has been recorded throughout history, but systematic group psychotherapy developed only after World War II. Because of a shortage of psychiatrists, the idea of treating clients in groups was attempted. The success of those first group therapies suggested that some psychological difficulties might be related to relationship problems with other people. Groups whose purpose is therapeutic are called healing groups or *change induction group*s. The central task of any therapeutic group is twofold: (1) to relieve emotional discomfort and human misery and (2) to cause psychological and behavioral changes.

Group therapy gatherings follow the medical model. Membership in the group is limited by the therapist. Group members are called "patients" who consider themselves "ill" and consequently exhibit "sick" behaviors. The goal of a professional therapist is to "cure" patients of their problems.

Self-help groups are limited to those people who share a common problem, symptom, or life situation. Examples include Alcoholics Anonymous (alcohol use problems), Synanon (drug use problems), Reach for Recovery (for postmastectomy women), and support groups for families of persons with mental illness.

T-groups evolved from systems theories. During the 1950s, basic skills training (BST) groups were formed by the National Education Association and the Research Center for Group Dynamics at M.I.T. to study the development, membership, leadership, and dynamics of group behavior. The name of the study groups was later changed to T-groups. Professionals from different disciplines began to adapt the T-group concept to their fields. Therapists with a client-centered clinical focus developed the *encounter group*, which uses a professional trainer to encourage intense group interaction. Other practitioners focused on small work groups and productivity. This area of interest eventually led to the "quality circle groups" and "total quality management" concepts.

Lastly, *consciousness-raising groups* use the interactions among its members as a vehicle for achieving behavioral changes. The group is supportive of change, allowing individuals to analyze their interactions, then "try out" new behaviors with people from varied backgrounds.

Group therapy causes changes in behavior through one or more change mechanisms (Table 6-2). The evidence compiled over 35 years demonstrates that many

Case Study

Larry, an alert 6-year-old, arrives at the clinic knowing that he would be on the receiving end of a "shot." He dreads the sight of the approaching nurse and begins to whimper. The nurse says, "I would like you, Larry, to hold still now and look very closely at that orange circle-square over there. Tell me whether it is getting bigger or smaller, and really look! Just look there and tell me . . ." By this time the injection has been given. "But I don't see it," says Larry. "That's right," says the nurse, "and you didn't feel it either!"

◆ What do you think made the outcome of this situation so positive?

Modified from Bierman SF: Medical hypnosis, *ADVANCES: The Journal of Mind-Body Health* 11(1):65, 1995.

Table 6-2	Group Change Mechanisms
Therapeutic mechanism	**Description**
Expressiveness	Group members share emotional expression of positive and negative emotions.
Experience of intense emotion	Generating intense group emotion activates individual issues.
Altruism	The experience of helping others improves low self-esteem and poor self-concept.
Self-disclosure	The sharing of deeply personal material involves risk and develops trust.
Cognitive factors	Intellectual knowledge leads to a deeper understanding of self.
Communion	Groups foster a sense of oneness and belonging.
Discovering similarities	Relief is experienced when individuals discover that their problems are not unique.
Experimentation	Working with new behaviors within the low-risk group setting encourages change.
Feedback	Receiving information about how one is perceived by others is unique to groups.
Feelings of hope	Groups help individuals feel and believe that they can change with the group's help.

groups do provide benefits for their members. The emotional support of one person for another appears to be an effective therapeutic tool.

Online Therapy

Along with the growth of the Internet, a number of therapists have established online therapy practices. Types of therapies offered are varied and services range from answering a single question to ongoing counseling. Critics feel online therapy may be unethical and ineffective. Proponents see it as a way to reach those individuals who are otherwise unable to seek counseling. Because Web therapy has sparked fierce debates about its usefulness, the American Psychological Association is studying the issue (Beckett, 1998).

SOMATIC THERAPIES

The word *somatic* refers to the body. Historically, therapies for people with psychological distresses have been divided into those that work primarily with the mind (psychotherapies) and those that affect the body (**somatic therapies**). This division will soon fade as our knowledge of the effects of emotion on the dynamics of human physiology evolves.

Today, the somatic treatment of mental illness is growing with the introduction of new therapies based on biochemical and physiological research. Drug treatment therapy *(pharmacotherapy)* and electroconvulsive therapy were established years ago and are still in use today. Biofeedback and phototherapy are relatively recent developments. Acupuncture as a therapy for addictions is the application of an ancient treatment method to modern problems.

Pharmacotherapy

The use of drugs to change behavior dates back centuries, but it was not until the 1950s that effective medications

for the control of mental illness were widely available. Currently, there are several groups of medicines that affect the mind. See Chapter 7 for a more detailed discussion of psychotherapeutic medications.

Other Somatic Therapies

Biofeedback

A technique that teaches clients how to control their physical responses is called **biofeedback.** It provides visual or auditory information about autonomic body functions. Bodily functions, such as respiration, pulse, or skin responses are monitored by machines. Clients practice relaxation techniques and change the monitored data. Changes in respiratory or pulse rates, for example, which can be seen on a graph provide clients with objective feedback and encouragement. Biofeedback has proven very useful in treating anxiety, hypertension, insomnia, and headaches.

Phototherapy

A relatively new development in somatic therapy is the use of bright lights for the treatment of depression. **Phototherapy,** also known as light therapy, has been used with success in the treatment of *seasonal affective disorder (SAD)*. During the winter months when the available daylight hours are fewer, many people become irritable, unable to concentrate, and even depressed. Researchers found that exposure to full-spectrum light for at least 20 minutes per day resulted in an improvement of depressive symptoms (Rosenthal, 1993). Phototherapy appears to be a promising form of treatment for some disorders, but further studies and research are needed to determine its long-term effectiveness.

Acupuncture

For more than 2000 years, acupuncture, a treatment in Oriental medicine, has cured disease and alleviated suffering. **Acupuncture** is defined as the inserting of fine needles into the skin along specific sites on the body. These sites travel along energy channels called *meridians*. Stimulating these points is thought to restore the energy or *chi* balance within the body. More Western explanations of acupuncture relate to the release and movement of neurotransmitters, neuropeptides, and hormones (Bennett, 1995). Acupuncture has been successfully used for the treatment of drug addictions and is proving to be a cost-effective and safe form of therapy.

FUTURE DEVELOPMENTS

During the new millennium, scientific knowledge will grow faster than our ability to make sense of it all. Evolving theories and their research activities now flow across many fields of study. Researchers are investigating many aspects of human consciousness and describing their effects on the body's physical systems. Investigations are being made into the area of extrasensory perception (ESP) and other phenomena outside our current realm of understanding.

Several innovative therapies have recently been introduced. Feminist and women's therapy grew from the feminist movement of the 1970s; creative aggression therapy arrived in the 1970s and taught clients to redirect their aggression and "fight fairly"; and movement therapy attempts to bring the body in tune with itself and restore balance. Aromatherapy treats emotional states through the use of certain odors, whereas reflexology focuses on releasing tension by stimulating certain points in the body. Theories about the nature of human beings and their environments will continue to evolve as will advances in therapies and treatments. We each must face the challenge and be open to new learning.

KEY CONCEPTS

- Systems theories view humans as functioning within a set of interacting and related units known as open or closed systems.
- Cognitive theories focus on the importance of intellectual factors in human development and function.
- Glasser's reality therapy attempts to teach people how to fill their needs in effective, satisfying, and appropriate ways.
- Sociocultural theories focus on the impact of a society on its people's behaviors and view mental illness as the result of social conditions.
- Szasz believed that mental illness is a culturally defined myth with which people cooperate.
- The concept of homeostasis was developed during the 1920s by Cannon, who found that the body has a tendency to achieve and maintain a steady internal state.

- The general adaptation syndrome, described by Seyle, consists of the stages of alarm, resistance, and exhaustion.
- If we are to be effective health care providers, we must consider clients' stress and anxiety levels.
- Procedures for crisis intervention focus on the concepts of immediacy, control, assessment, disposition, referral, and follow-up.
- Psychobiology is the study of the biochemical bases of thought, mood, emotion, and behavior.
- Psychoneuroimmunology is the study of the interactions among an individual's central nervous system, immune system, and personality.
- Research has demonstrated that anxiety, stress, and depression can decrease immune functions, whereas relaxation exercises and other positive emotional states increase the production of antibodies and stimulate immune system functions.
- Current treatments for mental health problems include psychotherapies and somatic therapies.

Suggestions for Further Reading
The article titled "Psycho—versus bio—medical therapy" by Kenneth J. Gergen (*Society* 35[1]:24, 1997) argues that both approaches complement each other when treating mental disorders.

References
Ader R: *Psychoneuroimmunology*, New York, 1981, Academic Press.
Bandura A: *Social foundations of thought and action: a social cognitive theory*, Englewood Cliffs, NJ, 1986, Prentice-Hall.
Beckett J: Online therapy raises red flags, *San Francisco Chronicle*, August 17, 1998.
Bennett C: The tao, acupuncture, and crack cocaine, *Capsules of Community Psychiatric Nursing* 1(4):2, 1995.
Bierman SF: Medical hypnosis, *Advances: The Journal of Mind-Body Health,* 11(1):65, 1995.
Cade B, O'Hanlon WH: *A brief guide to brief therapy*, New York, 1993, WW Norton.
Dillon KM, Minchoff B, Baker KH: Positive emotional states and enhancement of the immune system, *International Journal of Psychiatric Medicine* 15:13, 1985.
Glasser W: Reality therapy: a new approach to psychiatry, New York, 1965, Harper & Row.
Maltz M: Psycho-cybernetics: a new way to get more living out of life, Englewood Cliffs, NJ, 1960, Prentice-Hall.
Matheny KB, Kern RM: Cognitive therapies. In Corsini RJ, editor: *Encyclopedia of psychology*, ed 2, New York, 1994, John Wiley & Sons.
Mead GH: *Mind, self, and society from the standpoint of a social behaviorist*, Chicago, 1934, University of Chicago Press.
Meichenbaum D: Cognitive behavior modification: an integrative approach, ed 2, New York, 1989, Plenum.
Moore S: Meditation. In Corsini RJ, editor: *Encyclopedia of psychology*, ed 2, New York, 1994, John Wiley & Sons.
Raichle ME: Visualizing the mind, *Scientific American* 270(4):58, 1994.
Rosenthal N: *Winter blues: SAD—what it is and how to overcome it*, New York, 1993, Guilford Press.
Royce JR, Powell AD: *A theory of personality and individual differences*, Englewood Cliffs, NJ, 1983, Prentice-Hall.
Salk J: Biological basis of disease and behavior, *Perspectives of Biological Medicine*, 5:198, 1961.

Selye H: *Stress in health and disease,* Toronto, 1976, Butterworth Press.

Smoyak S: American psychiatric nursing: history and roles, *American Association of Hospital Nurses Journal* 41(7):316, 1993.

Szasz TS: *The myth of mental illness: foundations of a theory of personal conduct,* ed 2, New York, 1974, Harper & Row.

Taylor CM: *Essentials of psychiatric nursing,* ed 14, St. Louis, 1994, Mosby.

Wickramasekera IE: *Clinical behavioral medicine: some concepts and procedures,* New York, 1988, Plenum.

Wilson HS: The 1990s as the decade of the brain, *Capsules of Community Psychiatric Nursing* 1(1):1, 1994.

Chapter 7

Psychotherapeutic Drug Therapy

Learning Objectives

1. Briefly explain how psychotherapeutic medications affect humans.
2. Name four classifications of psychotherapeutic medications.
3. List three classes of antianxiety agents and identify the side effects associated with each.
4. Describe the health care implications for clients who are receiving both antidepressant and antimanic medications at the same time.
5. List the client care guidelines for monitoring antipsychotic (neuroleptic) drug therapy.
6. List five care guidelines for clients receiving psychotherapeutic drugs.
7. Discuss four nursing responsibilities for teaching clients about their medications.
8. Describe how informed consent and noncompliance relate to psychotherapeutic medications.

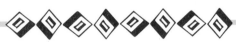

Key Terms

affective disorder

akathisia

akinesia

antipsychotics

autonomic nervous system (ANS)

central nervous system (CNS)

drug-induced parkinsonism

dyskinesia

dystonia

extrapyramidal side effects (EPSEs)

hypertensive crisis

informed consent

lithium

mania

monoamine oxidase inhibitors (MAOIs)

mood disorders

neurons

neuroleptic malignant syndrome

neurotransmitter

noncompliance

parasympathetic nervous system

peripheral nervous system (PNS)

psychotherapeutic drugs

sympathetic nervous system

tardive dyskinesia

Psychotherapeutic drugs are powerful chemicals that produce profound effects on the mind, emotions, and body (Keltner and Folks, 2001). The first psychotherapeutics were discovered as a result of exploring the side effects of other drugs, such as antihistamines for allergies. In 1949 lithium was found to be effective in treating the mania of bipolar illness, and the 1950s brought the use of chlorpromazine (Thorazine) into the therapeutic regimen.

The tranquilizer meprobamate (Miltown) became so popular in 1955 that drugstores were "required to place signs in the window when they sell out" (Keltner, Schwecke, and Bostrom, 1999). By the early 1960s tricyclic antidepressants, monoamine oxidase inhibitors (MAOIs), and haloperidol (Haldol) had been placed on the market. The antianxiety drug diazepam (Valium) became extremely popular, and soon it was the most often-prescribed medication in the world. Newer psychotherapeutic drugs have been introduced and even more will be available in the future. Health care professionals who work with these drugs must remember that psychotherapeutic medications are powerful chemicals with many, sometimes severe, side effects.

HOW PSYCHOTHERAPEUTIC DRUG THERAPY WORKS

Medications to treat people with mental health problems act mainly on the body's nervous system by altering the delicate chemical balance that continually exists within that system. Most psychotherapeutic medications interrupt the chemical messenger (neurotransmitter) pathways within the brain by suppressing major nerve pathways that connect the deeper brain to the frontal lobes and limbic system.

The *frontal lobes* of the brain are the source of the higher human functions, such as love, creativity, insight, planning, judgment, and abstract reasoning. The *limbic system* is responsible for emotions, motivation, memory, and the fight-or-flight response. When these areas of the brain have been affected by medications, profound changes in behavior result. People usually experience more stable moods, but many higher brain functions are impaired. As with all medications, there is a trade-off between therapeutic effects and unwanted reactions. One of the primary responsibilities of health care providers (especially nurses) is to recognize these differences.

The human nervous system consists of an "intensive, intricate network of structures that activates, coordinates, and controls all the functions of the body" (Anderson, Anderson, and Glanze, 1998). All parts of the nervous system work together. It is important to remember that if a drug affects one part of the nervous system, it will, without a doubt, have an impact on the other activities of that system.

The **central nervous system (CNS)** is composed of the brain and spinal cord, which together control all the motor and sensory functions of the body. Information about movement travels from the brain down through the spinal cord, reaches the appropriate muscle group, and results in movement. *Sensory information* (e.g., touch, temperature, position) is relayed in the opposite direction: from the muscles and other body areas, up through the spinal cord, and into the brain. Throughout this process, the CNS combines all incoming (sensory) and outgoing (motor) data.

The **peripheral nervous system (PNS)** is composed of the 31 spinal cord nerves plus the 12 pairs of cranial nerves. The peripheral nervous system is further divided into a "motor" system and an "autonomic" (automatic) system. Figure 7-1 illustrates the divisions of the nervous system.

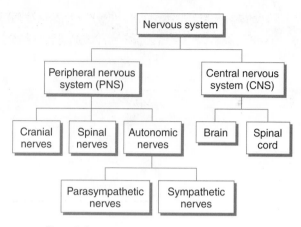

Figure 7-1 Divisions of the nervous systems.

Each spinal nerve contains motor and sensory **neurons** (nerve cells). The motor portion of the spinal nerve activates heart, muscles, and glandular secretions, whereas sensations of touch, temperature, pain, and spatial perception are transmitted by the sensory portion. The cranial nerves carry a mixture of information; some nerves are mainly motor, others carry mainly sensory information, and a few perform both motor and sensory functions.

The **autonomic nervous system (ANS)** is responsible for regulating the vital functions of the body. The activities of the heart muscle, smooth muscles, and glandular secretions are all controlled "automatically" by this remarkable system. Two divisions of the autonomic nervous system, the sympathetic and parasympathetic systems, work together to monitor and govern "automatic" body responses.

The **sympathetic nervous system** prepares the body for immediate adaptation through the fight-or-flight mechanism. The heart rate increases its output and moves blood into the muscles. Vessels to the stomach and other nonvital organs constrict and detour blood to the skeletal muscles. The pupils of the eyes dilate to improve visual acuity, and the bronchioles of the lungs expand to allow for greater exchange of airflow. Increases in blood sugar and fatty acid levels provide glucose for fuel, and all digestive and excretory processes are slowed. The result is greater cellular energy production and increased mental activity. Physically, the body is preparing to protect itself. People who are highly stressed demonstrate many sympathetic nervous system responses.

The **parasympathetic nervous system** is designed to conserve energy and provide the balance for the sympathetic system's excitability. The main functions of this system are to monitor and maintain control over the "regulatory" processes of the body, which it accomplishes by governing smooth muscle tone and glandular secretions. Parasympathetic stimulation slows the heart rate, decreases circulating blood volume, relaxes sphincters, and increases intestinal and glandular activity. Respira-

	Table 7-1 Autonomic Nervous System Actions	
Tissue	**Parasympathetic (cholinergic or muscarinic) response**	**Sympathetic (adrenergic) response**
Eye	Constriction (miosis)	Dilation (mydriasis)
	Accommodation (focus on near objects)	
Glands	Increased salivation (copious, watery)	Increased sweating*
	Increased tears and secretions of respiratory and gastrointestinal tract	Increased salivation (thick, contains proteins)
Heart	Decreased rate	Increased rate
	Decreased strength of contraction	Increased strength of contraction
	Decreased conduction velocity through the atrioventricular node	Increased conduction velocity through the atrioventricular node
Bronchioles	Smooth muscle constriction (restricts airways)	Smooth muscle relaxation (opens airways)
Blood vessels	Constriction of vessels in heart (not a prominent effect in humans)	Dilation of vessels in heart and skeletal muscle
	Dilation of vessels in salivary gland and erectile tissues	Constriction of vessels in skin, viscera, salivary gland, erectile tissues, kidney
Gastrointestinal tract		
Smooth muscle	Contraction	Relaxation
Sphincters	Relaxation	Contraction
Urinary bladder		
Fundus	Contraction	Relaxation
Trigone and sphincter	Relaxation	Contraction
Uterus		Contraction
Liver		Glycogenolysis

Modified from Clark JF, Queener SF, Karb VB: *The pharmacologic basis of nursing practice*, ed 5, St. Louis, 1997, Mosby.
*Acetylcholine is the neurotransmitter for this response.

tory, circulatory, digestive, excretory, and reproductive functions respond to parasympathetic messages. The parasympathetic nervous system uses the neurotransmitter acetylcholine to do its work and is often referred to as the cholinergic nervous system.

As you can see, the sympathetic and parasympathetic divisions of the autonomic nervous system act in opposite ways. Fortunately, this excite/calm interaction provides a balance. Organs are rich in both adrenergic (sympathetic) and cholinergic (parasympathetic) receptor sites, and this allows the organism to maintain itself in a state of balance or *homeostasis*. Table 7-1 lists the physical responses to parasympathetic and sympathetic nervous system stimulation. It is wise to be familiar with these responses because many clients receiving psychotherapeutic medications demonstrate side effects related to autonomic nervous system functions.

The basic unit of the nervous system is the **neuron** or nerve cell. The function of the neuron is to transmit electrical information to other neurons. Electrical information traveling through a neuron generates a chemical messenger called a **neurotransmitter** to inform other neurons of its arrival. Neurotransmitters are divided into four groups: monoamines, cholinergic group, amino acids, and neuropeptides.

Although nerve cells are found in great abundance throughout the body, they are not physically connected to one another. Each neuron is separated by a small space or gap called a *synapse*. Neurotransmitters travel across this gap, open a channel for the electrical information to pass, and then quickly become inactivated. Many psychotherapeutic drugs act in or around the synapse by altering the flow of message exchanges. The study of the neurochemistry of behavior has already altered the way in which mental-emotional problems are considered.

CLASSIFICATIONS OF PSYCHOTHERAPEUTIC DRUGS

There are four classes of psychotherapeutic medications: (1) antianxiety agents; (2) antidepressants and (3) antimanics, which are used to treat mood or emotional disorders; and (4) antipsychotics, which help curb the hallucinations and loss of reality suffered by individuals with psychotic disorders.

It is estimated that over 25 million people are currently being treated with psychotherapeutic drugs (Psychiatric News, 1998). People receiving psychotherapeutic (also called *psychotropic*) medications must be routinely monitored for effectiveness, side effects, and life-threatening adverse reactions. Because of this need for close monitoring, nurses and all caregivers must be knowledgeable about the roles that these powerful chemicals play in treating mental illness.

Antianxiety Medications

Anxiety is common to all of us. However, when it interferes with one's ability to function, it becomes an anxiety disorder. In today's world, anxiety disorders are a common mental health problem. A thorough discussion of anxiety and its treatments can be found in Chapter 20. Here we consider the antianxiety medications that are a usual part of the therapeutic treatment plan.

Antianxiety agents are drugs that reduce the psychic tension of stress. They are also referred to as *anxiolytics* or "minor tranquilizers." Medications in the antianxiety group are divided by chemical formulas into nonbenzodiazepines and benzodiazepines (Clark, Queener, and Karb, 1997). Today, the drugs of choice for the treatment of anxiety are the benzodiazepines.

The benzodiazepines have almost completely replaced other medications in the treatment of anxiety disorders. They are effective, generally well tolerated, and do not affect sleeping patterns (a common problem with many psychotherapeutic drugs). Benzodiazepines are prescribed to provide sedation, induce sleep (called a *hypnotic*), prevent seizures, and prepare clients for general anesthesia, but they are mainly used to decrease anxiety.

People with high levels of anxiety have low levels of a neurotransmitter called *GABA*. Benzodiazepines act by increasing GABA activity, which results in decreased anxiety (NAMI/NYC, 1999). They are fast acting, with the onset of action occurring within 1 hour. The drug exerts its action (duration) for about 4 to 6 hours. Thus clients experience relief from symptoms within hours.

Benzodiazepines are metabolized by the liver and excreted by the kidneys. People with impaired liver or kidney function must be carefully monitored if this drug class is prescribed. Pregnant and nursing women are usually not treated with benzodiazepines because these medications enter the breast milk. Caution must also be used when administering antianxiety agents to older or debilitated adults because of their slower metabolism. Box 7-1 lists commonly prescribed antianxiety agents.

Antianxiety drugs have several drug interactions, including central nervous system (CNS) depression when they are combined with other CNS depressants, such as alcohol and street drugs (Skidmore-Roth, 2001). The combination can produce serious, even fatal, reactions. Concentrations of the cardiac drug *digoxin* may be increased during treatment with antianxiety medications, so clients taking this medication must be routinely assessed for signs or symptoms of digoxin toxicity. Antacids should not be taken because they interfere with absorption of the antianxiety agent into the bloodstream.

Box 7-1 Commonly Prescribed Antianxiety Agents	
Generic name	**Trade name**
Benzodiazepines	
Alprazolam	Xanax, Apo-Alpraz
Chlordiazepoxide	Libritabs
Clorazepate potassium	Tranxene
Diazepam	Valium
Halazepam	Paxipam
Lorazepam	Ativan
Prazepam	Centrax
Nonbenzodiazepine	
Buspirone	BuSpar

The side effects of benzodiazepines are usually minimal, but they include fatigue, sedation, dizziness, and orthostatic hypotension (a drop in blood pressure on standing). Because long-term use of antianxiety drugs can result in dependence, therapy for clients is usually limited to a few months.

A new antianxiety agent, called *buspirone* (BuSpar), differs from benzodiazepines in several ways. First, it belongs to a different chemical class, the azapirones, and does not cause the sleepiness or muscle relaxation associated with benzodiazipines. Second, therapeutic effects are not seen for 3 to 6 weeks after beginning treatment. Buspirone has less potential for abuse; however, clients are still cautioned to avoid alcohol. Third, the potential for overdose is lessened because the drug has a wide dosage range. Side effects are few: lightheadedness, dizziness, headache, and nausea (Keltner and Folks, 2001).

Nursing care for clients receiving antianxiety agents includes frequent assessments for therapeutic actions and side effects. Many of these drugs are prescribed on an "as needed" (prn) basis. Medications used on this basis require accurate client assessments, good judgment, repeated evaluations of the medication's effects, and objective documentation.

Antidepressant Medications

Feelings of great joy and deep sadness are common human experiences. We are all familiar with these emotional extremes and think of them as the natural highs and lows of everyday life, but when one's mood begins to interfere with the ability to perform the routine activities of daily living, intervention is needed. **Mood disorders** are ineffective emotional states, ranging from deep depression to excited elation. They are also called **affective disorders** because the word "affect" means emotions. The major mood disorders are discussed in Chapter 21.

Box 7-2 Commonly Prescribed Antidepressants

Generic name	Trade name
Tricyclics	
Amitriptyline	Elavil
Amoxapine	Asendin
Clomipramine	Anafranil
Desipramine	Pertofrane
Doxepin	Sinequan
Imipramine	Tofranil
Nortriptyline	Pamelor
Protriptyline	Vivactil
Trimipramine	Surmontil
SSRIs	
Citalopram	Celexa
Fluoxetine	Prozac
Fluvoxamine	Luvox
Paroxetine	Paxil
Sertraline	Zoloft
MAOIs	
Phenelzine	Nardil
Tranylcypromine	Parnate
Miscellaneous	
Bupropion	Wellbutrin
Maprotiline	Ludiomil
Nefazodone	Serzone
Trazodone	Desyrel
Venlafaxine	Effexor

Basically, antidepressant medications exert their action in the body by increasing certain neurotransmitter activities. Based on their chemical formula, antidepressants are divided into categories: tricyclics, **monoamine oxidase inhibitors (MAOIs),** selective serotonin reuptake inhibitors (SSRIs), and miscellaneous agents (Box 7-2).

The physician's first choice for the treatment of depression is often an antidepressant. They are also indicated for bipolar disorders, panic disorders, obsessive-compulsive disorders, enuresis (bed wetting), bulimia, and neuropathic pain. Antidepressants have also been used with some success in posttraumatic stress disorder, organic mood disorders, attention deficit-hyperactivity disorder, and conduct disorders in children.

Antidepressants interact with a variety of other substances. Because they block the destruction of specific major neurotransmitters, higher levels of these chemicals circulate throughout the body. Ingesting foods or drugs that contain certain chemicals produce more neurotransmitters, which can result in overstimulation of the nervous system. Antidepressant drug interactions can produce serious cardiovascular and blood pressure reactions, as well as CNS depression. Table 7-2 gives a description of the more serious drug interactions encountered with the MAOI antidepressants.

Antidepressant medications require 1 to 2 weeks before symptom relief is noticed. However, side effects may be experienced soon after beginning therapy. Some side effects are a nuisance, like a dry mouth. Others, such as a **hypertensive crisis** (a sudden, severe elevation in blood pressure) can be life threatening. Anticholinergic side effects include dryness of the mouth, nose, and eyes, urinary retention, and sedation. These discomforts can be so bothersome that some people refuse to take their medications regularly. Clients should be routinely monitored for physical and behavioral changes. Those experiencing postural hypotension should be protected from falls. Kidney and liver function should be assessed and monitored monthly. Any signs of toxicity (e.g., headache, stiff neck, palpitations) should be reported to the physician immediately.

Clients should also be assessed for changes in attitudes and suicidal gestures. Frequently, depressed people attempt suicide when taking antidepressants because of increased energy levels, which can lead to a renewed interest in suicide. Take precautions to protect clients if you believe that they may be suicidal. Changes in a client's behavior may indicate a therapeutic improvement, a drug side effect, a drug/food interaction, or an emerging psychosis. Good communication with clients helps to assess subtle changes that may indicate problems.

Clients, no matter which medications they are taking, must be taught about their drug therapy. Instructions should include information about dosages, actions, and wanted and unwanted effects. Those who are taking MAOIs must understand their dietary and drug restrictions. Box 7-3 lists the foods and medications that must be avoided while taking MAOIs.

Selective serotonin reuptake inhibitors (SSRIs) are a relatively new class of antidepressants. They are the first choice in treatment for many physicians because their side effects are more manageable (Box 7-4). Because of this, SSRIs are indicated for both short- and long-term therapy.

Antimanic Medications

Mania is a state characterized by excitement, great elation, over talkativeness, increased motor activity, fleeting grandiose ideas, and agitated behaviors. Some therapists refer to mania as *agitated depression* because it frequently occurs with severe depression. Antidepressant drug therapy helps clients cope with their depression, but it has little effect during the manic stage of behavior.

Lithium is a naturally occurring salt. The word *lithium* is derived from the Greek word for *stone.* In 1949 lithium was found to be effective in the treatment of mania, but as a result of reports of fatal side effects, the drug was not

Table 7-2 Drug Interactions With Monoamine Oxidase Inhibitors

Type of interaction	Signs/Symptoms
Anticholinergic reactions	Dry mouth, decreased tearing, blurred vision, constipation, urinary hesitancy or retention, excessive sweating
Hypertensive crisis	Throbbing, radiating headache, stiff neck, palpitations, tightness in chest, sweating, dilated pupils, very high blood pressure and pulse rate
CNS depression	Changes in level of consciousness; sedation, increasing lethargy, disorientation, confusion, agitation, hallucinations, lower seizure threshold

CNS, Central nervous system.

Box 7-3 Dietary and Drug Interactions With Monoamine Oxidase Inhibitors

Medications to Avoid

Prescription and over-the-counter drugs: Nasal and sinus decongestants; cold, allergy, and hayfever remedies; inhalants for asthma; weight-loss pills, pep pills, stimulants; narcotics, local anesthetics
Any medication should be approved by the physician.

Illicit drugs: Cocaine, any amphetamine (uppers)

Foods to Avoid

Alcoholic drinks: Beer, ale, red wines (Chianti), sherry wines, liqueurs, cognac
Dairy products: Aged cheese, sour cream
Fruits and vegetables: Avocados, bananas, fava and broad beans, canned figs, any overripe fruit
Meats: Pickled or smoked, bologna, chicken or beef liver, dried fish, meat tenderizer, salami, sausage
Other foods: Large amounts of caffeinated coffee, tea, or cola; chocolate; licorice; soy sauce; yeast

Box 7-4 Side Effects of SSRI Antidepressants

Dry mouth, nausea, vomiting constipation, diarrhea, anorexia, differences in taste; headache, changes in alertness, tremor, dizziness, weakness, fatigue, increased sweating; sexual dysfunction; visual disturbances, urinary disturbances

Box 7-5 Commonly Prescribed Antimanics

Generic name	Trade name
Carbamazepine	Tegretol
Clonazepam	Klonopin
X Lithium carbonate	Carbolith, Duralith, Eskalith CR, Lithane, Lithotabs
X Valproic acid	Depakene

mood, it is indicated for the treatment of acute mania and as a prophylaxis (preventative) for clients with bipolar disorders. Lithium has also been investigated for the treatment of drug abuse, alcoholism, phobias, and eating disorders. Therapy is contraindicated (not prescribed) for pregnant women and people with kidney failure. Clients with physical health problems must be carefully monitored.

Lithium is well absorbed into the bloodstream and excreted faster than sodium by the kidneys. For this reason, clients who are taking lithium must be cautioned about balancing their salt intake, fluid intake, and activity. Lithium interacts with a variety of other drugs. For a list of significant drug interactions associated with antimanic drugs, consult a drug reference.

The difference between therapeutic and toxic levels of lithium is minimal. The drug is usually well tolerated by most clients, but how well the drug is excreted varies from client to client. The "narrow therapeutic index" of lithium requires close observation of client responses. If the blood levels are too low, manic behavior returns; however, if levels are too high, an uncomfortable and possibly life-threatening toxicity may result. Lithium levels above 1.5 mEq/L are considered toxic.

Clinical improvement commonly takes as long as 3 weeks. Clients in the acute manic stage usually require the addition of antipsychotic or sedative medications until the effects of lithium take hold. Clients are monitored monthly for thyroid and kidney function because long-term use of lithium can cause altered thyroid function (hypothyroidism) and loss of the kidney's ability to

available in the United States until 1970. Lithium is the mainstay treatment of the manic phase of bipolar depression. Newer products are currently under investigation for clients who do not respond or cannot tolerate lithium therapy. Box 7-5 lists the major antimanic medications.

Lithium is currently used in the United States for the treatment of manic episodes. Because lithium stabilizes

Box 7-6 Guidelines for Clients Taking Lithium

To achieve a therapeutic effect and prevent lithium toxicity, clients taking lithium should be advised of the following:

1. Lithium must be taken on a regular basis at the same time daily. If you miss a dose wait until the next scheduled time to take the lithium.
2. When lithium treatment is started, mild side effects may develop, such as fine hand tremor, increased thirst and urination, nausea, anorexia, and diarrhea or constipation. Some foods, such as celery and butter fat, may have an unappealing taste. Most side effects will pass with time.
3. Serious side effects of lithium include vomiting, extreme hand tremor, sedation, muscle weakness, and dizziness. The physician should be notified immediately if any of these effects occur.
4. Lithium and sodium compete for elimination from the body through the kidneys. An increase in salt intake increases lithium elimination, and a decrease in salt intake decreases lithium elimination. Thus it is important that the client maintain a balanced diet, liquid, and salt intake. The client should consult with the physician before making any dietary changes.
5. Various situations can require an adjustment in lithium doses; for example, the addition of a new medication to the client's drug regimen, a new diet, or an illness with fever or excessive sweating.
6. Blood for determination of lithium levels should be drawn in the morning approximately 8 to 14 hours after the last dose was taken.

Modified from Keltner NL, Folks DG: *Psychotropic drugs,* ed 3, St. Louis, 2001, Mosby.

Box 7-7 Commonly Prescribed Antipsychotics

Generic name	Trade name
Phenothiazines	
Chlopromazine	Thorazine
Fluphenazine	Prolixin
Mesoridazine	Serentil
Perphenazine	Trilafon
Prochlorperazine	Compazine
Promazine	Sparine
Thioridazine	Mellaril
Trifluoperazine	Stelazine
Triflupromazine	Vesprin
Butyrophenone	
Haloperidol	Haldol
Miscellaneous	
Clozapine	Clozaril
Loxapine	Loxitane
Molindone	Moban
Olanzapine	Zyprexa
Quietiapine	Seroquel
Risperidone	Risperdal
Thiothixene	Navane

Lithium → Polyuria

concentrate urine. Great care must be taken to frequently assess and monitor each client's responses to each medication as undesirable effects are present with every medication the client receives.

The major guidelines for safe and effective client care relate to three areas: helping with the prelithium workup, educating the client to maintain stable blood levels of the drug, and monitoring the client for side effects and possible toxic reactions.

The *prelithium workup* consists of a complete physical, history, electrocardiogram (ECG), and numerous blood studies. Nurses are responsible for obtaining a complete functional assessment that describes the client's habits and activities of daily living. They should also review of the results of all diagnostic tests. Data from these assessments allow nurses to plan appropriate care and forecast potential problems.

Stabilizing lithium levels involves teaching the client and family about: expected side effects, the difference between common side effects and those requiring imme-

diate notification of the physician, and coping with the lifestyle changes required by this medication. Box 7-6 lists the most important guidelines for clients who are receiving lithium.

Be sure the client and family understand each bit of information. Ask them to repeat what they have learned, apply it to several "what if" situations, and describe the appropriate actions for each side effect. Reinforce the information with written instructions. The informed client is a more willing participant in treatment.

Antipsychotic (Neuroleptic) Medications

Antipsychotics are also referred to as *major tranquilizers* or *neuroleptics.* Most antipsychotic medications are available in tablet, liquid, and injectable forms. Each class of antipsychotics has profound effects on the most complex of all the body's systems—the brain and nervous system.

Most antipsychotic drugs are used to treat the symptoms of major mental disorders, such as schizophrenia, acute mania, and organic mental illnesses. They are also used to treat some resistant bipolar (manic-depressive), paranoid, and movement disorders. A few antipsychotics are used to treat nausea, vomiting, and intractable hiccups. Box 7-7 lists commonly prescribed antipsychotic drugs.

The psychosis called *schizophrenia* is associated with two kinds of symptoms: Type 1, positive schizophrenic symptoms, and Type 2, negative schizophrenic symptoms (Table 7-3). Antipsychotic medications appear to be much more effective in controlling the positive symptoms of acute schizophrenia. Their use for clients with chronic brain disorders remains controversial because these drugs block already depleted dopamine (a neurotransmitter) pathways.

Antipsychotic medications interact with many other chemicals. For example, antacids hinder the absorption of antipsychotic drugs, so they must be administered 2 hours after the oral antipsychotic. Alcohol, antianxiety medications, antihistamines, antidepressants, barbiturates, mesperidine (Demerol), and morphine produce severe CNS depression when mixed with antipsychotics. As a health care provider, you are responsible for the safety of your clients. Research every medication that may possibly interact with the prescribed antipsychotic and monitor your clients' responses to each drug. If drug references do not contain enough information, consult the pharmacist or physician.

The side effects and adverse reactions of antipsychotic medications are numerous and troublesome for the client. Both the central and peripheral nervous systems are affected by antipsychotics. **Extrapyramidal side effects (EPSEs)** are CNS side effects described as abnormal movements produced by an imbalance of neurotransmitters in the brain. They include the following:

Akathisia, the inability to sit still

Akinesia, absence of physical and mental movement

Dyskinesia, the inability to execute voluntary movements

Dystonia, impaired muscle tone (rigidity in the muscles that control gait, posture, and eye movements)

Drug-induced parkinsonism, a term used to describe a group of symptoms that mimic Parkinson's disease

Neuroleptic malignant syndrome (NMS), a serious and potentially fatal extrapyramidal side effect

Tardive dyskinesia is a serious, irreversible side effect of long-term treatment. The word tardive means "appearing later," and many clients will exhibit the signs of tardive dyskinesia after several months of drug treatment. This condition is discussed in detail in Chapter 31. See Appendix C for the AIMS assessment tool.

Peripheral nervous system side effects include dry mouth, blurred vision, and photophobia (sensitivity to bright light), tachycardia, and hypotension. Caregivers must protect clients from falls during the first few weeks of therapy because the chance for low blood pressure (hypotension) is greatest when clients stand or change positions suddenly. These hypotensive episodes cause tachycardia (rapid heartbeat) as the body attempts to adapt to a lower blood pressure. Antipsychotic drugs affect each person uniquely. They are powerful medications that must be administered with great care.

CLIENT CARE GUIDELINES

Nurses and those who administer psychotherapeutic drugs have five basic responsibilities relating to these medications: (1) assess clients, (2) coordinate care, (3) administer medications, (4) monitor and evaluate client responses, and (5) teach clients about their medications. Each area of responsibility involves careful observation and an understanding of each drug's therapeutic and adverse actions. All caregivers should be aware of each client's medication regimen and report any unusual signs or symptoms to the nurse or physician.

Table 7-3 Positive and Negative Types of Schizophrenia		
	Type 1: Positive schizophrenia	**Type 2: Negative schizophrenia**
Signs and symptoms	Delusions, illusions, hallucinations	Anergia (lack of energy); anhedonia (inability to feel happiness or pleasure); apathy (does not care about anything); avolution (unable to choose or exert own will); flat affect (no emotional responses); will not speak unless spoken to
Anatomy and physiology	Hyperdopaminergic reactions (too much dopamine)	Nondopaminergic reactions (too little dopamine)
	Brain size and structure normal	Brain has structural changes: decreased blood flow, increased size of ventricles, decrease in size of brain
Response to antipsychotic medications	Usually good	Usually poor

Assessment

The first step of the (therapeutic) nursing process is the most important because an accurate and complete database enhances the quality and effectiveness of client care. Many nurses are very skilled with the psychosocial and mental status assessments necessary for the care of clients with mental-emotional problems. However, it is important to remember that physical difficulties are common companions of psychic problems. See the Case Study box for a vivid example of this principle.

A history should be completed for every client whether the presenting problems are of physical or mental origin. A complete health history includes a profile of the client's current living situation, family structure, and daily activities. Attention should also be paid to his or her past medical, family, and social histories. An investigation of the client's chief complaint (presenting problem) rounds out the basic database. Laboratory and other diagnostic studies may be ordered by the physician or nurse practitioner, and special medication assessments must be conducted for clients receiving psychotherapeutic medications (Stuart and Laraia, 1998). Table 7-4 offers an example of a medication history assessment tool. Assessing clients is a continual process. Good physical and psychosocial assessments add an important dimension to the client's overall plan of holistic care.

Coordination

Physicians prescribe treatments, psychologists recommend therapies, and social workers, psychologists and other health care team members propose plans of care based on their area of expertise. Nurses coordinate and ensure that each component of the treatment plan is carried out. They juggle scheduling for tests, treatments, and therapies; monitor responses to medications; teach clients and their significant others about treatments, medications, and other aspects of therapy; and encourage clients to become actively engaged in their treatment. Nurses also act as advocates, consult with other members of the treatment team throughout the client's stay, and provide care that encourages clients toward wellness.

Each health care team member coordinates client care with others. Multidisciplinary care planning meetings are held frequently to discuss client progress and problems from each specialist's viewpoint. Treatment goals are discussed and care plans are updated as client behavior changes.

Drug Administration

One traditional role of nurses is the administration of medications to clients. Today, in some facilities, this task has fallen to the certified medication aide (CMA). The term *certified medical technician (CMT)* is also used. CMAs or CMTs are usually nursing assistants with specialized training in the administration of certain oral

Case Study

Gary T., a 36-year-old man, was admitted to the mental health unit of the community hospital with a diagnosis of paranoid schizophrenia. He is considered a danger to others because of his aggressive and uncooperative behaviors. After receiving a major tranquilizer, he spent a relatively quiet night but cried out frequently. Today, Mary S. has been assigned to care for him.

After reviewing the change-of-shift report and Gary's record, Mary decided that he needed a thorough assessment so she went in search of her client. She was surprised to find a rather burly, bearded man lying curled on his side and whimpering quietly to himself. While knocking on the door, she introduced herself and requested a few minutes of his time. "Hardly matters," he grumbled softly.

Mary approached his bed carefully, remembering his tendency for physical aggression. As she seated herself near his bedside, she thought she caught an expression of pain. Acting on this nonverbal message, Mary gently questioned, "Where are you hurting?"

Gary, who had averted her gaze, looked straight into her eyes and said through clenched teeth, "I think it's my back or legs or something. Ever since this pain started, I've been unable to control myself. All I want to do now is make everybody who is messin' with me hurt as much as I do."

This was the clue that sent Mary on the path of assessing Gary's pain. She discovered in his past medical history that Gary had fallen off a roof about 3 months ago. The injuries had not resolved, and attempts at treatment were resulting in ever-increasing discomfort. Pain medications, even when combined with alcohol, had little effect on the pain. Mary's physical assessment revealed difficulties with walking, sitting, and changing positions. He was not able to lift his legs off the bed.

Mary knew something was physically wrong. Her first priority of care was to help Gary find some relief from his pain. After sharing her findings with her supervisor, Mary consulted the physician in charge of Gary's case who ordered several diagnostic tests. The results of the tests revealed a large herniated disc in his back. Gary was immediately transferred and prepared for surgery.

Weeks later, a large, burly man approached Mary in the hallway. He reminded her of someone familiar, but she couldn't quite place him. As he drew closer, she recognized Gary, who had come to thank her for listening to him. "I told the others that I was hurtin', but they didn't listen, so I got upset. I guess I can be pretty rowdy when I'm hurtin'. But you listened to me and I had surgery and the pain is gone. I can be a nice guy again. If you hadn't listened to me, I'd really be crazy by now. Thanks."

Mary felt great, but she reminded herself to carefully and thoroughly (physically, emotionally, socioculturally, and spiritually) assess each client as a unique individual. The answer to a complex problem may lie in a simple solution, but one must be alert enough to recognize the clues.

◆ What do you think may have happened if Mary had not assessed a physical problem with this client?

Table 7-4 Medication History Assessment Tool

Psychotherapeutic medications	Other prescriptions	Over-the-counter drugs	Substance use
			Alcohol, caffeine, street drugs
Each drug ever taken	Each drug in past 6 mo	Each drug in past 6 mo	
Drug name?	Drug name?	Drug name?	Substance(s)?
Reason for prescription?	Reason for prescription?	Reason for taking?	When used?
When started?	When started?	When started?	
Length of time taking drug?	Length of time taking drug?	Frequency of use?	Frequency of use?
Highest daily dose?	Highest daily dose?	Highest dose?	
Effectiveness?	Effectiveness?	Effectiveness?	Effects?
Side effects, adverse reactions?	Side effects, adverse reactions?	Side effects, adverse reactions?	Side effects, adverse reactions?
Any physical changes since starting medication?	Any physical changes since starting medication?		Any problems associated with use?
Was drug taken as prescribed (compliance)?	Was drug taken as prescribed (compliance)?		

Modified from Stuart GW, Laraia MT: *Quick psychopharmacology reference*, ed 2, St. Louis, 1995, Mosby.

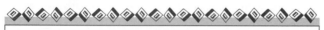

Think About

You are monitoring the responses of three clients who are taking Haldol. The first client is a 23-year-old female. The second is a 50-year-old male, and the last is a 76-year-old male.

◆ Which client is at greatest risk for developing side effects?

◆ What are your reasons for making this choice?

medications. However, it remains the responsibility of the nurse to monitor clients for drug effectiveness and adverse reactions. Other care providers should also become aware of the actions and side effects of their clients' medications.

It is not uncommon for a client to be taking two or more psychotherapeutic drugs at a time. In these instance, caregivers must be especially vigilant for side effects and signs of drug interactions.

Monitoring and Evaluating

Physicians evaluate client responses and adjust medical therapies, but care providers are in the best position to observe the physical and behavioral changes that accompany the administration of psychotherapeutic medications. All caregivers should be familiar with the major side effects and adverse reactions for each class of psychotherapeutic drugs used in their practice settings.

Interactions with other medications and substances can become life threatening. For example, when alcohol is combined with antidepressant drugs, severe CNS depression occurs. This, in turn, results in lethargy, progressing to respiratory depression, coma, and even death. Certain groups of people are at an increased risk for developing drug interactions, including older adults, the debilitated, people with immunosuppressed or compromised organ systems (especially liver and kidneys), and clients who have physical illnesses (see Think About box).

Monitoring clients' responses to their drugs is an important, potentially life-saving intervention. Do not take this responsibility lightly because your clients depend on your knowledge of their medications.

Client Teaching

Every individual has a right to be informed about his or her diagnosis and treatment plan. Each client must be prepared to safely take each medication, monitor for side effects daily, and know what course of action to take when side effects occur.

Nurses must be able to reach clients "on their own level" of understanding. To prevent miscommunication, the nurse must speak in terms that the client can understand and proceed at a pace that allows for understanding and the formulation of questions. Most psychotherapeutic medications slow the client's ability to follow and comprehend a line of thought. Therefore it is important to repeat essential points. Be sure the client understands by having him or her repeat the most important information. Provide important information in writing. Having a written explanation gives the client something tangible and real that can be reviewed and referred to when memory fails. Clients taking psychotherapeutic medications are likely to forget what has been taught. Preprinted drug information is helpful, but there is no substitute for individualized client teaching. If possible, such teaching should include the family or significant others. They can be very helpful in assisting the client to follow the medication regimen (Table 7-5).

Table 7-5	Teaching Clients About Psychotherapeutic Medications

Nursing process	Examples of actions

Assessment	Assess client for the following:
	    Level of understanding
	    Ability to self-administer medications
	    Willingness to take medications on a daily basis
	    Level of cooperation
	    Ability to obtain and purchase medications
	    Support of family
	    Past medication history including side effects of any drug taken

Planning	Nursing diagnoses:
	    Knowledge deficit: psychotherapeutic medications
	    Risk for noncompliance
	    Plan to teach use of *(specify)* medications

Interventions	For each drug, teach client to recognize the following:
	    Generic and brand names
	    Purpose and action
	    Therapeutic effects
	    Dosage, route, schedule of drug
	    Administration, what to do if a dose is missed
	    Specific precautions (driving, operation of power equipment)
	    Side effects and actions to take if they occur
	    Possible drug/food interactions
	    Signs of overdosage or underdosage
	    Drug storage, expiration dates
	Provide information in written form.
	Develop written medication schedule.
	Reinforce other data given by care team.

Evaluation	Observe client to evaluate effectiveness of teaching. Reassess if any areas of instruction were not understood by client or family.

Helping clients and their significant others to adapt to change is a health care provider responsibility. Psychotherapeutic medications are designed to produce behavioral changes, and these changes affect the client and people within the client's environment. A well-taught client and family are able to cope more effectively with the life changes that result from psychotherapeutic drug therapy.

SPECIAL CONSIDERATIONS

Because most psychotherapeutic medications affect the body's nervous system, they are potentially harmful chemicals. Professionals with prescriptive authority must weigh the benefits of therapy with the possible harm that may result from taking a medication.

Adverse Reactions

Health care providers, especially nurses, must constantly remain vigilant for the effects of psychotherapeutic medications. Clients who are taking psychotherapeutic drugs (especially antipsychotics) are at risk for developing the serious problems of neuroleptic malignant syndrome and tardive dyskinesia (Lader, 1999). Accurate identifica-

tion of the signs and symptoms of each may prevent many complications. Detailed descriptions of these reactions are found in Chapters 31 and 32.

Noncompliance

An informed decision, made by a client, not to follow a prescribed treatment program defines **noncompliance**. Many psychiatric clients choose to discontinue or reduce their medications because of the distressing side effects. Others have difficulty following treatment programs because of the nature of their problems. For example, paranoid or delusional people seldom cooperate with medication regimens or schedules. Many outpatient clients do not take their medications as prescribed. Even clients within inpatient settings do not take their medications consistently. It is not uncommon for people to hide drugs in the cheek or pretend to swallow and then discard or hoard them. The physician should be notified in these cases and a liquid form of the medication should be requested.

Informed Consent

Another consideration relating to psychotherapeutic medications is the issue of informed consent. **Informed** consent is the process of presenting clients with information about the benefits, risks, and side effects of specific treatments, thus enabling them to make voluntary and knowledgeable decisions about their care. With the treatment of physical disorders, the process is straightforward: treatments are described and the client makes the decision to accept or reject the plan. However, with mental disorders, the picture is not so clear. In the past, psychiatric clients who were considered a danger to themselves or others were routinely medicated without their permission.

Today, the Patient Self-Determination Act states that clients have the right to accept or refuse care and cannot be pushed, coerced, or talked into following a certain course. In 1986 the New York Court of Appeals held that "in nonemergency situations, involuntary patients cannot be forced to take psychotic medications" (Keltner, Schwecke, and Bostrom, 1999). This ruling has led to an uncomfortable compromise between client rights and people's needs to feel safe.

When a client becomes noncompliant with medications, the care guidelines center around ensuring safety and assessing for the return of symptoms. When caring for the client within an inpatient setting, caregivers should observe for any changes in behavior, be prepared for the client to become aggressive or act out, and protect the client and others from harm. If the setting is the clinic, the caregiver should instruct the client's significant others about the return of psychiatric symptoms, the signs and symptoms of side effects and adverse reactions, and the available community resources. Although nurses cannot manipulate or force a client into taking medications, they can use their rapport with clients to assist them in making decisions based on complete information and sound judgment.

KEY CONCEPTS

◆ Psychotherapeutic medications are powerful chemical substances that produce profound effects on the mind, emotions, and body.
◆ Most psychotherapeutic medications produce their effects by interrupting the chemical messenger (neurotransmitter) pathways within the brain.
◆ The drugs of choice for the treatment of anxiety are benzodiazepines, which are known as antianxiety agents.
◆ Antidepressant medications treat depression and other mood disorders by increasing certain neurotransmitter activity within the brain and CNS.
◆ Mania and bipolar depressive illnesses are treated with lithium, a naturally occurring mood stabilizer.

◆ Antipsychotic (neuroleptic) drugs are indicated for clients suffering from schizophrenia, acute mania, organic mental illnesses, some resistant bipolar disorders, paranoid disorders, some disorders of movement, nausea and vomiting, and intractable hiccups.
◆ Extrapyramidal side effects are CNS alterations that produce abnormal involuntary movement disorders, including akathisia, akinesia, dyskinesia, dystonia, and drug-induced parkinsonism.
◆ Clients who are receiving psychotherapeutic drugs (especially antipsychotics) are at risk for developing the serious problems of neuroleptic malignant syndrome and tardive dyskinesia.
◆ Nurses who work with clients who are receiving psychotherapeutic drugs have five basic responsibilities: assess, coordinate, administer, monitor and evaluate, and teach.
◆ A special medication assessment (drug history) must be conducted for clients receiving psychotherapeutic medications.
◆ A primary responsibility of nurses is to monitor the clients for drug effectiveness and adverse reactions.
◆ Client education is a major role of nurses.
◆ Noncompliance is defined as an informed decision, made by a client, not to follow a prescribed treatment program.
◆ Informed consent is presenting clients with the information about the benefits, risks, and side effects of specific treatments, thus enabling them to make decisions about their care.

Suggestions for Further Reading
The book titled *Psychotropic Drugs* by Norman Keltner and David Folks (St. Louis, 2001, Mosby) offers a thorough discussion of most medications for mental health problems.

References
Anderson KN, Anderson LE, Glanze WD: *Mosby's medical, nursing, and allied health dictionary,* ed 5, St. Louis, 1998, Mosby.
Clark JF, Queener SF, Karb VB: *Pharmacologic basis of nursing practice,* ed 5, St. Louis, 1997, Mosby.
Keltner NL, Folks DG: *Psychotropic drugs,* ed 3, St. Louis, 2001, Mosby.
Keltner NL, Schwecke LH, Bostrom CE: *Psychiatric nursing,* ed 3, St. Louis, 1999, Mosby.
Lader M: Some adverse effects of antipsychotics: prevention and treatment, *Journal of Clinical Psychiatry* 60(12):18, 1999.
National Alliance of Mental Illness: *Benzodiazepines,* New York, 1999, The Alliance.
Prescriptions for antidepressant, stimulants increase dramatically, *Psychiatric News,* March 17, 1998.
Skidmore-Roth L: *Mosby's 2001 nursing drug reference,* St. Louis, 2001, Mosby.
Stuart GW, Laraia MT: *Pocket guide to psychiatric nursing,* ed 4, St. Louis, 1998, Mosby.

Chapter 8

Principles of Mental Health Care

Learning Objectives

1. Describe three characteristics of a mentally healthy adult.
2. Explain how the phrase "do no harm" applies to mental health care.
3. Discuss the importance of mutual trust in the mental health caregiver–client relationship.
4. Identify the four components of any behavior.

5. Predict the outcome for a mental health client who develops more effective adaptive (coping) skills.
6. Describe the concept of consistency and its use in providing effective mental health care.
7. Explain the advantages of setting and enforcing limits when working with clients who are experiencing mental health problems.

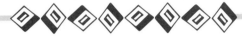

Key Terms

adaptation	consistency	principle
advocacy	empathy	responsibility
behavior	holistic health care	stigma
caring	mentally healthy adult	

A **principle** is a code or standard that helps people govern their conduct. Principles guide the decisions and actions of the people who choose to follow them. Professional principles provide guidelines for people who practice within certain professions. Helping professions, such as medicine, nursing, psychology, social work, and other health care specialists, all have established sets of principles. Most professions are guided by standards of care, state practice acts, and principles. This chapter examines seven basic principles for those who work with mentally or emotionally troubled clients.

The Mentally Healthy Adult

The concepts of mental health and mental illness are not easily defined. Health, by its very nature, is a changing state that is influenced by an individual's patterns of behavior and interactions with the environment (Haber and others, 1997). Mental health is just as dynamic—changing as the stresses of life are met.

Most people manage to adapt to the changes in their lives. They remain contributing members of their group, community, and society. Although problems may exist, they are content with who and where they are in life. They are able to love and express love freely without the fear of losing their independence. Flexibility and a willingness to try something different lead to an eagerness for learning. Life is considered important, and its special moments are cherished. Adversity is seen as a challenge or opportunity for growth. To simplify, a **mentally healthy adult** is a person who can cope with and adjust to the recurrent stresses of daily living in an acceptable way. Although mentally healthy adults experience unhappiness, anxiety, or other psychic distresses, they manage to pool their resources, rise above the negativity, and continue with their lives.

In our culture, *mental illness* results when the problems associated with an individual's life become so overwhelming that the person is unable to cope and develops maladaptive behaviors. They become unable to carry out the activities of daily living or function independently. Citizens of the industrialized cultures label a person as mentally ill only after the ability to function independently in society is impaired for a period (Giger and Davidhizar, 1999). Other cultures have different definitions of mental illness (see the Cultural Aspects box for an example of another viewpoint).

Mental Health Care Practice

Practicing the principles of mental health care is the responsibility of all health care providers. Every caregiver addresses the mental health needs of each person who becomes a client. One of the foundations of the helping professions is based on the care of the whole person. No matter which specialty is practiced or where the setting is located, every caregiver helps people cope with their problems. To do this effectively, clients' mental-emotional status, how they view their problems, and which resources and supports are available for resolving the difficulties must be considered (Starck and McGovern, 1992).

The world of health care is familiar and comfortable for those who practice within its realm. The sights, sounds, and smells of the health care environment become known and familiar. Daily routines are established, and the facility's employees all understand what behaviors are expected of them.

However, to a person who is ill (disabled, stressed) in some way, visiting a medical facility can be an uncomfortable experience. Anxiety results when illness or disability affects an individual. No matter how casual a client may appear, a heightened stress level is present every time interactions with health care providers take place. Some people are so intimidated by the thought of visiting a health care provider that they wait until their problems become severe and difficult to treat. Health care providers who remember that clients are "out of their element" when seeking health care are able to provide much needed emotional support and more effective care.

The skills developed when working with the mental and emotional needs of people will be used throughout your career, for yours is the profession of caring. May these seven principles of mental health care help guide you:

1. Do no harm.
2. Accept each client as a whole person.
3. Develop mutual trust.
4. Explore behaviors and emotions.
5. Encourage responsibility.
6. Encourage effective adaptation.
7. Provide consistency.

DO NO HARM

The first rule of medicine, nursing, and other helping professions states that if you cannot do something right, at least do not do something wrong. No matter what the circumstances, avoid any action that may result in harm to the client. The "do no harm" principle also relates to the "reasonable and prudent nurse (caregiver)" concept found in U.S. law. It is derived from the ancient writings of Hippocrates, whose principle of "do no harm" proves to be as true and valid today as it was in his era.

Caregivers' Tools and Arts

Every occupation has its tools. The carpenter finds the saw, drill, and level indispensable. The accountant cannot function without the computer, calculator, or calendar. The surgeon uses specialized instruments, and the cook is lost without pots and pastry cutters. Health care providers, however, are a bit different.

Care providers use several tools to practice their professions. We can identify the more obvious equipment, but beneath the visible tools lie skills of the individual. Caregivers use skills of the "self." The ways in which caregivers communicate, interact, and behave all require the use of therapeutic tools (techniques), which require study and practice to learn. These therapeutic tools include the use of eye contact, facial expressions, body movement, and other nonverbal behaviors. Other tools are developed when therapeutic communication skills are practiced. Interactions with people from various cultures and backgrounds help to refine the caregiver's tools.

Cultural Aspects

Laos is a country in southeast Asia. Its inhabitants, the Lao, believe that 32 spirits live within the body and govern its functions. Illnesses, including mental disturbances, are thought to be the result of an imbalance of the spirits, unhealthy air currents, or bad winds. Pinching or scratching parts of the body to produce red marks helps to let the bad winds out of the body and restore health. Strings are worn around the wrists, neck, ankles, or waist to prevent soul loss.

Remember that you are a therapeutic agent who guides clients toward wellness. Learn to "see" yourself working with clients, analyze your behaviors, and try new approaches. Work to improve your ability to become a "therapeutic tool," and clients will respond.

The "do no harm" principle serves as a guide for therapeutic actions. Care providers in every care setting have the responsibility to protect clients, but sometimes a well-intended action can result in a harmful situation. To illustrate, telling the client about therapy before the physician has spoken with him or her could alter the client's decision about treatment. The caregiver had good intentions—to help the client cope—but the outcome could result in the client refusing treatment.

For caregivers working with mental health clients, this principle is especially important because the main therapeutic tool of the mental health care provider is the "self." The therapeutic use of the self can result in great improvements in clients' behaviors when the "do no harm" principle is applied. When the principle is overlooked or forgotten, the one who loses is the client, the very person we are obligated to protect.

The Therapeutic Process

The therapeutic process is also called the *nursing process*. It serves as an organizational framework for giving care and consists of five steps: assessment, diagnosis, planning, implementation, and evaluation. Use of the process encourages us to consider the client and develop appropriate, as well as effective, care measures.

Assessment is the data-collection step. Information relating to the client is collected from every possible source. Both subjective and objective data are collected. *Subjective data* relate to clients' perceptions and abstract information that is difficult to measure or share. The experiences of pain, nausea, and anxiety, for example, cannot be measured by anyone but the individual experiencing them. *Objective data* refers to information that can be measured and shared. It is gathered through the senses of sight, smell, touch, and hearing. Test results and blood pressure readings are examples of objective data.

To gather data, medical records are reviewed, a history is obtained, and observations are made. When discussions with family members or friends take place, a picture of the client begins to emerge. Using this mass of information or database, care providers plan care based on the needs, abilities, preferences, and concerns of the client.

Next, data are sorted into related areas, and problems or concerns are identified. Each problem is then examined. Problem statements and nursing diagnoses are developed. Medical diagnoses and interventions relate to the client's physical or mental dysfunctions. Nursing diagnoses and interventions are concerned with how the client's problems affect his or her ability to carry out the activities of daily living. Client needs must be remembered whenever problem statements are being developed.

During the *planning* phase, the outcome of each problem is projected by identifying behaviors that indicate that the problem is solved. These "expected outcomes" are then used to monitor the client's progress. Specific short and long term goals are developed, and therapeutic actions (interventions) are planned.

Once actions are formulated, they are communicated through a written care plan and implemented. The *implementation* phase includes the actual delivery of the planned actions. Client responses to care are monitored. Work to keep an open mind when observing the client's responses to care and remember that many reactions are culturally determined.

The final phase of the nursing process, *evaluation*, determines the effectiveness of care. By comparing expected outcomes with actual results, care providers are able to note which actions met the goal and which did not. Those actions that did not result in improvement are reassessed, and the process of planning care is begun again.

Health care providers practice the "art" of caregiving by learning to perceive the meaning of clients' verbal and nonverbal messages. This ability can save lives and defuse potentially harmful situations. Experience will teach that your "sixth sense" is correct many more times than it is wrong. The Case Study box provides a vivid example of this concept.

◇ Case Study

Mike S. was in charge of the walk-in clinic on the evening shift at the community hospital. The shift began uneventfully, and nothing amiss was noted. However, Mike was stuck with an uncomfortable feeling about Mr. B., a 60-year-old man who was suffering from a high level of anxiety. Although Mr. B.'s vital signs and physical assessments were within normal, he was becoming increasingly anxious and restless as the evening progressed. He even admitted to Mike that he felt that "something was going to happen."

Mike had no physical data but decided to act based on his observations of Mr. B's increasing anxiety. He called the clinic physician, who listened politely and then ordered blood tests. As the lab technician entered the room, Mr. B. suddenly became cyanotic (blue) and unresponsive. Because of Mike's uneasy perception and his ability to grasp the meaning of the interactions with his client, Mr. B. received prompt, life-saving treatment for the pulmonary embolism (blood clot in the lung) he sustained that evening.

◆ What information do you think led Mike to act on his perceptions or feelings?

The artful care provider can establish a connection with the client that bridges the technology gap. Through the caregiver's behaviors and communications, an expressive capacity emerges that connects with the client as one human being to another. It is this connection, this relationship, that helps clients cope with the impersonal, technologically oriented world of modern medicine. Establishing this connection requires genuine caring expressed in both verbal and behavioral actions. It does not matter if the medical diagnosis is physically or psychologically based—every client needs to know that his or her caregiver really cares.

The caregiver's art includes the ability to perform activities with skill and proficiency. Because most therapeutic activities consist of a combination of verbal and manual skills, the artful caregiver is able to effectively implement actions while gaining client cooperation. This principle also states that caregivers can learn and grow through practice, repetition, and experience.

The ability to rationally choose an appropriate course of action is important. The nursing (therapeutic) process serves as a tool for defining and solving client problems, but use of the tool is only as effective as its practitioner. The art of choosing the best course of action must be practiced carefully. Let the "do no harm" principle guide you as you grow.

Last is the ability to practice your profession morally, with compassion, empathy, and patience (Abdenour, 1999). Health care professions are focused toward the good of the client. Caregivers must possess the personal beliefs, attitudes, and moral principles that support caring for others (Gaut, 1993). Moral practice also includes the duty to stay competent and up-to-date with new knowledge.

ACCEPT EACH CLIENT AS A WHOLE PERSON

People with mental problems suffer from a socially imposed stigma. The word **stigma** is defined as a sign or mark of shame, disapproval or disgrace, of being shunned and/or rejected. Because people feel uneasy about discussing behaviors that are different, they shy away from the mentally troubled. One of the barriers in recovering from a mental illness is the social stigma clients experience. Caregivers should set an example in acting as advocates for their clients and educating themselves about psychiatric illnesses (see Think About box).

The principle of acceptance is important in health care because you will care for many different people. Those differences do not have to be understood, but they must be accepted. You may even disapprove of clients' attitudes and behaviors, but you must accept the person because it is the *person* who is the focus of your health care activities. This section discusses a point of view that encourages the principle of acceptance.

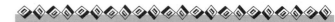

Think About

Your best friend was just released from the hospital after an episode of depression and a suicide attempt.
◆ How do you feel about visiting him or her?
◆ What will you talk about during the visit?

Holistic Framework

Remember the definition of *holistic care:* a concept designed to help clients achieve harmony within themselves (and with others, nature, and the world). **Holistic health care** is based on the concept of "whole." Understanding clients in relation to their work, family, and social environments encourages caregivers to consider their many needs. Interventions tailored to the individual can then be planned and implemented.

Health care providers who practice holistically realize that each person must also be accepted for who and what he or she is, no more no less. Accept the person, uncomfortable behaviors and all. Learn about their environment, lifestyle, and social interactions. Search for meaning in their behaviors because actions are attempts to fill needs. Your acceptance will be communicated to the clients, and your actions will eventually result in success. However, if you pass judgment, clients will sense your disapproval. Therapeutic actions in these cases usually fall on fallow ground.

Viewing clients holistically also involves an acceptance of their lifestyles, attitudes, and living conditions. Sometimes this can be difficult, especially when their environment or lifestyle is harmful. For example, a nurse once cared for a young woman who was addicted to heroin. Once the nurse accepted her, heroin addiction and all, she was able to meet the goal of providing the client with good prenatal care. At first, it was not easy to accept her destructive lifestyle, but as the nurse became more accepting and less judgmental, an intelligent, witty, and caring woman emerged.

People with mental or emotional difficulties may display some odd behaviors or verbalize unusual beliefs. These people need to be accepted just as much as clients with physical maladies. Their behaviors also have meaning, but our reactions can sometimes cloud their messages. Identify your reactions to clients who engage in unusual or bizarre behaviors. Work to develop an acceptance of each client by considering the whole individual. A holistic point of view helps us accept all people, regardless of how different from ourselves they are.

The traditional medical model of care views illness or dysfunction as a pathological condition: something is wrong with the client, and a repair or return to function constitutes a "cure." A health-oriented model, however, focuses on clients' abilities—what they *can* do—instead of on their disability or disease. In a health-oriented model, clients are assessed for their strengths and abilities. Goals of care are mutually developed. Interventions are designed for the individual, and clients receive the services most important and relevant to them. Responsibility for success is shared among clients and care providers.

Distress of the human spirit can be far more damaging than a medical diagnosis. A positive, health-oriented attitude alone may make a difference in functioning. Learn to approach problems with an attitude that employs the client's strengths, assets, and resources. A focus on the positive aspects of a situation stands a greater chance of success.

When it is assumed that the mental health client will succeed, clients usually live up to expectations and do just that—succeed. One small success fosters and breeds other triumphs. When enough small successes are experienced, dignity begins to return. Keep your focus on the "can do." It can have surprising results. Know that an intervention in one area of the client's life has an impact on all other daily activities, so keep the focus on the positive.

Caregivers may find that progress comes slowly when working with clients who are experiencing mental health problems. A health-oriented point of view and a focus on the positive encourages both care providers and clients to strive for success. It also allows psychiatric clients the respect and dignity that are not readily available to them within the medical model.

DEVELOP MUTUAL TRUST

Individuals who are unable to trust cannot rely on others for help. The word *trust* means assured hope and reliance on another. Erikson's theory (see Chapter 5) lists the development of trust as the first core task of the infant. Trust is an important concept for human beings, who are by nature social and group oriented. It implies cooperation, support, and a willingness to work together.

Trust occurs on many levels. For example, when you drive your vehicle onto a road, you are engaging in an act of trust—you have the trust that oncoming drivers will stay on their side of the small, painted yellow line that divides the road. When you buy an item, you trust that it will be repaired or replaced if it is defective. Numerous other small acts of trust occur throughout the day. We are just too busy to notice many of them. Yet, to care providers, the concept of trust holds much importance.

Many people with mental-emotional problems struggle with the problem of trusting others. Sometimes the person's internal conflicts result in suspicion, paranoia, and fear of the unknown. Care providers must routinely demonstrate that they can be trusted. To communicate the messages of trust, remember to *do what you say you will do*. If you tell a client that you will return in 10 minutes,

be back in 10 minutes (better yet, be there in 9). Clients soon learn which caregivers follow their words with actions. Trust begins to grow when clients know they can depend on their caregivers.

Trust is the foundation of the therapeutic relationship. It forms the basis for the success or failure of all actions. People who become your clients, no matter what their diagnoses, need to trust that they will be cared for in a safe and supportive manner. The development of trust between clients and caregivers involves three concepts: caring, empathy, and advocacy (Keltner, Schwecke, and Bostrom, 1999). When clients feel that their care providers understand and act with their best interests in mind, trust is established. The therapeutic relationship is more fully discussed in Chapter 10.

Caring, Empathy, and Advocacy

Illness or disability restricts a person's ability to perform daily work and social activities. Mental illness has the additional impact of negative cultural and social attitudes. People seem to readily accept the physically infirmed, but for those with mental-emotional difficulties, the road can be rocky and lonely. In addition, coping with mental illness is difficult and takes courage. Some people have written about their experiences with mental illness in an attempt to help others understand and accept them. Several authors have identified that the acceptance, caring, and support of their friends and care providers played a major role in their recovery.

Caring is the thread that connects people and moves them toward recovery. On occasion, when the client ceases to care, the caregiver has cared enough for both, which has pulled more than one client from despair. "The demonstrations of caring brought forth physical and mental changes, positive outcomes that resulted in a trusting relationship" (Starck and McGovern, 1993). For people with mental illness, caring plays an especially important role. They know, subconsciously, whether you actually care or regard them as just another client. Before trust can be developed, clients must truly believe that their nurses and other providers care.

Empathy is the ability to recognize and share the emotions of another person without actually experiencing them. It includes an understanding of the meaning and significance of that person's behavior. Empathy is the willingness to walk a mile in another's shoes, to see the world as he or she does. Although we may have never experienced the anxiety of having no home or being harassed by insulting voices inside our heads, we have all felt discomfort, pain, and insecurity. Clients with mental illnesses frequently live in a lonely world of personal suffering, detached from society. Empathy in these cases becomes a powerful therapeutic tool, one that can reestablish a person's self-worth and dignity. If clients believe that their caregivers are willing to share their discomforts, they become more interested in learning to help themselves.

Advocacy is the process of providing a client with the information, support, and feedback needed to make a decision (Keltner, Schwecke, and Bostrom, 1999). Client advocacy frequently goes a step further by adding the obligation to act in the client's best interest. People with mental-emotional difficulties are not always capable of making informed decisions. In cases like these, caregivers intervene to ensure that the client's basic needs are being met. For example, if a client decides not to eat, the care provider may act in the client's best interest by making the food easily available. The client cannot be forced to eat, but he or she can be encouraged to make more healthful choices.

Client advocacy involves the concept of *empowerment*. As changes in the health care system continue, a move toward mutual participation is replacing the traditional sick-role model in which clients are passive receivers of health care. For mental health clients, this remains difficult because of the long-standing cultural and social stigma attached to people with psychiatric problems. Many mentally ill people are quite capable of taking part in their care and treatment. Some are not, but all deserve the opportunity to make the decisions they are capable of making.

Nurses and other caregivers act as advocates by assisting clients through the decision-making process. Providing information and education assists clients in making appropriate decisions about their care. "There is no doubt that an educated patient can more successfully comply with the prescribed medical regimen, achieve more positive medical outcomes, and decrease readmission rates" (Weaver and Wilson, 1994).

EXPLORE BEHAVIORS AND EMOTIONS

All behavior has meaning. Actions are the result of attempts to fill personal needs and goals. Behaviors can be better understood when one considers the person's internal frame of reference and the context in which the behaviors occur. Each of us lives within a private world of our own. Most people's private worlds (internal frames of reference) are agreeable with others. However, people with mental-emotional difficulties have private worlds that may be difficult for the average person to understand.

"**Behavior** consists of perceptions, thoughts, feelings, and actions" (Stuart and Laraia, 2001) (Figure 8-1). A disruption in any one of these areas may result in behavioral problems. Distorted perceptions, impaired thought processes, and alterations of emotional expression lead to maladaptive actions.

Behaviors also must be understood in terms of the context or setting in which they occur. Most people are more comfortable in certain environments than they are in

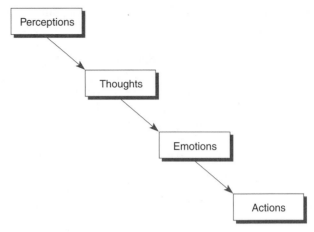

Figure 8-1 Components of a behavior.

others. Sometimes a particular environment is threatening because of uncomfortable experiences in similar settings. A nurse who once cared for wounded soldiers in a war zone and now experiences anxiety when she cares for trauma clients in the emergency room is an example of how the context or setting can influence behaviors.

Meanings to the Client

All behavior serves a purpose, and all behavior has meaning. However, it is sometimes difficult to accurately interpret or receive the message that a client's behavior is sending. Actions may be clouded with symbols, such as the client who is sure that the government has planted a microphone in his brain to read his thoughts. In this case, the individual feels so powerless that he knows he is being controlled by others with authority, such as the government.

Actions may also be influenced by chemical substances. Alcohol and other drugs affect perceptions, emotional expression, judgment, and behavior. People may behave in bizarre ways while under the influence of a chemical and then feel very remorseful and apologetic after the substance has been cleared from the body. The same can hold true for the chemicals that are called medications.

Meanings to Others

An often overlooked method of understanding the meaning of a client's behavior is to simply ask the individual. Many clients are willing to share the emotions attached to their behaviors when (1) they have trust in you and (2) you are willing to take the time to listen. When people with mental health problems can discuss their behaviors or share their emotions, they are not looking for approval or reproach. Acceptance and a gentle exploration of what the behaviors mean to them will help clients develop and practice insight. Recognizing ineffective behaviors and replacing them with more appropriate and effective actions is the first step toward gaining some control over one's situation.

Explaining how you view the client's behaviors allows for perception checks. Is the client sending the same message that you are receiving? Do each of you see the same communication in the client's symbols? If the client says he feels like a duck, do you know what he is really trying to portray? Sharing your perceptions helps clients see how their behavioral messages are being received by other people. It also allows caregivers the opportunity to gain insight into their clients' worlds.

Some clients are so caught up in their worlds that they are unable to verbally share the meanings of their behaviors. They speak with their actions only. With these individuals, caregivers must develop acute observational skills. Some repeated behaviors are attempts to undo or fix something. Other actions can be cries for help or forms of self-punishment for wrongful deeds. The meaning of a client's actions may be shrouded in mystery, but time, trust, and persistent observations will assist in discovering the real meanings that lie behind the messages.

ENCOURAGE RESPONSIBILITY

The fourth basic principle of mental health care relates to the concept of **responsibility.** Responsible people are capable of making and fulfilling obligations. They are answerable and accountable for their decisions or actions. Responsibility infers that a person is able to exercise capability and accountability. Individuals who are unable to make or keep an obligation are usually not considered to be responsible. People vary in their abilities to cope with the stresses of life, thus some people live more responsibly than others.

Health care providers work with clients who exhibit a wide variety of coping styles and behaviors. Encouraging responsibility is a primary intervention for clients with mental-emotional difficulties because it helps build self-worth, dignity, and confidence, while assisting clients in learning more successful coping behaviors. Responsibility is a cornerstone of modern societies and a goal of mental health care.

Responsibility for Self

As children grow and develop the necessary skills for living within a society, so do their responsibilities. Infants are not required to be responsible, but when the child begins to explore and manipulate the environment, responsibilities are shouldered. To illustrate, children associate with the responsibility of being cooperative by learning to play with other children, and understanding the concept of truth brings with it the responsibility not to lie.

Responsibility is learned early. The primary instructor is the family, but the social group and culture exert strong influences. As children learn about "right behaviors" (the culturally defined actions that are labeled right and wrong), they develop the responsibility to engage in them. There is a saying that states: If the family does not teach responsibility, the school will. If the school does not teach responsibility, then the group will. If the group does not teach responsibility, then society will, and society sends irresponsible people to jail.

Many people with mental-emotional problems have difficulty behaving in responsible ways. Some have never been taught about obligations and duty because of their dysfunctional family or childhood experiences. Others cannot remember or hold onto a logical picture long enough to discharge their responsibilities. However, every person has the capacity for growth and therefore some degree of responsibility. Nurses and other professionals who work with the mentally ill plan and implement specific interventions designed to help clients achieve their highest level of responsibility.

The first step in developing self-responsibility relates to care of the self. The basic physical needs of life (Maslow's lower-order needs) must be met, no matter what the circumstances. Every adult and sadly many children must procure food, clothing, and shelter for themselves daily. People with mental-emotional problems commonly have difficulty in meeting these basic needs, so the lessons of self-responsibility usually begin with something as fundamental as caring for one's daily personal hygiene needs.

Caregivers should assess their clients' abilities to perform the skills associated with the activities of daily living. For example, sometimes the reason for poor hygiene is a lack of knowledge. A person may never have been taught to bathe frequently or brush his or her teeth after every meal. In such cases, the responsibility is for the caregiver to teach and the client to learn the basic skills of personal cleanliness. When the client assumes responsibility for basic needs like personal hygiene, it leads to improved feelings of self-worth. When one looks good, one feels better. Small successes become positive steps that help equip clients with the skills necessary for functioning at their highest possible levels.

The next step in assuming self-responsibility is to be accountable for one's emotions. "I'm sorry. I lost my temper," does not excuse the action. Losing one's temper does not describe a rationale person. Mental health clients frequently have poor control over their emotions (called *poor impulse control*). They feel the emotion and then immediately act without considering the consequences of their behaviors. Becoming responsible for one's emotions involves the willingness to identify and then "own" the problems and emotions. It also requires a willingness and determination to try new and more effective behaviors when coping with emotional reactions.

When clients learn to replace an unacceptable behavior with a more effective action, they achieve a degree of control over their lives. As individuals become responsible, they begin to succeed. Those small successes help remove them from the role of victim and realize the value of taking responsibility.

Responsibility to Others

People who seek treatment for mental or emotional problems must assume the responsibility for cooperating with and following their therapeutic plan of care. This involves a commitment to become actively involved with a group of mental health care providers by sharing personal information, being open to new ideas, and being willing to try new ways of doing things. Caregivers have the obligation to help clients adapt and succeed and clients are responsible for working toward self-improvement.

Clients are also responsible for the effects of their actions on others. The enjoyment of social interactions is accompanied by the responsibility of behaving appropriately. People who have problems with emotional (impulse) control can become a threat to the safety of others when their behaviors are inappropriate. It is important for caregivers to assist clients in controlling their behaviors because people who act in irresponsible ways are soon removed from social settings.

Responsibility is a fundamental concept in mental health care. It is a key to developing more effective behaviors and building self-worth. Some psychiatric therapies are designed around the concept of responsibility. For example, William Glasser's reality therapy (1998) uses responsibility as a therapeutic tool (Box 8-1).

ENCOURAGE EFFECTIVE ADAPTATION

Mental health clients may be labeled with one or more psychiatric diagnoses, but all have one thing in common—unsuccessful (maladaptive) coping behaviors. The very nature of mental illness is characterized by actions that are not in keeping with society's definitions of appropriate behaviors. Mental health caregivers provide clients with education about and opportunities to engage in more effective behaviors. Encouraging effective adaptation is the sixth principle of mental health care.

Cure vs. Care

With some mental-emotional difficulties we can speak of cures. Situational depression, for example, is frequently cured when the client changes the situation that brought on the distress. Many cases of confusion or delirium are cured when a physical problem is discovered. However, some mental problems are chronic and force clients and their significant others to make permanent changes in how they live their lives.

Despite this reality, many people with chronic illnesses (physical and mental) adapt and progress to leading full, satisfying, and meaningful lives. **Adaptation** "in this context is not the same as the 'cure' of a medical illness. Instead it means sufficient improvement to carry on everyday activities" (Menninger Letter, 1995). In other words, if we can teach clients to replace maladaptive behaviors with more effective actions, they will improve their abilities to live more successfully.

Many mentally ill people find it difficult to cope with even minor changes. They require support and education to learn the skills that allow them to adapt. Clients who are able to adapt eventually become willing to take some risks and engage in new behaviors.. Slowly, the focus is changed from what cannot be done to what has been accomplished.

One Step at a Time

There is an old saying, "The longest journey begins with a single step." This was never so true as it is in mental health care. To people with mental-emotional problems, everything seems overwhelming. Even the simplest decisions, such as what to wear that day, are monumental to a person suffering from depression. People diagnosed with schizophrenia may not be able to differentiate one world from another long enough to follow a train of thought to a logical conclusion. Therefore it is important for caregivers to give instructions simply and repeat them often.

When planning therapeutic interventions, remember the importance of mastering the first item before proceeding onto more complex steps. This process involves

---

Box 8-1   Reality Therapy

Reality therapists do not accept the concept of mental illness. They believe that when people are unable to fulfill their needs, they behave unrealistically. Calling people "irresponsible" rather than "mentally ill" and describing how they are irresponsible helps clients develop the responsibility to satisfy their needs.

Reality therapy differs from psychoanalysis in six ways:

1. Because reality therapy does not accept the notion of mental illness, clients are not accepted into therapy as mentally ill people who have no responsibility.
2. Reality therapy works in the present with an eye on the future. It does not accept the limitations of the past.
3. Reality therapists personally relate to clients, not as aloof professionals or transference objects.
4. Reality therapists do not look for unconscious conflicts. Clients cannot excuse their behaviors based on unconscious motivations.
5. The morality of behavior is emphasized. Issues of right and wrong are defined and enforced.
6. The goal of reality therapy is to help clients help themselves fulfill their needs right now.

breaking down a task or concept into smaller and simpler units. For example, the goal is for the client to arrive on time for appointments. This may involve wearing a watch, being able to tell time, remembering the appointment, and transporting oneself to the building where the appointment takes place. The first step in meeting the goal may be the purchase of a watch.

There are two points to be made here. First, do not assume, assess. Using the example above, one assumes that every adult can tell time, but the results of this assessment revealed that the client could not tell time because of blurred vision. Unless the caregiver helps the client deal with the visual problems, he or she will not be successful in meeting the goal of routinely keeping all appointments. Second, remember that success is built on many small steps. Breaking each learning experience down into smaller units, increases the chances of mastering the skill or knowledge. Make sure that the client will succeed within the first few steps if at all possible. The taste of success is especially sweet in the early stages, and it encourages people to continue trying. One small, successful step soon becomes two, and those small triumphs can become symbolic of the client's potential for growth and change.

PROVIDE CONSISTENCY

The last principle for mental health care providers relates to the concept of **consistency.** People with mental illness often lack the security of someone who is there when needed. Without consistent parental guidance, children find ways to cope with the world, and some of these ways become ineffectual behaviors. In some cases in which individuals were not routinely guided as children, the consistency and reliability of mental health care providers are sometimes their only stability. The link that serves as a bridge between the client's world and the world of reality is frequently the reliability of the therapeutic relationship (McConnell, 1995).

The concept of consistency is usually addressed in the client's plan of care, but each therapeutic intervention must be routinely used by every member of the care team. Clients often test staff members by "playing one against the other" or attempting to manipulate the situation and gain control. However, when each care provider responds by giving the same message, clients learn that members of the care team can be relied on to do what they say they will do. Two general guidelines for providing consistency are to set limits and focus on the positive changes that clients are making.

Set and Enforce Limits
Children are taught from an early age which actions are acceptable in their society and which are not. When the behavioral messages are mixed or inconsistent, children

become confused and attempt to discover which actions best satisfy their needs in various settings. They learn that different rules apply to different situations. A good example of this is the mother who teaches her children to always tell the truth and then instructs them to tell the salesman on the telephone that she is not at home. In this case, the children have received the message that it is permissible to tell a lie under certain conditions. When enough of these double messages are received, children begin to devise their rules for living, which may not be in keeping with society's notions of right behavior.

Setting limits involves clients, staff members, and institutional policies (Chenevert, 1994). As the plan of care is developed by the care team and the client, each rule or limitation is established. Facility policies define some limitations. The remainder of the "rules" relate to therapeutic activities, social interactions, and personal behaviors. Whatever the limitations, the client must be informed and willing to cooperate with the plan of care.

Each member of the care team is responsible for understanding the purpose of each limitation and the methods for enforcing them. To illustrate, the facility's policy is for all clients to remain out of bed during the day. To accomplish this the staff informs each client every morning that the doors to the rooms will be locked by 9 AM. Then the aide makes 9 AM rounds and locks the door to each room. The clients were informed and then reminded of the rule. Last came the enforcement or actual action that demonstrated the limitation would be followed. Something as simple as providing a routine can teach clients about the value of reliability, consistency, and stability.

This brings us to a valuable point: Do not commit yourself unless you are able to fill the commitment. If your actions are not reliable, if you do not behaviorally demonstrate stability and consistency, then the therapeutic relationship will be established only with great difficulty. Clients are people, and they need to know if someone truly cares and is willing to make the connection that helps them to heal.

These seven principles are offered as guidelines for working with people who are suffering (Box 8-2).

> **Box 8-2 Principles of Mental Health Care**
>
> 1. Do no harm.
> 2. Accept each client as a whole person.
> 3. Develop mutual trust.
> 4. Explore behaviors and emotions.
> 5. Encourage responsibility.
> 6. Encourage effective adaptation.
> 7. Provide consistency.

Although the focus has been on the person labeled "mentally ill," every client in the health care system needs to be offered acceptance, trust, and emotional support. The whole person, not the pathological condition, is the focus of health care professionals.

KEY CONCEPTS

◆ A mentally healthy adult is a person who can cope with and adjust to the stresses of daily living in a socially acceptable way.

◆ The principle of "do no harm" provides a valuable guide for therapeutic actions.

◆ The therapeutic tools of the self and good skills, result in a practitioner of the health care arts.

◆ Understanding clients in relation to their work, family, and social environments encourages caregivers to practice holistic health care.

◆ Trust is the foundation of the therapeutic relationship and forms the basis for the success or failure of therapeutic actions.

◆ Behaviors can be better understood when caregivers consider the person's internal frame of reference (private world), the context in which the behaviors occur, and the meaning of the action.

◆ Encouraging responsibility is a primary intervention that helps build self-worth, dignity, and confidence; offers opportunities for learning to problem solve; and assists clients in learning more successful coping behaviors.

◆ In mental health terms, adaptation means sufficient improvement to carry out everyday activities.

◆ When therapeutic interventions are planned, the importance of mastering the first item before proceeding onto more complex steps must be kept in mind.

◆ The link that serves as a bridge between the client's world and the world of reality is frequently the consistency and reliability of the therapeutic relationship.

◆ Health care providers must be willing to set and reinforce clients' behavioral limits with gentle firmness and consistency.

Suggestions for Further Reading

Allie Laurie Chamberlain's article, "Abandoned to the Street," in *Hospitals and Health Networks* [7(14):18], offers a moving account of severe mental illness in today's society.

References

Abdenour JM: What makes a great nurse?, *RN* 62(10):47, 1999.

Chenevert M: *STAT: special techniques in assertiveness training,* ed 4 St. Louis, 1994, Mosby.

Coping with mental illness requires courage, *Menninger Letter* 3(4):3, 1995.

Gaut DA, editor: *A global agenda for caring,* New York, 1993, National League for Nursing Press.

Giger JM, Davidhizar RE: *Transcultural nursing: assessment and intervention* ed 3, St. Louis, 1999, Mosby.

Glasser W: *Choice theory,* New York, 1998, Harper-Collins.

Haber J and others: *Comprehensive psychiatric nursing,* ed 5, St. Louis, 1997, Mosby.

Keltner NL, Schwecke LH, Bostrom CE: *Psychiatric nursing,* ed 3, St. Louis, 1999, Mosby.

McConnell EA: Making the invisible visible, *Nursing 95* 25(4):53, 1995.

Starck PL, McGovern JP, editors: *The hidden dimension of human suffering,* New York, 1992, National League for Nursing Press.

Stuart GW, Laraia MT: *Principles and practice of psychiatric nursing,* ed 7, St. Louis, 2001, Mosby.

Weaver SK, Wilson JF: Moving toward patient empowerment, *Nursing Health Care* 15(9):480, 1994.

Chapter 9

The Therapeutic Environment

Learning Objectives

1. List two situations that indicate a need for hospitalization.
2. Describe three types of clients treated in the inpatient therapeutic environment.
3. State two goals of the therapeutic environment.
4. Discuss five environmental factors that must be assessed daily.
5. Explain the importance of setting limits on clients' behaviors.
6. Identify three ways the therapeutic environment helps clients meet their needs for love and belonging.
7. Examine how care providers' expectations influence clients' behaviors.
8. List three techniques to improve client compliance.

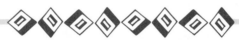

Key Terms

acceptance

chronicity

communication

crisis stabilization

expectations

involvement

limit setting

noncompliance

recidivism

self-actualized

therapeutic environment (milieu)

The history of the treatment of mentally troubled people has not been kind. In the United States, most of the mentally ill were housed in large, custodial care institutions until after World War II. With the introduction of psychotherapeutic drugs during the 1950s, a new interest in caring for the mentally ill developed, and researchers began to look at the environment in which people were treated.

In 1953 a small book by Maxwell Jones was published in England. In it, he described the value of the environment as a therapeutic tool. It was later published in the United States under the title *The Therapeutic Community* and soon fostered the development of treatment settings that promoted personal worth and dignity (Jones, 1953). Today, the therapeutic environment is an important part of clients' treatment plans.

The term **therapeutic environment (milieu)** describes certain settings or environments designed to help clients replace inappropriate behaviors with more effec-

tive personal and psychosocial skills (Stuart and Laraia, 2001). Therapeutic milieus can exist within hospital, home, or community settings, but each environment helps clients satisfy their needs and assists them with their problems.

Because most therapeutic environments require certain limits and controls, they are usually established in inpatient settings, as part of a community hospital, for example. Standards describing the therapeutic milieu are set forth by the Joint Commission on Accreditation of Hospitals, and several tools for assessing the therapeutic environment have been developed.

Most people with mental-emotional problems manage within their communities. However, there are times when a more secure and stable environment is needed. Admission to a psychiatric inpatient facility occurs after one of the following:

1. A person's behavior becomes a threat to the safety of self or others.

2. People within the environment are not able or willing to support the mentally troubled person.
3. The person perceives himself or herself as unable to cope or maintain behavioral control.

Admission to an inpatient facility can be on a voluntary or involuntary basis. Treatment plans are designed to return clients to their communities as soon as possible.

Caregivers who work in therapeutic inpatient settings provide the framework for the quality of the environment. Without a "staff with insight, understanding, personal warmth, and skill in directing groups, the concept of a therapeutic community could not have developed into a reality" (Taylor, 1994).

Psychiatric nursing practice has moved from custodial care to the management of complex therapeutic environments. Nurses, and other health care professionals, are now required to manage clients' environments, implement therapeutic interventions, coordinate and integrate multidisciplinary care delivery, and evaluate the outcomes of treatment for each client with whom they work.

USE OF THE INPATIENT SETTING

Before the 1960s, stays in psychiatric units often lasted for months or years. In contrast, today's psychiatric facilities offer shorter stays, more intensive therapies, and support during the transition from institution to community. Inpatient services are provided for three main groups of people: those experiencing crises, those with acute mental or emotional problems, and those with chronic mental illness.

Crisis Stabilization

People experiencing a crisis seek help when their discomfort becomes greater than their need to privately solve their problems. In many cases, **crisis stabilization** interventions are provided by placing clients in 1- or 2-day treatment settings where balance (homeostasis) can be reestablished. Clients undergo intensive counseling designed to solve their immediate problems. Medications, such as antidepressants or sedatives, may be prescribed. Stress management techniques are taught to help to modify stressful behaviors, and cognitive, relaxation, and behavioral therapies are often used to assist clients. The goal of inpatient crisis therapy is to help the client cope with the crisis. After clients are discharged from the crisis stabilization unit, they may be referred for assertiveness training; time, anger, or conflict management training; or problem-solving education.

Acute Care and Treatment

The inpatient environment is also needed when people cannot function sufficiently to satisfy their basic needs. By the time people seek voluntary admission to a treatment facility, they usually feel weakened and hopeless (Cohen, 1994). Frequently, clients are drug impaired or intoxicated. Some have experienced severe stress such as a job layoff, illness, or loss of support systems.

Admission to an inpatient psychiatric unit is a highly emotional experience for most people. Those who are hospitalized involuntarily experience an intense discomfort during their first hospital experience and a great sense of failure on subsequent admissions. Hospitalization can "dehumanize" an individual: personal items are taken away, and staff members often remember the diagnosis before the name. Care providers should try to "humanize" the hospital experience because the foundation of the client's success or failure lies with the first experiences in the therapeutic environment. Most people with acute psychiatric problems can be successfully treated if interventions are vigorous and well coordinated. Even with the best of therapies, however, some individuals progress to chronic maladaptive responses and cycles of repeated admissions.

The Chronically Mentally Ill

Many mental health problems are associated with a degree of **chronicity**, problems that tend to persist for a long time. People with chronic mental disorders may have periods of relative comfort and ease of functioning and then fall rapidly into acute psychiatric states. For these people, life grows into a see-saw existence between two worlds.

Often, people with chronic mental health problems are able to figure out when they are beginning to *decompensate* (or "lose it" as some clients say) and will voluntarily admit themselves to an inpatient facility. Many more, however, do not have the insight or judgment to know when they are acting in maladaptive ways. Others are *paranoid* (suspicious, afraid of others) and do not seek help or refuse treatment when it is offered. Last, there is the growing number of mentally troubled individuals who have never sought assistance or received treatment. They live with their distresses the best they can.

The inpatient therapeutic environment fills many needs for troubled individuals. It provides the physical

---

Think About

Many clients with chronic mental problems will admit themselves to an inpatient unit because they are looking for "three hots and a cot."
◆ What is the meaning of the statement?
◆ How does this statement relate to Maslow's hierarchy of needs theory? (Hint: see Chapter 5.)
◆ How do you think it affects the client's attitude toward the therapeutic treatment plan?

necessities of clean water, wholesome food, clean clothing, and a comfortable bed (see Think About box).

An inpatient facility also provides protection, safety, and security from a harsh world, and a staff of mental health care providers who offer individual attention and emotional support. From the chronically troubled person's point of view, life in the inpatient facility may actually be better than the lonely existence they face in the community.

Recidivism (repeated inpatient admissions) has become a way of life for many of the chronically mentally troubled. This is especially true for clients with cycles of assaultive behaviors. Recidivism is a frustrating aspect of inpatient mental health care for both clients and care providers. Clients feel like failures and caregivers become frustrated that their efforts during past admissions were not more successful. Several suggestions for managing feelings associated with return clients are listed in Box 9-1.

Recidivism, also called the *revolving-door syndrome,* continues to be a problem, especially for individuals with schizophrenia and those who use illicit chemicals. The primary reason clients return to the inpatient environment is refusal to take their prescribed psychotropic medications (noncompliance).

One of the most important factors in preventing recidivism is adequate community resources. Delaney (1998) recommends psychosocial rehabilitation clubhouses where clients receive support and educational and vocational opportunities. With the focus on the "least restrictive environment," many chronically mentally ill clients now live in small, homelike, sheltered group settings within the community, but there are many others who are homeless and/or continually involved in the revolving-door syndrome of admission and discharge.

GOALS OF A THERAPEUTIC ENVIRONMENT

Dr. Peter Breggin, author of *Toxic Psychiatry* (1991), defines mental illness as "overwhelm" and believes that people should be offered mental health care in small, local "sanctuaries" (rather than in psychiatric institutions) until they are able to cope with the demands of everyday life once again. Effective therapeutic environments provide the safety, security, and time to cope with difficulties. Members of the health care team offer therapeutic human contact designed to assist clients in learning about themselves and how they relate to others.

The goals of a therapeutic environment (milieu) are to provide protection, support, and education. A treatment team, composed of several specialists, is assigned to work with each client. On admission, a thorough assessment is done and a therapeutic plan of care is developed with the client. Figure 9-1 illustrates the roles of the mental health treatment team members. Nurses are more involved with direct care and management; however, all care team members communicate, collaborate, and teach.

Help Clients Meet Needs

People are admitted to inpatient psychiatric settings because they are unable to maintain their activities of daily living. Care providers assist inpatient clients in meeting their most basic needs first (see Chapter 5). Food, shelter, safety, and security are provided. Socialization needs are fulfilled during therapy and interactions with staff and other clients. Treatment plans provide opportunities for satisfying self-esteem needs through vocational training.

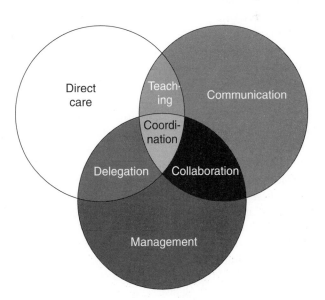

Figure 9-1 Mental health practice. (Redrawn from Stuart GW, Laraia MT: *Principles and practice of psychiatric nursing,* ed 7, St. Louis, 2001, Mosby.)

Box 9-1 Coping With Recidivism

Relating to Clients

Accept clients for themselves. They are doing the best they can at this time.

Learn about their lives outside of the inpatient setting.

Explore after-discharge resources in the community.

Maintain a positive attitude. Clients do better when they are encouraged, rather than discouraged.

Relating to Caregivers

Remember who "owns" the problem. Caregiver roles are to support, educate, and assist.

Attend a support group regularly. Discuss ways to stay positive.

Keep client problems "at the office."

Teach Psychosocial (Adaptive) Skills

People use behaviors that tend to work. When actions result in success, behaviors are more likely to be repeated whether they are socially acceptable. Admission to an inpatient therapeutic treatment environment allows people with maladaptive behaviors the opportunity to learn more acceptable ways of behaving. With the help of the treatment team members, clients can learn to replace their usual ways of behaving with more effective and adaptive actions.

THE THERAPEUTIC ENVIRONMENT AND CLIENT NEEDS

Maslow's theory of a hierarchy of needs (Figure 9-2) states that if a basic physical need goes unmet, it will be fulfilled before other, higher level needs. People who are suffering from mental and emotional troubles frequently are unable to obtain even the most basic of life's requirements.

We all feel hunger and thirst, but the person with a mental illness may not be able to recognize or act on the body's signals. Sometimes their reality makes no provisions for the care of the body. For example, some people may believe that it is inappropriate to eat or practice good hygiene, some do not care about the condition of the body, and others are just not aware of their bodies. The therapeutic environment offers a constructive setting for people to learn how to meet their own needs and the support and encouragement to practice new and more effective behaviors.

Remember that a change in one area of functioning brings about a response within the whole person. Therefore assisting clients in satisfying their more basic needs prepares the way for changes in other areas of life. Using Maslow's hierarchy of needs as a guide, consider how the therapeutic environment relates to meeting human needs.

Physical Needs

All people need to breathe. This is the first and most basic need. Without *air* or the ability to exchange it, a person will not survive for more than a few minutes. For most people, breathing is not a problem, but for those with lung disease, for example, the simple act of exchanging air can be their first and major priority throughout each day.

Many clients who are experiencing hallucinations or paranoid (suspicious) thoughts will refuse to eat or drink for fear of being poisoned, drugged, or controlled by the use of *food*. Some clients have eaten poorly before admission and welcome the opportunity to receive wholesome food and clean drinking water, whereas others may require special diets because of their medical conditions or medications. The Drug Alert box is a reminder of the importance of monitoring diets.

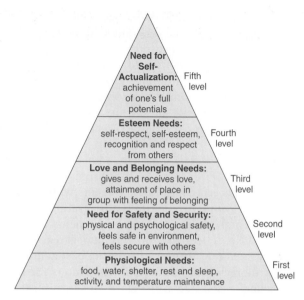

Figure 9-2 Maslow's hierarchy of needs. (Data from Maslow A: *Motivation and personality*, ed 2, New York, 1970, Harper & Row.)

 Drug Alert

Remember that clients who are taking monoamine oxidase inhibitors (MAOIs) are not allowed to eat certain meats (bologna, liver), dairy products (aged cheeses, sour cream, yogurt), vegetables (fava beans, avocados), fruits (bananas, figs), and alcoholic beverages (beer, ale, red wines, sherry). Clients should eat no chocolate and avoid caffeine in large amounts.

Monitor clients' food and fluid intake daily. Also routinely monitor vital signs, especially the pulse and blood pressure. Report any complaints of chest tightness, stiff neck, or throbbing headache to the physician immediately because these symptoms may herald the onset of hypertensive crisis.

The act of eating and sharing food is a social event in many cultures. Numerous customs have evolved around the obtaining, preparation, and consuming of food and drink. Learn about clients' perceptions associated with food. How does the cultural background of your clients influence the foods they consume? What are their food preferences? How do their mental health problems involve food? Assessing client behaviors associated with food allows caregivers to intervene at a basic level, prevent further problems, and evaluate the effectiveness of therapeutic actions. Table 9-1 lists client problems and therapeutic actions related to food.

Hygiene needs are important in the therapeutic environment. Clients are frequently admitted in various states of cleanliness ranging from obsessively tidy to

Table 9-1	Mental Health Problems and Nursing Interventions Associated With Food
Problem	**Nursing intervention**
Client believes food is poisoned or tainted.	Serve each food item in single-serving, disposable containers.
	Allow client to casually observe other people eating same food items.
Client has no interest in food or eating.	Serve meals at regular intervals.
	Leave food within easy reach of client.
	Offer frequent snacks.
	Use odors of certain foods to encourage client to eat.
Client uses food as emotional substitute.	Provide opportunities for interactions with other people that do not relate to eating.
	Work with client to discover which needs are being met through use of food.

extremely neglected. People who are experiencing acute episodes of schizophrenia, for example, seldom relate to their physical appearance or state of hygiene. Some individuals will dress inappropriately, putting on several shirts at one time or wearing undergarments over their coats.

Encourage good hygiene habits. Discover if the client has a preference or ritual for bathing or dressing. Compliment clients on their appearance when efforts have been made. Good hygiene practices help fill more than one basic physical need; they also communicate a willingness for social contact.

The physical surroundings of the therapeutic environment are important. Today, the architecture of the old asylum has been replaced by a more normalized environment, which includes provisions for personal space and privacy. Physical properties of an environment have an effect on the people who live within that space. The physical properties of a therapeutic environment include temperature, lighting, sound, cleanliness, and aesthetics. Nurses are responsible for monitoring how each aspect of the physical environment affects clients.

The temperature, air circulation, and humidity of the unit all have an effect on clients. People respond to these factors in highly individual ways. For example, an agitated or hyperactive individual may find the environmental temperature too high and react by becoming even more distressed. Hot days and high humidity can increase aggressiveness or make clients lethargic. People who are depressed and hypoactive may be more affected by cooler temperatures. Caregivers must be aware that the environmental temperatures and humidity levels have an impact on behavior. Therefore the daily assessment of the therapeutic environment should include temperature and humidity.

Next, the environment's lighting should be assessed. Lighting includes the "amount of light, its diffusion, and the reflection of light waves off environmental surfaces combined with the impact of surface colors" (Haber and others, 1997). Lighting should be constant and of the right intensity. Flickering lights can trigger delusions or hallucinations, whereas lighting that is too bright can result in overstimulation and aggressive behaviors. Lighting that is too low can present inaccurate stimuli, resulting in misperceptions of actual objects. For example, it becomes easier to perceive an animal where a chair is located when the room's lighting distorts environmental cues. Sunlight has an effect on clients who are receiving psychotherapeutic medications. When outdoors, these people must wear protective clothing, sunscreen lotion, and a large-brimmed hat. They also require extra fluids.

Some clients experience hypersensitivity to color, especially if they are confused, agitated, or hyperactive. Colors are very symbolic for human beings. Bright colors are stimulating, whereas dark colors are depressing. Neutral colors tend to calm emotions and behaviors. Certain colors hold meaning for some clients. Care providers should assess the impact of color and lighting for each client and observe client behaviors in various lighting and color settings.

The acoustical or sound environment is composed of noises generated by people and equipment. Walls, floors, and objects within the environment have sound-absorbing or acoustical qualities. Floors with carpeting, for example, absorb sound waves and quiet the environment, whereas hard tile floors tend to magnify sounds. Upholstered furniture absorbs more sound than wooden or plastic furniture.

Environmental noise can have a calming or agitating effect on clients. High noise levels can lead to distorted perceptions, altered thinking, and sensory overload. High noise levels in inpatient environments are common and result in "negative physical effects because of increased physiological stress on the body. Excessive sound also interferes with cognitive functioning" (Holmberg, 1999). Calm music, the sound of ocean waves, or a light rain can produce relaxation.

People experiencing mental illness are commonly hypersensitive to sounds. When noise levels become too intense, clients tend to become distracted and agitated.

This does not imply, however, that each staff member must walk around in silence, but it does alert you to the important role that sound plays in the therapeutic environment (Table 9-2).

The hygiene associated with the environment refers to the state of cleanliness of the physical space and the objects within it. Because many clients live close to one another, the likelihood of infection is increased. The stresses of mental illness can also decrease clients' resistance to infection. In addition, the potential for nuisances such as mice, cockroaches, and other vermin is increased if the physical surroundings are not kept clean.

People with mental or emotional difficulties can have little regard for the cleanliness of their surroundings. Sometimes people with lice, scabies, or crabs are admitted to the therapeutic environment, and if allowed to continue unchecked, every client within the immediate environment will require treatment. Nurses and direct care providers assess the state of the unit's cleanliness on a daily basis. Clients should be protected from communicable health problems. Small assessments today prevents large problems from developing tomorrow.

Last is the issue of aesthetics. Is the space pleasing to the eye? Does the environment make one want to stay and relax or leave quickly? The condition of the furniture and other objects within a setting leaves people with a certain impression. An environment that is tidy and in good condition sends a message of caring and pride in appearance. The careful use of color and texture can also produce an environment that communicates a sense of hospitality and belonging.

It is important for health care providers to remember that we go home every night to our own homes. Clients who are living within the therapeutic setting do not. They are there 24 hours of every day. If you were in this situation, you would appreciate the efforts of others to make the physical environment as pleasant as possible.

Safety and Security Needs

The safety and security offered by the therapeutic environment is one of the most important factors in mental health care. Safety and security needs within the therapeutic environment include the feeling of physical safety, the security of a limited setting, and the ability to feel secure with others. For clients who are depressed or suicidal, the therapeutic environment offers special protection from self-harm. Clients with aggressive behaviors are offered protection from themselves and assurance that limits will be placed on their actions.

Safety also includes a freedom from hazards. Objects that have the potential for harm are removed, and the design of electrical fixtures, doors, and other equipment helps to promote safety. Paging systems with identification codes allow help to be summoned when needed. Often, a client will act out or behave impulsively. When this occurs, members of the treatment team set limits on the maladaptive actions and then attempt to identify the feelings that motivated the response.

People also need to feel secure within their environments. The inpatient therapeutic environment provides the comfort of order and organization in the form of a daily routine, a set of rules, schedules, and activities. For many psychiatric clients, knowing what is going to happen tomorrow adds to their sense of security today.

The use of space is important in maintaining a therapeutic environment. The design of the physical setting has an influence on how space is used for daily activities. Factors such as the location of the recreation room, medication area, and clients' sleeping areas define how physical space is used. Caregivers are also concerned with the concepts of space that relate directly to client care: territory and distance.

Chapter 4 discusses distance and territory in detail, but the importance of these two concepts to the therapeutic environment is emphasized here. Each person needs personal space with defined boundaries (Goren and Orion, 1994). Mental health clients in an inpatient setting establish a territory that "belongs to them." Usually clients claim their rooms, dressers, and sleeping areas as their own. Every person who works with clients or their environments (e.g., housekeepers) must be aware of invading clients' territories. Behaviors such as knocking or announcing oneself before entering client's rooms demonstrates respect for personal space.

The physical distance between people affects clients. People with suspicious feelings usually feel more comfort-

Table 9-2 A "Sound" Exercise	
Action	**Evaluation**
Listen to a short composition of classical music.	Record how you felt as soon as the piece was finished.
Listen to a hard rock musical selection.	Record your feelings as soon as the song is finished.
Compare your immediate feelings associated with both musical selections.	Did one composition make you feel more excited, calmer? How do you think different types of music affect your mental health clients?

able when caregivers are outside their intimate space. Depressed persons may need touch and physical contact, an excellent opportunity for therapeutic touch. Aggressive clients may interpret the close presence of a caregiver as threatening. Touch must be used cautiously, as a therapeutic tool and with the client's best interest in mind. Inappropriate use of touch can lead to charges of sexual harassment and possible litigation (legal proceedings). Each client must be observed carefully; it is usually possible to tell which distances are most comfortable for interacting.

Limit setting allows the therapeutic environment to be consistent and predictable. Every human being must function within certain limits established by one's culture, social group, and laws that govern one's society. Many clients with mental problems have difficulty behaving within these limits. Clients know that care providers will enforce the external controls that keep everyone within the environment safe. Knowing that aggressive actions will be contained fosters a sense of safety and security.

Two important therapeutic interventions for setting limits are:

1. Reinforce the established structure (rules, routine) of the therapeutic setting.
2. Be consistent.

When the environment is controlled, clients have an opportunity to safely explore their feelings and learn new, more effective behaviors (see Case Study box).

The concept of *time* is impaired for many psychiatric clients, which causes various degrees of disorientation and insecurity about the environment. The perception of the passage of time may be altered, and time may pass very quickly or too slowly. Some individuals do not pay attention to time. As a result, clients have problems with appointments, scheduled events, and tasks—anything that involves the concept of time (Table 9-3). Interventions for clients with a distorted sense of time focus on routinely orienting clients to time through the use of clocks, written schedules, and diaries kept by clients.

Love and Belonging Needs

The fact that a person is struggling with a mental health problem does not dismiss the need to be accepted and find one's place within a group. Life in the community can be a lonely existence, with no friends, few acquaintances, and fewer resources. The isolation of mental illness is intense.

◈ Case Study

Ned was admitted 4 days ago and proved to be quite a manipulator. When other clients were involved with therapy or other group activities, Ned would be found lying on his bed, reading comic books. He often offered the excuse that another caregiver had given him permission to be in his room. The staff agreed to limit his behavior by keeping him involved in physical activities. By 10:00 AM Ned was complaining of a headache and wanted to lie down. He asked three caregivers, and they all tried to refocus him into an activity. His request to the fourth staff member was feeble, and by noon he was no longer complaining of a headache.

◆ What message(s) did the staff's behavior toward Ned send?
◆ How did Ned react to the situation?

Table 9-3 Examples of Impaired Time Concepts	
Disorder	**Change in concept of time**
Organic mental disorders (Alzheimer's disease and others)	Difficulty understanding passage of time *Example:* Clients ask frequently about date, day, schedules. Clients think they were just admitted when they have been there for several days. Clients are poor historians.
Substance abuse Hallucinogenics	Time passes quickly, space is smaller. *Example:* Clients arrive early, write larger than usual.
Tranquilizers	Time passes slowly, space is larger. *Example:* Clients arrive late, writing is small, cramped. Ignore past, focus on present, and are unrealistic about future.
Depression	Time passes slowly. Clients tend to focus on past, ignore present, and show little interest in future.

Modified from Haber J and others: *Comprehensive psychiatric nursing,* ed 5, St. Louis, 1997, Mosby.

Sometimes, the lack of human contact, combined with an existing psychiatric problem and the roadblocks created by stigmas, overwhelms the individual and results in more intense or frequent psychotic episodes.

The therapeutic environment offers clients many opportunities to appropriately fulfill their needs for companionship and group identification. Clients' love and belonging needs are fulfilled within the therapeutic setting through the use of communication, social interactions, and relationships.

Communication is the method by which one person interacts with another. It takes place on several levels, and not all aspects of every communication are obvious. In the inpatient setting, clients are respected as individuals who have the right to express themselves as long as their behaviors are appropriate. Caregivers communicate respect by encouraging clients to interact with each other and staff members. Through their caring, sensitive communications and interest in each person, care providers help their clients fill their needs for human companionship.

Love and belonging needs are also fulfilled through the social group to which one chooses to belong. Whenever people are together, they tend to form groups. Clients with mental health problems are no different in this respect. If their illness is not too severe, clients will attempt to form relationships with others. Activities as simple as walking together to an appointment help clients meet their belonging needs.

Social relationships can contribute greatly to meeting clients' needs for belonging, but the potential for abuse does exist. Caregivers need to be alert to the social relationships that are forming within the therapeutic environment. They must observe, monitor, and evaluate the appropriateness of certain relationships and discuss their concerns with the treatment team. Social relationships within the therapeutic environment have the same potential for positive growth or negative adaptation as any other relationship and clients can become too dependent on other clients for social support. Many inpatient units have visiting regulations for clients after they are discharged. Therefore caregivers must protect the more vulnerable and easily led clients from becoming dependent on more aggressive or manipulative people.

The caregiver-client relationship is another major tool for meeting clients' love and belonging needs. All members of the treatment team interact therapeutically with clients, but it is the direct caregivers who assist clients with the activities of daily living. They are in the special position of always being there, demonstrating consistency, reliability, and acceptance. It is the energy exchange of the therapeutic relationship that helps clients move from the overwhelming aspect of their illness, to the dependency of the therapeutic environment, and then to

the independence of autonomy. Chapter 10 explores the therapeutic relationship in greater detail.

Self-Esteem Needs

Respect, esteem, and recognition must be given by the self first, then by others. Self-respect, self-esteem, and self-recognition must be internalized or realized first. To state it simply: You must love and respect yourself before others can love and respect you. In the therapeutic setting, caregivers assist clients in building self-esteem needs through acceptance, expectations, and involvement.

Acceptance, in the mental health context, means that the nurse acknowledges clients as human beings worthy of respect and dignity. Although clients may behave in maladaptive or unacceptable ways, they are still worthy of respect. It is very important to *separate the behavior from the person.* You may not approve of the client's actions, behaviors, or attitudes, but you do accept the person. If a client must be corrected or reminded, focus on the behavior rather than on the person. For example, the statement "I have trouble following your thoughts when you speak so loudly" communicates more acceptance than "Stop yelling." Correcting or refocusing the behavior spares the self-esteem of the person.

Expectations play a role in the development of clients' abilities to meet self-esteem needs. When caregivers communicate what is expected, clients commonly live up to those expectations. This can work both ways. There is a valuable lesson here: Do not limit clients with your own expectations. Assume that they will succeed, but keep observations and assessments based in reality. You may be surprised at what clients are capable of achieving.

Clients also need involvement to meet their self-esteem needs. **Involvement** is the process of actively interacting with the environment and those persons within it. When clients are involved, they are actively sharing. These experiences foster ego strength and feelings of worth and importance. Involvement also offers opportunities to modify ineffective behaviors and try out new ones. Therapeutic treatment settings that focus on involvement use cooperation, compromise, and confrontation to foster behavioral control, effective social interactions, and a sense of self-worth in clients.

Self-Actualization Needs

The need to achieve one's full potential lies within us all. However, not all people will become **self-actualized.** Remember Maslow's basic point: Lower order needs must be met before the person can take steps to meet higher order needs. Consequently, people who cannot meet their basic physical needs will have little success in addressing their self-esteem or self-actualization needs. As clients in the inpatient psychiatric setting begin to stabilize, they become more able to cope. With the treatment team's assistance, new ways of coping are developed and tried. The process of trying and of becoming actively engaged leads clients in the direction of self-actualization. Living up to one's full potential means being the best one can be. People with mental-emotional problems deserve the opportunity to strive for this goal no less than the rest of us.

HEALTH CARE IN THE THERAPEUTIC ENVIRONMENT

Psychiatric hospitalization is a traumatic experience. Before being admitted to the inpatient environment, people often experience intense discomfort with the activities or details of their lives. Individuals who are admitted for the first time to an inpatient treatment setting report a sense of panic and lack of control over their situation. Those clients who are facing readmission most often express a sense of failure and worthlessness (Joseph-Kinzelman and others, 1994). Health care providers in the inpatient setting can do much to relieve the discomforts faced by clients. The mental health treatment team develops the therapeutic treatment plan, and each specialist plays a role in caring for the client. However, each staff member assists clients with the activities of daily living and monitors each step made toward the goals of treatment.

Admission and Discharge

The process of admitting a client to a health care facility is usually detailed but fairly straightforward. However, when clients are admitted to a psychiatric setting, their emotional state plays a large role in the actual process of admission. During admission, caregivers try to explain the rules, routines, and rituals of the unit. Clients, however, are almost always too anxious to understand or remember anything in detail. They are then expected to follow the rules and engage in the appropriate activities even though the memory of the first few days at the facility is absent or blurred.

People with high anxiety levels seldom remember what was said, especially when they are in unfamiliar settings. Approach clients in a calm and respectful manner. Give simple but clear explanations and repeat them as necessary. Give written instructions. They allow clients to read about the rules after their anxiety decreases. Answer any questions the client may have. Make sure that the client is more important than the admission form you must complete. Take the time to behaviorally communicate that you are concerned for his or her welfare. Make efforts to support the client in adapting to the therapeutic environment.

Most inpatient facilities have an established procedure for admitting clients and standard forms for data collection (Box 9-2). During the admission process, a person may be interviewed by several members of the treatment team, all of them asking the same questions. This situation causes unnecessary anxiety for clients and is a poor use of therapist time. Having one person perform the initial admission interview prevents confusion and added stress for the client. Once the client is emotionally stabilized, additional information is easily obtained.

The experience of being admitted to an inpatient setting establishes the tone for the client's entire stay. The first experience and the first impression with the therapeutic environment are often lasting ones.

The process of preparing for discharge begins on admission. The length of stay for mental health clients has decreased dramatically as the goal of inpatient treatment has shifted from custodial care to actively returning people to their communities. Because of this, discharge planning has assumed an important role in treatment as the bridge from the sheltered therapeutic environment to the reality of life in the community. Little research has been done to discover how well clients reintegrate themselves into their communities. Care providers who work with mental health clients are in excellent positions to assist clients in applying the new behaviors learned within the therapeutic setting to the less predictable world of the community.

By the time most clients are ready for discharge, they are actively participating in their treatment program. Decisions about housing, employment, treatment, and management of their mental health problems are made with the treatment team's assistance. A multidisciplinary discharge care plan is developed. Appropriate referrals to various agencies are made and follow-up care in the community is planned. A case manager is assigned to work with the client after discharge.

Returning to the community is a hopeful but demanding time. The support of the treatment team, as well as family and friends, is needed to ease the transition. As one researcher stated, the mentally ill "have no formal ceremonies to transform them back to 'normal' status" (Herman, 1993). The activities of the treatment team are needed to reinforce and strengthen clients' adaptive abilities throughout the discharge process.

Compliance

Clients who follow prescribed treatments are said to be in compliance. The term **noncompliance** refers to not cooperating with the treatment plan. Assisting clients to comply can be caregivers' biggest challenge, especially when working with troubled people. It is estimated that "40% to 80% of patients don't comply with their prescribed therapeutic course" (Wichowski and Kubsch, 1995).

Box 9-2 Admission Assessment

Demographic data: Full name, sex, age, date of birth, address, marital status, family members' names and ages, and (sometimes) religious preference.

Admission data: Date and time of admission, type of admission (voluntary or committed).

Reason for admission: Current problems as perceived by the patient. These include stressors, difficulty with coping, and "emergency behaviors" (suicidal or homicidal ideas/attempts, aggression, destructive behaviors, risk of escape).

Previous psychiatric history: Dates, inpatient/outpatient, reasons for and types of treatment, and their effectiveness.

Drug and alcohol use/abuse: Amount, frequency, duration of past and present use of legal/illegal substances, date and time of last use.

Disturbances in patterns of daily living: Sleep, intake, elimination, sexual activity, work, leisure, self-care, and hygiene.

Support systems: Amount of contact, nature/quality of relationships, and availability of support.

General appearance: Type and condition of clothing, cleanliness, physical condition, and posture.

Behaviors during the interview:
Expression of anger: covert, overt, verbal, or physical.
Degree of cooperation, resistance, or evasiveness.
Social skills: Positive/unpleasant habits, shyness, withdrawal.

Amount/type of motor activity: Psychomotor retardation, agitation, restlessness, tics, tremors, hypervigilance, lack of activity.

Speech patterns: Amount, rate, volume, pressure, mutism, slurring, or stuttering.
Degree of concentration and attention span.

Orientation: To time, place, and person; level of consciousness.

Memory: Recent/remote, amnesia, blackouts, confabulation.

Thought processes reflected in speech: Blocking, circumstantiality, loose associations, flight of ideas, perseveration, tangential ideas, ambivalence, neologisms, or "word salad."

Thought content: Helplessness, hopelessness, worthlessness, guilt, suicidal ideas/plans, homicidal ideas/plans, suspiciousness, phobias, obsessions, compulsions, preoccupations, antisocial attitudes, blaming of others, poverty of content, or denial.

Hallucinations: Visual, auditory, or other.

Delusions: Of reference, influence, persecution, grandeur, religious, or somatic.

Intellectual functioning: Use of language and knowledge, abstract vs. concrete thinking (proverbs), or calculations.

Affect/mood: Anxiety level; elevated or depressed mood; labile, blunted, or flat affect; or inappropriate affect.

Insight: Degree of awareness of problems and their causes.

Judgment: Soundness of problem solving and decisions.

Motivation: Degree of motivation for treatment.

From Keltner NL, Schwecke LH, Bostrom CE: *Psychiatric nursing,* ed 3, St. Louis, 1999, Mosby.

Table 9-4 Reasons for Noncompliance

Problem	Intervention
Lack of one or more of the following	
Understanding	Education, support
Finances to pay for treatment	Refer to Social Services
Access to treatment services	Refer to Social Services
Support from family and significant others	Involve family, support groups
Ability to understand or follow treatment plan	Education, involve family
Client suffering from	
Physical side effects	Refer to physician; monitor client's response to medication
Mental-emotional side effects	Communication, therapy, support

To improve clients' compliance, care providers must understand the reasons for clients' unwillingness to follow the treatment plan (Table 9-4).

A complete assessment of clients, their daily activities, their attitudes toward treatment, and their coping resources will help identify the overt (outward) causes of noncompliance. However, many times the reasoning for noncompliance lies within clients' negative attitudes toward treatment and recovery. Alert caregivers help their clients change many self-defeating attitudes that bind them to their problems.

Challenging client's expectations is one technique for increasing compliance. Helping clients to remove self-imposed boundaries offers them the hope that improvement is possible or even attainable. Other techniques involve using a positive outlook and redirecting negative attitudes into more constructive ones. A genuine concern is a powerful tool. These techniques are designed to help your clients improve their outlooks on life. When one believes that success is attainable, it becomes easier to

Sample Client Care Plan — Noncompliance

Assessment

History: Tom is a 24-year-old male with a history of paranoid schizophrenia and several admissions to the unit. Following his last discharge, he refused to take his medications or seek follow-up therapy and, consequently, began to hallucinate and behave inappropriately. He is being admitted today in order to adjust his medications and devise a plan of treatment.

Current Findings: A disheveled young adult who refuses to eat or drink because people "are trying to poison my brain."

Multidisciplinary Diagnosis

Noncompliance, related to suspiciousness

Planning/Goals

Tom will eat three meals a day by June 22.

Therapeutic Interventions

Intervention	Rationale	Team Member
1. Offer prepackaged foods.	Tom may think there is less likelihood that food is poisoned.	Nsg, Diet
2. Monitor food and fluid intake	Prevents malnutrition; to find which foods and fluids Tom is willing to consume.	Nsg
3. Offer fluids (prepackaged) every 2 hours	Prevents fluid imbalance; to gain trust.	Nsg, Diet
4. Leave snacks within reach.	Tom may eat when he thinks that he is not being watched.	Nsg, Diet
5. Allow Tom to see what other clients are eating and drinking.	Helps lessen suspiciousness.	Nsg

Evaluation

By the fifth day of hospitalization, Tom was drinking 1000 ml of prepackaged liquids. He was still refusing to eat but would occasionally take a bite of bread if someone else started eating it first.

A complete client care plan includes several other diagnoses and interventions.

comply with the therapies and medications prescribed in the plan of care. The Sample Client Care Plan offers some specific interventions to improve compliance.

KEY CONCEPTS

◆ The term therapeutic milieu is used to describe an environment that is structured to assist clients in controlling inappropriate behaviors and learning more effective adaptive (coping) personal and psychosocial skills.

◆ The inpatient psychiatric settings of today provide services to three main groups of people: those experiencing crises, those with acute mental or emotional problems, and those with chronic mental illness.

◆ The basic goals of a therapeutic environment (milieu) are to protect the client and others during periods of maladaptive behaviors, help individuals develop self-worth and confidence, and teach more effective adaptive (coping) skills.

◆ Clients are assisted to meet the physical needs associated with nourishment, personal hygiene, and clean surroundings.

◆ The physical properties of a therapeutic environment include temperature, lighting, sound, cleanliness, and aesthetics.

◆ Setting limits allows the therapeutic environment to be consistent and predictable because clients know that external controls will be enforced.

◆ In the therapeutic setting, caregivers assist clients in building their self-esteem needs through acceptance, expectations, and involvement.

◆ The process of being admitted to an inpatient setting establishes the tone for the remainder of a client's stay.

◆ Discharge planning is the bridge from the sheltered therapeutic environment to life in the community.

◆ An important responsibility of the inpatient staff is to educate and encourage clients to play an active and responsible role in their own care.

Suggestions for Further Reading

A Right to Mental Illness?, by E. Fuller Torry and Mary Zdanowicz (*New York Post,* May 28, 1999) offers insight to a pressing mental health problem.

References

Breggin PR: *Toxic psychiatry,* New York, 1991, St. Martins Press.

Cohen LJ: Psychiatric hospitalization as experience of trauma, *Archives of Psychiatric Nursing* 8(2):78, 1994.

Delaney C: Reducing recidivism: medication versus psychosocial rehabilitation, *Journal of Psychosocial Nursing and Mental Health Services* 36(11):28, 1998.

Goren S, Orion R: Space and sanity, *Archives of Psychiatric Nursing* 8:237, 1994.

Haber J and others: *Comprehensive psychiatric nursing,* ed 5, St. Louis, 1997, Mosby.

Herman NJ: Return to sender: reintegrative stigma-management strategies of ex-psychiatric patients, *Journal of Contemporary Ethnography* 22:295, 1993.

Holmberg SK: Ambient sound levels in a state psychiatric hospital, *Archives of Psychiatric Nursing* 13(3):117, 1999.

Jones M: *The therapeutic community,* New York, 1953, Basic Books.

Joseph-Kinzelman A and others: Clients' perceptions of involuntary hospitalization, *Journal of Psychosocial Nursing and Mental Health Services* 32:11, 1994.

Stuart GW, Laraia MT: *Principles and practice of psychiatric nursing,* ed 7, St. Louis, 2001, Mosby.

Taylor CM: *Essentials of psychiatric nursing,* ed 14, St. Louis, 1994, Mosby.

Wichowski HC, Kubsch S: Improving your patient's compliance, *Nursing 95* 25(1):67, 1995.

Chapter 10

The Therapeutic Relationship

Learning Objectives

1. Describe the difference between a social relationship and a therapeutic relationship.
2. Explain the five dynamic concepts of the therapeutic relationship.
3. List three components of a therapeutic rapport.
4. Explain the meaning of "therapeutic use of self."
5. State two ways to use oneself therapeutically.
6. Identify the four phases of the therapeutic relationship.
7. Describe four roles of the caregiver in the therapeutic relationship.
8. Discuss three problems that may be encountered in the therapeutic relationship.

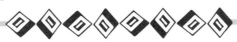

Key Terms

autonomy
countertransference
dynamics
empathy
genuineness

hope
limit setting
mutuality
noncompliance
rapport

resistance
secondary gain
therapeutic relationship
transference
trust

The **therapeutic relationship** is a directed energy exchange between two people, a flow that moves clients toward more effective behaviors. A poem of Native American tradition by Strong Spirit Path (Spencer, 1991) sums up the essence of a therapeutic relationship:

> UNIVERSE
> is Space
> which contains Energy
> Energy
> of its nature moves
> and produces Change
> Change is
> it was <> it is <> it will be
> sometimes we call this past, present, future
> and we say it is Time
> it is not Time
> it is Change

> you see how everything in Universe
> is Energy
> flowing from one place to another
> what we call Matter
> is merely a relatively stable form
> of Energy
> which is also changing
> only more slowly
> like Earth and Ocean
> each at its own pace
> all things that contain Energy
> are alive
> and all things are *related*
> each to the other
> *always*

The energies of care providers are used to direct clients toward more constructive ways of thinking and more effective ways of coping with their problems. Caregivers use their abundance of health-directed energies to first balance or stabilize clients. Then they assist clients to mobilize and direct their own energies into more life-fulfilling directions.

The art of helping others involves an energy exchange that takes place every time caregivers interact with their clients. This chapter focuses on how health care providers use their energies to establish and direct the therapeutic relationship.

DYNAMICS OF THE THERAPEUTIC RELATIONSHIP

Dynamics refers to the interactions that occur among various forces. For example, a social relationship includes such dynamics as having fun together, supporting each other through difficult times, and enjoying each others company. A social relationship is a two-way energy exchange based on the sharing of personal opinions, attitudes, and tastes.

A work relationship has the purpose of achieving certain goals. It includes the dynamics of motivation, performance, and evaluation. People within a work relationship are there to achieve a goal, produce a product, make a profit, or deliver a service.

The therapeutic relationship differs from other relationships. First, the focus of energies is primarily on the client. Second, the therapeutic relationship is consciously directed. Friendships and other social relationships happen mostly by chance. In therapeutic relationships, however, care providers consciously establish a connection with clients to help them cope with their particular life demands.

The dynamic components of the therapeutic relationship include the concepts of trust, empathy, autonomy, caring, and hope. Using these concepts as a framework encourages caregivers to develop the skills and sensitivity necessary to direct their energies into effective helping relationships.

Trust

Trust is defined as "a risk-taking process whereby an individual's situation depends on the future behavior of another person" (Anderson, Anderson, and Glanze, 1998). Without trust, people become isolated and incapable of relying on other people. Attitudes regarding trust are based on past experiences, which have the power to influence the present and future.

Within the therapeutic relationship, trust is "the assured belief that other individuals are capable of assisting in times of distress and will probably do so" (Travelbee, 1971). Trust is an important part of any therapeutic relationship. Each and every person for whom we care needs to be able to trust that their caregivers will act in their best interests.

Illness or dysfunction of any kind requires much energy. When clients arrive for care, their energies are usually very low. The role of "receiver of care" fosters a dependency on caregivers and feelings of vulnerability. Care providers who recognize this situation work to establish a sense of trust with each client.

There are several ways in which caregivers direct their energies toward establishing trust with clients. They first assess the client's ability to trust others. Each therapeutic behavior is then designed to promote trust. For example, a caregiver who says she will return in 10 minutes arrives at the appointed time. This one simple action reassures clients that caregivers will follow through on their verbal statements.

Second, care providers must be honest with their clients. To tell a child, for example, that the injection will not hurt makes him or her less likely to believe the next health care provider's explanations or instructions. If these experiences are repeated often enough, people develop a mistrust of the entire medical care system (see Think About box).

The third focus in the establishment of trust is clear communication. Give information to clients slowly, using terms that can be understood by the average person. Clients cannot learn to trust if they cannot understand. Offer clients the time to share their feelings and apprehensions. "Without the establishment of trust, the helping relationship will not progress beyond the level of mechanical provision for tending to superficial needs" (Sundeen and others, 1998).

Empathy

Empathy is the ability to walk a mile in another person's shoes. It enables caregivers to enter into the life of

---

Think About

Mary J. is a 42-year-old woman who has been treated for severe depression for 21 years. She has received several electroconvulsive therapy treatments, which she was told would relieve her depression; they did not. Various psychotropic medications, on several occasions, have had little success. Currently, you, as one of the staff at the community mental health center, have been following Mary's care.

Although Mary is required to return to the clinic weekly for medication monitoring, she keeps her appointments only when she wants more medication. When questioned about her refusal to keep her appointments, she tells you that no one really cares about her so why go through the motions. "Just fill the prescription, keep your mouth shut, and let me go," she replies to your statement of concern.

◆ How could Mary be encouraged to return to treatment?

a person and to share his or her emotions, meanings, and attitudes. Empathy is communicated verbally, nonverbally, and behaviorally. It is the interconnectedness between caregiver and client that improves the effectiveness of the therapeutic relationship. In short, empathy is the ability to share in the client's world.

Unfortunately, there are no specific directions for the development of empathy. However, you can become more empathetic by focusing your attention (energies) on what clients are trying to communicate. Learn to listen with more than just your ears. Concentrate on the speaker and listen objectively, without passing judgment. Accept what is being said. You do not have to agree with anything the client says, but you need to demonstrate acceptance of the client's communications.

The development of empathy can also be nurtured by becoming secure in your therapeutic actions. When care providers are confident with their abilities, their energies can be devoted to clients and their situations, instead of being concerned about performance. The caregiver's confidence sends a message that encourages clients to share more of themselves.

Last, learn to consciously focus on your client. Enter into each interaction expecting to learn something new. Become aware of the entire message the client is sending. Observe body motions, gestures, eye movement, facial expressions, and vocal tones. Together, these small cues send powerful messages.

Autonomy

The concept of **autonomy** relates to the ability to direct and control one's activities and destiny. When people seek health care, they risk losing their autonomy because health care delivery is a specialized, complex world, full of the unknown.

Frequently, care providers think that clients are incapable of making good health care decisions. They assume an attitude of paternalism in which care providers become the judge of what is best for the client. This attitude limits the client's ability to make decisions and increases dependency on others. People with mental health difficulties have problems with autonomy because the nature of their illness sometimes results in their making inappropriate decisions. However, autonomy is just as important for these individuals. Autonomy is encouraged by the caregiver through the use of the concept of mutuality.

The concept of **mutuality** relates to the process of sharing with another person. When a therapeutic relationship has mutuality, both client and caregiver focus their unique strengths on fulfilling health care needs. The care provider has theoretical knowledge that can assist the client in identifying specific problems and possible solutions, and the client has the knowledge of self and needs that are important to him or her. Both contribute to the plan of care.

Because clients are unique individuals, therapeutic interventions are modified to meet each person's needs. For example, clients who are unable to remember their appointments are reminded. Mutuality also helps both clients and care providers meet goals. When goals are based on the client's needs, they are more apt to be achieved because clients have a role in establishing them.

Caring

Caring is a vital part of the therapeutic relationship; its thread is interwoven through every aspect and interaction. Caring is the energy that allows caregivers to unconditionally accept each person, even when they are most unlovable.

Clients will often question caregivers about their ability to truly care. Statements such as "You are just doing this because it's your job" or "You don't really care—you're getting paid to be nice to me" express the need to be accepted , cared for, and loved. People who have had negative experiences with the health care delivery system can become cautious and suspicious of the intentions of their care providers. They "can tell" when someone is sincere or merely concerned with the diagnosis, test, or function rather than the person. Caregivers who demonstrate a high degree of caring are able to enjoy the rich uniqueness of each individual. They are able to give of themselves without losing their own identity. To develop and nurture your caring abilities, practice these four steps:

1. Become aware of the client as an individual.
2. Learn to respect the uniqueness and individuality of each person for whom you care.
3. Increase your knowledge of the client's needs.
4. Develop mutual sharing.

Caring is an energy that communicates concern, sensitivity, and compassion. Cherish and nurture your ability to care because it is a connection that enhances the therapeutic relationship.

Hope

The concept of hope involves the future. For many people, especially those who are ill or distressed, the future can appear bleak. Hope is not easily defined; however, from a therapeutic point of view, we can say that **hope** is "a multidimensional dynamic life force characterized by a confident yet uncertain expectation of achieving a future good" (Dufault and Martocchio, 1985). For a hope to be achievable, it must be realistic, possible, and personally significant. Hope is a highly personal concept, and it can be the energy that motivates people toward health.

For caregivers, hope is a therapeutic energy tool that can have a powerful effect on client care outcomes. The emotions and behaviors relating to hope are many,

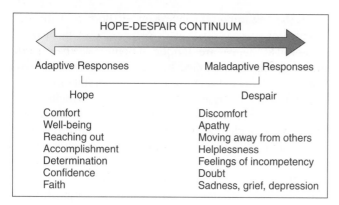

Figure 10-1 The hope-despair continuum.

Table 10-1	Interventions Related to the Dimensions of Hope
Dimension	**Therapeutic interventions**
Affective	Provide an opportunity for expression of feelings
	Respond empathically
	Assist in coping with feelings
Affiliative	Support helpful relationships
Behavioral	Encourage appropriate dependent, independent, and interdependent actions
	Enhance self-esteem to decrease feelings of helplessness
Cognitive	Clarification
	Provide information
Temporal	Help to see the relationship between past experiences and hope
Contextual	Help to create a supportive, hopeful environment

Modified from Dufault K, Martocchio BC: *Nursing Clinics of North America* 20:379, 1985.

ranging from feelings of despair to inspiration and determination. They can be illustrated on a continuum or range (Figure 10-1), with the behaviors of despair on one end and the behaviors of great hope on the other.

Dufault and Martocchio (1985) have described six dimensions related to the concept of hope. The first is known as the *affective dimension*. It includes all the feelings that one has about hope such as anticipation, the desirability attached to the outcome, and dread. It is the emotional aspect of hope.

The second area, the *affiliative dimension,* addresses how hope is related or interwoven. It includes spirituality—how one relates to life and other people. Behaviors in this dimension include the seeking or receiving of help, using others as a source of hope, and seeking support and encouragement.

Third is the *behavioral dimension,* which consists of the actions or behaviors that may make the hoped-for situation come true. For example, people who begin an exercise program hoping that they will prevent heart problems are operating in the behavioral dimension.

Fourth is the *cognitive dimension* or the thinking area. It is the process of thinking through and analyzing the hope. Some people operate within this dimension by defining what their hopes are. Others explore all the factors that relate to the hoped-for situation, whereas some compile facts to encourage a successful outcome. The acts associated with problem solving are in the cognitive dimension.

Fifth is the *temporal dimension* of hope; the experience of time as it relates to hope. Because hope is accompanied by time, one's past, present, and future interact. One may hope to repeat the pleasant experiences of the past and use them as a frame of reference to avoid problems in the future.

Last is the *contextual dimension* of hope, which includes one's personal life situation as it relates to hope. It becomes much easier to have hope if one's environment is stable. Inadequate resources (physical,

Box 10-1	Components of the Therapeutic Relationship

T = Trust
E = Empathy
A = Autonomy
C = Caring
H = Hope

financial, emotional) provide a context in which hope may be difficult to muster. Hope conforms to an individual's point of view.

There are several therapeutic interventions relating to hope. Table 10-1 lists an intervention for each dimension of hope. The concept of hope is a basic component of the therapeutic relationship because without it, no movement or progress toward a goal is real.

The dynamics of the therapeutic relationship are not overt. They lie quietly, waiting to be energized by the therapeutic agent. Trust, empathy, autonomy, caring, and hope are the techniques with which caregivers build the foundation of the therapeutic relationship. Look closely at the first letters of each word, which when aligned together, spell the word *teach*. With these tools, caregivers can guide the therapeutic relationship and move (teach) their clients toward their highest levels of wellness (Box 10-1).

CHARACTERISTICS OF THE THERAPEUTIC RELATIONSHIP

Therapeutic relationships vary in importance to clients. For clients who are hospitalized or institutionalized, the therapeutic relationship assumes a greater importance. People with chronic conditions usually place a high degree of importance on their relationships with caregivers. People with emotional or mental problems often need the therapeutic relationship to serve as the bridge between mere existence and success. To successfully establish a therapeutic relationship, the qualities of acceptance, genuineness, and rapport must be communicated to the client.

Acceptance

The verb *accept* means to receive or take what is being offered. People entering the health care system arrive as complex individuals with past histories, internal needs, and external realities. Each person must be accepted exactly as they are. Most people are cooperative and interested in working toward relieving the problems for which they have sought health care. However, some people are more difficult to accept, especially when their behaviors are unusual or not socially appropriate. "It is difficult to fully understand the overwhelming experience of having to live with mental illness" (Vellenga and Christenson, 1994), but the importance of accepting these individuals cannot be stressed enough in the therapeutic relationship.

Whereas care providers may be concerned with the long-term aspects of a client's mental illness, distressed individuals are more concerned with their present pain and the need for relief. Not only must they cope with the discomforts of their illness, but they must also deal with the alienation forced on them by others. The stigma of being mentally ill follows them into the home and workplace and results in the loss of emotional relationships and vocational opportunities. Many individuals experience distress, which is described as feelings of hopelessness, fright, and an inability to function. "Clients believed that acceptance lent them a sense of strength and value and made them feel more normal" (Vellenga and Christenson, 1994). For people with mental-emotional problems, acceptance is of prime importance.

Caregivers can develop acceptance by remembering that it is the person (the individual) who must be accepted, not the behaviors or the attitudes. The very purpose of mental health care is to replace inappropriate behaviors with more effective actions. However, if the client feels accepted for who he or she is, then treatment strategies will be far more effective.

Rapport

The second ingredient that care providers need for an effective therapeutic relationship is **rapport**—the ability to establish a meaningful connection with clients. Rapport is a dynamic process, an energy exchange between caregiver and client that provides the background for all therapeutic actions. Rapport is an individual, personal concept. It is the person of the caregiver therapeutically interacting with the person of the client.

Rapport is characterized by a concern for others and an active interest in the well-being of one's clients. A belief in the worth and dignity of each individual, along with an accepting attitude is essential for forming rapport. Every care provider has a certain degree of skill in establishing rapport with clients. Actively work to improve your abilities to establish meaningful connections with clients. Rapport is not a scientific tool but an application of our willingness to care.

Genuineness

Something that is genuine is real. **Genuineness,** in the therapeutic relationship, "implies that the nurse is an open, honest, sincere person who is actively involved in the relationship" (Stuart and Laraia, 2001). The quality of honesty is a part of being genuine. However, the goal of the therapeutic relationship is to move the client toward wellness. Sharing yourself must be done while remembering that the client is the primary focus. In this way, caregivers can be genuinely involved without using the therapeutic relationship to meet their own needs.

Therapeutic Use of Self

The most therapeutic tool of any care provider is the self: the ways in which we interact, attend to, and encourage clients. Caregivers are role models for health and coping, especially with people who are mentally or emotionally troubled. Care providers' behaviors set examples for successful actions.

Caregivers direct themselves therapeutically by focusing energies on the client. Sometimes they share small bits of personal information, but that sharing always has a purpose that benefits the client. For example, a client asks how many children the caregiver has. The care provider answers the question and then focuses on the client by asking him how many children he has. This technique allows caregivers to maintain the focus on the client while sharing information about themselves.

To improve your skills in using "self" therapeutically, remember two important thoughts. First, feel good about yourself. You cannot be therapeutically effective when your personal life is in turmoil. Clients can sense a caregiver's emotional discomfort. Work to become aware of your own feelings and attitudes and how they affect the therapeutic relationships with clients.

Second, work to develop an awareness of how your actions, gestures, and expressions affect other people. During each interaction, "step out" of the situation and consider how the client is reacting. With experience and effort, the majority of your actions will be therapeutic, no matter what the practice setting or type of client you encounter.

PHASES OF THE THERAPEUTIC RELATIONSHIP

The therapeutic relationship, like plants and people, needs time to grow even though it is a time-limited, purposeful series of interactions. Every therapeutic relationship moves through four phases, and each phase has identifiable tasks and goals (Table 10-2). As these tasks are accomplished, a readiness to move onto the next phase is experienced. Interventions are guided by the therapeutic goals of the client's treatment plan throughout the relationship. The four stages or phases of the therapeutic relationship are called the preparation, orientation, working, and termination phases.

Preparation Phase

This is the data-gathering stage in which the caregiver prepares for the relationship. Although complete information about the client is usually unavailable, it is very important to learn as much as possible about the client before meeting him or her. This is also the time for you to look at your own possible reactions. The therapeutic goals for this phase are to establish a client database and assess your own feelings regarding the client.

To establish a database, review all possible information relating to the client. Past medical records, current records, and interactions with significant others in the client's life are excellent sources of information. Once the information is gathered, look for the recurring patterns of behavior to develop a picture of the client. Armed with this knowledge, you can now begin to form ideas about the relationship and hopefully forecast possible problems. A word of caution: Do not accept labels as fact. Keep an open mind. Because a client is labeled psychotic, do not expect him or her to behave as other people with the same label. People are individuals with their own unique behaviors.

Next, look inward to your own reactions. Caregivers are also unique individuals, and their attitudes and behaviors affect the therapeutic relationship. First identify your initial reactions to the client. Is there anything that may block your ability to help? For example, a caregiver's attendance at an Alanon support group for the spouses of alcoholics may have an influence on his or her ability to help a client being treated for alcoholism.

Next, assess for stereotyping: If the client is a member of a particular group or culture, will he or she will behave in a certain way? The belief that people with mental illness cannot behave responsibly is an example of a stereotype that can impact the therapeutic relationship. For this reason, be aware of any preconceived ideas or attitudes about the client.

Finally, recognize the anxiety that is generally present in the caregiver during this phase. Mild anxiety is common and sharpens the senses. High anxiety levels can affect a nurse's judgment, so seeking assistance from one's supervisor is advised when anxiety may affect the therapeutic relationship.

During this phase caregivers also begin to think about the termination phase. Because the therapeutic relationship is based on helping clients with their problems, it is time limited and caregivers reinforce this throughout each phase of interaction.

The last step in the preparatory phase is to make plans for the first interaction with the client. Find a quiet setting—free from interruptions. Plan for sufficient time, and identify what information must be covered during the first interaction. Make a mental outline, and your preparations are complete.

Table 10-2 Goals of and Caregiving Behaviors in Each Phase of the Caregiver-Client Relationship		
Phase of nurse-client relationship	**Goals**	**Caregiver behaviors**
Orientation	Develop mutual trust	Establishes mutually acceptable contract
	Establish caregiver as significant other to client	Responds to testing behavior of client by adhering strictly to terms of contract
Maintenance	Identify and address client's problems	Highly individualized to nature of client's problems
		Empathic, nonpunishing limit setting
Termination	Assist client to review what was learned and to transfer this learning to interactions with others	Understands client's sense of loss
		Helps client express and cope with feelings
		Encourages client to channel feelings into constructive activity, such as farewell party
		Recognizes own feelings of loss

Modified from Taylor CM: *Essentials of psychiatric nursing*, ed 14, St. Louis, 1994, Mosby.

Orientation Phase

During the orientation phase, caregiver and client become acquainted, agree to work with each other, and establish the purpose for the relationship. The first meeting establishes the tone and forms the impressions that both people will carry with them throughout the entire relationship. The basic goals for this phase are to build trust and establish the caregiver as significant in the life of the client.

The first and most important step at this time is to identify each other by name. Introduce yourself by name and position. Establish how the client wishes to be addressed. When the client responds, an exchange begins. Next, explain your role, particularly as it relates to the client. This gives the client an idea of what may be expected in the relationship. Once client and caregiver are comfortable, an agreement to work with each other is established.

Establishing a working agreement or caregiver-client contract is the next step in the orientation phase of the therapeutic relationship. The contract is simply an agreement that describes the nature of the relationship. Both client and care provider discuss their expectations and then agree on the goals they want to meet. The contract, which includes a description of each person's roles and responsibilities, is then written or verbally established. The word *contract* may provoke anxiety in some persons, so it is not often used when interacting with clients. The term is less important than actually gaining the client's agreement. Once arrangements have been made, it is extremely important for the nurse to keep his or her end of the bargain, or, as Taylor (1994) states, "to respond to the client's behavior with meticulous consistency."

During the orientation phase, both the client and the caregiver carry out assessments or "size up" each other. It is the time when the care provider becomes aware of the client as a real person, unique and individual. Work to keep a nonjudgmental attitude. The label of "client" soon falls by the wayside, and a genuine person-to-person energy exchange begins to evolve into a therapeutic relationship.

Clients will often test the reliability of their caregivers. Testing is an important step in establishing trust in the therapeutic relationship. Although clients may not appear for scheduled appointments, use profane language, or resist sharing their feelings, the caregiver must demonstrate a willingness to continue the therapeutic relationship by doing what was promised in the contract. This reliability is important because many troubled people have never had a reliable or consistent relationship. When the care provider has established reliability and the client has gained enough trust to no longer test, the therapeutic relationship is ready for the next stage.

Working Phase

The focus of the working phase of the therapeutic relationship is to achieve the goals that were agreed on in the client-caregiver contract. This is the time for solving problems and trying out new behaviors. During this phase, care providers are guided by their knowledge of human behavior, the client's plan of care, and the agreed-on goals.

The working phase consists of periods of growth and resistance. If the relationship is moving toward its goals, the client's behavior changes. At this time it is important to explore the meaning of the change with the client and mutually decide if the behavioral change is meeting the agreed-on goals. Periods of growth are accompanied by episodes of resistance. Changing one's behavior is very hard work. It requires energy and self-disclosure. Clients often feel self-conscious, shameful, and vulnerable during this time. The caregiver's gentle acceptance and reliability help clients move through their periods of resistance.

An important technique for care providers is knowing when to set limits. **Limit setting** is an intervention designed to prevent clients from harming themselves or others. The necessity for setting limits often occurs during the working phase because the client may be experiencing many painful emotions. When setting limits, do so in a calm, non-threatening manner. The client is not being punished, just protected until self-control can be regained. Clients often feel a sense of relief and trust when they know that someone cares enough to protect them, even if the threat is from themselves.

Client and caregiver continue to work on meeting the goals of the relationship. Other members of the treatment team may also be involved in specific areas of the client's therapy. Therefore it is important to understand how each member of the team functions and shares responsibility in relation to the client. During the working stage, caregivers frequently assess for behaviors that indicate the goals are being met. Clients are educated about exploring community resources. Preparations for ending or terminating the relationship are made. The time finally arrives when the goals are accomplished or one of the people is no longer able to maintain the relationship. It is the signal for the final phase, termination.

Termination Phase

When the goals of the therapeutic relationship are achieved, both the client and caregiver share a sense of accomplishment. However, this is balanced by the loss of a meaningful person in the client's life. When the mutual goals have not been met, termination can be difficult. This is a major reason why it is important to set realistic goals at the beginning and frequently monitor the client's progress.

Steps toward termination should begin *before* the last meeting. Both parties need time to prepare the client for

Table 10-3	Behavioral Responses to Termination	
Regression	**Withdrawal**	**Continuation**
Return to previous maladaptive behavior	Denial of caregiver's help	Tries to continue relationship
Increased anxiety	Demands to stop relationship now	Brings up new problems
Tardiness or absence from appointments	Absence from appointments	Becomes helpless
Expresses doubts about value of relationship	Superficially interacts with caregiver	Wants caregiver to solve his or her problems

Modified from Sundeen SJ and others: *Nurse-client interaction: implementing the nursing process,* ed 6, St. Louis, 1998, Mosby.

independence. During this phase, the caregiver reviews the steps taken toward achieving the goals. Clients feel a sense of pride and accomplishment when they can review their progress. This is also an opportunity to encourage clients to apply their more effective behaviors to other situations.

People respond to the loss of a therapeutic relationship as they would any loss. Some may show signs of regression or withdrawal or engage in behaviors to continue or intensify the relationship (Table 10-3). The feelings behind these behaviors should be identified and shared. Looking toward the future and reminding clients of their progress helps ease the transition to independence. Saying goodbye is never easy, but a client who is able to function more effectively as a result of your interventions is the reward of a successful therapeutic relationship.

ROLES OF THE CAREGIVER

Throughout the course of the therapeutic relationship, caregivers play several roles, each designed to assist clients in meeting specific therapeutic goals. Care providers who work with mental health clients assume the roles of therapeutic change agents, teachers, technicians, and therapists. Together, these roles move clients toward more successful and adaptive coping behaviors.

Change Agent

The therapeutic environment is more than a physical space. The psychological atmosphere created by caregivers is one of the major contributions toward successful recovery. Caregivers provide an accepting atmosphere that values the contributions of every individual. They accept the fact that some client behaviors may not be appropriate, but they never discredit the person. Individuals are supported and encouraged to exchange their unsuccessful actions for more effective behaviors. Caregivers' attitudes foster a climate that anticipates, expects, and promotes positive change. Hopefully, each staff member acts as a role model for successful living, thus demonstrating to clients that there are other ways of

Table 10-4	Teaching Opportunities for Caregivers	
Topic	**Health team member**
Activities of daily living	All members
Mental illness and its treatments	Nursing, Therapists
Effects, side effects, adverse reactions of medications	Nursing
Early signs and symptoms of return to maladaptive functioning	All members
How to cope with stressors of daily living	All members
What to say to others about the mental illness	Nursing, Therapists
Teaching the public about mental health and illness	All members

behaving. When the atmosphere promotes change and provides the security to practice those changes, clients are more likely to improve.

Care providers also function as socializing agents. They assist clients to participate in group activities and various social interactions. They introduce clients to each other, encourage conversations, and help clients focus on the healthy aspects of their lives. Interactions with others are seen as opportunities to encourage successful social experiences for their clients.

Teacher

Members of the mental health care team are constantly alert for opportunities to teach. In the mental health care setting, teaching opportunities range from instructions about daily living activities to major lifestyle changes (see Table 10-4).

All clients must be instructed about areas such as their medications and diet, but equally important opportunities for instruction exist with every client interaction.

Through these interactions, nurses are able to assess and monitor existing problems, plan for corrective learning opportunities, and forecast possible difficulties. Clients and their families trust caregivers, and they often confide in them. These times of sharing become great teaching opportunities. Teaching is an important part of care because it provides a solid bridge for the passage from existence to effective adaptation.

Technician

The technical roles of the mental health team members focus on holistic care. Attention is given to the whole client. Caregivers should be informed about the physical conditions of their clients, as well as their mental status. Too many times, providers involved with the client's care focus on the mental-emotional status of the client and exclude the physical realm. For this reason, caregivers must remain alert to the physical problems that may be present with mental health clients. Remember Maslow's hierarchy of needs—physical needs are satisfied first. Many mental health clients suffer from physical problems, just as many medical clients suffer from psychological problems. The technical role for nurses in the mental health setting includes administering, monitoring, and evaluating medications; managing medical problems within the mental health environment; assessing the difference between physical and psychiatric conditions; maintaining safety; and managing environmental factors. Other team members have technical roles related to their specialties.

Therapist

Although all care providers use every opportunity to assist their clients in developing more effective behaviors, nurses who function as therapists are usually educated at the master's level in the principles of psychotherapy. Nurses who formally engage in the therapist role routinely consult with a more experienced therapist who acts as a resource and provides guidance.

Caregivers function in many roles when working with mental health clients. Through "practiced awareness," they are able to use a variety of roles to assist clients toward their goals. The therapeutic use of self is applied each time caregivers interact with their clients, and every interaction is seen as a learning opportunity.

PROBLEMS ENCOUNTERED IN THE THERAPEUTIC RELATIONSHIP

Throughout the therapeutic relationship, caregivers are continually assisting their clients toward more effective functioning. However, problems or barriers arise and challenge us to devise creative solutions. The most common problems can be grouped into three broad areas: the environment, the care provider, and the client. By

> ### Case Study
>
> It took Marguerite 3 weeks for her client to engage in a meaningful conversation with her. Today, as the discussion progressed, Marguerite could see that her client was about to share something important. Suddenly three people entered the room and began to demand that the client join them for coffee. The moment was lost, the client mumbled something about "later" and left.
> ◆ How could Marguerite have prevented this interruption from happening?

remaining alert for these potential areas of difficulty, caregivers are able to prevent larger problems and increase their effectiveness when interacting with clients.

Environmental Problems

Problems with the environment include such things as a lack of privacy, an inappropriate meeting place, or uncomfortable furniture, lighting, or temperature. Noise and frequent interruptions disrupt interactions and become troublesome, especially if clients are attempting to share personal information. See the Case Study for an example of this situation.

To minimize environmental problems, caregivers should make appropriate arrangements for interactions with the client. Find an area within the environment where interruptions and distractions will be minimal. Next, spend the allotted time focusing on the client as being interrupted stops the communication flow between caregiver and client and does little to foster the relationship. Be alert to how the environment affects the therapeutic relationship, and problems will be easier to prevent.

Problems With Care Providers

The barriers relating to care providers in the therapeutic relationship include difficulties with attitude, setting helping boundaries, and countertransference.

Care providers are human beings with attitudes, opinions, and problems of their own. Working within a therapeutic relationship requires energy, time, and persistence. If the caregiver is expending his or her energies in coping with personal difficulties, there is little left for the client. Historically, health care providers were taught to leave their personal lives at the door and to ignore them during working hours. Now we know that it is not possible to separate the caregiver from the person. They are one, and it is the "person" aspect of the caregiver that is so effective in helping clients. Personal health is a primary ingredient of effective client care.

Attitude is also important in how the caregiver views the client. Care providers who are skeptical about the

Modified from Pilette PC, Berck CB, Achber LC: *Journal of Psychosocial Nursing and Mental Health Services* 33:40, 1995.

Box 10-2 Self-Assessment of Helping Boundaries

1. Have you ever felt too involved with a client?
2. Have you ever received feedback that you are overly intrusive or involved with clients or their families?
3. Do you have difficulty setting and enforcing limits?
4. Do you spend more than the allotted time with the client or arrive early or stay late for appointments?
5. Do you relate to clients as you do family members?
6. Do you feel that you are the only one who "really understands" the client?
7. Do you feel that other staff members are too critical of "your" client or jealous of the relationship you have with the client?
8. Do you find it difficult to handle the client's unreasonable requests or behaviors?
9. Do you look forward to the client's praise, appreciation, or affection?

A "yes" answer to any question indicates a need to identify the behaviors that are blurring the boundaries of the therapeutic relationship.

---

client's willingness or ability to change are already dooming the relationship to failure. Discomfort with the feelings expressed by the client can also slow the relationship. To be an effective mental health caregiver, one must know thyself.

Compassion is a key quality; however, when that compassion leads one to "rescue" clients, the caregiver is becoming too involved. "Owning" client problems wears the caregiver out and does nothing to promote the client's abilities to solve problems. To prevent this situation, establish your own professional boundaries. Professional boundaries define the limits of the client-caregiver relationship. Behaviors that, "well intentioned or not, could lesson the benefit of care" (AARN, 1998) for clients is considered outside professional boundaries. The focus of the therapeutic relationships is the client. Clients must be allowed to own their problems or the therapeutic relationship loses its effectiveness. Caregivers' actions must always be designed to move clients toward the goals of therapy (Box 10-2).

Countertransference is a barrier in the therapeutic relationship based on the caregiver's emotional responses to the client. It is an inappropriate, emotional response on the part of the caregiver, who identifies with someone from the past, or personal needs on the part of the caregiver begin to inhibit the effectiveness of the therapeutic relationship. Common reactions usually include intense feelings of caring, involvement, disgust, hostility, or anxiety. To prevent countertransference, remember that the focus of the relationship is the client's needs. Recognizing when one's personal needs are beginning to overshadow the client's needs is a good way to prevent countertransference.

Problems With Clients

The progress of the therapeutic relationship can also be slowed or blocked by the client. Not infrequently, clients engage in various behaviors to stall or block the effectiveness of therapeutic actions. Client activities that block progress of the therapeutic relationship fall into three basic categories: resistance, transference, and compliance.

Resistance was first defined by Freud as a client's attempts to avoid recognizing or exploring anxiety-provoking material. These attempts are further classified into primary and secondary types of resistance. Clients who demonstrate primary resistance are unwilling to change even when they are aware of the need for change. Behaviors include attempts to thwart the therapeutic process, a refusal to work toward the therapeutic goals, and attempts to manipulate the situation. Clients may also resist in reaction to the caregiver's interventions. Also, if the caregiver is not an appropriate role model for therapeutic behavior, primary resistance may occur.

Secondary resistance is seen when the client is motivated by drives other than the need to regain mental health. Many times the payoff for remaining ill outweighs the advantages of recovery. Some clients actually profit or avoid unpleasant situations by remaining ill. This situation is known as **secondary gain.** For example, the client who is facing legal problems on discharge attempts to remain in the therapeutic environment because he or she does not want to go to jail. Secondary gain can be a powerful motivation for resisting the treatment team's therapeutic efforts.

Transference is a client's emotional responses, based on earlier relationships, to the caregiver. The most outstanding characteristic of transference is the inappropriateness of the client's response. Because the client is generalizing the emotions associated with one person to another (the caregiver), little opportunity for self-awareness exists. Clients may become hostile and express their feelings by demanding an end to the relationship or showing no interest in the caregiver's interventions. Other clients can become dependent, submissive, and passive; with transference cases, clients overvalue the caregiver's characteristics and place unreachable expectations on the relationship.

To prevent or cope with transference, first listen. Hear what the client is trying to communicate. Recognize areas of resistance and then clarify them with the client. Explore behaviors and try to identify possible reasons for their use. With time and experience, you will become adept

Sample Client Care Plan — Therapeutic Relationship

Assessment

History: Heather is a 14-year-old girl who is being treated for an eating disorder. She and the members of the treatment team have set a goal for a weight gain of 2 pounds a month. Sue, the treatment team's nurse, has assumed responsibility for seeing Heather weekly and monitoring her weight gain.

Current Findings: Heather keeps her appointments but tends to display negative reactions to every suggestion offered by the treatment team. Discussions with other care providers are superficial with little meaning. When interacting, Heather assumes a challenging attitude. Her weight has remained stable for the past 3 weeks.

Multidisciplinary Diagnosis

Ineffective individual coping related to a disturbance in self-concept.

Planning/Goals

Heather will establish a trusting relationship with a member of the treatment team by September 23.

Therapeutic Interventions

Interventions	Rationale	Team Member
1. Prepare for first meeting by researching data about Heather, her family, and her past history.	Helps define the client as an individual with particular strengths and problems.	All
2. Plan time, setting, and outline of goals for each meeting.	Helps to define and focus on the goals of the relationship.	All
3. Establish an atmosphere of warmth and acceptance during first meeting.	Communicates respect and a willingness to become involved with Heather.	All
4. Help Heather define her problems.	Helps reduce emotional reactions and break her problems into smaller, more manageable units.	Psy, Nsg
5. Develop a contract (working agreement) for a self-motivated weight gain of 6 pounds per month.	Defines limits, expectations of goals; helps to plan steps for meeting goals.	Psy, Nsg
6. Assist Heather to learn positive thinking techniques.	Helps replace self-defeating thoughts and actions with more effective ways of coping.	All

Evaluation

Heather remained silent during the first two interactions with Sue. By September 10, she was willing to talk to Sue. By September 19 Heather began the interaction and stated that she would be willing to work on gaining weight and discussing her problems.

A complete client care plan includes several other diagnoses and interventions.

---

when working with the uniquely human behavior of transference.

Noncompliance is the behavior of not following the prescribed treatment regimen. For individuals with mental-emotional problems, noncompliance is very high. According to Forman (1993), the main reasons for noncompliance are a lack of knowledge, medication side effects, and the caregiver-client relationship. Throughout the therapeutic relationship, caregivers are continually assessing and monitoring the progress of their clients. Identifying and sharing problems of compliance with the client helps to remove another barrier from recovery.

When clients are prescribed medications for the control of their symptoms, all caregivers must remain especially alert for side effects. Many clients stop taking their psychotropic medications because of distressing side effects. Other clients simply feel that they do not need their medications. Whatever the reasons, caregivers are in excellent positions to improve their clients' compliance through the use of the therapeutic relationship.

The therapeutic relationship provides health care providers with a powerful tool for client care. Interventions are designed to promote the client's growth and movement toward self-awareness and independent functioning. Throughout each phase of the relationship, clients are encouraged to focus their energies toward more effective and adaptive ways of living. The Sample Client Care Plan describes several therapeutic interventions for establishing a therapeutic relationship.

KEY CONCEPTS

◆ The therapeutic relationship is a directed energy exchange between two people that guides clients toward more effective behaviors.

◆ The dynamic components of the therapeutic relationship include the concepts of trust, empathy, autonomy, caring, and hope.

◆ The four stages or phases of the therapeutic relationship are the preparation, orientation, working, and termination phases.

◆ To successfully establish a therapeutic relationship, the nurse communicates the qualities of acceptance, genuineness, and rapport to the client.

◆ Care providers who work with mental health clients function as therapeutic change agents, teachers, technicians, and therapists.

◆ The most common problems in the therapeutic relationship relate to the environment, the caregiver, and the client.

Suggestions for Further Reading

The Alberta Association of Registered Nurses' September, 1998 position statement relating to professional boundaries offers a short discussion that is relevant for all health care providers.

References

Alberta Association of Registered Nurses (AARN): Professional boundaries for registered nurses, position statement, September, 1998.

Anderson KN, Anderson LE, Glanze WD: *Mosby's medical, nursing, and allied health dictionary,* ed 5, St. Louis, 1998, Mosby.

Dufault K, Martocchio BC: Hope, its spheres and dimensions, *Nursing Clinics of North America* (2):379, 1985.

Forman L: Medication: reasons and interventions for noncompliance, *Journal of Psychosocial Nursing and Mental Health Services* 31(10):23, 1993.

Pilette PC, Berck CB, Achber LC: Therapeutic management of helping boundaries, *Journal of Psychosocial Nursing and Mental Health Services* 33:40, 1995.

Spencer PU: A native American worldview. In McNeill B, editor: *Noetic Sciences Collection 1980-1990,* Sausalito, Calif, 1991, The Institute of Noetic Sciences.

Stuart GW, Laraia MT: *Principles and practice of psychiatric nursing,* ed 7, St. Louis, 2001, Mosby.

Sundeen SJ and others: *Nurse-client interaction,* ed 6, St. Louis, 1998, Mosby.

Taylor CM: *Essentials of psychiatric nursing,* ed 14, St. Louis, 1994, Mosby.

Travelbee J: *Interpersonal aspects of nursing,* Philadelphia, 1971, FA Davis.

Vellenga BA, Christenson J: Persistent and severely mentally ill clients' perceptions of their mental illness, *Issues in Mental Health Nursing* 15:359, 1994.

Chapter 11

Therapeutic Communication

Learning Objectives

1. Describe two theories of communication.
2. Identify two types of communication.
3. List the five components or parts of any communication.
4. Compare the characteristics of verbal and nonverbal communications.
5. Identify three interventions for communicating with people who do not speak English.
6. List eight principles of therapeutic communication.
7. Describe eight therapeutic communication skills.
8. Name three techniques for communicating with clients who have mental-emotional problems.

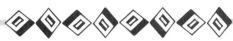

Key Terms

aphasia
communication
communication style
disturbed communications
dyslexia
feedback

incongruent communications
interpersonal communications
intrapersonal communications
nontherapeutic communications
nonverbal communication
perception

responding strategies
speech cluttering
therapeutic communications
verbal communication

Communication is an essential component of survival for all creatures. Research has demonstrated that when a tree is attacked by insects, it sends a chemical message to other trees in the area. Animals communicate in subtle and complex ways using both sound and movement; but the master communicator, the user of language, is the human being. Infants are born communicating with their first squall, and the elderly die listening to the last communications in a world they are about to leave. The fulfillment of human basic needs requires interactions with others. To meet even the most basic needs for food and water requires the cooperative efforts of people, which is achieved through communication and understanding. "**Communication** refers to the reciprocal exchange of information, ideas, beliefs, feelings, and attitudes between two persons or among a group of persons" (Taylor, 1994). All people communicate, but members of the health care professions modify ordinary

communications to promote the health of their clients and practice therapeutic communications based on certain principles. Those who work with the mentally and emotionally troubled refine their therapeutic communication skills to become highly skilled listeners "who can plan and carry out interactions specifically designed to achieve client outcomes" (Rawlins, Williams, and Beck, 1993). In this chapter we explore the elements and skills of therapeutically designed communication techniques.

The study of interactions between human beings has been a source of interest for centuries. Paintings on the walls of caves attest to prehistoric man's desire for communication. The introduction of the printing press during the fifteenth century made mass production of the written word possible. As people learned to read and write, learning evolved from an oral form to a visual one. Communications became more complex and a step removed from face-to-face interpersonal contact.

The inventions of the telegraph, telephone, radio, and television made information available to everyone. Today, satellite communications, interactive computers, and "the Internet" are moving communications and information exchanges into new and unknown realms. Tomorrow's technological developments will move us further, but the need for effective verbal and nonverbal communication skills will never be replaced by technology.

THEORIES OF COMMUNICATION

Probably one of the earliest theorists on therapeutic communications was Florence Nightingale, whose book *Notes on Nursing* emphasized the need to effectively understand and communicate with patients. However, the rest of the medical world placed little focus on the value of interacting therapeutically until the 1950s, when the publication of several theories sparked an interest in client-caregiver communications.

Ruesch's Theory

A theory of communication that considers communications as the social matrix (framework) for health care was developed by J. Ruesch in the late 1950s. He believed that communication was a circular process in which messages traveled from within one person to another person and back again.

Events within the sender prompt the sending of a message. The message is then transmitted to another who receives it, processes it internally, and responds. Successful communications occur when agreement about the meaning of the message has been reached. Communications are unsuccessful when there is a lack of agreement or understanding about the message. Ruesch (1961) coined the term **disturbed communications** to describe unsuccessful interactions resulting from an interference in the sending or receiving of messages, inadequate mastery of the language being used, insufficient information, or little or no opportunity for feedback.

Therapeutic communications are distinguished from ordinary communications by the intent of one of the participants to bring about a positive change. According to Ruesch's point of view, a therapist is one who directs the exchanges to bring about more satisfying social relations. Therapists seek to find the nature of clients' distresses and develop an understanding of their problems. Then, with the use of therapeutic communication techniques, both the client and the therapist agree on the nature of the problem and what should be done about it. Many of Ruesch's ideas are useful for interacting with clients.

Transactional Analysis

In 1964 Dr. Eric Berne, a physician with training in psychoanalysis, published *Games People Play*, which became a best seller even though it was not intended for the general public (Berne, 1964a). In the book Berne used the term *transactional analysis* to refer to the process of investigating what people say and do to each other. Berne also believed that three ego states exist within all of us: the parent (P) who focuses on rules and values, the child (C) who focuses on emotions and desires, and the adult (A) who bases his or her approach to the world on previous observations. These ego states make up one's individual personality, and Berne coined the term *structural analysis* to refer to the study of the personality. See Box 11-1 for an example of each communication type.

Many of the interactions in which people engage, Berne noticed, have ulterior or hidden motives used to manipulate others. He labeled these manipulations psychological *games* and *rackets* and offered his game analysis to refer to the hidden interactions that lead to a payoff.

The main goal of transactional analysis, according to Berne, is to "establish the most open and authentic communication possible between the affective (feeling) and intellectual components of the personality" (Berne, 1964b). Analyzing one's structure, transactions, and games encourages people to gain insight and determine what changes are most desirable. Because Berne (like Maslow) believed that every person needs positive feedback or "strokes" to thrive, he encouraged communications that are positive in nature. This approach is particularly valuable for nurses and other health care professionals. The focus on one's abilities (instead of disabilities) fosters more effective and satisfying communications for everyone involved with the client.

Neurolinguistic Programming

Much of the basis for neurolinguistic programming lies in the work of Milton H. Erickson who, until his death in 1980, was considered a great medical hypnotist. To find the keys to his success, Richard Bandler and John Grinder spent several years doing careful analyses of Erickson's work and extensive writings. Using their observations as a framework, they developed a method for analyzing an individual's system of communication based on the theory that any effective communication is a state of hypnosis. Effective communications alter a person's state of consciousness. The Think About box presents an exercise that demonstrates this point.

Box 11-1 ◈ **Transactional Analysis Communications**

Parent: I told you that was a foolish thing to do.
Child: I just was trying get what I wanted.
Adult: In the past, this is what worked for me.

If your answer is "yes" to any of these questions, then the communication was successful. The pattern of communication in the paragraph altered your state of consciousness, which allowed you to share an experience. This is the "hypnosis" of neurolinguistic programming.

By learning an individual's communication patterns, one is able to achieve more effective and fulfilling interactions. Patterns include eye-accessing clues (ways in which people move their eyes while thinking), different language patterns, and the pace and rhythm of speech. Health care providers are finding neurolinguistic programming to be a powerful tool for communicating.

Other theories of communication focus on the use of body language (kinesics), how people use their space (proxemics), and channels of communication. Becoming familiar with several theories allows caregivers to expand and improve their communication skills and abilities.

CHARACTERISTICS OF COMMUNICATION

Communication is the act of sending and receiving information. When this definition is applied to a computer or some other mechanical mover of data, the interaction is simple. One machine contacts the other, data are

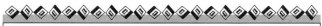

Think About

Picture yourself in the forest, surrounded by tall, stately trees. You look up to see the sun filtering through the dense canopy of tree branches. Below you the forest floor is dappled with sunlight and shade patterns dance slowly across your shoes. The air is cool and musty, damp from the mist left from the night. The world is silent except for the chirping of a lone songbird.

◆ What did you experience when you were reading the above paragraph?
◆ Did you actually experience a moment in the forest?
◆ Do you wish that you could go there yourself?

exchanged, and the interaction is over. With people, however, the information exchange is much more complex. Human behaviors have strong influences on communications.

Types of Communication

People engage in two types of communications: intrapersonal and interpersonal. Each may occur singly or in combination, and each may be used in effective or maladaptive ways.

Intrapersonal communications take place within oneself and are commonly referred to as our "self-talk" or "self-dialogue." They are conversations that we have with ourselves when solving problems, making plans, and reacting emotionally. Intrapersonal communications are adaptive when they help us cope or focus our energies in specific directions. When dysfunctional, they can result in altered states of functioning. Hallucinations are an example of dysfunctional intrapersonal communications.

Our intrapersonal communications affect our interactions with others. If your intrapersonal communications are upbeat and optimistic, then your interactions with clients will be too. If your self-talk is negative and glum, your communications will reflect this.

Interpersonal communications are interactions that occur between two or more persons. They are the verbal and nonverbal messages that are sent and received during every interaction. Symbols, language, culture, and behaviors have an impact on communications among people. As a result, interpersonal communications are complex and sophisticated. No matter what the communication, the importance of each message lies in its clarity. Clear communications offer a greater chance of success in every interaction.

Process of Communication

For a successful communication to occur, five elements must be in place (Figure 11-1). There must be a *sender* who forms the *message* and *transmits* it. A *receiver* is necessary to accept the message and respond in return. **Feedback** refers to the responses of each person

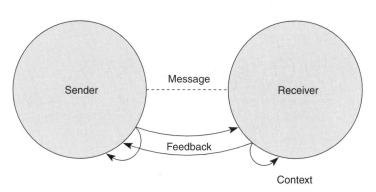

Figure 11-1 Components of the communication process. (Redrawn from Sundeen SJ and others: *Nurse-client interactions: implementing the nursing process*, ed 6, St. Louis, 1998, Mosby.)

when messages are being sent and received. Last, though not an actual part of the message, the *context* or setting in which the communication takes place must also be considered.

When a message is sent, a whole chain of events is triggered. First, *perception* is needed to recognize the presence of a message. **Perception** refers to the use of the senses to gain information. Vision, hearing, and touch are used to sense the meaning of the communication. A person's perceptions can be affected by many factors, including past experiences, emotional states, and physical problems.

The second step in the process of communicating is *evaluation,* the internal assessment of the message. All overt and hidden messages are considered and then compared with past experiences. The result is an emotional reaction to the message and preparation to return a message to the sender.

Transmission (a response) is the last step in the communication process. It includes conscious and unconscious responses to the message received. As the receiver of the message responds with a message of his or her own, the cycle begins again and is repeated with every interaction. If a person has difficulty with any step of the communication process—perceiving, evaluating, or transmitting messages—a communication problem may exist. Alert caregivers are aware of each client's process of communication and are prepared to intervene when clients are having communication difficulties.

Factors That Influence Communication

The process of interacting with others is influenced by many factors, but among the most important are culture (see Chapter 4), social class, relationships, perceptions, values, and parts of the message.

The *social class* to which one belongs has a profound influence on communications. People of various social classes interact using their own terminology, slang, cliches, rate of speech, gestures, and appearances. This variation in communication patterns can create problems for health care providers who interact with clients from social classes different from their own. Caregivers should be careful not to label clients based on their communications.

Communicating with clients from different social classes requires effort and patience. Both the care provider and client will feel misunderstood and attempt to withdraw unless steps are taken to establish effective communication exchanges. Box 11-2 lists several nursing interventions for interacting with people from different social classes.

Relationships affect communications because of the level of relatedness of each person involved in the interaction. Levels of relatedness refer to the degree of intimacy, authority, and role status of the communicators.

Box 11-2 🔷 **Communicating With Clients From Different Social Classes**

Show acceptance and respect for the person.

Consider the environment in which clients must cope, especially those from social classes of poverty.

Assess the client's patterns of communication, verbal and nonverbal.

Use terms the client can understand. Avoid using medical terminology.

Do not talk "up" or "down" to clients.

Ask clients to clarify any terms that are not understood.

Invite the client to take an active part in the treatment plan and its activities.

People communicate differently with strangers than they do with family members.

Perception*s* and values color one's communications. One's internal experiences (an individual's view of the world), when combined with the personal rules by which one lives *(values),* results in a unique frame of reference for communicating. It is important for caregivers to remember that it may be their perceptions that are impeding effective communication.

The content and context of a message have a strong impact on communications. The *content* of a message is the information being sent. The receiver of the message is affected by its content and must choose an appropriate reaction. The receiver can recognize the communications, ignore it, or change the subject. An awareness of the emotional impact related to the content of messages helps caregivers communicate more effectively with clients, especially those with mental-emotional difficulties.

Communications are also affected by the *context,* or environment, in which they take place. Care providers who expect clients to share personal information about themselves must provide an environment that fosters privacy. The day room or lounge is not a place for self-disclosure. Becoming aware of the context helps to send and receive messages with greater success. Many other factors, such as one's appearance, expressions, and body movements also have an impact on communications.

LEVELS OF COMMUNICATION

Communicating is an energy exchange that takes place on several levels. Each person involved in the sending and receiving of messages is a unique personality who interacts on verbal and nonverbal levels at one time. Communications at both levels occur with every person-to-person interaction.

Verbal Communication

Verbal communication relates to anything associated with the spoken word. Verbal communications include speaking, writing, the use of language and symbols, and the arrangement of words or phrases.

For many clients with mental-emotional problems, communicating with others can be difficult. Certain clients have difficulties in perceiving. The person who is experiencing hallucinations, for example, may be unable to understand a message is being sent because the communications within his or her inner world are drowning out the messages from the reality outside.

Understanding verbal messages involves the ability to form abstract ideas and concepts. People with schizophrenia often have great difficulty with abstraction and using words that are reality oriented. Transmitting messages is a problem for many depressed clients; identifying and verbalizing how they feel is commonly stated in one or two words.

Although verbal communication is the most overt or obvious form of interaction, it actually represents only a small part of an entire communication. Words are only symbols; they do not have the same meaning to all people. To make matters more complicated, the problem intensifies as words become more abstract. Emotions are an excellent example of abstractions that cannot be easily communicated on the verbal level. This is an important point for caregivers to remember. If communications are to be effective, you must understand the client's meaning of the word.

Nonverbal Communication

Messages sent and received without the use of words define **nonverbal communication.** The nonverbal level includes one's messages created through the body's motions; eye contact and movement; gestures; and use of touch, space, and sight.

Messages sent at the nonverbal level are expressed in at least one of four ways: appearance, body motions, use of space, and nonlanguage sounds. One's appearance can convey strong nonverbal messages. The state of hygiene and personal grooming habits, choice of clothing and accessories, hairstyle, and jewelry send messages. Facial expressions, gestures, posture, and use of the body can communicate one's emotions more easily than words. Caregivers who are aware of this are careful to use their nonverbal behaviors therapeutically. For example, notice the position of your body when you are interacting with someone you find unpleasant. Are your arms crossed? Is your body position open and inviting communication or closed with crossed legs or an angled stance? The use of space and distance (see Chapter 4) communicates concepts such as authority and intimacy. Nonlanguage sounds are verbalizations without words. The scream of a woman and the grunt of someone lifting

Cultural Aspects

Sidney Jourard (1971) studied the cultural differences relating to the use of touch by observing the behaviors of pairs of people in coffee shops throughout the world. Observations revealed that more touch occurred in certain cities.

City	Couples touched (times/hr)
San Juan, Puerto Rico	180
Paris, France	110
Gainesville, Florida	2
London, England	0

a heavy load do not rely on words to convey their messages.

In short, the nonverbal level of communications include everything outside the realm of speaking, writing, or singing. It is a subtle world, rich in variation. The more caregivers are able to recognize and use the nonverbal level of communication, the more effective their interventions will become. Each level of communication, verbal and nonverbal, sends and receives messages during every interaction. If messages are successfully sent and received, the results are communications rich in variety and complexity.

INTERCULTURAL COMMUNICATION

When communicating with people from other cultures, care providers must take special considerations to ensure understanding. How people communicate is based on their cultural backgrounds, language systems, and social patterns. Cultures are transmitted through communication, and cultures define how emotions are expressed and shared. The use of touch and other nonverbal forms of communication varies considerably with different cultures (see Cultural Aspects box).

Cultures, and the social groups within them, have variations in the use of verbal and nonverbal communications. Caregivers who work with clients from culturally different backgrounds should resist the tendency to stereotype people and to learn the most culturally appropriate methods for communication.

Intercultural Differences

To fulfill basic needs, people must interact and communicate with each other. For people of differing cultures, this interacting with others can be a difficult process. Communication styles, nonverbal behaviors, and values, as well as the use of the language, are areas in which cultural communications basically differ.

Case Study

Sarah had been working with clients on the reservation for almost 6 months. During her interviews with clients, she had great difficulty in obtaining information, although she knew she was practicing good interviewing skills and attending behaviors.

One morning, she was discussing her problem with the reservation physician, who had been working with her clients for several years. He asked, "How is your eye contact?" "Good," she replied. "I always look clients in the eye when interviewing and express interest in what they say—when I can get them to talk to me." "That is your problem, then," her physician replied. "These people believe that it is an invasion of privacy to give direct eye contact, especially if you are not a member of their group. Try looking at their feet. It will convey respect and they may be more likely to communicate with you."

Sarah followed the suggestion and soon her clients began sharing important health information.

◆ How could Sarah have prevented this situation from occurring?

Communication style refers to the rituals connected with greeting and departure, the lines of conversation, and the directness of communication (Giger and Davidizar, 1999). Greeting rituals should be assessed by considering the process of the greeting interaction, including the use of compliments and physical behaviors such as touching, handshaking, or kissing. The Case Study demonstrates this point.

Are the lines of communication linear or circular? *Linear communication styles* come directly to the point. To illustrate, most Anglo-American men favor an open and frank conversation style, whereas Thai Americans favor a more circular line of communication known as *kreng jai,* a consideration for the feelings and needs of others.

Circular communication styles direct the conversation in circles around the main point. Often, the main point is left unstated. Once the important information has been communicated, it is assumed that the receiver got the point. This style is often found in Oriental and far Eastern cultures. "There's a fire in the wastebasket" is an example of a linear message, whereas "I saw someone drop a match in the wastebasket earlier; now it appears to be smoking" illustrates a circular style of communication.

The directness and openness with which people solve their problems influence communications. Are problems communicated directly, communicated in a circular manner, or denied and ignored? How appropriate is it to state an opinion or offer help?

Cultural differences affect the nonverbal tone of the receiver. Body language, such as eye contact, gestures, and distance, are culturally determined. Much of the message is lost when one does not understand the communications of the body.

Values guide many communications within cultures. They help determine whether the individual or the group is more important and how individuals of various statuses should be treated. How individuals from various cultures use time is an example of cultural value that affects communications.

Religious beliefs and practices can also affect communications. For example, followers of Buddhism may not share that they are in pain because they believe their suffering is due to a failure of righteousness.

Cultures that place a high value on nonverbal communications practice "high-context" communications whereby nonverbal cues and sensitivity play a larger role than the actual verbal message. Cultures that practice "low context" communications tend to focus more on the words rather than the emotional tone of the message.

Another major cultural communication difference is the use of a society's language. Language use considers a culture's use of names and titles; the structure of grammar; the use of vocabulary, jargon, and slang; and vocal qualities such as tones, pronunciation, rhythm, and speed of communications. The meaning of silence also varies from culture to culture (Pore, 1995). Caregivers need to be aware of the meanings of culturally different communications. The effectiveness of the therapeutic relationship depends on it.

Improving Communication

Communications are improved by the following (Bennett, 1994):

1. Recognize what is different from your own cultural style.
2. Adapt your behavior to accommodate the difference.
3. Call attention to the difference to explain the confusion in communication.

The most important intervention for communicating with culturally different clients is an acceptance of the client as a person and a willingness to work toward the therapeutic goals of care.

THERAPEUTIC COMMUNICATION SKILLS

The goals of **therapeutic communications** are to focus on the client and foster the therapeutic relationship. Therapeutic communication techniques are skills that assist care providers to effectively interact with clients. Each therapeutic communication skill is based on the eight principles of therapeutic communication: acceptance, interest, respect, honesty, concreteness, assistance, permission, and protection (Table 11-1). The principles of therapeutic communication serve as guidelines for effective interac-

Table 11-1	Principles of Therapeutic Communication	
Principle	**Illustration**	**Example**
Acceptance	Accepting caregivers communicate a favorable reception of another person by implying, "You have a right to exist, to live your life, to have somebody care about you." One does not have to approve of another's behavior to be accepting. It is only when people feel accepted for what they are that they will consider changing.	*Client:* I know it's been destructive for me to live with my parents, and I get irresponsible living there, but I feel like that's where I need to go after I leave the hospital. *Caregiver:* I may not agree with your decision about where to live, but I accept your choice to do that and will work with you to evaluate how it works out for you.
Interest	Caregivers communicate interest when they express a desire to know another person. Interest is conveyed by asking about those aspects of a person's life that others often reject. Caregivers communicate by their attitude that "everything can be talked about here."	*Client:* I'm so ashamed of what I've done, I can't tell you about it. You won't ever talk to me again! *Caregiver:* Sandy, I'm interested in everything about you, the good, the bad, the sad, the happy. This is not just a "good times only" relationship. You and I have committed to working on a number of issues of importance, and I have a feeling that this is one of them. So why not go ahead and begin?
Respect	Caregivers show consideration for another by communicating their willingness to work with the client and accept the client's ideas, feelings, and rights. It is communicated by listening attentively, expressing belief in the client's ability to solve personal problems with assistance and assume responsibility for his or her own life, collaborating on shared goals, calling the client by name, arriving and leaving on time, and keeping one's word. False reassurance and critical judgment are to be avoided.	*Client:* I know it's silly for me to feel so frightened about living alone, but I'm terrified. *Caregiver:* I could tell you that you have nothing to worry about, that you'll do just fine. But, I hear your terror, your voice is shaking, and you're all perspired. It must be hard to imagine being able to survive on your own after being married for 30 years.
Honesty	Caregivers are honest when they are consistent, open, and frank. They communicate with the client as an authentic person. They use tact and timing in judging the use of honesty so that clients are not burdened with information or feedback they are not ready to hear. Caregivers are honest and nondefensive about their thoughts and feelings that they discover through self-assessment.	*Client:* I hate the way he treats me; he takes me for granted, leaving and not telling me when he's coming home. It will never change. *Caregiver:* Carol, we've discussed this pattern before, and the alternative ways for dealing with the situation. Quite honestly, I think a major reason for Lou's not changing his behavior is that you allow him to continue it. *Client:* What do you mean? *Caregiver:* I mean that unless or until you let him know that his behavior is unacceptable, why should he change? This way he doesn't have to be accountable to anyone, even his wife.
Concreteness	Concrete caregivers are specific, to the point, and clear when they communicate. They use understandable language and avoid the use of jargon. Clients who speak in vague, general, unfocused ways are helped to be more specific and focused.	*Client:* I feel sort of uneasy, I get a feeling like . . . that every so often . . . (perspiring, wringing hands, tapping feet) *Caregiver:* Describe the feeling for me in detail.
Assistance	Caregivers assist clients by committing time and energy to therapeutic relationships. They convey that they are present and available and have tangible aid to offer that will help the client choose and develop more functional ways of living.	*Caregiver:* While you're in the hospital, you and I will be meeting every day at 2 PM for 45 minutes. I am available to you to help you work out the problems that are bothering you. I'll also see you lots of other times, since I work on the unit. I hope you'll feel free to approach me if you need something.

From Haber J and others: *Comprehensive psychiatric nursing*, ed 5, St. Louis, 1998, Mosby.   *Continued*

Table 11-1 Principles of Therapeutic Communication—cont'd		
Principle	**Illustration**	**Example**
Permission	Caregivers communicate permission by conveying the message that it is acceptable to try new ways of behaving. Often clients are afraid to choose freely and act autonomously. They are bound by misconceived archaic rules and magical thinking and need to be given permission and encouragement to see and do things in new ways.	*Client:* How can I suddenly trust people when I've been hurt so badly in the past? *Caregiver:* Clarify for me who hurt you? *Client:* Well, my brother, you know how he hurt me. *Caregiver:* Yes, I do know that. What about other people. Can you tell me about them? *Client:* Well, I can't tell you any others specifically. It's just the way I feel about people. *Caregiver:* I think you may be looking at other people and seeing your brother in them. You might be bringing the past into the present.
Protection	Caregivers protect clients by ensuring clients' safety. Caregivers assume responsibility of working with clients to anticipate trouble spots with new behavior and develop effective ways of dealing with anticipated or actual problems, thus maximizing the possibility of success.	*Client:* I'm really scared to go home on my pass this weekend. What will people say? How will they expect me to behave? *Caregiver:* I hear that you're scared, and that's very natural for you to feel. Let's work together to try to anticipate what will happen over the weekend and see if, together, you and I can come up with some strategies for dealing with those "hot spots."

From Haber J and others: *Comprehensive psychiatric nursing,* ed 5, St. Louis, 1998, Mosby.

tions. Refer to them often as they will help you cope with the complexities of communication.

Therapeutic communication techniques are divided into two equally important areas: listening skills and interacting skills. Each is vital if communications are to be clearly understood and therapeutic actions are to be successful.

Listening Skills

In our fast-paced, time-oriented world, people are so intent on sending their messages that they seldom take the time to listen, to truly hear what the other person is trying to communicate. The art of listening is a necessary ingredient for every health care provider, not just those who work in psychiatry. Effective listening improves caregivers' abilities to meet their clients' needs. In addition, effective listening can identify hidden messages and agendas, minimize misunderstandings, and clarify messages. Although it may require time and practice to perfect your therapeutic listening skills, the rewards are worth the efforts (Box 11-3).

To polish your listening skills, first concentrate on the speaker. Next, listen objectively. Many words call forth emotional responses that can color communications. Learn which words trigger your emotional responses. This awareness helps you to remain tuned in and attentive to the speaker even when an emotional button has been pushed. Use appropriate eye contact and body language. Remember the speaker's cultural background. Maintaining a relaxed body position at eye level with the speaker

---

Box 11-3 Therapeutic Listening Skills

Concentrate on the speaker and the message.
Keep distractions and interruptions to a minimum.
Change the setting (environment) if necessary.
Assess nonverbal communications and metacommunications.
Listen objectively.
Discover which words trigger emotional responses in you.
Use eye contact and body language that is culturally appropriate.
Do not interrupt. Let the speaker finish delivering the message.
Jot down notes if needed.
Do not assume that you have understood another person's thoughts.
Clarify any message about which you are unsure.

---

communicates acceptance and interest. Make sure that your nonverbal messages match the verbal messages. If at all possible, do not interrupt. Let the speaker be fully expressive. Jot down notes for clarification later, but let the speaker finish. If time becomes a problem and you must interrupt, explain that the conversation is important but your time is limited. Follow up with telling the speaker when you will return to finish the conversation.

Box 11-4 Therapeutic Communication Techniques

Listening

Definition: Active process of receiving information and examining reaction to messages received
Example: Maintaining eye contact and receptive nonverbal communication
Therapeutic value: Nonverbally communicates caregiver's interest and acceptance
Nontherapeutic threat: Failure to listen

Broad Openings

Definition: Encouraging client to select topics for discussion
Example: "What are you thinking about?"
Therapeutic value: Indicates acceptance by caregiver and value of client's initiative
Nontherapeutic threat: Domination of interaction by nurse; rejecting responses

Restating

Definition: Repeating main thought the client expressed
Example: "You say that your mother left you when you were 5 years old?"
Therapeutic value: Indicates that caregiver is listening and validates, reinforces, or calls attention to something important that has been said
Nontherapeutic threat: Lack of validation of caregiver's interpretation of message; being judgmental; reassuring; defending

Clarification

Definition: Attempting to put into words vague ideas or unclear thoughts of client to enhance caregiver's understanding; asking client to explain what he or she means
Example: "I'm not sure what you mean. Could you tell me about that again?"

Therapeutic value: Helps to clarify feelings, ideas, and perceptions of client and provide explicit correlation between them and client's actions
Nontherapeutic threat: Failure to probe; assumed understanding

Reflection

Definition: Directing back client's ideas, feelings, questions, and content
Example: "You're feeling tense and anxious and it's related to a conversation you had with your husband last night?"
Therapeutic value: Validates caregiver's understanding of what client is saying and signifies empathy, interest, and respect for client
Nontherapeutic threat: Stereotyping client's responses; inappropriate timing of reflections; inappropriate depth of feeling of reflections; inappropriate responses to cultural experience and educational level of client

Humor

Definition: Discharge of energy through comic enjoyment
Example: "That gives a whole new meaning to the word nervous," said with shared kidding between caregiver and client
Therapeutic value: Can promote insight by making conscious repressed material, resolving paradoxes, tempering aggression, and revealing new options; is socially acceptable form of sublimation
Nontherapeutic threat: Indiscriminate use; belittling client; screen to avoid therapeutic intimacy

Informing

Definition: Skill of information giving
Example: "I think you need to know more about how your medication works."

Modified from Stuart GW, Laraia MT: *Principles and practice of psychiatric nursing*, ed 7, St. Louis, 2001, Mosby.

Continued

The last and most important guideline for becoming an effective listener is to clarify what the speaker said. If you are uncertain about what was communicated, ask for clarification. Clarification is a primary therapeutic communication technique that, when used in combination with good listening skills, enhances every caregiver's abilities to successfully interact with clients.

Interacting Skills

Therapeutic techniques that relate to the care provider's actions while communicating are called **responding strategies** or interaction skills. These are the verbal and nonverbal responses that encourage clients to communicate in a way that will encourage their growth. When

using therapeutic interactions, caregivers use words that have meaning to the client. Communications are direct and related to the situation. Messages have a clear meaning, are easily understood, and allow enough time for a response. Questions do not contain the word *why* because it requires a response that justifies one's actions or opinions.

There are twelve commonly used therapeutic communication techniques (Stuart and Laraia, 2001). They are often referred to as responding strategies because their use encourages clients to continue communicating. Carefully study the information in Box 11-4.

Practice these techniques with clients, peers, and even people outside the health care environment, and note the results. With patience and practice, these techniques

Box 11-4   Therapeutic Communication Techniques—cont'd

Therapeutic value: Helpful in health teaching or client education about relevant aspects of client's well-being and self-care
Nontherapeutic threat: Giving advice

Focusing

Definition: Questions or statements that help client expand on topic of importance
Example: "I think that we should talk more about your relationship with your father."
Therapeutic value: Allows client to discuss central issues; keeps communication process goal-directed
Nontherapeutic threat: Allowing abstractions and generalizations; changing topics

Sharing Perceptions

Definition: Asking client to verify caregiver's understanding of what client is thinking or feeling
Example: "You're smiling, but I sense that you are really very angry with me."
Therapeutic value: Conveys caregiver's understanding to client and has potential for clearing up confusing communication
Nontherapeutic threat: Challenging client; accepting literal responses; reassuring; testing; defending

Theme Identification

Definition: Underlying issues or problems experienced by client that emerge repeatedly during course of caregiver-client relationship
Example: "I've noticed that in all of the relationships that you have described, you've been hurt or rejected by a man. Do you think this is an underlying issue?"
Therapeutic value: Allows caregiver to best promote client's exploration and understanding of important problems
Nontherapeutic threat: Giving advice; reassuring; disapproving

Silence

Definition: Lack of verbal communication for therapeutic reason
Example: Sitting with client and nonverbally communicating interest and involvement
Therapeutic value: Allows client time to think and gain insights; slows pace of interaction and encourages client to initiate conversation, while conveying support, understanding, and acceptance
Nontherapeutic threat: Questioning client; failure to break nontherapeutic silence

Suggesting

Definition: Presentation of alternative ideas for client's consideration relative to problem solving
Example: "Have you thought about responding to your boss in a different way when he raises that issue with you? For example, you could ask him if a specific problem has occurred."
Therapeutic value: Increases client's perceived options or choices
Nontherapeutic threat: Giving advice; inappropriate timing; being judgmental

Modified from Stuart GW, Laraia MT: *Principles and practice of psychiatric nursing,* ed 7, St. Louis, 2001, Mosby.

become important tools for effectively interacting with all clients.

NONTHERAPEUTIC COMMUNICATION

Messages that hinder effective communication are called **nontherapeutic communications.** They are interactions that slow or halt the development of the helping relationship. Nontherapeutic communications include barriers that arise within the environment, the caregiver or the client, and the responses that block further communications.

Barriers to Communication

Barriers to effective interactions can arise during each step of the communication process. They are protective behaviors when one feels threatened. The problem with their use is that they are likely to increase the client's "self-exposure, insecurity, and helpless-

ness" (Haber and others, 1997). If allowed to go unchecked, the use of barriers will smother the therapeutic relationship and prevent the client from reaching the treatment goals.

Because the environment is difficult to control, it can often have a negative effect on communications. It may be too noisy or crowded for the sharing of personal information. Sometimes the client will attempt to send an important message in an inappropriate setting. For example, while waiting in line at the lunchroom, your client announces that he is leaving his wife. In this instance, the environment acts as a barrier to further exploration because of the noise level and lack of privacy.

Problems with the individuals involved in the communication can arise. The caregiver may be physically tired or would prefer not to interact with the client. Such feelings may lead to **incongruent communications,** in which the verbal messages being sent do not match the nonverbal communications. Incongruent communications can be sent by either the client or the caregiver, but it is the caregiver's responsibility to match each level of his or her communication with the message.

On occasion, a client will refuse to communicate or cooperate. This lack of cooperation erects a large barrier and prevents other people from attempting to interact. Such a client requires extra patience and repeated messages of acceptance. With time and persistence, clients usually become more willing to interact because no person likes to be cut off from their fellow human beings.

The following are methods for coping with the barriers to communications:

1. Recognize that a problem exists.
2. Identify what purpose or need the problem is filling.
3. Explore appropriate alternative behaviors.
4. Implement the alternative behaviors when interacting.
5. Evaluate whether therapeutic communications have improved. If they have not, reassess and try another approach. Being aware of communication barriers allows caregivers to intervene early and effectively.

Nontherapeutic Communication Techniques

According to Sundeen and others (1998), nontherapeutic communications are problems of omission or commission. Nontherapeutic communication techniques of *omission* relate to the caregiver's failure to do something (e.g., to use a therapeutic technique) when the moment is right. Communication acts of omission include failure to listen, probe, elicit descriptions, or explore the client's point of view. Giving vague descriptions and inadequate answers, parroting, and following the standard forms too closely are also considered in this category.

Those nontherapeutic techniques in which the caregiver communicates in an undesirable manner fall into the category of nontherapeutic communications of *commission*. They include giving advice or disapproval, being defensive, making judgments, patronizing, making stereotyped responses, reassuring, or rejecting client messages. Table 11-2 lists several nontherapeutic communication techniques.

Become an observer of your own communications. See if your verbal and nonverbal communications send the same message. Evaluate your use of different techniques and enhance your ability to effectively communicate.

PROBLEMS WITH COMMUNICATION

For many people, communicating with others can be a difficult process. *Sensory-impaired clients* have difficulty receiving or sending messages because of problems with sight, hearing, or understanding. The first step in interacting with sensory-deprived individuals is to achieve a successful introduction. If the client knows your name and purpose, cooperation is more likely. If possible, learn how the client communicates (signing, writing, touch), then encourage him or her to become actively involved in the communication process. Maintain good eye contact and attentive nonverbal behaviors. Communicate directly with the client. Do not try to finish the client's sentence or fill in words. Allow extra time for the client to think and form responses. Last, do not forget the importance of the use of touch. For people who have diminished sight or hearing, touch is a powerful method of communication.

Some people may have problems with sending messages. Persons with **aphasia** (inability to speak), **dyslexia** (impaired ability to read sometimes accompanied by a mixing of letters or syllables in a word when speaking), and **speech cluttering** (rapid, confused delivery of unrhythmic speech patterns) cannot focus on verbal communications as their main form of human interaction. Therefore it is important for the caregiver to tune into the client's nonverbal behaviors and become extra alert for the messages being sent. For clients with communication problems, the speech therapist can be a valuable member of the multidisciplinary treatment team.

Communicating With Mentally Troubled Clients

Problems with communication are a common feature in many forms of mental illness. People with mental-emotional difficulties find it difficult to develop trust in other people. Loneliness is the companion of mental illness. Sincere, respectful caring of another person can help remove the barrier that isolates the mentally ill from the world.

To communicate effectively with mentally and emotionally troubled clients, caregivers realize that every interaction is a part of the total therapeutic process. A climate of trust and respect must be established before clients feel safe enough to honestly share themselves. Establishing this trusting climate requires patience, persistence, and, most important, consistency. Mental health clients need routine, the security of a dependable environment, and care providers with calm, reliable temperaments. This consistency satisfies basic needs and allows clients to focus on communicating.

Caregivers begin their interactions with mental health clients by introducing themselves and explaining their purpose. The caregiver then starts the conversation by introducing a neutral subject, such as weather, sports, or entertainment events and then waits quietly for the client to comment, using the opportunity to assess nonverbal behaviors or barriers to communication.

Once the client is communicating, the caregiver should avoid a verbal assault of questions. Data may have to be obtained but not at the expense of threatening the fragile communication line so recently established. As long as the client is interacting, necessary data will eventually be revealed and recorded.

Table 11-2　Nontherapeutic Communications

Nontherapeutic technique	Description	Example
Failure to listen	Placing own thoughts above client, not being involved in communication	Yawning when client is speaking, looking at watch frequently, missing client's messages
Failure to explore client's point of view	Does not ask client to describe abstract words such as *pain, angry, sick*	*Client:* "My head hurts." *Caregiver:* "You're just getting used to your new medication." *Better:* "Tell me more."
Failure to probe	Does not seek clarification or validation from client	*Client:* I've had bad experiences with doctors." *Caregiver:* "That's too bad." *Better:* "Would you like to explain?"
Eliciting vague descriptions	Does not encourage client to explain or expand on message	*Client:* "I keep hearing voices." *Caregiver:* "O.K." *Better:* "What do they say?"
Giving inadequate answers	Does not collect enough data to answer client's question accurately	Instructs client about medication then finds out he is allergic to it
Parroting	Continuous repeating of client's words	*Client:* "I haven't slept in 2 nights." *Caregiver:* "You haven't slept in 2 nights?" *Better:* "What do you think is causing this?"
Following standard forms too closely	Using a question-and-answer format to elicit specific information	*Caregiver:* "Do you have any problems chewing?" *Client:* "No, but I have this pain in my jaw at night." *Caregiver:* "Do you have any problems with indigestion or constipation?" *Better:* "Tell me about your jaw pain."
Being judgmental: giving approval, agreeing or disagreeing	Many responses that tell clients that they must think as you do	*Client:* "I saw my wife today." *Caregiver:* "You should be nicer to her." *Better:* "How did it go?"
Giving advice	Telling clients what to do; gives message that they are inferior and not able to make good decisions	*Client:* "I'm nervous about meeting Dr. Dow." *Caregiver:* "You just march in there and say what you want, but don't raise your voice." *Better:* "I can understand that."
Being defensive	An attempt to protect something or someone; prevents clients from communicating	*Client:* "That last nurse is a dope." *Caregiver:* "All of our nurses here are highly trained." *Better:* "What makes you think that?"
Challenging	Inviting or daring client to explain, act, or compete	*Client:* "I'm really dead, you know." *Caregiver:* "If you are really dead then why is your heart still beating?" *Better:* "You're dead?"
Giving reassurance	Messages that negate feelings of client and offer false hope	*Client:* "I'll never get out of here." *Caregiver:* "Everything will turn out for the best." *Better:* "You feel that you have been here a long time?"
Rejecting	Refusal to discuss feelings or areas of concern	*Client:* "You know that I raped my sister." *Caregiver:* "Let's not talk about that." *Better:* "Would you like to talk about it?"
Using stereotyped responses	Using cliches, popular sayings, or trite expressions	*Client:* "I feel so depressed today." *Caregiver:* "Everyone gets the blues now and then." *Better:* "What's making you feel so blue?"

Modified from Sundeen SJ and others: *Nurse-client interactions: implementing the nursing process,* ed 5, St. Louis, 1998, Mosby.

One of the most important tools for communicating with mentally ill clients is therapeutic listening. Attentive listening alone communicates acceptance and respect, messages not often received by mental health clients. Once the client believes that you sincerely care about him or her as a person, a flow of communications will come easily. A Sample Client Care Plan based on the use of therapeutic communication principles is presented below.

Assessing Communication

Because the flow of information between people occurs naturally, we seldom take the time to assess a client's abilities to communicate. However, a communication assessment is an important part of the mental health workup.

First, assess the client's ability to hear and speak. Second, note the content, quality, and pace of the client's speech. Is it coherent, logical, or easy to follow? Is the pace fast or slow? Is the volume loud, too soft, or whispered? Are there any physical speech problems, like stuttering? Are the number of words used excessive or few? How much time lapses before the client responds to your message? Can the client read or write? Is a *cultural communication* assessment necessary? The answers to these questions provide the caregiver with a solid database and offer valuable information that is used by the

---

⟫⟫⟫ Sample Client Care Plan — Communication

Assessment

History: Amy, a 30-year-old married woman, is suffering from depression. Currently, she refuses to speak or acknowledge anyone, including her husband and children. Today she is being admitted for evaluation and treatment of her depression.

Current Findings: An untidy woman who stares at the floor and does not respond to staff members' questions. Sighs frequently. Sits immobile in chair for long periods.

Multidisciplinary Diagnosis

Impaired verbal communications related to emotional state.

Planning/Goals

Amy will communicate her wishes and feelings with at least one staff member by April 22.

Therapeutic Interventions

Interventions	Rationale	Team Member
1. Present a calm, patient attitude rather than attempting to make Amy speak.	Helps decrease fears and anxieties; demonstrates respect and acceptance.	All
2. Actively listen, observe for verbal and nonverbal cues and behaviors.	Helps piece together communication methods in an effort to understand Amy's messages.	All
3. Encourage other ways of communicating, such as drawing or writing.	Demonstrates empathy, helps develop trust, and encourages communication.	All
4. Anticipate needs until Amy can communicate them.	Provides safety, comfort, and support; helps develops trust.	Nsg
5. Spend time (at least 15 minutes twice a day) with Amy in a private, quiet setting.	Promotes trust and interest; helps promote self-esteem.	Nsg
6. Praise any attempt to communicate.	Encourages communication and demonstrates interest.	All

Evaluation

The second day after admission, Amy began to draw. By the fourth day of hospitalization, she answered "yes" or "no" questions. On April 17, Amy was able to discuss her feelings with one nurse.

A complete client care plan includes several other diagnoses and interventions.

Table 11-3 Speech Patterns Associated With Psychiatric Problems

Speech pattern	Description	Example
Blocking	Loses train of thought, stops speaking because of unconscious block	"Then my father . . . what was I saying?"
Circumstantiality	Describes in too much detail, cannot be selective	When asked "How are you?" replies "My left hand aches a bit, my nose has been leaking, my hair won't stay in place . . ."
Echolalia	Repeats last word heard	"Please wait here" is responded to with "Here, here, here . . ."
Flight of ideas	Shifts rapidly between unrelated topics	"My cat is grey. The food here is good."
Loose associations	Speaks constantly, shifting between loosely related topics	"Martha married Jim who is a cook. I can cook. Cows are something that we can cook."
Mutism	Able to speak but remains silent	
Neologism	Coins new words and definitions	"Zargleves are good to eat" referring to any candy snack
Perseveration	Repeats single activity, cannot shift from one topic to another	Answers new question with previous question's answer
Pressured speech	Speech becomes fast, loud, rushed, and emphatic	Persons with mania often move and speak very rapidly with great urgency
Verbigeration	Repeats words, phrases, sentences several times over	*Nurse:* "It's time to take your pill." *Client:* "Take your pill, take your pill, take your pill . . ."

multidisciplinary treatment team to establish appropriate therapeutic goals. Table 11-3 describes some of the more common abnormal speech patterns demonstrated by clients with psychiatric problems.

The ability to effectively communicate is a most important therapeutic skill. Good communication skills must be practiced and evaluated frequently. To evaluate the effectiveness of your communications, assess each interaction. Ask yourself, "Was the interaction appropriate to the goals of care? Was there enough communication and feedback to meet the goals? Was the interaction flexible enough to allow for a balance between spontaneity and control? Was the communication effective?" Practice, patience, and a continual willingness to evaluate your interactions are the keys to developing effective communication skills. Work hard to become a good communicator. Your clients' well-being depends on it, no matter what the diagnosis.

KEY CONCEPTS

◆ Communication is the exchange of information between two persons or among a group of persons.
◆ In the 1960s Dr. Eric Berne coined the term *transactional analysis* to describe the process of investigating what people do and say to each other.
◆ Neurolinguistic programming focuses on learning the patterns of an individual's communications, which

include eye accessing clues, different language patterns, and the pace and rhythm of speech.
◆ For communication to occur, there must be a sender, a message, a receiver, feedback, and context.
◆ The process of communicating involves perception, evaluation, and transmission.
◆ Communications occur on verbal and nonverbal levels.
◆ Health care providers who work with clients from culturally different backgrounds must resist the tendency to stereotype people and learn culturally appropriate methods for communication.
◆ Therapeutic communication techniques are skills that assist caregivers to effectively interact with clients.
◆ The goals of therapeutic communications are to focus on the client and foster the therapeutic relationship.
◆ The art of listening is a necessary ingredient for every health care provider.
◆ Responding strategies are the verbal and nonverbal responses that encourage clients to communicate in ways that help them to grow.
◆ Messages that hinder effective communications are referred to as *nontherapeutic communications*.
◆ Sensory-impaired clients have difficulty receiving or sending messages.
◆ Problems with communication are a common feature of many forms of mental illness.

◆ To communicate effectively with psychiatric clients, the caregiver remembers that every interaction is a part of the total therapeutic process.

◆ Practice, patience, and a continual willingness to evaluate your interactions are the keys to developing effective communication skills.

Suggestions for Further Reading

Transcultural nursing: assessment and intervention by Giger and Davidizar, (ed 3, St. Louis, 1999, Mosby) is an excellent book, full of practical tips for communicating with people from different cultural backgrounds.

References

Bennett MJ: *Checklist for intercultural communications,* Portland, Oreg, 1994, The Intercultural Communication Institute.

Berne E: *Games people play: psychology of human relationships,* New York, 1964a, Grove Press.

Berne E: *Principles of group treatment,* New York, 1964b, Oxford University Press.

Giger JN, Davidizar RE: *Transcultural nursing: assessment and intervention,* ed 3, St. Louis, 1999, Mosby.

Haber J and others: *Comprehensive psychiatric nursing,* ed 5, St. Louis, 1997, Mosby.

Jourard S: *The transparent self,* New York, 1971, Van Nostrand.

Pore S: I can't understand what my patient is saying, *Advances in Nurse Practice* 3(7):47, 1995.

Rawlins RP, Williams SR, Beck CK: *Mental health-psychiatric nursing: a holistic life-cycle approach,* ed 3, St. Louis, 1993, Mosby.

Ruesch J: *Therapeutic communications,* New York, 1961, WW Norton.

Stuart GW, Laraia MT: *Principles and practice of psychiatric nursing,* ed 7, St. Louis, 2001, Mosby.

Sundeen SJ and others: *Nurse-client interactions: implementing the nursing process,* ed 6, St. Louis, 1998, Mosby.

Taylor CM: Essentials of psychiatric nursing, ed 14, St. Louis, 1994, Mosby.

Chapter 12

The Most Important Skill: Self-Awareness

Learning Objectives

1. List three characteristics of caring.
2. Describe how failure contributes to the development of insight.
3. Explain the concept of helping boundaries.
4. Identify three ways to prevent overinvolvement and codependency.
5. Discuss the importance of personal and professional commitments.
6. Describe three techniques for developing a positive mental attitude.
7. List six principles for nurturing yourself and other caregivers.
8. Identify four practices that help develop self-awareness.

Key Terms

acceptance
caring
commitment
compassion
confidence

conscience
courage
failure
insight
introspection

nurture
risk taking
self-awareness

Caregiving is seen by the public as a selfless service offered by knowledgeable and caring people. The actions that connect us as people are what clients remember about their caregivers. The care provider who sat with the grieving parent or comforted the anxious client is remembered long after the one who was friendly but casual.

For people with mental-emotional problems, the interactions of caregivers may serve as a vehicle for improved functioning and more satisfying relationships. Caregivers serve as therapeutic instruments, with each interaction designed to move clients toward the goals of care. They also serve as role models for good mental and physical health. They are expected to help solve problems while graciously coping with the varied personalities of many individuals. Caregivers work to instill confidence in their clients and encourage them to change, trying new behaviors within the security of the therapeutic relationship.

To practice effectively, a caregiver's approach to clients must continually be monitored and adjusted. Thought and consideration must be given to each therapeutic action. Making a positive, therapeutic use of your personality requires "a consistent, thoughtful effort directed toward developing an awareness of self and others" (Taylor, 1994).

126

SELF-AWARENESS

Simply defined, **self-awareness** is a consciousness of one's personality. It is the act of looking at oneself: considering one's abilities, characteristics, aspirations, and concepts of self in relation to others. It is an alertness to one's personal and social behaviors and their impact on others (Morrison, 1993). In short, self-awareness is the ability to objectively look at oneself.

The development of self-awareness does not occur overnight. It requires time, patience, and a willingness to routinely consider your behaviors, attitudes, and values. The rewards, however, are worth the efforts because both clients and caregivers benefit when therapeutic goals are achieved. Personally, self-awareness allows individuals to direct and mold the pattern of their lives, to be in charge of their own growth and development. Caregivers encourage the development of self-awareness in their clients and must be ready to practice it themselves. To improve self-awareness requires insight, caring, acceptance, a consideration of values, a positive outlook, and the willingness to nurture yourself. If you are willing to put effort into these areas, you will evolve into a person who is able to use your personality to achieve therapeutic change and personal fulfillment.

Caring

Every person has the universal human need for love. Maslow's hierarchy of needs lists the need for love and belonging as the first nonphysical requirement after safety. Infants who do not receive enough loving touch fail to grow and thrive. Adults who do not meet their needs for love become isolated, lonely, and depressed. Human beings are gregarious creatures. They are meant to live with others. Although physical appearances, behavioral patterns, and communication styles may differ, each person carries with him or her the need to belong and be loved.

Caring is the energy on which the health care professions are built. It is defined as a concern for the well-being of another person and includes such behaviors as accepting, comforting, honesty, attentive listening, and sensitivity. Caring is the glue that binds individuals to each other. It is energy of the soul, freely given in hopes of helping another human being. Caring cannot be taught as a procedure or skill. It must be developed and encouraged, and it must be molded into the therapeutic behaviors that make up the personality of the caregiver.

Characteristics

Theorists have tried to explain the concept of caring, but its nature defies description. In 1987 the theorist M. Roach identified attributes of caring and labeled them the five Cs. They are commitment, compassion, competence, confidence, and conscience. The attributes of commitment and competence are discussed later in the chapter. Here we focus on the qualities of compassion, confidence, and conscience.

The quality of **compassion** relates to feeling the sorrows, sufferings, or troubles of another. It includes empathy, the willingness to try to understand how another person is feeling and tolerance for the many differences of individuals. Compassion enables us to share in the emotional state of another person. When used therapeutically, it helps caregivers understand and guide clients toward more effective and satisfying lives. Become aware of your feelings of compassion. They are powerful motivators.

Confidence is "the quality which fosters trusting relationships" (Roach, 1987). It is a belief in the caregiver's ability to assist clients in coping with the difficulties and implications of their health problems. Confidence is also trust and belief in your own abilities. Self-awareness grows as long as one has the confidence to investigate one's own thoughts and actions.

The word **conscience** describes a knowledge or feeling of what is right and wrong. It is often accompanied by a strong desire to do the right thing. People with well-developed consciences act based on firm values and beliefs. They are aware of their definitions of right and wrong. They do not hesitate to follow their moral principles and attempt to correct what they perceive as wrong.

To the five attributes of caring, one more can be added: the quality of **courage,** the response that allows us to face and cope with the dangerous, difficult, or painful aspects of life. Courage is the quiet companion of caring that enables care providers to take the first step in establishing connections with each client. It is also a part of the energy engine that supplies us with the motivation to learn and grow.

The interconnectedness of people is demonstrated through the act of caring, which can be as personal as an embrace or as removed as stopping your car for someone to cross the street on a busy day. For health care providers, caring serves as the vehicle for interacting with people, for making the connection with clients that communicates respect and dignity. Box 12-1 lists therapeutic actions that demonstrate caring.

When the caregiver and client experience connectedness, "the intensity of the work accomplished seems to be enhanced, benefiting both" (Heifner, 1993). Caring acts as the connection that binds each human being to the other. The quality of caring, when combined with insight, acceptance, and a positive outlook on life, helps us develop the self-awareness that leads to becoming an effective therapeutic personality. See the Case Study for an example of one nurse's attempt to connect.

Insight

We all are responsible for our own growth and development, both professionally and personally. We gain insight

Case Study

Leo was admitted to the unit because the police found him wandering in the traffic, talking to himself. He was unshaven, hadn't bathed for many days, and appeared exhausted. The look in his eyes was wild, as if he were being tormented by an unknown assailant. Leo was diagnosed with paranoid schizophrenia. The staff was at a loss for how to cope because Leo refused to communicate with anyone.

Bart, the nurse who was assigned to monitor Leo, decided to meet his most basic needs first. With Leo watching his every move, Bart began to offer him food. He opened a single-serving container of juice and slowly moved it across the table toward Leo, who slapped it away and muttered "Poison." After a short time, Bart opened another juice container and, once he was sure that Leo was watching, took a sip. Again, he slowly pushed the container toward the thirsty-appearing Leo. This time, Leo picked up the container, tasted the juice, then greedily consumed it. Within a few days Leo was eating and drinking—as long as Bart tasted everything first. He still refused to speak, but Bart knew that he had connected with Leo and that was at least a beginning.

◆ What did Bart do that communicated caring to this client?

and wisdom through experience. **Insight** is the ability to clearly see and understand the nature of things. Insight relies on the skills of common sense, good judgment, and prudence. Self-awareness is expanded when one strives to learn and become competent. Although not always comfortable, our insights provide us with new opportunities to take risks, explore our own potential, and fail, as well as

succeed. For care providers, it includes a sensitivity to people, the ability to make keen observations, and the willingness to seek new knowledge.

Insight refers to two types of knowledge: the wisdom to know oneself and the clear-sightedness to learn about others. The first duty of a health care provider is to *know thyself*. The very success of one's professional practice depends on it. If health care providers are unable to assess their learning needs or communications skills, for example, they will remain stagnant and refuse to grow or evolve. The same holds true for all people.

Self-awareness is developed through the practice of **introspection,** which is the process of looking into one's own mind. Introspection is an analysis of self, including one's feelings, reactions, attitudes, opinions, values, and behaviors. It is also a process for observing and analyzing one's behavior in various situations. Introspection allows us to "step out" of the interaction and watch our own behaviors. This process is assisted when caregivers can view themselves interacting with various clients on videotape or television.

Introspection allows caregivers to identify both personal and professional learning needs. Seeking new knowledge is a fundamental requirement of the health care profession. Caregivers are responsible for remaining knowledgeable. Only the confidence of a strong knowledge base can ease the anxiety of the "What shall I do now?" syndrome.

Practice professional introspection by keeping a small notebook with you. Throughout the day, jot down any questions or subjects that relate to the care of your clients—anything about which you feel you need to know more. After work, make it a point to research at least one question or topic every day. This practice will serve as a valuable aid for routinely gaining new knowledge. Knowledge breeds competence, and from competence grows the confidence to provide the best possible care.

Personal introspection is the process of learning who you are: your likes, dislikes, habits, and behavior patterns. This type of introspection may be accompanied by the emotional discomfort of an unexpected discovery about yourself. However, for those individuals who can overcome their own emotional defenses, introspection serves as a valuable tool for developing self-awareness.

Risk Taking and Failure

Developing self-awareness is also based on enlarging one's experiences. Purposefully engaging in unfamiliar activities and observing your responses allow you to expand your knowledge, examine your reactions, and reconsider your beliefs.

The process of developing self-awareness includes the elements of risk and failure. If one is to grow, then one must take risks. Without a willingness to take chances and possibly fail, a person remains tied to the same pattern of life. One engages in **risk-taking** behaviors when

Box 12-2   Developing Risk-Taking Skills

Plan the risk-taking activity only after thorough assessment of the situation and consideration of all possible outcomes.

Eliminate fear and other roadblocks to risk-taking.

Give yourself permission to fail, to make mistakes, and to learn from them.

Reward yourself for trying something new regardless of the outcome.

Review your history of successes to build the self-confidence to take risks.

Find a mentor who is a successful risk taker and learns from previous mistakes.

Support others who are engaging in risk-taking behaviors.

Think About

To use failure positively, do the following:

1. Realize that failure is a necessary part of growth.
2. Give yourself permission to fail.
3. Consider failure as a learning experience.
4. Discover new options and opportunities created by the failure.
5. Expect to succeed with the next attempt.

◆ How do you think following the above steps could help you become a better health care provider?

the rewards of success are larger than the consequences of failure. Several hints for taking risks are presented in Box 12-2.

Risk taking implies the possibility of **failure.** For most of us, the word failure has a negative meaning. It implies defeat, a "you lose" attitude, and a lack of success. However, failure can be filled with positive, growth-promoting experiences. *Failure provides the opportunity for change.* It encourages creativity, stimulates learning, and sharpens one's judgments. Failure is a price that must be paid for improvement. When used as a learning tool, the experience of failure can provide the foundation for the next step toward success. The person who never fails cannot savor the rewards of success.

How do we grow from our failures? The first and most important step is to understand that failure is a necessary part of change. Biologist Lewis Thomas (1979) maintains "that humankind is set apart from the rest of creation by our unique ability to make mistakes. If we were not provided with the knack of being wrong, we could never get anything useful done." Failure is a part of the growth experience and thus self-awareness.

The second step is to give yourself permission to fail. The guilt associated with failure can generate feelings of inadequacy that can paralyze you into denying yourself valuable opportunities for learning. The odds of a person living a lifetime without a failure are about zero. Failure, learning, and growth are all partners in the development of self-awareness.

The third step is to consider your failure as a learning experience. Examine the elements of the failure: the "what, how, when, who, where, and why" aspects. Discover what could have been done differently and what improvements could be made. This examination is an important part of one's self-education because more effective actions in the future avoid the failures of the past.

The fourth and last step in using failure as a tool for developing self-awareness is to discover the opportunities

that are created by failure. Many times a failure opens new doors or presents a problem in an entirely different light. To illustrate, the gold miners in the hills of Virginia City, Nevada, used to throw "that darned blue stuff" into piles outside their poorly producing gold mines. It was only after a young miner began to think about the blue material in a different way (and had it chemically analyzed) that the miners realized that "the cursed blue stuff" was actually high-grade silver ore, worth millions of dollars. Examining and learning from failure can create new options and opportunities. The Think About box lists several suggestions for using failure as a positive experience. Remember, one fails only when one refuses to grow from the experience.

VALUES AND BELIEFS

To briefly review, a value is something that is held dear or a belief about the worth of an item, idea, or behavior (Stuart and Laraia, 2001). Individuals who choose the health care professions usually arrive with a strong set of personal values and beliefs, many of which are shared with other members of the profession. For example, caregivers value human dignity and the right of clients to make their own decisions.

People's belief systems strongly affect their behaviors and provide the comfort of stability and knowing what to expect. However, a static, unquestioning attitude is not enough for those health care professionals who truly want to be effective. Because one's values and beliefs can influence behavior and color judgments, caregivers should strive to develop a level of self-awareness that encourages an exploration of their values. Exploring one's values is not always easy because, by their very nature, values are cherished and difficult to change. Using the values clarification process of choosing, prizing, and acting (see Chapter 3) allows caregivers to evaluate their own values and beliefs.

Guidelines for Therapeutic Actions

Every nurse has a right to his or her values and beliefs. The value a nurse places on a client's behaviors influences the relationship. If the nurse values the client as an individual and expresses faith in his or her abilities to change, then the client will strive for greater achievements. Do not limit clients with the force of your own values. Set expectations high and provide frequent encouragement. Clients have the right to achieve and to fail, just as we do. Limiting your clients by placing expectations on them, based on your values and beliefs, deprives them of opportunities for growth and achievement.

Guidelines for many values can be found in the philosophical beliefs statement of psychiatric nursing practice (Box 12-3). These beliefs can serve as a guide for discovering your values and belief systems. Their exploration is an essential step toward achieving the self-awareness that makes nurses the therapeutic instruments of healing.

Acceptance

Several beliefs of caregivers relate to acceptance of the person we call "the client." Although people may engage in behaviors that are considered inappropriate, each individual has worth and some degree of dignity. Each client must be given respect and the opportunity to participate in care if treatment is to be successful. **Acceptance** in this context means the receiving of the entire person and the world in which he or she functions.

Accepting clients does not necessarily include approving of their behaviors. This is an important distinction; you must accept the person but you do not have to accept the behavior. Many caregivers who work with mentally and emotionally troubled clients will not hesitate to tell a client when his or her behavior is inappropriate, but no mental health caregiver should ever directly attack or correct the *person*. Table 12-1 presents examples of communications that focus on the difference between correcting the behavior and correcting the person. The very reason clients with mental-emotional problems have sought help is to correct their ineffective behaviors. We, as their care providers, work with them to replace these behaviors with more successful and satisfying ways of functioning, but to do this we must accept the entire person as a complete package, regardless of our own reactions. This acceptance then becomes the foundation on which other therapeutic actions are based.

Helping Boundaries

Caregivers are expected to give of themselves in the care of others. Today they realize that to effectively care for others, they must care for themselves and recharge their batteries, if they are to maintain the necessary energy to therapeutically work with clients. One of the ways in which caregivers maintain their energy levels is to define their helping boundaries (Heinrich and Killeen, 1993).

We all have limits or boundaries over which we will not cross. Personal boundaries provide order and security

Box 12-3 **Beliefs of Psychiatric Nursing Practice**

The individual has intrinsic worth and dignity.
The goal of the individual is one of growth, health, autonomy, and self-actualization.
Every individual has the potential to change and the desire to pursue personal goals.
The person functions as a holistic being who acts on, interacts with, and reacts to the environment as a whole person.
All people have common, basic, and necessary human needs.
All behavior is meaningful. It arises from personal needs and goals and can be understood only from the person's internal frame of reference and within the context in which it occurs.
Behavior consists of perceptions, thoughts, feelings, and actions. Disruptions may occur in any area.
Individuals vary in their coping capacities. All individuals have the potential for both health and illness.
Illness can be a growth-producing experience for the individual.
All people have a right to an equal opportunity for adequate health care regardless of gender, race, religion, ethics, sexual orientation, or cultural background. Care is based on the needs of individuals, families, and communities and mutually defined goals and expectations.
Mental health is a critical and necessary component of comprehensive health care services.
The individual has the right to participate in decision making and the right to self-determination. It is the decision of the individual to pursue health or illness.
An interpersonal relationship has the potential for producing change and growth within the individual. It is the vehicle for the attainment of the goals of care.

Modified from Stuart GW, Laraia MT: *Principles and practices of psychiatric nursing*, ed 7, St. Louis, 2001, Mosby.

because they help to establish the limits of one's behavior. To illustrate, theft is an example of a personal boundary. You would not think of stealing from your friends because a personal boundary limits you from doing so.

Professional boundaries define the needs of the caregiver "as distinctly different from the needs of the patient: what is too helpful and what is not; and what fosters independence vs. unhealthy dependence" (Pillette, Berck, and Achber, 1995). Once clients are stabilized, they are expected to begin functioning independently with guidance and encouragement from the members of the health care team. When caregivers become overhelpful or controlling, professional (helping) boundaries have been crossed. We all want our clients to succeed, adapt, and function happily, but sometimes that drive motivates us to exclude or ignore our clients' needs. In the end, the

Table 12-1	Focus on Correcting Behavior vs. Person	
Focus on behavior		**Focus on person**
"Sam, undressing in the dayroom is inappropriate."		"Sam, I've told you not to undress in the dayroom."
"Mary, stop! No slapping is allowed here."		"Mary, stop that! Why are you slapping him?"
"I find it difficult to be here when you . . . "		"You're disgusting when you do that."

caregiver may feel good, but do the clients function any better as a result of his or her interventions?

The need for professional (helping) boundaries must be continually balanced with one's needs to be caring. To do this, care providers establish their own set of professional (helping) boundaries. They define the limits of both their personal and professional lives, and usually the two remain quite separate. The focus of the professional aspect of the caregiver's life is the client, but the focus of the caregiver's personal life is him or herself. The boundaries of each remain distinct because one cannot focus on the client and the self at the same time.

To maintain their professional boundaries, caregivers assess relationships with their clients often. If they find themselves having difficulty in setting limits or feel that they are the only one who "really understands" a certain client (the beginnings of codependency), then cause for concern exists and help should be sought. Discussing the situation with appropriate persons helps provide perspective and increases one's therapeutic effectiveness. The therapeutic relationship is anchored in the effective management of professional (helping) boundaries. When the focus of interaction is the client and progress is being made toward the therapeutic goals, the relationship is effective and satisfying for both client and caregiver.

Detecting boundary violations is often difficult because "a person's own needs stimulate and maintain the violation" (Pillette, Berck, and Achber, 1995). However, early detection helps prevent larger problems in the future. Frequent self-assessments assist in monitoring for problems. A delicate balance exists between knowing when to help and when not to help clients. Caregivers who are aware of this balance keep the client as the major concern of focus and maintain the professional boundaries that help individuals progress toward their therapeutic goals.

Overinvolvement and Codependency

We have all had (or will have) special clients, those who have touched us so deeply that we have become too emotionally involved. Becoming overinvolved is not difficult to do. However, to thrive and grow ourselves, care providers must learn to walk the fine line between compassion and overinvolvement.

Years ago, care providers were taught to always maintain a "professional distance" from clients. Today, however, we recognize the power of the therapeutic relationship and its effect on clients. We realize that caregivers are people too, complete with their own set of attributes and problems. It is easier to form a rapport with some clients than others. Sometimes that rapport leads to an overinvolvement because the client touches the caregiver in some special way. This initial attraction can soon result in conflict because the caregiver begins to have difficulty separating the professional relationship from the growing friendship with the client. When the relationship begins to fulfill the caregiver's needs, codependency results. Soon the relationship loses its therapeutic effectiveness, and the caregiver or client withdraws, left with a mixture of unresolved feelings and unmet goals (Yates and McDaniel, 1994).

To protect yourself from becoming codependent with certain clients, remember this one rule of thumb: *If you show a significantly greater level of concern for one client than for others, then you are running the risk of becoming overinvolved.* Recognize this risk early, and discuss it with your supervisor. Exploring your feelings in relation to the client helps to regain the balance between professionalism and compassion. Often just the personal awareness of the potential of becoming overinvolved is enough to prevent it from occurring. Compassion, empathy, and acceptance are vital elements of health care, but they must be balanced by professionalism, judgment, and therapeutic actions that meet the client's needs.

Commitment

A **commitment** is a personal bond to some course of action or cause. The health care professions are undergoing radical changes. Many of these changes are influenced by sources outside the helping professions. If provision of high-quality care for every person is to remain a primary goal of our society, then a strong commitment from each health care provider will be needed to maintain the focus on our clients. Caregivers must be committed to providing competent health care, no matter what the setting or circumstances.

Personal Commitments

The first and most important commitment is to yourself, the commitment to consciously take charge of your personal and professional growth. A refusal to grow within the self cannot encourage growth or self-awareness in others. Self-commitment involves a promise to do the best you can in every situation and to be the best that you can be.

Each person has a unique set of talents, an individual personality, and areas of their lives that need improvement. People who are committed to improving themselves are able to consider both the positive and negative characteristics of their personalities without guilt or remorse. They realize their mistakes and attempt to profit from them by extracting the lessons hidden in each error. They then commit themselves to applying those hard-earned lessons to new situations, thus enhancing self-awareness and expanding their ability to cope with new experiences. Commit to your personal growth and consider who you are. What attitudes or behaviors would you like to change? Accept and love who you are, but commit to strive for greater learning.

Commitments to Others

Health care providers have strong commitments to other people. As with most people, they are committed to their family units, social circles, and communities. However, caregivers have a commitment larger than that of the community—the commitment to caring about the welfare of humankind. They demonstrate dedication to their clients by continually seeking out new knowledge, keeping up-to-date with the latest professional developments, and striving to improve their therapeutic effectiveness.

You are committed, otherwise you would not be reading these words. Take the time to discover what you feel is most important in life. Then look behind the topic, and you will find yourself committed to a certain course of action. The exercise of describing one's commitments helps to expand self-awareness and remind us of the interconnectedness of all human beings.

POSITIVE OUTLOOK

One of the most effective and important tools for developing self-awareness is a positive or optimistic attitude. One's outlook on life affects every perception, every thought, and every emotion. A person with a positive outlook radiates energy and well-being that cheers up everyone in the vicinity. People are attracted to individuals with positive attitudes. They hope that a bit of that radiant energy will be somehow passed on to them. On the other hand, individuals with negative attitudes tend to discourage other people from interacting with them. Their attitude of doom and gloom actually fosters the development of many physical and mental problems.

Researchers have found that "negative thoughts about self and future have been found to predict future depression" (Lightsey, 1994). Science is now attempting to discover the role of positive thinking on health. This new knowledge is significant, especially for providers of health care.

Positive attitudes and thoughts can act as buffers against stress and conflict. They can prevent caregiver's burnout, the syndrome that results when care providers give too much without renewing their energies. In addition, caregivers who practice positive thinking can act as role models for those clients who have not learned to cope effectively within their worlds.

A positive outlook does not require caregivers to be continually upbeat and exclude everything unpleasant or objectionable. The reality of each situation must be considered objectively, but there is no reason to harbor a negative attitude when a positive one is much more fulfilling.

Achieving and maintaining a positive outlook is especially important for caregivers who work with the mentally and emotionally troubled individuals of society. Much unhappiness and misfortune plagues these people, and remaining upbeat in the face of continuing adversity can be a challenge for anyone. A positive attitude is the secret weapon for coping with the adversity of life. It is the key to maintaining physical and emotional health, especially for those who share their energies therapeutically. To develop a positive outlook on life, one needs only to become aware: of existing attitudes, of the need to add positive thinking to one's point of view, and of the therapeutic effectiveness that results from a positive outlook.

Daily Awareness

Developing a positive attitude is a process that requires persistent and patient efforts because our current attitudes and habits are deeply ingrained. However, the process can be assisted by following these five tips:

First, *listen to your self-talk*. Pay attention to the words you use. Each word has an emotional attachment to it. The human brain is programmed by thought patterns. Thoughts can become feelings, which, in turn, evolve into words and actions. Many people complain of being under too much stress or pressure. No one denies that modern life contains its share of stresses. However, it is how each stressor is perceived or defined that determines your point of view. If you do not define the event as stressful, then it is not. Practice listening to yourself. You may be surprised at what you discover.

Second, *change recurrent negative themes*. Any thought, emotion, word, or action that is self-defeating

To Develop a Positive Attitude

1. Recognize the negative thoughts, emotions, and attitudes. Reject them and throw them out of your personality.
2. Replace each negative attitude by frequently repeating positive statements.
3. Repeat upbeat and enthusiastic words that help to build a feeling of success.

To Nurture Caregivers

1. Be knowledgeable.
2. Value each individual as a human presence.
3. Be responsible and accountable for your actions.
4. Be open to new ideas.
5. Connect with others. Support your colleagues.
6. Take pride in yourself.
7. Like what you do.
8. Recognize the moments of joy in the struggles of living. Take time to smell the roses.
9. Recognize and accept your own limitations but strive to improve. At the end of the day, focus on your accomplishments rather than the things left undone.
10. Rest each day and begin anew.

Modified from Sherwood G: The responses of caregivers to the experience of suffering. In Starck PL, McGovern JP, editors: *The hidden dimension of illness: human suffering,* New York, 1992, National League for Nursing Press.

needs to be replaced with a positive, empowering one (Box 12-4).

Releasing and replacing one's negative attitudes lead to greater self-esteem, awareness, confidence, and happiness, not to mention the added benefits of a highly effective immune system. Practice changing your negative themes because your outlook determines the success or failure of an action.

Third, *be your own cheerleader.* Give yourself a pep talk every morning and whenever you are coping with stresses. Present yourself with positive, inspiring thoughts. Your brain does not question your thoughts. It only stores information for future use. Those stored thoughts then become the basis for actions. Positive statements uplift the spirits and help to convince you of your value.

Fourth, *visualize future successes.* Take a few moments during each day to picture yourself achieving a goal. Fantasize about the feelings associated with achieving the goal, and think about the steps that lead to the goal. Picture yourself as a dynamic person and capable caregiver; it will help to provide the blueprint for future growth. Besides, it is fun to do.

Fifth, *act the part.* Visualize yourself as a person with confidence and ability. You will find that your actual level of confidence grows each time you project an image of self-assurance.

Developing a positive outlook will serve you well. Positive mental attitudes help to develop self-esteem, which in turn helps to build self-awareness, self-respect, and self-acceptance.

Nurturing Yourself

A critical first step in the development of self-awareness is to recognize and tend to your needs. To **nurture** someone encourages their development. Caregivers are expected to work hard for the welfare of their clients, but they must also care and nurture themselves because energy cannot be continually spent without being renewed. Care providers function at a high level of wellness to provide the energy required by their clients. You have chosen to care for others. Part of the responsibility you accepted when making this decision was to care for

yourself. To nurture your clients you must first nurture yourself.

Principles and Practices for Caregivers

Health care providers seek to "instill hope, empower others, encourage independence, and help improve the other's condition. When we are unable to achieve that, unable to alleviate suffering, we often experience a sense of frustration and failure" (Sherwood, 1992). When this frustration occurs over and over, we become emotionally worn or *burned out,* as many caregivers call it. Somehow each of us must find the balance between the moral duty to care amidst the stress of constant suffering and the concern for one's well-being. In Box 12-5, Sherwood (1992) offers us basic principles for maintaining the self in caring for others.

Using these principles as guidelines will assist you in finding the balance between giving and renewing. Remember these principles because they are guidelines for replenishing the energies that you so freely share with others.

To nurture yourself requires more than the ingestion of food and water or the needs for sleep and activity. To nourish the part of the self from which one's therapeutic energies are drawn requires special renewal. Caregivers nurture themselves in different ways. Some turn to a special source of comfort, whereas others find renewal in the adventure of trying new things. Spending time alone, removed from the stimuli of the day, recharges some nurses. Others need the challenge of physical activities, travel, or new relationships.

Recently, research has pointed out the many benefits of daily meditation for stress reduction, relaxation, and renewal (Kabot-Zinn, 1994). Basically, meditation, termed the *relaxation response* by Western medicine, is the practice of becoming still and quiet. First, one assumes a comfortable body position within a quiet environment. Then one concentrates on just breathing. As the mind begins to wander elsewhere, it is gently escorted back to the breath. This focus allows one's energies to become calm and concentrated instead of wandering through scattered bits of self-talk. Soon an inner stillness and peace are experienced, stress is relieved, and energies are renewed. Health care professionals who practice meditation for as little as 15 minutes a day find it a valuable source of renewal and stress reduction.

In this busy world, it is easy to lose sight of one simple fact: your ability to care for your clients depends on how well you care for yourself. How you choose to nurture and renew yourself is a matter of personal preference. The important thing is that you do it regularly and without guilt. A good diet, adequate exercise, and restful sleep must not be ignored, but the essence of caring must also be applied to the self. Caregivers need to be willing to accept, love, and nourish themselves as much as they do their clients.

KEY CONCEPTS

◆ Self-awareness is a consciousness of one's own individuality and personality.

◆ Caring is a concern for the well-being of another person; it includes accepting, comforting, honesty, attentive listening, and sensitivity.

◆ The characteristics of caring are commitment, compassion, competence, confidence, conscience, and courage.

◆ Caregivers are responsible for their own growth and development, both professionally and personally.

◆ Insight is the ability to clearly see and understand the nature of things.

◆ Introspection is an analysis of self, including one's feelings, reactions, attitudes, opinions, values, and behaviors.

◆ To successfully cope with failure, one must realize that failures are a necessary part of change.

◆ Caregivers have the power to shape their clients' successes or failures, based on their own personal values and beliefs.

◆ The exploration of one's values and beliefs is an essential step toward achieving self-awareness.

◆ Professional boundaries define what is too helpful and what is not.

◆ A commitment is an intellectual or an emotional bond that moves the individual to action.

◆ One of the most effective tools for developing self-awareness is a positive or optimistic attitude.

◆ A critical first step in the development of self-awareness is to recognize and tend to your own needs.

◆ Meditation is the practice of becoming still and quiet.

◆ Your ability to care for your clients depends on how well you care for yourself.

Suggestions for Further Reading

"Nurse-Patient Boundaries: Crossing the Line" by Linda Smith and others (*American Journal of Nursing* 97(12):36, 1997) provides sound advice to all caregivers.

References

Heifner C: Positive connectedness in the psychiatric nurse-patient relationship, *Archives of Psychiatric Nursing* 7(1):11, 1993.

Heinrich K, Killeen ME: The gentle art of nurturing yourself, *American Journal of Nursing* 93(10):41, 1993.

Kabot-Zinn J: Meditate! . . . for stress reduction, inner peace . . . or whatever, *Psychology Today* 26(4):36, 1994.

Lightsey OR: "Thinking positive" as a stress buffer: the role of positive automatic cognitions in depression and happiness, *Journal of Counseling and Psychology* 41:325, 1994.

Morrison M: *Professional skills for leadership: foundations of a successful career,* St. Louis, 1993, Mosby.

Pillette PC, Berck CB, Achber LC: Therapeutic management of helping boundaries, *Journal of Psychosocial Nursing Mental Health Services* 33:40, 1995.

Roach M: *The human act of caring,* Ottawa, 1987, Canadian Hospital Association.

Sherwood G: The responses of caregivers to the experience of suffering. In Starck PL, McGovern JP, editors: *The hidden dimension of illness: human suffering,* New York, 1992, National League for Nursing Press.

Stuart GW, Laraia MT: *Principles and practice of psychiatric nursing,* ed 7, St. Louis, 2001, Mosby.

Taylor CM: *Essentials of psychiatric nursing,* ed 14, St. Louis, 1994, Mosby.

Thomas L: *The medusa and the snail: more notes of a biology watcher,* New York, 1979, Viking Press.

Yates G, McDaniel JL: Are you losing yourself in codependency? *American Journal of Nursing* 94(4):32, 1994.

Chapter 13

Mental Health Assessment Skills

Learning Objectives

1. Identify two purposes of the mental health treatment plan.
2. List and define each step of the nursing process.
3. Describe three methods of data collection.
4. Explain the importance of performing physical assessments on clients with psychiatric diagnoses.
5. List five parts of a holistic nursing assessment.
6. Identify four guidelines for conducting effective psychiatric interviews.
7. Explain the purpose of the mental status examination.
8. List the five general categories of the mental status examination.
9. Describe the process for conducting a mental status examination.

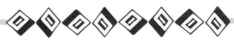

Key Terms

affect	interview	perceptions
assessment	judgment	risk factor assessment
calculation	memory	sensorium
data collection	mood	thought content
insight	nursing (therapeutic) process	thought processes

The ability to obtain and effectively use information about clients is the foundation of the nursing (therapeutic) process and a vital part of the multidisciplinary treatment plan. Learning about clients' problems requires special abilities. Physical examination skills, for example, provide information regarding clients' physiological state. Special communication and interaction skills are needed for learning about the cultural, psychosocial, and spiritual aspects of individuals. This chapter provides the starting point for the practice of making thorough mental health assessments. Good assessment skills are critical to quality health care. Caregivers must first learn about the person before they can provide effective care or judge the effectiveness of any therapeutic action.

MENTAL HEALTH TREATMENT PLAN

People enter the health care system because they are distressed, disabled, or suffering. When problems are physical, a diagnosis is made, the client is treated, and the disorder is either resolved or becomes chronic. The diagnosis and treatment of people with mental-emotional problems are challenging because problems cannot be as easily identified and defined. According to the *Diagnostic and Statistical Manual of Mental Disorders* (DSM-IV–TR), "no definition adequately specifies precise boundaries for the concept of mental disorder" (American Psychiatric Association, 2000) because the relationship between the physical and psychological self is difficult to separate. It is important to remember, though, that every

Table 13-1	DSM-IV–TR Axes	
Axis	**Category**	**Example**
I	Clinical disorders	Mood, substance abuse, schizophrenic disorders
II	Personality disorders and mental retardation	Dependent, antisocial personality disorders
		Mild, moderate, severe retardation
III	General medical conditions	Heart, digestive diseases
IV	Psychosocial and environmental problems	Educational, housing, legal, economic, social environment problems
V	Global assessment of functioning (GAF)	Overall level of psychological, social, and occupational functioning

psychological illness has physical effects and every physical illness is accompanied by psychological effects. The wise care provider is aware of both.

When individuals first enter the mental health care system, a comprehensive assessment is usually performed. Clients may be interviewed by several members of the multidisciplinary health care team. Physical and psychological diagnostic testing is done, and data are gathered from as many sources as possible. Team members meet to compare data, identify problems, and develop treatment approaches. The team and the client then agree on the treatment goals, and a course of action is planned. Usually a combination of medical treatments (medications) are combined with psychotherapies, behavioral therapies, and various social approaches. The overall health care treatment plan is then developed especially for the individual client. Therapeutic actions are implemented, and the client's progress toward each goal is routinely evaluated.

The mental health treatment plan serves several purposes. First, it is a guide for planning and implementing client care. Nurses are guided by the treatment plan when they develop specific nursing care plans. Psychologists, social workers, and other therapists use the mental health treatment plan as a framework for implementing their specialized therapeutic actions.

Second, the plan serves as a vehicle for monitoring the client's progress and assessing the effectiveness of the therapeutic interventions. Clients meet often with treatment team members to discuss problems or difficulties that may be hampering attempts to meet their goals. Therapeutic interventions are evaluated, and the treatment plan is revised to include new information.

Third, the mental health treatment plan serves as a means for communicating and coordinating client care. It prevents costly duplication of services and provides a focus for all therapeutic activities, regardless of specialty, which increases the effectiveness of each member of the treatment team. Developing the mental health treatment plan is not a complex process, but it is a dynamic (changing) one that allows clients and care providers the opportunity to work together.

DSM-IV–TR Diagnosis

Most therapists who work with mental or emotionally troubled individuals use the DSM-IV–TR (see Appendix B) to aid in diagnosis and help guide clinical practice. Clients are assessed and then classified according to five categories or axes (Table 13-1).

Table 13-2 explains the global assessment of functioning (GAF) scale.

Using a multiaxial (many category) system helps care providers gain a more complete understanding of the complexity of each person and promotes therapeutic interventions based on individual clients. The diagnosis of mental health problems remains the responsibility of the physician, but nurses and other care providers should be familiar with the multiaxial system of psychiatric assessment.

Nursing Process

Each step of the **nursing (therapeutic) process** is designed to support goal-directed care for clients (Stuart and Laraia, 2001). Nurses perform holistic assessments, develop nursing diagnoses, and work with mentally troubled clients to set and achieve realistic treatment goals. Because the nursing profession is concerned with the impact of illness and dysfunction on clients' activities of daily living, many nursing diagnoses fit well with the multiaxial diagnoses of the DSM-IV–TR. Therapeutic interventions, which are carried out by all mental health care team members, guide clients toward their goals. Evaluations of both clients' and caregivers' actions allow for adjustments to be made in the dynamic process that is known as "treatment."

Clients are involved as partners in care. Although some individuals are unable or too discouraged to make decisions, most clients are capable of participating in some part of their care. Caregivers help clients problem solve by involving them in the care planning process.

Use of the nursing (therapeutic) process allows health care providers to share information important for the client's care and treatment. Client responses to various treatments and therapies are assessed and documented,

Table 13-2	Global Assessment of Functioning Scale
Score	Level of function
100-91	**Superior functioning** in a wide range of activities; no symptoms; handles life's problems; sought out by others for many positive qualities
90-81	**Absent or minimal symptoms;** everyday problems and concerns; socially effective; generally satisfied with life
80-71	**Transient, expectable symptoms;** normal reactions to psychosocial stressors; Example: difficulty focusing following an argument
70-61	**Some mild symptoms** or some difficulty in social, occupational, or school functioning; has some meaningful interpersonal relationships
60-51	**Moderate symptoms** or moderate difficulty in social, occupational, or school functioning; has few friends, conflicts with peers or co-workers
50-41	**Serious symptoms;** serious impairment in social, occupational, or school functioning; no friends; unable to keep a job
40-31	**Impaired reality testing, communication;** major impairment in several areas (work, school, family relations, mood, thinking); Example: depressed man avoids friends, can't work, neglects family
30-21	**Seriously impaired judgment, communication;** inability to function in almost all areas; behavior influenced by hallucinations, delusions
20-11	**Some danger to self or others** or gross impairment in communication or occasionally fails to maintain personal hygiene; suicidal; violent; manic excitement
10-1	**Persistent danger of hurting self or others** or persistently does not maintain minimal personal hygiene; serious suicidal acts with expectation of death; recurrent violent acts

Modified from American Psychiatric Association: *Diagnostic and statistical manual of mental disorders,* ed 4, text revision, Washington, DC, 2000, The Association.

allowing care to be adjusted and adapted as goals are reached and clients improve. The process requires knowledge, experience, and the use of good judgment. Experience grows with each application of the therapeutic process, whereas sound judgment is learned by looking at every possible side of a problem before arriving at a decision.

ABOUT ASSESSMENT

Assessment includes the "gathering, verifying and communicating of information relative to the client" (Anderson, Anderson, and Glanze, 1998). Clients are viewed as dynamic (changing) individuals affected by more than an illness or disorder. For this reason the holistic assessment includes the gathering of information about the physical, intellectual, social, cultural, and spiritual sides of each person. The more complete the picture of the client, the more effective the treatment approaches will be.

Data Collection

The term **data collection** refers to a variety of activities designed to gather information about a certain subject. Data (information) relating to clients are grouped into two types: objective and subjective data. The term *objective data* refers to information that can be measured and shared. This kind of information is gathered through the senses of sight, smell, touch, and hearing. Blood pressure readings, pulse rates, and laboratory reports that

are compared with "normal" illustrate the use of objective data. When working with mental health clients, care providers obtain objective data through the use of physical examinations, daily assessments, diagnostic testing results, and repeated observations of behaviors (Potter and Perry, 1998).

Subjective data relate to clients' perceptions. They include information that is abstract and difficult to measure or share. The experiences of pain, nausea, and anxiety, for example, cannot be measured by anyone but the individual experiencing them. Feelings, emotions, and mental states are all subjective and difficult to measure. As a result, it is extremely important for all health care providers to document subjective information as descriptively and accurately as possible. Do not include interpretative statements (judgments). To document that the client is angry (unless he states that he is angry) is an interpretative statement or judgment. It is better to state that the client was pacing about the room while slamming his fist into the wall and swearing. When documenting subjective data, quote the client as much as possible. Subjective information is collected during the initial health history interview and during every interaction with clients. The simple question "How do you feel?" usually elicits much subjective information.

Data collecting methods for care providers include interviews, observational techniques, and rating scales and inventories. Each method overlaps the other. For instance, during the health history interview with the client, the nurse uses observational techniques and interviewing skills.

An **interview** is a meeting of people with the purpose of obtaining or exchanging information (Keltner, Schwecke, and Bostrom, 1998). Interviews can be formal and highly structured, or informal and casual. Information gathered from formal interviews is usually documented on a standardized form. The interview is an excellent method for accomplishing assessments. It also serves as the starting point for building the therapeutic relationship. Informal interviews usually occur casually or by chance, but they provide great opportunities to learn more about clients and their families. Caregivers use informal interview techniques when they investigate client problems or explore certain topics.

Data gathering through the use of observational techniques is commonly used. *Observation* is the process of purposeful looking. When using observation as a data-gathering technique, caregivers must be careful to be objective. Personal bias or attitudes can alter the caregivers' perceptions and affect the objectivity of the observations. The use of observation is an excellent method for gathering information when the caregiver can remain impartial and does not pass judgment.

Physical examination skills are important to the data-gathering process for nurses. They include specialized methods for obtaining information about the body's level of physiological functioning. The technique of observation is called *inspection,* which means a purposeful examination of the body. The skills of *auscultation* and *percussion* use the examiner's sense of hearing to detect sounds within the body. Finally, the technique of *palpa-tion* requires the sense of touch to draw out information about temperature, texture, and pulsations of the body. Physical examination skills are used to gather data during the initial assessment, to investigate whenever a change in a client's physical condition is noted, and to evaluate the effectiveness of a therapeutic intervention.

Rating scales and inventories are frequently used by social workers, psychologists, and other therapists. They are data-gathering tools specifically designed to bring out certain kinds of information. The results are then compared with standardized measurements. Rating scales and inventories can be very useful for focusing on certain aspects of client problems.

Assessment Process

To gain an understanding of clients, caregivers learn to become observant and alert for information that may have an impact on clients' care. The process of assessing clients is ongoing. It begins with the clients' admission to the facility or service and ends only after the clients' relationship with the health care system has ended.

Holistic Assessment

A person's cultural, social, intellectual, emotional, and spiritual areas have an impact on the physical body and its functions. Without a knowledge of these five aspects of a client, health care providers become narrowed and limited in their effectiveness. The holistic assessment for those who work with mentally and emotionally troubled clients is the same as that used by caregivers in any setting. In psychiatric treatment situations, however, the emphasis is on mental-emotional functioning rather than physical

Table 13-3 Summary: Psychiatric Assessment Tool	
Area of assessment	**Example**
Appraisal of health/illness	Events leading to problem, definition of problem, client's goal, regular health care received
Previous psychiatric treatment	Diagnosis, type of treatment, medications, compliance, psychiatric history in family
Coping responses, physical status	Review of function in each body system, physical assessment, diet history, sleep patterns, exposure to toxic substances, activities of daily living
Coping responses, mental status	Appearance, speech, motor activity, mood, affect, interactions, perceptions, thought content and process, memory, concentration, calculations, intelligence, insight, judgment
Coping responses, discharge planning, needs	Client's ability to provide for food, clothing, housing, safety, transportation, supportive relationships, work needs, financial needs
Coping mechanisms	Adaptive mechanisms, maladaptive mechanisms
Psychosocial and environmental problems	Educational, occupational, economic, housing problems; difficulties with support group, culture, access to health care services
Knowledge deficits	Understanding of psychiatric problem, coping skills, medications, stressors

Modified from Stuart GW, Laraia MT: *Principles and practice of psychiatric nursing,* ed 7, St. Louis, 2001, Mosby.

functioning. The psychiatric assessment tool is focused on obtaining data about the problems, coping behaviors, and resources of clients (Table 13-3).

The information collected from assessment activities serves as part of the database from which medical, nursing, and other treatment decisions are made. For clients suspected of being capable of violence toward themselves or others, a risk factor assessment should be done first.

Risk Factor Assessment

A **risk factor assessment** helps "formulate a nursing diagnosis based on the identification of risk factors that potentially present an immediate threat to the patient" (Stuart and Laraia, 2001). With this assessment tool, eight areas of potential risk are identified (Figure 13-1). Positive findings lead to more specific assessments or appropriate safety precautions. Although the risk factor assessment is usually completed by a registered nurse, other health care providers assist by gathering important information and making objective observations.

THE HEALTH HISTORY

Each client should be interviewed on admission to the health care service. The purpose of the history interview is to obtain data about the unique individual who is the client. It offers care providers an opportunity to introduce themselves and serves as a starting point for establishing the therapeutic relationship. During the interview, insight into client concerns, worries, and expectations is gained, and the interview offers the opportunity to obtain clues that may require further investigation. When used appropriately, the interview is a powerful method for gathering important information about clients.

Effective Interviews

The success of any client interview rests on the caregiver's ability to listen objectively and respond appropriately. To enhance your interviewing skills, follow these guidelines.

Remember that *personal values must not cloud professional judgments.* Reacting to a client's personal appearance or behaviors can stereotype him or her and result in a negative impact on the effectiveness of the therapeutic relationship.

Do not make assumptions about how you think the client must feel. Discover what each event means to the client and how he or she views the situation. The experience of losing a loved one, for example, depends on how an individual interprets or perceives an event.

Always *take into account the client's cultural and religious values and beliefs.* With mental health clients, this point cannot be emphasized enough. Caregivers must learn about their clients' cultures if they are to understand their points of view. With clients from unfamiliar cultures, it is wise to research information about the culture and its religious practices before conducting the interview.

Pay particular attention to nonverbal communications. Much can be learned if one is observant. Note which subjects are avoided or quickly passed over during the interview. These behaviors can be clues that indicate a need for further investigation. Observing methods of self-expression helps the caregiver to focus on the client's unspoken signals and the messages they communicate.

Have clearly set goals. Know the purpose of the interview. Is this an initial assessment interview or the investigation of a specific condition? The assessment interview is not a random discussion; it is a purposefully planned interaction with the client.

Finally, *monitor your own reactions* during the interview. Use self-awareness to signal when you are becoming too emotionally involved. A caregiver may identify with certain clients with similar interests or situations, but self-awareness allows one to understand the emotional responses generated by certain clients.

Interviewing skills are used throughout the nursing (therapeutic) process. Work to develop and refine your interviewing skills because they are an important tool.

Sociocultural Assessment

The health history includes obtaining information about both the physical and psychological functions of an individual. Sociocultural assessment focuses on the cultural, social, and spiritual aspects of an individual. During the history interview, the care provider obtains information about a client's background. This time also offers an opportunity to observe the client's appearance, behaviors, and attitudes (areas also included in the mental status examination).

The sociocultural assessment includes six areas. Clients are asked questions about their age, ethnicity (culture), gender, education, income, and belief system. The client's risk factors and stressors are defined during the sociocultural assessment (National Depressive and Manic-Depressive Association, 1995). This information helps care providers develop accurate and appropriate plans of care.

Review of Systems

The holistic assessment also includes a review of each body system and its functioning. Clients are first questioned about their general health care, past illnesses and hospitalizations, and family health history. Questions then are focused on the function of each body system. Last, the lifestyle and activities of daily living are assessed.

RISK FACTOR ASSESSMENT

DIRECTIONS

The purpose of this assessment is to identify risk factors that potentially present an immediate threat to the patient. An RN must complete this assessment within the **FIRST HOUR** of the patient's encounter with the health care system.

The space labeled "Informants" should identify by name any source of information used to assess the patient. The "Reason for This Encounter" should quote the patient when possible.

The tool comprises eight (8) areas of potential risk. Positive findings in any area direct the nurse to initiate a more specific assessment or to initiate appropriate precautions. At the end of the risk factor assessment, the nurse must list the nursing diagnoses and total number of risk factors identified. A nursing care plan must be initiated immediately to address any nursing diagnosis that reflects an identified risk factor.

RISK FACTOR ASSESSMENT TOOL

Date: _____

INFORMANTS: _____

REASON FOR THIS ENCOUNTER: _____

_____

_____

RISK FACTORS:

1. Potential for Suicide/Self-Harm:

☐ yes ☐ no   Active or recent suicidal or self-harm ideation or attempt?
☐ yes ☐ no   History of suicidal or self-harm ideation or attempt?

• If yes to either question, initiate a Suicide/Self-Harm Assessment.

2. Potential for Assault/Violence:

☐ yes ☐ no   History of assaultive, destructive, or violent behavior?
☐ yes ☐ no   Does the patient express feelings of anger or aggression?

• If yes to either question, initiate a Assault/Violence Assessment.

3. Potential for Substance Abuse Withdrawal (alcohol, illicit drugs, prescription drugs, or inhalants):

☐ yes ☐ no   Have you ever felt the need to cut down on your drinking or drug use?
☐ yes ☐ no   Have people annoyed you by criticizing your drinking or drug use?
☐ yes ☐ no   Have you ever felt bad or guilty about your drinking or drug use?
☐ yes ☐ no   Have you ever had a drink first thing in the morning (eye opener)?

• If yes to either question, initiate a Assault/Violence Assessment.

4. Potential for Allergic Reaction/Adverse Drug Reaction:

☐ yes ☐ no   Food
☐ yes ☐ no   Medication
☐ yes ☐ no   Other

• If yes to either question, initiate a Assault/Violence Assessment.

5. Potential for Seizure:

☐ yes ☐ no   Is there a history of seizures?

• If yes to this question, initiate a Seizure Assessment.

6. Potential for Falls/Accidents:

☐ yes ☐ no   Ages 70 or older/5 or under
☐ yes ☐ no   History of confusion
☐ yes ☐ no   History of falls/accidents
☐ yes ☐ no   Sensory deficits
☐ yes ☐ no   Impaired mobility/balance
☐ yes ☐ no   Medications (check as many as apply)
　　　　　☐ yes ☐ no   Sedatives/tranquilizers/narcotics
　　　　　☐ yes ☐ no   Anesthetics
　　　　　☐ yes ☐ no   Diuretics/antihypertensives
　　　　　☐ yes ☐ no   Laxatives
　　　　　☐ yes ☐ no   Substance abuse
　　　　　☐ yes ☐ no   Psychotherapeutics

• If yes to two or more items, initiate Fall Precautions.

7. Potential for Elopement:

☐ yes ☐ no   Does the patient wish or intend to leave?
☐ yes ☐ no   Does the patient have a history of elopement?

• If yes to either question, initiate Elopement Precautions.

8. Potential for Physiological Instability:

☐ yes ☐ no   Existing unstable physical problem?

Vital signs: T _____ P _____ R _____

BP Stand _____ BP Sit _____ Weight _____ Height _____

• If yes to unstable problem or data out of normal range, intiate Physical Assessment.

Total number of risk factors identified (1-8) _____

IDENTIFIED NURSING DIAGNOSES:

☐ yes ☐ no   Potential for violence (self-directed)
☐ yes ☐ no   Potential for violence (other-directed)
☐ yes ☐ no   Risk for self-mutilation
☐ yes ☐ no   Potential for injury, related to_____

RN Signature_____ Date:_____ Time:_____

Figure 13-1 Risk factor assessment. (Courtesy Division of Psychiatric Nursing, Medical University of South Carolina.)

Box 13-1　Health History for Mental Health Clients

Health Care History

General Health Care

Regular health care provider

Frequency of health care visits

Last medical examination and test results

Any unusual circumstances of birth, including mother's preterm habits and condition

Hospitalizations and surgeries: When, Why indicated, Treatments, Outcome

Diagnosed brain problem

Head trauma: Details of any accidents or periods of unconsciousness for any reason—blows to the head, electrical shocks, high fevers, seizures, fainting, dizziness, headaches, falls

Endocrine disturbances: Thyroid and adrenal function particularly, Diabetes, Stability of glucose levels

Lifestyle

Eating: Details of unusual or unsupervised diets, appetite, weight changes, cravings, and caffeine intake

Medications: Full history of current and past psychiatric medications in self and first-degree relatives

Substance use: Alcohol and drug use

Toxins: Overcome by automobile exhaust or natural gas, Exposure to lead, mercury, insecticides, herbicides, solvents, cleaning agents, lawn chemicals

Occupation (current and past): Chemicals in workplace (farming, painting)

Cancer: Full history, particularly consider metastases (lung, breast, melanoma, gastrointestinal tract, and kidney are most likely to be affected), Results of treatment (chemotherapy and surgeries)

Lung problems: Details of anything that restricts flow of air to lungs for more than 2 minutes or adversely affects oxygen absorption (brain uses 20% of oxygen in body) such as with chronic obstructive pulmonary disease, near drowning, near strangulation, high-altitude oxygen deprivation, resuscitation

Cardiac problems: Childhood illnesses such as scarlet or rheumatic fever, History of heart attacks, strokes, or hypertension

Blood diseases: Anemia, Arteriosclerotic conditions, HIV, Work-related accidents, Military experiences

Injury: Safe sex practices, Contact sports and sports-related injuries, Exposure to violence or abuse

Presenting symptoms and coping responses: Description—nature, frequency, and intensity, Threats to safety of self or others, Functional status, Quality of life

From Stuart GW, Laraia MT: *Stuart and Sundeen's pocket guide to psychiatric nursing,* ed 4, St. Louis, 1998, Mosby.

Box 13-1 lists the topics covered by the health history for physical functioning.

When the results of the history interview are added to the database, a clear picture of the individual begins to emerge. Data obtained from physical assessments and various diagnostic examinations add even more information and help to complete the picture of the individual client.

PHYSICAL ASSESSMENT

Clients receive a physical examination on admission to a psychiatric service. The purpose of the examination is to discover physical problems that can be treated medically. Many alterations in behavior can often be traced to a physical cause. For example, low blood sugar levels can result in confused and uncooperative behavior. Hormone imbalances, exposure to toxic substances, and severe pain can also affect behavior.

A complete physical examination is most often performed by a physician or nurse practitioner. The client's current health status is explored, and then each system is examined. Nurses have an obligation to assess each client's health status on a routine basis. A complete physical assessment is not needed every day, but nurses must be alert to changes in their clients' conditions. To do

this, many nurses use a head-to-toe assessment, which takes less than 5 minutes and can be performed any time information about physical functions is needed.

Diagnostic studies for clients with mental-emotional problems include standard blood and urine tests, evaluation of electrolytes, and hormone function examinations. Many clients are screened for tuberculosis, human immunodeficiency virus (HIV), and sexually transmitted diseases. Studies, such as x-ray examinations, electrocardiograms (ECGs), and electroencephalograms (EEGs) and brain imaging studies (computed tomography [CT], magnetic resonance imaging [MRI], positron emission tomography [PET] scans) may be ordered. The physical assessment, along with the health history and diagnostic test results, helps to form a picture of the individual. The mental status examination offers important additional information about the client's current mental and emotional state.

MENTAL STATUS ASSESSMENT

The mental status examination allows care providers to observe and describe a client's behavior in an objective, nonjudgmental way. It is a tool for assessing mental health dysfunctions and identifying the causes of clients' problems. Understanding each part of the examination enables

Table 13-4	The Mental Status Examination
General description	Appearance; speech; motor activity; interaction during interview
Emotional state	Mood; affect
Experiences	Perceptions
Thinking	Thought content; thought processes
Sensorium and cognition	Level of consciousness; memory; level of concentration and calculation; information and intelligence; judgment

From Stuart GW, Laraia MT: *Stuart and Sundeen's pocket guide to psychiatric nursing,* ed 4, St. Louis, 1998, Mosby.

care providers to plan and deliver the most appropriate care for each of their clients.

The mental status examination explores the following areas: general description, emotional state, experiences, thinking, and sensorium and cognition (Table 13-4).

General Description

Under the category of general description, the client's general appearance, speech, motor activity, and behavior during the interaction are assessed.

The general appearance category includes everything that can be readily observed about a client, such as physical characteristics, dress, facial expressions, motor activity, speech, and reactions. To assess a client's physical characteristics, observe each part of the client's body, noting anything unusual. Describe the person's body build, skin coloring, cleanliness, and manner of dress. Does the person appear neat and tidy or careless and unkempt? Note any body odors. If cosmetics are used, are they appropriately applied? Does the client's appearance match his or her sex, age, and situation? People with depression, for example, may look unkempt and neglected. It is not uncommon for manic clients to dress in colorful, but bizarre, clothing and wear many cosmetics and jewelry. Document all findings.

Facial expressions, eye contact, and pupil size should be noted. Do the client's facial expressions match his or her emotions and actions? Is eye contact avoided or held for long periods of time? Note the size of the client's pupils. Large, dilated pupils are seen in people with drug intoxication, whereas small pupils are associated with narcotic use.

The client's speech is then assessed and described by its rate, its volume, and its characteristics. Note any abnormal speech patterns (see Chapter 11).

Next, turn your attention to the client's motor activity, gestures, and posture. Observe the client's physical movements for the level of activity, the type of activity,

Think About

Cybil is being admitted to the clinic's day treatment program. She insists that she feels fine, but she will not speak, except to answer yes or no and refuses to give her caregiver eye contact.
◆ What messages is Cybil's behavior sending?
◆ How do her verbal and nonverbal messages agree or disagree?

and any unusual movements or mannerisms. Is the client agitated, tense, restless, lethargic, or relaxed? Are there any tics, grimaces, repeated facial expressions, or tremors present? Excessive body movements are seen in individuals with anxiety or mania. They can also result from the use of stimulants or other drugs. Repeated movements or behaviors are seen in clients with obsessive-compulsive disorders, and picking at one's clothing is often seen in clients with delirium or toxic reactions.

To complete the general description, assess the client's behavior during the interaction (see Think About box). How did the client relate to you? Was he or she cooperative, hostile, or overly friendly? Did the client appear to trust you? Note if the client's verbal messages matched the behavior. Clients who use unconnected gestures may be having hallucinations.

Emotional State

To assess the client's emotional state, the care provider considers the client's mood and affect. **Mood** is defined as the individual's overall feelings. Mood is a subjective factor that can be explained only by the person experiencing it. Usually people will have a basic mood, although it may change sometime during the day. To illustrate, a basically relaxed and happy person may feel disappointed by an incident during the day but soon forgets and returns to his or her commonly happy mood.

Affect is the client's emotional display of the mood being experienced. Table 13-5 explains several kinds of affect. A person's mood can range from overwhelming sadness to great elation and joy. These variations are referred to as one's range of emotion. Affect can be categorized as appropriate, inappropriate, pleasurable, or unpleasurable. To assess a client's mood, ask what he or she is feeling and then observe the reactions. Do the responses to your questions match with the subjects being discussed? Is the client overreacting, not reacting at all, or responding inappropriately? Document objective descriptions of the client's behaviors. Descriptions communicate much more information than a single medical term does.

Experiences

This category explores the client's **perceptions,** the ways in which he or she experiences the world. An individual's

Table 13-5 Common Emotional Responses (Affects)

Name of affect	Description
Inappropriate Response	
Labile	Rapid, dramatic changes in emotions
Inconsistent	Affect and mood do not agree
Flat	Unresponsive emotions
Pleasurable Response	
Euphoria	Excessive feelings of well-being (feeling too good)
Exaltation	Intense happiness, often with feelings of grandeur
Unpleasurable (Dysphoric) Response	
Aggression	Anger, hostility, or rage that is out of keeping with situation
Agitation	Motor restlessness, often seen with anxiety
Ambivalence	Having both positive and negative feelings
Anxiety	Vague, uneasy feeling, often from unknown cause
Depression	Sadness, hopelessness, loss that is present over time
Fear	Reaction to recognized danger

Table 13-6 Disorders of Thinking

Disorder	Description
Thought Processes (How One Thinks)	
Blocking	Thoughts stop suddenly for no reason
Flight of ideas	Rapid changes from one thought to another related thought
Loose associations	Poorly organized or connected thoughts
Perseveration	Repeating same word in response to different questions
Thought Content (What One Thinks)	
Delusions	False beliefs that cannot be corrected by reasoning or explanation
Obsession	Thought, action, or emotion that is unwelcome and difficult to resist
Phobias	Strong fears of certain things, places, or situations
Preoccupations	All experiences and actions are connected to central thought that is usually emotional in nature
Others	
Amnesia	Inability to remember past events
Confabulation	Using untrue statements to fill in gaps of memory loss

perceptions are often referred to as one's *frame of reference*. In short, a person's perceptions help determine his or her sense of reality.

People who are having mental health problems may have difficulty in perceiving the same reality as the rest of society. *Hallucinations* are perceptions that have no external stimulus. The client may hear voices or see things that are not perceived by other people. Hallucinations involving taste, touch, or smell may indicate a physical problem. Visual and auditory hallucinations are associated with schizophrenia, the acute stage of alcohol or drug withdrawal, and organic brain disorders. Alterations in perceptions that have a basis in reality are called *illusions*. External stimuli are present, but they are perceived differently by the client. For example, a client perceives the person walking down the hall as a wolf.

To assess clients' perceptions, ask them if they can hear voices or see things when other people are not present. If the answer is yes, ask them to describe the experience. Questions that may be asked include the following:

How many different voices (images) do you hear (see)?
What do the voices say (images do)?
Do you recognize any of the voices (images)?

When did the voices (images) first begin? What was happening in your life at the time?
How do you feel about the voices (images)?

Remember that hallucinations or illusions are very real to the person experiencing them. Caregivers cannot "talk them out of it" or tell them to ignore what they are perceiving. However, because they are so real, clients usually are willing to describe them when asked.

Thinking

The "thinking" section of the mental status examination focuses on the client's thought content and process. **Thought content** relates to *what* an individual is thinking. Clients may be experiencing delusions, obsessions, phobias, preoccupation, amnesia, or confabulations.

Disturbances in **thought processes** relate to *how* a person thinks—how he or she analyzes the world and connects and organizes information. Disorders of thought process include blocking, flight of ideas, loose associations, and perseveration (Table 13-6).

Another problem of thinking is *depersonalization,* a feeling of unreality or detachment from oneself or one's environment. The unreal feelings produce a dreamlike atmosphere that overtakes the individual's consciousness. One's body does not feel like one's own. Events that are dramatic or important are perceived with a detached calmness, as if the person were watching instead of participating in reality. With functional people, feelings of depersonalization can occur when one is anxious, stressed, or very tired. Depersonalization disorders are commonly seen in clients with severe depression and in some forms of schizophrenia.

Assessment of the client's thought content and process is carried out throughout the entire mental status examination. Are the client's thoughts based in reality? Are ideas communicated clearly? Do the client's thoughts follow a logical order? Are there any unusual thoughts, preoccupations, or beliefs present? Does the client have any suicidal, violent, or destructive thoughts? (Forster, 1994). Are there any persistent dreams? Does the client believe that someone is intent on harming him or her (feelings of persecution)? Observe the client closely and listen intently. Much of this information will be revealed during the course of the interaction.

Sensorium and Cognition

The **sensorium** is that part of the consciousness that perceives, sorts, and combines information. People with a clear sensorium are able to orient to time, place, and person. They are also able to use their memories to recall recent and remote information. Levels of consciousness and memory recall help to assess a person's sensorium.

Level of consciousness can be determined by observing the amount of stimuli it takes to arouse the client (Table 13-7).

If the client cannot be awakened by verbal stimuli, notify your supervisor immediately. If the client is awake, note his or her responses to your questions, the degree of interaction, and the amount of eye contact that is being made.

Memory is the ability to recall past events, experience, and perceptions. For the purpose of testing, memory is divided into three categories: immediate, recent, and remote memory. Immediate memory is sometimes referred to as *recall.* To assess immediate memory (recall), ask the client to remember three things (e.g., a color, an address, and an object). Later in the conversation (at least 15 minutes), ask the client to repeat the three items. Recall can also be tested by having the client repeat a series of numbers within a 10-second period.

Recent memory includes events within the past 2 weeks. Caregivers test recent memory by asking the client to recall the events of the past 24 hours. Loss of

recent memory is often seen in people with Alzheimer's disease, anxiety, and depression.

Assessing *remote memory* involves asking the client questions about his or her place of birth, schools attended, ages of family members, and other questions about the person's background. This part of the mental status examination can easily be done during the nursing health history interview. It is sometimes difficult to tell if the client has accurate memories. Long-term memory loss is seen in clients with organic (physical) problems, conversion disorders, and dissociative disorders.

The level of concentration focuses on the client's ability to pay attention during the conversation. **Calculation** tests the ability to do simple math problems. Have the person count rapidly from 1 to 20; perform simple addition, multiplication, and division problems; and subtract 7 from 100, then 7 from 93, and so on. Then ask practical questions such as the number of dimes in $1.90. Note how easily the client becomes distracted during the tasks. People with mental-emotional problems commonly have difficulty with concentration and calculations. These difficulties are also seen in people with physical disorders, such as brain tumors, so it is important to assess the client's ability to concentrate and do simple calculations.

During this phase of the mental status examination, the client's education level, general knowledge, ability to read, use of vocabulary, and ability to think abstractly are assessed. General knowledge can be tested by asking the person to name the past five presidents, five large cities, or the occupations of well-known people in

Table 13-7	Levels of Consciousness
Comatose/unconscious	Unresponsive to any verbal or painful stimuli
Stuporous	Responds only to strong physical stimuli; falls asleep if not stimulated
Drowsy/somnolent	Wakens with strong verbal stimuli; falls asleep if left undisturbed
Lethargic	Can be verbally aroused; shows decreased wakefulness; may have periods of excitability alternating with periods of drowsiness
Alert	Awake and responsive; oriented to time, place, and person
Hyperalertness	Increased state of alertness or watchfulness (hypervigilance)
Mania	State of extreme excitement, elation, and activity

the community. Ask the client about the last grade completed in school.

To determine reading ability, print a command, such as "Close your eyes," on a piece of paper. Ask the client to read it and follow the directions. During the conversation, note the client's choice of words and their use.

Assess the client's ability to think abstractly by having him or her explain the meaning of several well-known proverbs, such as a stitch in time saves nine; a rolling stone gathers no moss; when it rains, it pours; or people in glass houses shouldn't throw stones.

Many people with mental health problems give concrete answers such as "Moss only grows on the north sides of stones" or "People who live in glass houses shouldn't throw stones because it breaks the glass."

Judgment refers to the ability to evaluate choices and make appropriate decisions. During the health history interview, observe how the client explains personal relationships, his or her job, and economic responsibilities. Assess the client's judgment by asking such questions as "What would you do if you . . .

found an addressed envelope on the ground?"
ran out of medication before the next appointment?"
won $25,000?"

Judgment is often impaired in people with chemical dependence, intoxication, schizophrenia, mental retardation, and organic mental disorders. Document the client's responses using the client's own words whenever possible.

Insight refers to the client's understanding of the situation. What is the client's understanding of the disorder? Questions that help the caregiver assess insight include "Have you noticed a change in yourself recently?" and "What do you think is the cause of your anxiety (discomfort)?" Expect clients to have different degrees of insight. For example, a person with an alcohol problem may realize that he or she drinks too much but does not think that it is interfering with family life. Again, be sure to document the client's statements rather than your opinions.

Although the mental status examination may appear to be a lengthy process, much of it can be performed during the history interview. Checklists that address each area of the examination are available (see Box 13-2 and Appendix D for a copy of the Mental Status Assessment at a Glance).

Care providers often use parts of the mental status examination to assess clients whose mental state changes frequently. For example, the caregiver assesses the

---

Box 13-2 Mental Status Assessment at a Glance

1. Appearance
   _____ Manner of dress
   _____ Personal grooming
   _____ Facial expressions
   _____ Posture and gait
2. Speech
   _____ Manner of response (frank, evading)
   _____ Choice of words (to assess general intelligence, education, levels of function, thought)
   _____ Speech disorder
3. Level of consciousness
   _____ Level of alertness
   _____ Orientation (time, place, person)
4. Attention span
   _____ Ability to keep thoughts focused on one topic
   _____ Repeat a series of numbers
   _____ Serial 7s (ask client to subtract 7 from 100, 7 from 93, etc.)
5. Memory
   _____ Immediate memory (ask client to repeat words after 15 minutes)
   _____ Recent memory (ask client about yesterday's activities)
   _____ Remote memory (ask client about dates of birth, marriage, schooling)

6. Understanding abstract relationships
   _____ Understanding of proverbs (concrete or abstract)
   _____ Ability to understand similarities (e.g., "How are a bicycle and an automobile alike?")
7. Arithmetic and reading ability
   _____ Simple addition, subtraction, multiplication, and division (ask client to make change)
   _____ Ability to read newspaper, magazine
8. General information knowledge
   _____ Discuss newspaper or magazine article
   _____ General information questions (e.g., "How many days in a year? Where does the sun set?")
9. Judgment
   _____ Responses to family, work, financial problems
   _____ Responses to "What would you do if . . ." questions
10. Emotional status
   _____ Ask "How do you feel today?" or "How do you feel about . . ." questions
   _____ Affect
   _____ Current situation and coping behaviors

Modified from Jess LW: *Nursing 88* 18(6):42, 1988.

hallucinating client for thought content and process at intervals throughout the day.

Work to develop your powers of observation. Do not pass judgment or let your opinions interfere with data gathering. Remember, the results of the mental status examination can be affected by attitudes and beliefs. Learn to use assessment skills because they will serve you well in all practice settings.

KEY CONCEPTS

◆ The ability to effectively obtain and use information about clients is a vital part of the multidisciplinary treatment plan.

◆ Every psychological illness has physical effects, and every physical illness is accompanied by psychological effects.

◆ Therapists who work with mentally and emotionally troubled individuals use the DSM-IV–TR to aid in diagnosis and help guide clinical practice.

◆ The nursing (therapeutic) process is a purposeful and organized approach to solving client problems that requires knowledge, experience, and the use of good judgment.

◆ Data collection refers to a variety of activities that are designed to elicit, gather, or discover information about a certain subject.

◆ The process of assessing a client is ongoing. It begins with the client's admission and ends only after the client's relationship with the health care system has ended.

◆ The psychiatric assessment tool includes an appraisal of the client's health, previous psychiatric treatment, physical and mental coping responses, discharge planning needs, psychosocial and environmental problems, and needs for knowledge.

◆ The purpose of a risk factor assessment is to formulate a nursing diagnosis based on the identification of risk factors that may present an immediate threat to the client or others.

◆ The history interview is an organized conversation with a client that has the purpose of bringing out certain information about the client's health status.

◆ The sociocultural assessment focuses on the cultural, social, and spiritual aspects of an individual.

◆ Head-to-toe assessments are a quick way to gather data about a client's current condition.

◆ The mental status examination explores general appearance, level of consciousness, behavior, speech, mood, affect, thought content, intellectual performance, insight, judgment, and perception.

◆ Caregivers often use various parts of the mental status examination to assess clients whose mental state changes frequently.

Suggestions for Further Reading

"Asking Questions Effectively," written by Susan Smith (*Nursing 95* 25[3]:83, 1995), offers some excellent hints for improving your interviewing skills.

Internet Mental Health (www.mentalhealth.com) dispenses information, diagnostic tools, news, articles, and editorials about common mental disorders.

References

Anderson KN, Anderson LE, Glanze WD: *Mosby's medical, nursing, and allied health dictionary,* ed 4, St. Louis, 1998, Mosby.

American Psychiatric Association: *Diagnostic and statistical manual of mental disorders,* ed 4, text revision, Washington, DC, 2000, The Association.

Forster P: Accurate assessment of short term suicide risk in a crisis, *Psychiatric Annals* 24:571, 1994.

Jess LW: Investigating impaired mental status: an assessment guide you can use, *Nursing 88* 18(6):42, 1988.

Keltner NL, Schwecke, Bostrom CE: *Psychiatric nursing,* ed 3, St. Louis, 1998, Mosby.

National Depressive and Manic-Depressive Association: Patient's cultural background important in diagnosis and treatment, *DMDA Newsletter* 7(3):3, 1995.

Potter PA, Perry AG: *Basic nursing: theory and practice,* ed 4, St. Louis, 1998, Mosby.

Stuart GW, Laraia MT: *Principles and practice of psychiatric nursing,* ed 7, St. Louis, 2001, Mosby.

Stuart GW, Laraia MT: *Stuart and Sundeen's pocket guide to psychiatric nursing,* ed 4, St. Louis, 1998, Mosby.

Chapter 14

Problems of Childhood

Learning Objectives

1. Identify three common problems of childhood and list two therapeutic interventions for each.
2. Describe the impact of homelessness and violence on children.
3. Identify two therapeutic interventions for the child with anxiety.
4. Name four behaviors that are seen in children with attention-deficit hyperactivity disorder.
5. Explain the importance of early diagnosis of disruptive behavioral (conduct) disorders.
6. State three therapeutic actions for children with mental retardation.
7. Identify three types of learning disorders.
8. Describe the behaviors seen in children with pervasive developmental disorders.
9. List three general interventions for children with mental health problems.

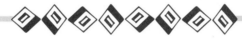

Key Terms

abuse

anxiety

attention-deficit hyperactivity
    disorder (ADHD)

autism

cephalocaudal

communication disorders

conduct disorders

development

dyslexia

encopresis

enuresis

growth

homelessness

learning disorder

mental retardation

neglect

pervasive developmental disorders

pica

posttraumatic stress disorder (PTSD)

proximal-distal

schizophrenia

somatoform disorder

victimization

G rowth and development are a vital part of life. Each individual is involved in a lifelong process of learning and mastering life's developmental and situational tasks. Children develop with great speed and constantly changing mental, social, and emotional abilities. Each child develops at an individual rate and may master the skills in one area of development while lagging in another. Behaviors considered normal in one age group become worrisome when they occur at another age. Health care providers who work with children must have an understanding of normal de-

velopment, as well as an awareness of the child's individual pace.

This chapter presents an overview of normal growth and development patterns for children, the mental health problems that can arise during childhood, and therapeutic actions for the care of mentally, emotionally, and developmentally troubled children.

Many theories about the growth and development of children exist. Table 14-1 lists the most common theories of childhood development, Chapter 5 provides a more thorough explanation of each theory.

Table 14-1	Theories of Childhood Growth and Development
Theory	**Explanation**
Freud—psychosexual development	Individuals grow and develop by taming their primitive libidinal (sexual, pleasurable) energies as they move through the stages of childhood.
Piaget—intellectual (cognitive) development	Growth is the ability to organize and integrate experiences.
Erikson—psychosocial development	Each person has a core task or problem that must be resolved before he or she can successfully move on to the next stage.

Maslow's hierarchy of needs, although not a developmental theory, is also important to consider when working with children. Essentially Maslow states that a child's most basic physical needs (air, water, food, elimination, and sleep) must be met before higher level needs (such as security, love, belonging, and esteem) are considered. Children must master skills that move them from complete dependence to independent functioning in only a few short years. It is the responsibility of every nurse to nurture and foster the growth of their youngest clients—the children.

NORMAL CHILDHOOD DEVELOPMENT

Growth is the increase in physical size. It can be measured in pounds, inches, kilograms, or centimeters. **Development** refers to the increased ability in skills or functions. Although each child grows and develops at an individual pace, each follows organized and orderly patterns throughout the growth process. The first pattern is known as **cephalocaudal** direction, where growth occurs from head to tail. Infants learn to control head movements before those of the trunk and arms. Growth also occurs in a **proximal-distal** (near-far) pattern. For example, the child's central nervous system develops before the peripheral nervous system. Last, growth moves from simple to complex (differentiation). Children learn to control the body's large muscle groups, such as walking, before mastering the fine motor skills of writing or building.

Growth is a continuing process. Recognizing the general patterns and principles of growth and development allows nurses to accurately assess, assist, and guide young clients (Box 14-1).

Development is the result of growth, learning, and the ability to combine the two. Children with growth or learning problems may mature later than other children. Development proceeds from simple to complex, from gross to fine, and from large to small. Physically, children learn to control the large muscles of their bodies first (walking, running), then move on to develop the finer movements (writing, reading). A child's reasoning is simple and uncomplicated until the nervous system develops the more complex organization required for abstract thinking. Social and emotional development also move from simple to complex. The younger the child, the more simple the emotions and the ability to communicate.

The emotional development of children is an ongoing process. During each stage, the child must learn to solve a central problem or task, which lays the basis for the next stage of development. If the child is unable to cope with the task or central developmental problem, then mental health difficulties may arise (Table 14-2).

The process of growth includes sensitive periods. During the growth process, children have certain times at which they are more affected by influences (positive or negative) in the environment. For example, according to Erikson, without a consistent adult caregiver during infancy, the child could develop problems trusting other people. Without nurturing, a child is ripe for developing mental health problems that may last a lifetime. For example, the child who was raised in an institutional setting often has difficulties bonding with a significant other as an adult. Nurses and other caregivers often provide the only consistency in these children's young lives.

Common Behavioral Problems of Childhood

Most children experience problems during each developmental stage. Some of the most common behavioral difficulties during the early years of childhood are colic, problems with feeding and sleeping, temper tantrums, and breath-holding spells.

Colic is a set of behaviors most commonly seen in middle-class infants. Severe periods of late-afternoon crying are first noticed when the infant is about 2 weeks old. The infant cries with clenched fists and pained looks and refuses attempts by adults to soothe him or her. Behaviors usually peak around 2 or 3 months, but they can persist until the infant is 4 or 5 months old. A colicky infant is defined as a healthy and well-fed child who cries for more than 3 hours every day for more than 3 weeks (Wong, 1998). Interventions designed to calm both parents and child appear to help. Nurses can help parents manage colic by helping them learn about the normal characteristics of crying and recognizing their infant's cues. Changing the feeding procedure and allowing adequate time for burping and cuddling helps to control symptoms. Other effective measures include creating a

Box 14-1 Developmental Periods

Prenatal Period: Conception to Birth

Germinal: Conception to approximately 2 weeks
Embryonic: 2 to 8 weeks
Fetal: 8 to 40 weeks (birth)

A rapid growth rate and total dependency make this one of the most crucial periods in the developmental process. Adequate prenatal care is extremely important for a healthy child.

Infancy Period: Birth to 12 Months

Neonatal: Birth to 28 days
Infancy: 1 to approximately 12 months

The infancy period is one of rapid motor, cognitive, and social development. Through bonding with the caregiver (parent), the infant establishes a basic trust in the world and the foundation for future interpersonal relationships. The critical first month of life is filled with major physical adjustments to life outside the womb and psychological adjustment of the parents.

Early Childhood: 1 to 6 Years

Toddler: 1 to 3 years
Preschool: 3 to 6 years

This period, which extends from the time the child attains upright locomotion until he or she enters school, is characterized by intense activity and discovery. It is a time of marked physical and personality development, while motor development advances steadily. Children acquire language and social relationships, learn role standards, gain self-control, develop increasing awareness of dependence and independence, and begin to develop a self-concept.

Middle Childhood: 6 to 10 Years

Frequently referred to as the "school age," this period is one in which the child is directed away from the family group and is centered around the wider world of peer relationships. There is steady advancement in physical, mental, and social development with emphasis on developing skill competencies. Social cooperation and moral development take on more importance. This is a critical period in the development of a self-concept as peers' and teachers' evaluations become part of the child's self-assessments.

Later Childhood: 10 to 19 Years

Prepubertal: 10 to 13 years
Adolescence: 13 to approximately 19 years

The period of rapid maturation and change known as adolescence is considered to be a transitional period that begins at the onset of puberty and extends to the point of entry into the adult world. Biological and personality maturation are accompanied by physical and emotional turmoil, and there is a redefining of the self-concept. In the late adolescent period, the child begins to internalize all previously learned values and begins to focus on an individual identity.

From Wong DL: *Whaley and Wong's nursing care of infants and children,* ed 6, St. Louis, 1998, Mosby.

Table 14-2 Emotional Developmental Tasks of Childhood

Stage	Age	Core task
Infancy	Birth–1 year	Trust vs. mistrust
Early childhood	1-3 years	Autonomy vs. shame and doubt
Preschool years	3-6 years	Initiative vs. guilt
School age	6-12 years	Industry vs. inferiority
Puberty	12-18 years	Identity vs. diffusion

quiet, restful environment, aromatherapy with lavender, and avoiding overhandling of the infant. Massage can soothe, relax, and calm some infants. Most children outgrow their colicky behavior by 5 months, but parents need a great deal of emotional support and encouragement during this stressful time.

Feeding disorders range from overeating, which leads to obesity, to undereating, which leads to malnutrition.

Infants may refuse to eat if the feeding experience is not satisfying. Young children who have had an unpleasant experience with food (being force-fed or choking) or are engaged in a conflict (power play) with caregivers may refuse to eat. Physical problems, such as poor oral motor control or swallowing problems, can cause unpleasant experiences with food. Children suffering from depression often refuse to eat, and adolescents may engage in destructive eating behaviors, such as anorexia or bulimia.

Problems with sleep are common to many children and include night terrors, problems falling asleep, and nighttime awakenings. In the past, the usual course of action was for the parents to let children "cry it out" until they fell asleep. Today each child's sleeping characteristics are considered, the parents' expectations and fears are addressed, and treatment is designed to assist both parents and child in establishing a restful pattern of sleep. Following bedtime rituals, such as reading a book or limiting television viewing, are often helpful measures.

Temper tantrums are a common expression of anger and frustration for children between 1 and 4 years of age.

In fact, temper tantrums are seen in 50% to 80% of children in this age group (Hagerman, 1995). In the young child, temper tantrums are considered normal behavior. Children are attempting to master their environments and become frustrated when they are unable to achieve control. Tantrums become a problem when children use them to express more emotions than just frustration or when the tantrums occur so frequently that they disturb family functioning.

Temper tantrums are the result of a loss of control. Most children feel a blow to their self-image, and some children are quite upset about the experience. Adults in the environment should remain calm during the tantrum. Therapeutic interventions for temper tantrums are listed in Box 14-2.

Mental Health Problems of Childhood

Each stage of life flows into the other. In reality there are no clear divisions of development. Many of the mental-emotional problems diagnosed in adulthood find their roots in the experiences of childhood. Health care providers play an important role in the recognition and treatment of children's mental health problems because without love and assistance, many children are doomed to failure.

The major mental health problems of childhood are grouped into seven categories (Table 14-3). Clients may be labeled with one diagnosis yet engage in behaviors that belong to another diagnostic category. Remember, each person is an individual. The diagnosis is less important than the person.

Many children have "mental health problems" sometime during the journey from infant to adult. Emotional difficulties arise during periods of change in one's life. The birth of a sibling or a move to a new city can disrupt a routine, create new demands, or make children more vulnerable. Stresses can push children to behave in worrisome ways. Peers can have influences that are not always desirable. How do parents know when their children's problems are a part of the normal process of growing up and when they are serious enough to require professional assistance? When a child demonstrates an absence of growth, an inability or refusal to change, or a failure to achieve the developmental tasks of his or her age group, mental health help should be sought.

Box 14-2 Nursing Actions for Children With Temper Tantrums

Prevent Tantrums

1. Childproof the environment: Remove anything that the child is not allowed to touch. Fewer restrictions lessen the chances for conflict.
2. Present choices and options: Allow the child to choose (within acceptable limits). Offer the opportunity to practice autonomy and mastery skills.

Control Tantrums

1. When frustration increases, use distraction. Focus the child's attention on calmer activities and reward positive behaviors.
2. Protect the child during the tantrum. Do not allow a child to hurt himself or herself or others.
3. Do not abandon the child during the tantrum. Stay close, but do not intrude on his or her space.
4. Point out to the child that he or she is out of control. Do not react negatively or try to discipline the child. Praise when control is regained.
5. Fight only those battles that must be won. The conflicts that serve no important purpose should be avoided. However, do not give into the demands that led to the tantrum.

After the Tantrum

1. Do not hold a grudge or hold on to negative emotions. Recognize that the child probably feels worse than you do.
2. Praise the child for gaining control.
3. Keep reinforcing desired behaviors. Do not overreact to undesirable actions.

Table 14-3 Categories of Mental Health Problems in Childhood

Category	Examples
Environmental problems	Poverty, homelessness, child abuse, child neglect, violence
Problems with parent-child interactions	Primary caregiver dysfunction, parent-child conflict
Emotional problems	Anxiety, depression, somatoform disorders (physical signs/symptoms with psychological causes), posttraumatic stress disorder
Behavioral problems	Attention-deficit hyperactivity disorder, disruptive behavior (conduct) disorder, antisocial disorder, oppositional defiant disorder
Eating or elimination problems	Anorexia, bulimia, enuresis, encopresis
Developmental problems	Mental retardation, learning disorders, communication disorders
Pervasive developmental disorders	Autism, childhood disintegrative disorder, schizophrenia

ENVIRONMENTAL PROBLEMS

Many children must cope with more than just developmental tasks. For children who are poor, homeless, abused, or neglected, growing up can be difficult. Problems associated with environment can have a strong impact on mental health. Poverty, for example, influences the growth and development of children more than one would expect. In 1998, the U.S. Census Bureau reported that more than 20% of the nation?s children lived in poverty-stricken families. The rate of poverty for children in the United States is greater than those rates in Canada and Western Europe.

Poverty and mental health problems go hand in hand. By age 5, poor children scored much lower on IQ tests and demonstrated higher rates of anxiety, unhappiness, and fearfulness. Programs such as Head Start help prepare children for school and attempt to improve thinking, communication, and social skills. However, more remains to be done if we are to prevent the many mental health problems that accompany the lack of an adequate income.

Homelessness

The lack of a permanent residence (**homelessness**) affects children in many ways (Figure 14-1). Studies (Rafferty and Shinn, 1991) revealed that homeless children had very high infant mortality rates; twice the normal incidence of illness and disease; and elevated lead levels in the blood. They also experienced hunger (or routinely did not have enough to eat); behavioral problems, developmental delays, speech delays, sleep disorders, and immature motor actions; short attention spans, withdrawal, aggression, return to toddler behaviors; inappropriate social interactions with adults, and immature peer interactions. The problem described in the Case Study box is unfortunately all too common.

Case Study

Carol had come to us as a very lost, exhausted, young girl, dressed in tattered jeans and with sad, red eyes that seemed to cry every time she opened her mouth to talk to us.

For her first few weeks at Covenant House, we could not really get her to talk about herself . . . who she was, why she was here, where she came from, how we could help her. The only words she spoke were cried out unconsciously in her nightmares, which crept up on her while she was vulnerable and alone at night, unable to run away.

"You don't want to know about me." "It hurts too much," she would say. "I . . . I can't talk about it."

Finally though, one night after another nightmare, her lonely pain got to be too much, and she began to open up. She was born in South Carolina but ran away because her parents beat her. "They were on drugs," she shrugged. "I guess they couldn't help it," she said. Frightened for her life and unable to stand the abuse any longer, she had run away to the city. Penniless and alone, she soon began to sell the only worldly possession she had— her body.

Then one night she met "him." He was 70, like a grandfather. "He said he would take care of me. I was so alone. And those first few days were great. He gave me everything—money, clothes. He made me feel good. Then he started crawling in bed with me at night . . . and doing terrible things. He began to give me cocaine and stuff to make it easier. He . . . I . . . I had no place to go. And then he started to beat me too . . ."

◆ In which behaviors did Carol engage to fulfill her basic needs?

◆ How do you think Carol behaves when she becomes angry?

Modified from McGeady MR: *"Does God still love me?": letters from the street,* New York, 1995, Sr Mary Rose McGeady.

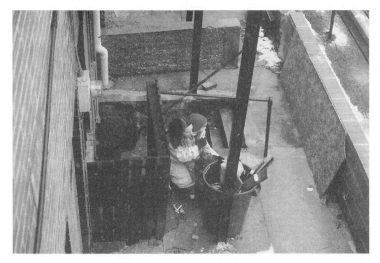

Figure 14-1 Many of the homeless are young mothers with young children. (Copyright © Cathy Lander-Goldberg, Lander Photographics.)

Table 14-4   Special Nursing Actions for Homeless Clients

Topic	Nursing actions
Psychological	Know your own feelings about homeless people.
	Approach clients with a positive attitude.
	Greet clients and communicate that they will be treated as people worthy of care and respect.
Client interview	Delay asking questions about occupation, address, next of kin, educational level until later in the interview.
	Promise that information is confidential.
	Ask simple, concrete questions:
	Where do you get your money?
	When did you have your last drink?
	Relate to homelessness in matter-of-fact way.
Health assessment	Educate as you assess.
	Assess children for signs of malnutrition, abuse, or neglect.
Discharge planning	Ask these questions:
	Do you understand what your problem is?
	How will you get your prescriptions filled?
	Where will you sleep tonight?
	Help client to keep follow-up appointments.
	Write down all instructions.

Modified from Hunter JK: *RN* 55(12):48, 1992.

Nurses must learn about the lifestyles of their clients and families, use good communication skills, and remain nonjudgmental. Table 14-4 offers a few special guidelines for nurses who work with homeless clients of all ages.

Abuse and Neglect

A victim is defined as someone who has been caused harm. **Victimization** is the process of causing harm. **Abuse** is defined as causing harm to or maltreating another. **Neglect** is not meeting a child's basic needs for food, clothing, shelter, love, and belonging. According to the U.S. Census Bureau (1998), over 51% of documented maltreatment cases are due to neglect. Child abuse and neglect are hitting crisis levels. The problems of abuse and neglect are becoming threats to the lives of infants and small children in America The actual statistics are grim, as Box 14-3 illustrates.

The victimization of children comes in many forms. Physical abuse is commonly associated with burns, bruises, fractures, and head and abdominal injuries. Sexually abused children have been violated through inappropriate sexual activities. Emotional or psychological abuse erodes children's self-esteem through rejection, criticism, isolation, or terrorism. Children also suffer from neglect—the failure to provide for their physical, emotional, and medical needs. Childhood abuse and neglect also have long-term effects. Today a wide variety of behavioral and physical disorders seen in adulthood, such as chronic anxiety and depression, and are thought to be associated with childhood abuse.

Box 14-3   Abuse and Neglect in Children

Five children die each day at the hands of their parents.

Although unintentional injuries are the leading cause of death in all children over 1, deaths caused by abuse or neglect in children ages 4 and younger outnumber those from falls, car accidents, suffocation, drowning, or choking on food.

18,000 children a year are permanently disabled by abusive caregivers.

142,000 children suffer serious physical injuries at the hands of their parents or other caretakers.

U.S. Advisory Board on Child Abuse and Neglect, 1995.

Factors that influence the potential for abuse and neglect include parental characteristics, such as social isolation, teenage motherhood, and difficulty controlling aggressive impulses. Children who are unwanted or disabled are at a higher risk for abuse and neglect, and environments filled with chronic stress may lead to child maltreatment. By recognizing these problems and referring families to appropriate services, health care providers may help prevent abuse and neglect from occurring.

Preventing and treating child abuse and neglect is the responsibility of every single health care provider, no matter what training or title. Education is a powerful first step. Programs such as "Don't Shake the Baby" (Showers, 1992) and materials from the National Clearinghouse on

Child Abuse and Neglect ([800] 394-3366) are increasing awareness of this international tragedy.

Helping the victims of child abuse also requires nurses to look at their own feelings about abuse. Being objective and supportive can be difficult in these situations, but it is important. Health care providers are in positions to recognize abuse and help provide early intervention. The problems of our children are the problems of us all.

PROBLEMS WITH PARENT-CHILD INTERACTIONS

A healthy family is able to cope with most of its emotional problems and knows when to seek help. Every child faces difficult emotional adjustments throughout childhood as change creates many new demands for children and their parents. One of the most common parent-child problems is conflict.

Parent-Child Conflicts

Children require consistent guidance and unconditional acceptance. Relationships with their caregivers serve as a testing ground for learning right from wrong and which behaviors result in reward or punishment. Parents who set limits and enforce them consistently provide the stability for children to test their limits in healthy ways. Conflicts between children and parents frequently occur and can take the form of verbal arguments or silent power struggles. No child or parent escapes childhood without conflict; however, when conflicts are constant and worsen over time, mental health assistance should be sought.

Primary Caregiver Dysfunction

When a parent is unable to meet the needs of a child, a disturbance in the parent-child interaction exists. The parent is commonly a person who has had difficult times in the past with personal relationships, psychiatric disorders, or behavioral problems. Perhaps the pregnancy was unwanted, or the child seems unresponsive. In this situation, the child is frequently described by the caretaker as difficult, defective, or disappointing.

The signs and symptoms seen in the child that suggest primary caregiver dysfunction include feeding and sleeping problems, delays in development, failure to thrive, signs of inadequate physical care or abuse, frequent visits to the physician, and excessive parental worry. Treatment is focused on supporting and educating the parents and helping them develop more effective and appropriate child care skills. With aggressive intervention, the long-term outlook for the children of these parents improves.

EMOTIONAL PROBLEMS

Emotional problems occur in children when they cannot successfully cope with their situations. They can range

---

Drug Alert

When children are prescribed antidepressant medications, the child and family should be taught to:

1. Drink plenty of fluids, especially water
2. Eat foods that are high in fiber to prevent constipation
3. Exercise regularly to help prevent constipation
4. Ensure the child's safety because he or she may experience dizziness

---

from anxiety to severe depression and suicide. Fortunately, most children are able to cope successfully with life's anxieties when they are nurtured and supported. This section focuses on the emotional problems of children that are most likely to be encountered by nurses in everyday treatment settings: anxiety, depression, somatoform disorders, and posttraumatic stress disorders.

Anxiety

Anxiety is a vague, uneasy feeling that occurs in response to a threat, and most children experience fear and anxiety as a part of growing. One of the most frequent anxieties of infants and toddlers, called separation anxiety, is a fear of being separated from their parents. Eventually, the fear decreases as children broaden their worlds to include others. However, if a child older than 4 years has separation anxieties lasting for more than a few weeks, a problem may exist. Severe levels of anxiety in children may result in obsessive-compulsive behavior, a condition that is discussed in Chapter 20.

Anxiety-based school refusalor school avoidance is a behavioral pattern in which the child refuses to attend school. Causes include anxiety, fear of leaving home (separation anxiety), fear of being ridiculed or embarrassed at school (social phobia), or fear of some aspect of school (school phobia). The main goal of treatment for children with school-related anxiety is to help the child confront and overcome the anxiety by returning to school. Many times, health care providers work with school personnel and parents to develop a plan for returning the child to school in a supportive manner. Antidepressants are sometimes prescribed for severe symptoms of anxiety or depression (see Drug Alert box).

Most children's bouts of anxiety are relieved when they receive reassurance and emotional support. If anxiety does not interfere with family, friends, or school, the child is coping effectively. However, when the anxiety is so pronounced that it is impossible for the child to function, then help should be sought.

Depression

Mood disorders, such as depression, are increasing in children. The term *depression* is used to describe a symptom, an emotional state, and a clinical syndrome. It is now known that depression can occur in children and adolescents. Children who have one or more depressed parents are more likely to be depressed themselves. Depression is seen more frequently as children grow older, and it occurs equally in boys and girls.

The clinical findings of depression arise from "an intense, persistent state of unhappiness and misery that interferes with pleasure or productivity"(Clark, 1995). Behaviors associated with depression vary little with age, except that school-age children tend to "act out," whereas adults withdraw. The clinical signs and symptoms of depression are discussed in Chapter 21. Treatment is designed to relieve the child's discomforting symptoms and help those in the environment to respond to the child's needs. Therapeutic interventions focus on reducing the problems that are causing the depression and providing the child with the emotional support to cope effectively.

Somatoform Disorders

A **somatoform disorder** is one in which the child (or adult) has the signs/symptoms of illness or disease without a traceable physical cause. The individual does not consciously take on the signs or symptoms, but he or she truly feels ill. Children often complain of headaches, upset stomach, or pain.

Somatic symptoms are not unusual in school-age children. They are thought to be expressions of stress or underlying conflict. Sometimes the child's signs or symptoms resemble those seen in another family member. In most cases, when the stress is relieved, the child returns to a healthy level of functioning. Somatoform disorders are covered in greater depth in Chapter 22. Here it is important to remember that children with somatoform disorders need understanding and reassurance.

Posttraumatic Stress Disorder

When children are repeatedly exposed to or participate in acts of violence, their psyches take steps to emotionally protect them. **Posttraumatic stress disorder (PTSD)** usually develops following an extreme traumatic event that involves injury or threat to the child, such as experiencing a fire or witnessing a shooting death. The child feels intense helplessness, fear, or horror. In younger children, behaviors become agitated and disorganized. Traumatic events are repeatedly relived, and the child goes to great lengths to avoid anything associated with the trauma. The traumatic event becomes generalized into nightmares of monsters or threats to the self. The past is relived through playing out of events related to the trauma. Somatic complaints, such as upset stomachs and other discomforts, may occur. Treatment is focused on early recognition and emotionally supportive care.

BEHAVIORAL PROBLEMS

Children experiment with various behaviors to test the limits of their environments and the people within them. Every child goes through periods of misconduct: refusing to do as told, lying, cheating, stealing, bullying others. Most often, these behaviors decrease with time and consistent guidance. For some children, however, undesired behaviors become more difficult to manage. These children clash with friends and classmates. They may develop a reputation for being unruly bullies or, worse yet, dangerous. When a child's conduct becomes inappropriate over a period of time, a disruptive behavioral disorder is usually diagnosed. Sometimes behavioral problems are linked to a physical cause, such as a lack of neurotransmitter production in the brain. The two disruptive behavioral disorders most commonly encountered by nurses are attention-deficit hyperactivity disorders and conduct disorders.

Attention-Deficit Hyperactivity Disorder

During the 1850s a German nursery rhyme told the story of "Phillip," a bad boy who could not sit down. A century later the children who exhibit Phillip's behaviors are diagnosed as having **attention-deficit hyperactivity disorder,** commonly called ADHD, which is now the most commonly diagnosed mental health problem in childhood. It affects about 3% of American children, and its symptoms can persist into adulthood. Attention-deficit hyperactivity disorder is seen more frequently in boys, with a ratio of about seven boys to one girl. Although ADHD was thought to be primarily a problem of childhood, it is often seen in adolescents and adults. It is a syndrome—a cluster of behaviors relating to inattention and impulsive actions. Within the ADHD category, a variety of subgroups exist: ADHD with learning disabilities, ADHD without hyperactivity, ADHD with speech disorders, ADHD with other psychiatric disorders, and ADHD with disorders of brain function. Box 14-4 lists the diagnostic criteria for ADHD.

There are two common clinical histories for children with ADHD. The first is the child who has been "fussy" or "a difficult child" from birth. As infants, they were difficult to soothe, and they have behaved impulsively as far back as family members can recollect. They are remembered as being "a handful." The second type of child is referred to as an *immature child* who displays silliness, distractibility (short attention span), restlessness, and clumsiness. Both types of children have problems with behavioral self-control, hyperactivity, relating to others, and focusing their attention. On entry into school, children with ADHD have difficulty in completing their schoolwork because they are easily distracted. They are usually academic underachievers, although they may have

Box 14-4 Attention-Deficit Hyperactivity Disorder

A. A disturbance of at least 6 months during which at least eight of the following are present:
    1. Often fidgets with hands or feet or squirms in seat (feelings of restlessness in adolescents)
    2. Has difficulty remaining seated when required to do so
    3. Is easily distracted by outside stimuli
    4. Has difficulty awaiting his or her turn in games or group situations
    5. Often blurts out answers to questions before they have been completed
    6. Has difficulty following through on instructions from others (e.g., fails to finish chores)
    7. Has difficulty sustaining attention in tasks or play activities
    8. Often shifts from one uncompleted activity to another
    9. Has difficulty playing quietly
    10. Often talks excessively
    11. Often interrupts or intrudes on others (e.g., butts into other children's games)
    12. Often does not seem to listen to what is being said to him or her
    13. Often loses things necessary for tasks or activities at school or at home (e.g., toys, pencils, books, assignments)
    14. Often engages in physically dangerous activities without considering possible consequences (e.g., runs into street without looking)
B. Onset before the age of 7 years
C. Does not meet the criteria for a pervasive developmental disorder

Modified from Wong DL: *Whaley and Wong's nursing care of infants and children,* ed 6, St. Louis, 1998, Mosby.

 Drug Alert

Psychotherapeutic medications are powerful chemicals. When prescribed for children, parents must be taught to routinely monitor for side effects, adverse reactions, any unwanted effect, and interactions with over-the-counter medications, such as cold medications (see Chapter 7). Nurses have an important responsibility to provide parents with written information about the medication(s) the child is receiving, how to monitor the child's response to the drug, and what side effects to report. They should be willing to monitor the child throughout the period he or she is receiving psychotherapeutic drugs.

normal or above-average intelligence. They may also have problems making friends because of their excitable and impulsive behaviors. Almost half the children with ADHD show symptoms of anxiety, aggression, depression, and resistance to any authority.

Treatment for children with ADHD requires a multidisciplinary approach Families are educated about the problem, and many children receive special education. Positive reinforcement programs help children choose more socially appropriate behaviors and reduce impulsive actions. Therapeutic interventions for children with ADHD focus on providing a consistent and structured therapeutic approach. Caregivers must be prepared to set limits on clients' behaviors and then be consistently willing to enforce them. They should also strive to acknowledge and reward the child for appropriate

behaviors. In cases in which the child is receiving drug therapy (i.e., Ritalin, antidepressants, such as imipramine or desipramine, and clonidine), nurses must carefully monitor each child's response to the medications (see Drug Alert box).

Disruptive Behavioral (Conduct) Disorder

Misconduct is common in every child, but when a persistent pattern of unacceptable behaviors is present, a conduct or disruptive behavioral disorder is established. Children with **conduct disorders** are defiant of authority. They engage in aggressive actions toward other people, refuse to follow society's rules and norms, and violate the rights of others. Many come from broken homes and backgrounds of violence, drug abuse, alcoholism, poverty, and lack of consistent caregivers.

The typical picture of a child with a conduct disorder is described as a boy with social and academic problems, truancy, and failure in school. He is defiant of authority and often engages in temper tantrums, running away, and fighting. Treatment focuses on providing a stable environment and consistently enforced limits. Associated neurological, educational, or psychiatric problems are also treated. The long-term outlook for children with conduct disorders is poor if the problems are present before the child is 10 years old or if antisocial behavior is displayed by the adults in the environment. Nearly half these children grow up to have antisocial or conduct disorders in adulthood. This makes early diagnosis and treatment very important if these children are to become productive members of society.

Oppositional Defiant Disorder

A recurring pattern of disobedient, hostile behavior toward authority figures describes this problem. Children with oppositional defiant disorder frequently lose their tempers, argue with adults, deliberately annoy other people, and refuse to compromise. They blame others for

Loss of temper on a daily basis
Frequent physical fighting
Vandalism or damage to property
Carries a weapon
Announces threats or plans to hurt others
Use of drugs and/or alcohol
Enjoys hurting animals
Carries a weapon
Engages in risk-taking behaviors
Details plans to commit acts of violence

their misbehaviors and continually test their limits by arguing, ignoring, or becoming aggressive. Treatment includes family therapy where limit setting and consistency are stressed.

Because of the increase in school-related violence, the American Psychological Association has developed a checklist for the warning signs of violence (Box 14-5). Children who demonstrate these behaviors are at risk for engaging in violent behaviors.

PROBLEMS WITH EATING AND ELIMINATION

The most common mental health problems seen in children that relate to eating are feeding disorders, pica, anorexia nervosa, and bulimia. Disorders of elimination include encopresis and enuresis. Eating disorders are most often encountered in adolescents, but young children can also use food inappropriately to cope with their emotions. Early recognition and treatment helps prevent greater problems later in life. Anorexia nervosa (a severe disturbance in eating behavior that results in a body that is much lower than its ideal weight) and bulimia (uncontrolled ingestion of large amounts of food followed by inappropriate methods to prevent weight gain) are discussed in the next chapter.

Eating Disorders

Children with eating disorders either do not eat enough or eat the wrong things. The diagnostic category of feeding and eating disorders of infancy or early childhood describes children who routinely fail to eat adequately. Weight loss or a failure to gain weight for at least 1 month in a child with no gastrointestinal tract problems is the most significant sign. Food is available, but the child does not eat. Most feeding disorders occur in children under 1 year, but they are seen in some 2- and 3-year olds. The long-term complications are malnutrition and delays in development.

Feeding disorders can result from repeated unsuccessful attempts to feed an irritable infant. Infants may be difficult to console, apathetic, or withdrawn during feedings. Some infants may have difficulty regulating their nervous systems, resulting in altered periods of alertness. Other factors associated with feeding disorders are parental mental health problems, abuse, and neglect. Treatment focuses on ruling out any physical cause, teaching parents appropriate feeding techniques, and monitoring the child's weight and developmental gains. In some cases, family therapy is helpful.

Pica is the term used to describe persistent eating of nonfood items for more than 1 month. The nonfood items chosen seem to vary with age. Infants and younger children will typically eat paint, hair, string, plaster, or cloth. Older children may eat sand, pebbles, insects, animal droppings, or leaves; adults may consume clay, soil, or laundry starch. Pica is often seen in children with mental retardation and pervasive developmental disorders (e.g., autism). Treatment includes ruling out any physical problems, such as vitamin or mineral deficiencies; removing the item from the child; and helping the child to replace the unacceptable items with more acceptable foods.

Rumination disorder is an uncommon feeding disorder in which the infant regurgitates (brings up) and rechews food. It is most often seen in infants from 3 to 12 months old but may occur in older children or adults with mental retardation. Characteristically, the infant will arch the back, hold the head back, make sucking movements with the tongue and give the impression of receiving satisfaction when the food is regurgitated. Malnutrition may occur because the food is brought back to the mouth soon after it is eaten. The disorder often disappears as the child grows older.

Elimination Disorders

The two most common elimination problems of childhood are enuresis and encopresis. **Enuresis** is the involuntary urinary incontinence of a child 5 years or older. It often has a tendency to run in families. Enuresis is divided into three categories: primary nocturnal enuresis (wetting the bed at night), diurnal enuresis (daytime wetting), and secondary enuresis (develops after child has achieved bladder control for a period of time).

Primary nocturnal enuresis common in children. It occurs three times more frequently in boys and often disappears without intervention. The actual cause of nighttime wetting is not known, but it is believed that a developmental delay in the sleep-wake mechanism or bladder capacity of the child may be a factor. Daytime (diurnal) wetting is less common. It is usually seen in shy children or those with ADHD. Daytime wetting occurs equally between boys and girls. Approximately 60% to 80% also wet the bed at night.

Secondary enuresis develops when a bladder-trained child becomes incontinent. Usually it follows a stressful

Table 14-5	Classification of Mental Retardation Levels			
Mild (85% incidence)	**Moderate (10% incidence)**	**Severe (3%-4% incidence)**	**Profound (2% incidence)**
Develops social and communication skills; has academic skills to sixth-grade level; has skills adequate for self-support; may need supervision and guidance but is able to successfully live in community	Develops communication skills; has academic skills to second-grade level; profits from vocational training; can attend to personal care with supervision; can work in sheltered setting or work in community under supervision; adapts well to community life in supervised environments	May learn to talk and do basic self-care skills; can learn key "survival" words (e.g., stop, bus, police); performs simple tasks with close supervision; adapts well to life with families or group homes	Exhibits associated neurological conditions, delays in development; has impaired sensorimotor function; is unable to care for self independently; may improve in highly structured environment; will always require sheltered environment with close supervision

Modified from American Psychiatric Association: *Diagnostic and statistical manual of mental disorders,* ed 4, text revision, Washington, DC, 2000, The Association.

event, such as the birth of a sibling or a divorce. Both diurnal and secondary enuresis are associated with high levels of emotional stress and anxiety.

Treatment for children with enuresis ranges from simple reassurance to various mental health therapies. Medications (desmopressin, imipramine) may be prescribed. Nurses can help parents cope by obtaining an accurate history of the child's problems, helping parents to establish a bedtime routine for the child, and providing emotional support. When mental health therapy is required, the focus is on helping the child verbally express the feelings associated with the symptoms.

Encopresis is defined as "the repeated, usually voluntary, passage of feces in inappropriate places" (Clark, 1995) in a child over 4 years of age with no physical abnormalities. It affects boys four times more than girls and is rarely seen in adolescence. After any physical problems are ruled out, treatment focuses on establishing a routine bowel care program. Praising the child for continent periods and having him or her assume the responsibility for rinsing the soiled clothing is often effective. Children who show little concern or distress about their incontinence are more difficult to treat.

DEVELOPMENTAL PROBLEMS

Children develop by mastering increasingly more difficult and complex tasks. Because each child is unique, some lags in certain areas of development are common and to be expected. However, if the child persistently falls behind in a developmental area, a disorder of intellectual functioning, learning, or communication is suspected. The developmental problems most often seen by health care providers include mental retardation, various learning disorders, and several types of communication disorders.

Mental Retardation

Children who function significantly below the average intellectual level for their age group and are limited in their abilities to function are said to be mentally retarded. The diagnosis of **mental retardation** is a powerful label and too often applied in haste. For a child to be considered retarded, he or she must have problems in general intellectual and adaptive functioning.

The degree of intellectual functioning is established by having the child complete one or more standard intelligence (IQ) tests. Children who repeatedly score lower than 70 are defined as retarded. The more important measure is the child?s adaptive functioning: how well the child copes with the demands of life. It includes the skill areas relating to self-care, home living, communication, social skills, use of community resources, academic skills, self-direction, and the child's work, leisure, safety, and health activities. Table 14-5 describes the various levels of retardation.

Fetal alcohol syndrome is the leading known cause of retardation in children. Inborn errors of metabolism, Down syndrome, birth injuries, shaken baby syndrome, high fevers in childhood, hormonal imbalances, poisonings, accidents, and falls are known causes of retardation. Heredity, fetal development, problems of pregnancy or infancy, and environmental influences are thought to be related factors, but for 30% to 40% of all children, no clear cause of mental retardation can be found. Treatment is individually developed and focuses on encouraging the child to function at the highest levels possible. Therapeutic actions focus on meeting the child's basic needs, providing a safe environment, and encouraging the development of life skills.

Learning Disorders

Formally called *academic skills disorders,* the category for problems with learning is broad. A **learning disorder** is diagnosed when a child with normal intelligence achievements on standard reading, mathematics, or written tests routinely falls below the results of other children in the same age and grade groups. Learning disorders can affect the child's thinking, reading, writing, calculation, spelling, and listening abilities. Approximately 5% of children in the U.S. public school system have learning disabilities (American Psychiatric Association, 2000).

Children with learning disabilities often feel low self-esteem and lack the social skills of other children. Many become discouraged and drop out of school early. Although no specific cause has been found for learning disorders, they have been associated with conditions such as fetal alcohol syndrome, lead poisoning, and fragile X syndrome (a genetic problem). Learning disorders are diagnosed only after the child has been assessed for physical disorders, such as hearing, speech, and visual problems. Cultural influences are also considered. A child is said to have a learning disorder only if the specific problem interferes with academic achievement or the activities of daily living.

Children with a reading disorder may have problems reading, understanding the written word, reading out loud, or writing. Individuals with **dyslexia** have problems with reading because although they can see and recognize letters, they have difficulty integrating visual information and thus tend to twist, substitute, distort, or omit many words. Children are seldom diagnosed before they have received several years of reading instruction in school. Early intervention is important because special education often results in great improvement. Reading disorders, if not addressed, may follow the child into adult life.

Many learning disorders are seen in children with ADHD. Other children with learning disabilities are quiet, with low activity levels. They are frequently overlooked because of their quiet manners or are mistaken for being retarded. Most children with learning disabilities respond well to special education classes and encouragement.

Communication Disorders

In children, the most common **communication disorders** relate to problems with expression, receiving messages, the pronunciation of words, and stuttering. Communication disorders may be the result of neurological or other medical conditions, but most often the cause is unknown.

Problems with language are usually seen in children around age 3. The child may fail to use expected speech sounds for his or her age group (phonological disorder); speak at a rapid or slow rate, with strange rhythms and word use (expressive language disorder); or have a disturbance in the pattern of speech in which sounds are frequently repeated (stuttering). Each is considered a disorder only if the problem interferes with the child's activities of daily living or ability to academically achieve.

Children with developmental problems must struggle more than other children for their learning. They need love, patience, and encouragement on a daily basis. Too often, adults fall into the "label trap" and condemn these children to performing at levels far below their actual abilities. Caregivers must remember that working with developmentally different children comes with a commitment to help them achieve to the best of their abilities.

PERVASIVE DEVELOPMENTAL DISORDERS

The word *pervasive* is defined as a tendency to spread throughout. When applied to mental health, the word means that a problem is severe enough to affect several areas of functioning. Children who are suffering from **pervasive developmental disorders** have difficulty with social interaction skills, communication skills, and learning. Their behavior is definitely different from that of other children of the same age and developmental level. Actual causes for these disorders remain unknown, but they are often seen with mental retardation, congenital infections, and abnormal central nervous system functions.

Pervasive developmental disorders include the following:

Autism: A disorder of communication, social interactions, and behavior

Rett syndrome: The development of motor, language, and social problems and loss of previous skills that occurs between 5 months and 4 years of age, where head growth declines, hand movements resemble hand-wringing, loss of social interest occurs, and severe speech impairments occur

Asperger's syndrome: Severe and long-lasting impairments in social interactions with repeated patterns of behavior, interest, and activities

Childhood disintegrative disorder: A period of severe regression in many areas following 2 years of normal development

Rett syndrome and childhood disintegrative disorder appear after a period of normal functioning, whereas autism and Asperger's syndrome are present in infancy. Autism is the most often encountered pervasive developmental disorder of childhood. It shares many of the same characteristics with the other listed disorders and serves as an example for learning about the behaviors of children with pervasive developmental disorders.

Autism

Autism is not a disease but a syndrome of associated behaviors. It results from some condition that affects the development of the nervous system, and it can remain with the individual throughout life. Autism is diagnosed when the child has serious problems with social interactions, communication, use of imagination, and demonstrates a markedly restricted scope of activities and interests.

The onset of autistic signs and symptoms begins in infancy or early childhood. Autistic disorders affect children from all classes and groups. Typically, autism is seen four times more frequently in boys. The majority of autistic children measure low on IQ tests. Motor skill development may be good, but the child's use of motor skills is inappropriate. Many autistic children become functioning adults, whereas others are totally dependent for care. Children who are able to develop language skills before the age of 5 years have better outcomes. If the child has seizures around puberty, the outlook for improvement is generally poor.

No single behavior or symptom is diagnostic of autism. Behaviors must be considered in relation to the whole child and his or her functioning. Monitoring children's early social responses, communication skills, and behaviors allows health care providers to intervene early when a problem is suspected.

The outstanding feature of autism is its different behaviors. Autistic children tend to use people in the environment like objects; they are unable to imitate others or make social contact. Other characteristics of autistic disorder include abnormal speech and communications, abnormal play activities, preoccupation with certain objects and routines, restricted body movements, and a very narrow range of interests.

Nurses who work with children must become keen observers and careful history takers. Parents should be questioned about the child's birth, developmental history, social responses, and communications. The picture of an autistic child begins to emerge when it is learned that the child does not act appropriately for his or her mental age, even with family members and other familiar people. Once the disorder is suspected, the child receives a complete physical examination to rule out central nervous system problems. The child is then referred to a treatment team that specializes in children with autistic problems. Parents are encouraged to work with physicians, nurses, several types of therapists, and special educators. A program is designed to meet the individual child's unique needs. Then parents, child, and treatment team work together for each small gain in functioning.

Schizophrenia

Schizophrenia is a condition associated with disturbing thought patterns and a distorted reality. Considerable disagreement exists concerning the onset of schizophrenia in childhood. Schizophrenia usually develops during late adolescence or early adulthood, but it has been seen in children. Recent research has demonstrated that schizophrenic children may have attention and memory problems that interfere with their ability to carry information into the short-term or working memory. As a result, many are unable to monitor the responses of other people or they interact and respond with illogical or disconnected statements (McClellan J and others, 1997).

The signs, symptoms, and behaviors of children with schizophrenia vary widely, but the core disturbance lies in a lack of contact with reality and the child's retreat into his or her own world. Common behaviors include bizarre movements; alternating periods of hypoactivity and hyperactivity; inappropriate emotions, language, and use of their body; distorted sense of time; treating self and others as nonhuman; compulsions; phobias; and temper tantrums. Early recognition and treatment are important because schizophrenia is often a long-term disorder.

THERAPEUTIC ACTIONS

Therapeutic interventions for children with mental health problems are first directed toward early identification and

Table 14-6	Pediatric Mental Health Screening Tool		

Assessment	Subject
Childhood history	Ambulation, behavior problems, bowel and bladder training/habits, communication (problems in speech or learning), discipline, eating habits, playmates (social interactions), psychiatric history (treatments, medications, suicide potential), school (reactions, experiences), sleep habits, unusual illnesses or injuries, current problem (with description of events that led to current situation)
Family history	Current household (members, relationship to child), mother and father, type of family (birth, blended, adopted, foster), mental health history of family (e.g., drug, alcohol use, arguments, violence, suicide attempts)
Mental status examination	General appearance, communication, emotion (mood, affect), intellectual level, orientation, thought processes

treatment. Health care providers fill a valuable role by performing health screening and routine examinations for healthy children in a variety of settings (Table 14-6).

Once a disorder is diagnosed, special treatment programs and specific goals are developed for each child. Nurses routinely assess and monitor the child's progress toward meeting each goal. In addition, they provide the emotional support and encouragement that is much needed by the parents and other family members.

The care for each child is special and is based on individual needs. Nursing diagnoses for children with mental health problems are listed in Box 14-6. Therapeu-

tic actions are basically focused on providing holistic care within an environment that fosters growth and development. The Sample Client Care Plan offers an example of a client care plan for a child with mental retardation. General interventions are focused on meeting basic needs, providing opportunities, and encouraging self-care activities.

Meet Basic Needs

Meeting the child's basic physical needs can range from a gentle reminder to providing total personal care. Caregivers are responsible for making sure the child adequately

---

⟫⟫ Sample Client Care Plan — Mental Retardation

Assessment

History: BJ is a 6-year-old boy with moderate mental retardation. His birth and the first 6 months of life were uneventful. At 7 months, BJ contracted "a virus" and since then has shown little developmental progress.
Current Findings: A slightly overweight 6-year old boy who is screaming uncontrollably at the time of interview. Mother reports that BJ is able to speak but prefers to

communicate by pointing at the desired object and grunting. When needs are not immediately met, BJ begins to scream in shrill voice. He feeds himself finger foods and refuses to use a spoon. He is not bowel or bladder trained and follows no daily routine at home. Eating and sleeping routines are nonexistent.

Multidisciplinary Diagnosis

Altered growth and development related to physical dysfunctions as evidenced by impaired developmental abilities

Planning/Goals

BJ will develop a daily routine for eating, sleeping, and activities by October 2.

Therapeutic Interventions

Intervention	Rationale	Team Member
1. Supervise closely for first 7 days on unit.	To assess strengths, abilities and needed interventions.	All
2. Approach BJ in a calm, peaceful manner.	Promotes self-esteem, decreases anxieties.	All
3. Introduce no more than two new people into the environment per week.	Decreases anxiety, provides security.	All
4. Establish a daily routine for food, naps, activity.	Prevents anxiety, provides security.	Nsg
5. Name each object that BJ points to and encourage him to repeat the name.	Encourages the use of speech and control over enviornment.	All
6. Assist with personal care as needed; praise for any attempt at self-care.	Promotes comfort, acceptance. Praise encourages further attempts at self-care.	Nsg, OT

Evaluation

By the tenth day in the unit, BJ was able to follow a simple daily routine with frequent coaching. Sleep at night progressed from 3-hour periods to 9-hour periods.

A complete client care plan includes several other diagnoses and interventions.

eats, sleeps, eliminates, and maintains personal cleanliness. Helping a child to meet basic needs includes the provision of love and acceptance, no matter how unusual or odd the behaviors. Many children with mental health problems have a special need to be nurtured. Often, the family and the child's caregivers are the only persons in environment who provide that energy.

Box 14-6 Nursing Diagnoses for Children With Mental Health Problems

Adjustment, impaired
Anxiety
Body image disturbance
Communication, impaired verbal
Coping, defensive
Coping, ineffective family
Coping, ineffective individual
Denial
Environment, impaired
Family process, altered
Fear
Growth and development, altered
Health maintenance, altered
Hopelessness
Infant behavior, disorganized
Infant feeding pattern, ineffective
Injury, risk for
Knowledge deficit
Loneliness, risk for
Nutrition, altered
Parent/infant/child attachment, altered
Parental role conflict
Parenting, altered, risk for
Personal identity disturbance
Posttrauma response
Powerlessness
Protection, altered
Rape-trauma syndrome
Self-care deficit

Provide Opportunities

Even the most profoundly retarded or mentally troubled child will achieve if given the opportunity, instruction, and support. Assessment tools, such as those listed in Table 14-7, allow nurses to screen for developmental levels, school readiness, and potential problems.

Each child is capable of something. Encourage young clients to grow and to reach for higher levels of function. Provide opportunities for small successes, which encourage everyone (especially the child) to strive for more.

Encourage Self-Care and Independence

Mentally troubled children grow and develop just as ordinary children do. Despite their problems, many become productive adults, able to live successfully within their communities. Health care providers who work with these children help them learn the important skills of daily living. Daily hygiene skills, such as how to dress, bathe, brush teeth, and comb hair are taught and reinforced. Caregivers coordinate with teachers, occupational therapists, and physical therapists to help teach the more complex skills of living, such as how to take a bus, spend money, or pay bills. Many will not be able to engage in the more complicated activities of daily life, but each child deserves the encouragement to function as independently as possible.

Caring for children with mental health problems is challenging work, but the rewards are many and worth the efforts. Our children are our priceless gifts to the future, and even the most troubled deserve our best efforts.

KEY CONCEPTS

◆ Health care providers who work with children must have an understanding of normal development and an awareness of the child's individual pace of growth and development.

◆ Common behavioral difficulties during the early years of childhood are colic, problems with feeding and sleeping, temper tantrums, and breath-holding spells.

Table 14-7 Assessment Tools for Children

Tool	Ages	Focus
Denver II	Birth to 6 years	Gross and fine motor skills; language; social skills
Preschool Readiness Screening Scale	4 to 5 years	Maturation; school readiness
Early Language Milestone Scale	Birth to 36 months	Speech and language development
Infant Temperament Questionnaire	1 to 2 months	Temperament
Toddler Development Scale	1 to 3 years	Temperament
Behavioral Style Questionnaire	3 to 7 years	Temperament
Middle Childhood Questionnaire	8 to 12 years	Temperament

◆ Many children must cope with the mental health problems that are a result of poverty, homelessness, abuse, or neglect.

◆ Primary caregiver dysfunction is diagnosed when a parent is unable to meet the caretaking or developmental needs of a child.

◆ The most common emotional problems of children include anxiety, depression, somatoform disorders, and posttraumatic stress disorders.

◆ The two disruptive behavioral disorders most commonly encountered by caregivers are attention-deficit hyperactivity disorders and conduct disorders.

◆ The most common pediatric mental health problems that relate to eating are feeding disorders, pica, anorexia nervosa, and bulimia.

◆ Disorders of elimination include encopresis and enuresis.

◆ The developmental problems most often seen include mental retardation, various learning disorders, and several types of communication disorders.

◆ Children who are suffering from pervasive developmental disorders have serious problems with social interaction skills, communication skills, and learning.

◆ Autism is diagnosed when the child has serious problems with social interactions, verbal and nonverbal communication, the use of imagination, and a restricted scope of activities and interests.

◆ The signs, symptoms, and behaviors of children with schizophrenia vary widely, but the core disturbance lies in a lack of contact with reality and the child's retreat into his or her own world.

◆ Therapeutic actions for children with mental health problems are basically focused on providing holistic care within an environment that fosters each child's growth and development.

◆ General interventions include meeting basic physical and emotional needs, providing opportunities for each child to grow and develop, and encouraging self-care activities.

Suggestions for Further Reading

Read your local newspaper daily for one week. Note the articles relating to children. What picture do you get of children in your community? What problems in your community are associated with children?

The American Psychological Association (helping.apa.org) offers interesting information about the prevention of violence in our schools.

References

American Psychiatric Association: *Diagnostic and statistical manual of mental disorders*, ed 4, text revision, Washington, DC, 2000, The Association.

Clark RB: Psychosocial aspects of pediatrics and psychiatric disorders. In Hay WH and others, editors: *Current pediatric diagnosis and treatment*, ed 12, Norwalk, Conn, 1995, Appleton & Lange.

Hagerman RJ: Growth and development. In Hay WH and others, *Current pediatric diagnosis and treatment*, ed 12, Norwalk, Conn, 1995, Appleton & Lange.

Hunter JK: Making a difference for homeless patients, *RN* 55(12):48, 1992.

McClellan J and others: Practice parameters for the assessment and treatment of children and adolescents with schizophrenia, *Journal of the American Academy of Child and Adolescent Psychiatry* 36(10):177, 1997.

McGeady MR: *"Does God still love me?": letters from the street*, New York, 1995, Sr Mary Rose McGeady.

Rafferty Y, Shinn M: The impact of homelessness on children, *American Psychologist* 46(11):1170, 1991.

Showers J: "Don't shake the baby": the effectiveness of a prevention program, *Child Abuse and Neglect* (16):11, 1992.

U.S. Advisory Board on Child Abuse and Neglect, April 26, 1995.

U.S. Bureau of the Census: *Statistical abstract of the United States: 1998*, ed 118, Washington, DC, 1998 U.S. Government Printing Office.

Wong DL: *Whaley and Wong's nursing care of infants and children*, ed 6, St. Louis, 1998, Mosby.

Chapter 15

Problems of Adolescence

Learning Objectives

1. Describe three common problems of adolescence.
2. Discuss three problems faced by adolescents with troubled family lives.
3. Identify the diagnostic criteria for behavioral disorders.
4. Explain how the signs/symptoms of adolescent depression differ from those seen in adult depression.
5. Define two eating disorders and describe the associated signs/symptoms and behaviors.
6. Describe the stages of chemical dependency in adolescence.
7. List four signs/symptoms indicating a potentially suicidal teen.
8. Identify four therapeutic interventions designed specifically for adolescent clients.
9. Explain how nurses and other health care providers help adolescents develop effective coping skills.

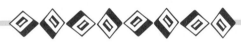

Key Terms

adolescence

adolescent suicide

anorexia nervosa

bulimia

chemical dependency

gangs

introspection

maturation

obesity

peer group

personality disorder

puberty

schizophrenia

sexual disorder

surveillance

Adolescence is a time of great change. Generally, **adolescence** begins at age 11 to 12 years and ends between 18 and 21. Physical and sexual growth are usually complete by 16 to 18 years of age, but in Western societies "the adolescence period is prolonged to allow for further psychosocial development before the young person assumes adult responsibilities" (Kaplan and Mammel, 1996). Because adolescence includes the ages 13 and 19, adolescents are also called teenagers or teens. All adolescents share the same growth and developmental processes, but each person's society and culture strongly influence that process of "growing up" (see Cultural Aspects box).

ADOLESCENT GROWTH AND DEVELOPMENT

The journey from child to adult is a time of physical and psychosocial growth. Adolescents undergo great changes in the physical, intellectual, emotional, social, and spiritual areas of their lives. Nurses must understand how adolescents grow and change if they are to assist them through this important developmental stage. Many adult problems find their roots in adolescence.

Physical Development

Changes in the body during adolescence occur in two general areas: (1) physical maturation and (2) sexual development.

Maturation is the process of attaining complete development (Wong, 1998). Physical maturation is the process of developing an adult body. Many physical changes occur during adolescence. Weight and height increase, and muscles grow. The major organs of the body double in size, and one's voice and appearance change.

Adolescence is also a time for sexual development. As changing bodies begin to secrete certain hormones known as gonadotropins, the process of puberty is begun. **Puberty** is defined as the stage during which an individual becomes physically capable of reproduction. With girls, puberty begins between 8 and 14 years of age. Today the average girl in the United States experiences the 24- to 36-month puberty growth spurt around 9 years of age and begins to menstruate (menarche) at about 12 years and 9 months. Menarche may begin as early as 10 or as late as 16 years of age. Breast development, body fat distribution, and the other physical changes that prepare the teen's body for adulthood are usually complete by ages 16 to 18 years.

Boys develop more slowly. The first signs of puberty are seen in boys around ages 10 to 12 years. The testicles enlarge, pubic hair develops, and the penis increases in length and width. The male growth spurt begins at age 11 and continues until about 14. Puberty lasts until about 18 years of age, but most male adolescents as young as 12 years old are capable of fathering children. Puberty is a time of many changes for both boys and girls. For a more thorough review of the growth and development of

adolescents, you are encouraged to consult a text on pediatric nursing.

Psychosocial Development

The term *psychosocial* refers to the nonphysical realms of human functioning. Adolescents undergo many changes in each area of functioning during their passage into adulthood. There are periods in teens' lives when they feel awkward, inadequate, and unworthy. Adults who are aware of these changes are better able to offer the emotional support and acceptance so needed by an adolescent. This section briefly explores the major developmental tasks for each psychosocial area of functioning.

Intellectual changes (cognitive development) involve learning to use abstract thinking. Children's thinking is concrete, that is, based on what is observed or experienced in the present time. Young adolescents (10 to 13 years) have trouble thinking realistically about the future. However, as teens mature, thinking moves from what is actually present and concrete to the future and what is possible. To illustrate, an 8-year old makes a judgment based on what he or she sees; a 17-year-old makes a judgment based upon reasoning. Teens begin to look at the world in new and exciting ways, to think beyond the present time, to consider a sequence of events or relationships, and to solve problems through the use of scientific reasoning and logic.

By the middle teens (14 to 17 years), abstract thinking (adaptable, flexible thinking that uses concepts, generalizations, and problem solving) is well entrenched, along with a feeling of power and self-centeredness. Many believe that they can change the world by just thinking about it. At about 17, teens' abstract thinking becomes more realistic, and they are able to plan reachable actions, goals, and careers.

Emotional development during adolescence is marked by rapid periods of change and adjustment. By 10 to 13 years of age, the emotional stability of childhood is replaced with a preoccupation about bodily changes, which bring about changes in self-esteem, body image, and self-concept. Coping with these changes becomes confusing to the adolescent. Behaviors swing rapidly from the pleasant, cooperative child to the moody, unpredictable, and emotional teen. Early adolescence is marked by rapid shifts between disturbed behavior and relative calm. Moods swing from upbeat and happy to withdrawn and depressed. Reactions to small events can trigger outbursts of acting out and aggressive behavior. Adolescents also daydream much of the time. Daydreaming is important for adolescents because it allows them to try out new roles and place themselves in "what if" situations. Because of this, they often miss many of the messages from other people and become labeled as sullen or withdrawn.

The emotions and mood swings of puberty become intense when teens are between 14 to 17 years of age. At

---

🌍 Cultural Aspects

Researchers at the University of Michigan studied the frequency of stressed and anxious feelings in more than 4000 U.S., Taiwanese, and Japanese teenagers and found some interesting results. Japanese adolescents were found to have the fewest reports of physical problems and depressed moods, whereas Taiwanese teens displayed more physical complaints and depressed moods. Students in the United States and Taiwan thought of school as a source of stress, but only U.S. teens mentioned out-of-school activities and sports as sources of stress. Japanese teens felt that peers were a greater source of stress.

Parents in the United States expected lower academic performance of their teens than the parents of Japanese and Taiwanese adolescents. Doing well in school was more supported and encouraged by the families of Asian teenagers. High achievers in the United States reported that they were frequently torn between their desires to put extra time into their studies and to follow other activities, such as dating, working, playing sports, and socializing.

this age they tend to stay alone, looking at themselves and how they fit into the world. For many adolescents, this is a troubled, lonely time. By about 18, most adolescents are in control of their emotions and have an established self-concept.

Social development is an important area for adolescents. Younger teens struggle to establish a group identity, as well as a personal identity. Most teenagers feel the need to belong to a group. Many needs are fulfilled by peer groups at this age, but the most important function of the group is to help adolescents define the differences between themselves and their parents. Dress, music, dancing, and language are all designed to display differences and to show how unique the group really is. Unless the standards set by the peer group place the teens in danger, they should be tolerated by adults. Belonging to a group serves as a stepping-stone in the process of establishing an individual identity and separating from the family.

Middle teens establish their identities by experimenting with different images of themselves. By this time, the peer group determines new standards for dress, behavior, and activities. Teens at this stage begin to see themselves as others might see them. A 14- to 16-year-old's social relationships are usually self-centered. Sexuality becomes more important, and by age 18 the majority of adolescents have engaged in sexual intercourse. Social relationships for adolescents over 17 years shift from the group to the individual. Caring more about others than oneself begins, and dating becomes more personal and intimate.

Spiritual development for adolescents begins with questioning family values and beliefs. Some teens may cling furiously to family values during periods of conflict, whereas others completely disregard them. Adolescents also use their abilities of abstract thinking to question their childhood religious and spiritual practices. Often they will stop attending church services, change churches, or choose to worship within the privacy of their rooms or other special space. Many teens are attracted to new religious sects or movements that suggest promises of unconditional acceptance and love during a time when the adults in their environment are seen as critical and intolerant. Most teenagers experience a great degree of inner emotional turmoil. Fearing that nobody will understand, teens become extremely private. Most adolescents have deep spiritual concerns and require acceptance, understanding, and patience as they struggle to find the spiritual rock that will anchor them in adulthood.

Adolescence is a time of rapid and uncontrollable change. Between the ages of 10 and 20, adolescents grow, develop, and mature within each area of functioning. Table 15-1 offers a brief explanation of the major changes experienced throughout adolescence. As adolescents ma-

Table 15-1 Growth and Development During Adolescence		
Early adolescence (11-14 yr)	**Middle adolescence (14-17 yr)**	**Late adolescence (17-20 yr)**
Growth		
Rapid growth	Growth slowing in girls	Physically mature
Reaches peak	Reaches 95% of adult height	Structure and reproductive
Sexual growth begins	Sexual growth well advanced	growth almost complete
Cognition (Intellect)		
Explores ability for limited abstract thought	Developing abstract thinking	Established abstract thought
Groping for new values and energies	Enjoys intellectual powers, often in idealistic terms	Can perceive and act on long range operations
Compares "normal" with peers of same sex	Concern with philosophical, political, and social problems	Able to view problems comprehensively
		Intellectual and functional identity established
Identity		
Preoccupied with rapid body changes	Modifies body image	Body image and gender role definition nearly secured
Trying out of various roles	Very self-centered	Mature sexual identity
Measures attractiveness by acceptance or rejection of peers	Tendency toward inner experience and self-discovery	Brings together identity
Conformity to group norms	Has rich fantasy life	Stability of self-esteem
	Idealistic	Comfortable with physical growth
	Able to perceive future implications of current behavior and decisions	Social roles defined

Modified from Wong DL: *Whaley and Wong's nursing care of infants and children*, ed 6, 1998, St. Louis, Mosby.

Continued

Table 15-1	Growth and Development During Adolescence—cont'd	
Early adolescence (11-14 yr)	**Middle adolescence (14-17 yr)**	**Late adolescence (17-20 yr)**
Relationships With Parents		
Defining independence-dependence boundaries	Major conflicts over independence and control	Emotional and physical separation from parents completed
Strong desire to remain dependent on parents while trying to detach	Low point in parent-child relationship	Independence from family with less conflict
No major conflicts over parental control	Greatest push for emancipation; disengagement	Emancipation nearly secured
	Final and irreversible emotional detachment from parents; mourning	
Relationships With Peers		
Seeks peers to counter instability generated by rapid change	Strong need for identity; self-image	Peer group fades in importance in favor of individual friendships
Close idealized friendships with members of the same sex	Behavioral standards set by peer group	Testing of male-female relationships; possibility of permanent alliance
Struggles for mastery within peer group	Acceptance by peers extremely important—fear of rejection	Relationships characterized by giving and sharing
	Explores ability to attract opposite sex	
Sexuality		
Self-exploration and evaluation	Multiple relationships	Forms stable relationships and attachments
Limited dating, usually group	Decisive turn toward heterosexuality (if is homosexual, knows by this time)	Able to give and take
Limited intimacy	Exploration of "self appeal"	Dating as a male-female pair
	Feeling of "being in love"	Intimacy involves commitment rather than exploration and romanticism
	Begins to establish relationships	
Psychological Health		
Wide mood swings	Tendency toward inner experiences; more introspective	More constant with emotions
Intense daydreaming	Tendency to withdraw when upset	Anger more apt to be concealed
Anger outwardly expressed with moodiness, temper outburst, verbal insults and name-calling	Wide emotions swings in time and range	
	Feelings of inadequacy common; difficulty in asking for help	

Modified from Wong DL: *Whaley and Wong's nursing care of infants and children,* ed 6, 1998, St. Louis, Mosby.

ture, they begin to move away from the family and function independently. Society welcomes them as adults, with all the rewards and obligations of the adult role.

COMMON PROBLEMS OF ADOLESCENCE

The world is large and complex. Even the most successful people feel overwhelmed by the sheer amount of information and experiences that are currently available. Adolescents, who are just beginning to emerge from the security of childhood, must gain understanding and control of themselves and, at the same time, learn to cope with living within an uncertain world. Most of the common problems of adolescence fall into two categories: problems that arise from within oneself (internal sources) and those that are rooted outside the teen's personal sphere of control (external sources).

Internal (Developmental) Problems

Most difficulties of early adolescence arise from within the individual. Physical changes are beginning to take place, and new sensations are being experienced. One's own body ceases to cooperate at times, and floods of intense emotions bring on dramatic emotional ups and downs.

An important developmental problem of adolescence is defining oneself— establishing an identity separate from one's family. At this stage, teens need to look into themselves and to engage in **introspection** (the process of examining one's own thoughts, emotions, reactions, attitudes, opinions, values, and behaviors by looking at the inner self). They consider who they are, how they see themselves, how they think others may see them, and how relationships with various people affect them. This process of looking inward helps teens to define themselves, but it also brings about many changes in mood, attitude, and behavior. Problems that threaten self-esteem or confidence routinely arise during the journey to adulthood. It is important for teens to feel secure and emotionally supported by adults during these confusing periods. Just knowing that someone accepts and cares goes a long way toward helping teens through troubled times.

External (Environmental) Problems

Problems that arise outside the thoughts and feelings of the teen are called external problems. External problems fall into three basic areas: family, social, and environmental. Even teens who are blessed with the best of everything experience difficulties in these areas of functioning.

Family problems change as the adolescent develops independence. During early adolescence (11 to 14 years) teens experience the pull between wanting to stay dependent and moving toward independence. They begin to seek their freedom. but still require the emotional ties provided by the family structure.

By midadolescence (14 to 17 years) the push for independence is in full swing, and major conflicts over control motivate the teen to detach from the family. Conflicts slowly fade as the adolescent matures into an independently functioning adult. Separating from the family and establishing independence are problems faced by every teen, but difficulties often arise from within the family that are not related to the adolescent's developmental stage. Families can range from the overprotective parents who limit their children's experiences and do not allow them to make decisions to those whose children grow up on the streets with little or no sense of belonging.

Children have no control over the methods of child rearing chosen by their parents, living conditions, or the environment in which they must grow. Many adolescents must cope with physical violence, sexual abuse, neglect, and/or parents who abuse alcohol or drugs. About 7 million children and adolescents have a parent in jail or on parole (Inmates' Kids, 1999). These are the types of problems that cannot be solved by just waiting for the adolescent to outgrow them. They must be faced every day, and they require energy that should be spent in self-discovery.

Adolescents who are not fortunate enough to have a caring, supportive family are considered to be at risk because the conditions to which they are currently exposed may threaten further development (see the Case Study box).

Every adolescent has some family problems because that is the nature of the maturing process. Those teens who are not blessed with a nurturing family face problems that would test the strongest adult.

Adolescents are also challenged with numerous social problems. Early teens seek out their peers and form intense bonds with certain groups. Peer groups are important for the social growth of adolescents. They serve

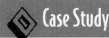

Case Study

Carol was a bright, energetic 5-year-old when her parents divorced, forcing her mother to live on a welfare income. Between the ages of 6 and 13, Carol experienced a series of "fathers" who lived with them for various periods of time. Some were kind to Carol, but one physically and sexually abused her. Her mother was usually away from home or with other adults, and Carol soon learned to fend for herself. By age 12 Carol had already experimented with different drugs, but found alcohol more to her liking. By the time she was 14, Carol was uncontrollable. She had learned to drive and would often steal her mother's car after she was asleep for the night. Unprotected sex happened frequently. Soon Carol dropped out of school because "it really doesn't matter."
◆ List the factors in Carol's life that put her at risk.
◆ Identify two of her problems.
◆ What do you think could help Carol?

many purposes and help teens cope with their life changes (Table 15-2).

Peer groups and gangs both consist of adolescents of about the same age and circumstances. The difference between the two groups lies in the behaviors or actions of the members. **Gangs** are usually associated with negative behaviors or destructive actions, whereas **peer groups** focus their energies in more constructive ways, such as volunteer work and projects that benefit their communities. Peer groups are often influenced by adults, as with coaches for sports teams or leaders for youth church groups. Although adolescents choose to join groups, concerned parents should support their teen's choice of a group but remain aware of the powerful influences groups exert on the developing individual.

Other social problems encountered by most adolescents relate to establishing their sexuality. Intimacy (emotional closeness) is limited in early adolescence. Same-sex friends are still of primary importance. As time passes, interest in people of the opposite sex begins to increase. By age 14 teens explore the concepts of "sex appeal" and "being in love." More than 50% of them have experienced sexual intercourse by this age. Dating may be limited to one person at a time, but many relationships are experienced as adolescents struggle to define themselves, both socially and sexually. Around 20 years of age, people begin to form stable, attached relationships that are based on a sense of giving rather than receiving.

Finally, environmental conditions have an impact on adolescent development because problems in the environment can threaten basic needs. The dirty air of so many cities, the quality and quantity of foods eaten, and the purity of the water have an impact, however subtle, on developing human beings. Exposure to drugs, crime,

Table 15-2	Peer Groups and Adolescents

Functions of Peer Groups

Helps to loosen family ties

Provides stability during times of change

Helps adolescents define present and future social roles; test their views of themselves; learn to trust their own choices; learn to make and stand by their commitments

Establishes behavioral and dress standards

Positive aspects	Negative aspects
Provides emotional support, a sense of belonging	Rules and standards of the group may be too rigid
Helps teens establish values and behavioral standards	Values and behaviors may not be in keeping with society's definition
Provides protection, safety	
Allows teens to test and try out new behaviors	May encourage self-destructive behaviors and disregard for others outside the group

prostitution, corruption, and violence are very real environmental problems for many teens. Activities that glamorize sex and violence through music, television, and the movies and adults who push children into becoming adults too soon are all environmental influences with which teens must cope.

Most adolescents, though, are concerned with the more immediate problems of learning to effectively function within their physical and social environments—the problems that "come with the territory" and are a part of one's daily life. Environments that foster growth offer fewer problems than surroundings that require a constant state of awareness just to live through the day. Environmental conditions and the problems that go along with them must be recognized and acted on by health care providers if we are to provide our teenagers with the tools for a successful transition to adulthood.

MENTAL HEALTH PROBLEMS OF ADOLESCENCE

Adolescence is the time for teens to develop the personal strengths and social skills that promote effective functioning in the adult world. It is a period that involves great emotional swings, a focus on oneself, and increasingly active sexual and aggressive drives. In an effort to cope with these changes, adolescents engage in a wide variety of behaviors. Some of these actions help adolescents to successfully adapt, whereas others result in negative outcomes. This is a period of "trying out" new behaviors, and adults need to consider this fact.

Adolescent mental health also includes the concept of well-being, which is the "presence of personal and interpersonal strengths that promote optimal functioning" (Kadzin, 1993). Well-being includes the ability to do the following:

Function well socially (social competence)

Have positive interactions with others

Cope with stress and troubled times

Become involved in activities and relationships with others

The word *dysfunction* means an impairment in everyday life. It means that the problems faced by the adolescent are so severe that he or she cannot or will not partake in the activities of daily living. When an adolescent's problems or emotions impair performance (school, social, or work) or threaten physical well-being, a mental health problem exists. Table 15-3 lists several categories of mental health disorders that affect adolescents.

Mental health services for adolescents focus on promoting positive life skills, prevention, and treatment of dysfunctions. Nursing interventions focus on health education, assisting with group and individual therapy, medication management, setting limits, and providing emotional support.

Behavioral Disorders

Every child goes through periods of misconduct, of refusing to do as told and of "being bad." However, for some teens the misconduct continues to occur. Their behaviors begin to disrupt their families, social interactions, and performance at school. They may clash with classmates, developing a reputation for being unruly, mean, or even dangerous. When a persistent pattern of disruptive behaviors is present, mental health interventions are usually necessary. The disruptive behavioral disorders category consists of two basic diagnoses: attention-deficit hyperactivity disorder and conduct disorders.

Attention-deficit hyperactivity disorder (ADHD) is usually diagnosed earlier in childhood, but its impact lasts through adolescence and into adulthood (Box 15-1). The two key features of ADHD are inattention and impulsivity. Teens with ADHD experience problems in focusing their attention, behavioral self-controls, and relating to

Table 15-3	Adolescent Mental Health Disorders
Classification of disorders	**Examples**
Behavioral disorders	Conduct disorder, attention-deficit hyperactivity disorder
Emotional disorders	Anxiety disorder, mood disorders (e.g., depression, posttraumatic stress disorder, suicidal thoughts and attempts)
Eating disorders	Anorexia nervosa, bulimia
Chemical dependency	Abuse of alcohol, amphetamines (speed), caffeine, cannabis, cocaine, nicotine, hallucinogens, inhalants, opiates, prescription drugs
Personality disorders	Antisocial disorder, borderline disorder, dependent disorder, obsessive-compulsive disorder, paranoid personality disorder
Schizophrenia	Paranoid type schizophrenia, disorganized type schizophrenia, delusional disorder
Sexual disorders	Gender identity disorder, inappropriate sexual behaviors
Other disorders of adolescence	Adjustment disorder, impulse-control disorders, problems related to abuse or neglect

Box 15-1 Adolescents With Attention-Deficit Hyperactivity Disorder

"Only about one-third of children with ADHD reach mid-adolescence with no diagnosable psychiatric disorder" (Clark, 1996). Teens with ADHD often have low self-esteem and poor socialization skills. Impulse control is usually a problem.

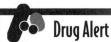

Drug Alert

Be sure to obtain a complete history of all drugs, herbs, medicines, or tonics taken. Write the names of each substance as they are given by the client. Many different names are used for the same item. Remember to ask about over-the-counter items too. Assess the teen's understanding of the prescribed drug, especially the side effects.

others. Because of these difficulties, many teens become chronically unhappy. They may begin to abuse chemicals or go on to develop conduct disorders.

Treatment for adolescents with ADHD requires a multidisciplinary approach. Small, structured classes and firm, but nonjudgmental, teachers are needed in the school environment. Positive reinforcement programs, which reward appropriate behaviors and task completion are helpful at home and school. Behavioral therapy assists both teens and their parents. Parents are taught how to structure and enforce limits on the teen's behaviors without becoming overly harsh, inconsistent, or angry. If the adolescent has specific learning disabilities, special education may be necessary. Medications to treat ADHD include stimulants, tricyclic antidepressants, and clonidine (see Table 15-4 and Drug Alert box). Adolescents who are taking their prescribed medications may also be using various other substances. Serious drug interactions can occur when street and pharmaceutical drugs are mixed. Do not judge the teen, but be sure to obtain a complete history of past and current use of chemically active substances

Conduct disorders are characterized by a defiance of authority and aggressive behaviors toward others. Often teens with conduct disorders violate the rights of other people or defy society's norms and standards. A common factor in the development of conduct disorders appears to be harsh parental discipline with physical punishment. Early harsh discipline tends to foster more aggressive behaviors later in a child's life.

The typical adolescent with a conduct disorder is a boy with a history of social and academic problems. Common symptoms include fighting, temper tantrums, running away from home, destroying property, problems with authorities, and failure in school. Stealing and fire setting may occur. Truancy, vandalism, and substance abuse are frequently encountered. Many teens with conduct disorders, especially those with violent histories, also have various physical and mental health problems, such as anxiety disorders and depression.

Treatment for adolescents with conduct disorders is focused on first stabilizing the teen's home environment and then working to improve family interactions and disciplinary techniques. Individual and family therapy is used to help the family learn to communicate and problem solve effectively. A combination of behavioral, emotional, and cognitive therapies helps the teen learn self-control. Success hinges on including the family, teachers, and other adults who are involved with the teen. Efforts are made to treat the adolescent within the home environment;

Table 15-4 Drugs for Teens With Attention-Deficit Hyperactivity Disorder

Drug examples	Dose	Client teaching
Stimulants		
Methylphenidate (Ritalin)	0.3-1.5 mg/kg, 1-3 doses daily	Watch for effects on growth; behavior
Pemoline (Cylert)	0.5-3.0 mg/kg/day	deteriorates when drugs are stopped abruptly.
Antidepressants		
Imipramine (Tofranil)	No more than 5 mg/kg/day	May cause dry mouth, blurred vision,
Clomipramine (Anafranil)	No more than 5 mg/kg/day	constipation, insomnia.
Antipsychotics		
Chlorpromazine (Thorazine)	6-8 mg/kg/day	May cause dry mouth, blurred vision, weight gain, low blood pressure. Report any
Haloperidol (Haldol)	0.05-0.15 mg/kg/day	abnormal muscle and body movements to physician.

however, residential (inpatient) treatment may be necessary when the teen becomes a danger to himself or herself or others.

The outlook for adolescents with conduct disorders is poor. Nearly half the children with antisocial behaviors or conduct disorders become antisocial as adults (Clark, 1996). These teens need health care providers with patience, a willingness to set limits, and the courage to always enforce them.

Emotional Disorders

Disturbed feelings or moods from time to time are a normal part of everyday living. Adolescents, because of their many developmental tasks, experience frequent emotional changes. Periods of feeling "down" or "blue" are not uncommon with teens. However, when the moods or feelings have an impact on the teen's daily activities, mental health care may be needed.

Problems that affect the emotional realm of human functioning are divided into two basic categories: anxiety disorders and mood disorders. Although each is discussed in detail in later chapters, a brief description of how these problems affect adolescents is important here.

Anxiety disorders result when the adolescent's ability to adapt is overwhelmed. When teens are overstressed, anxiety (that vague, uneasy feeling of tension) may balloon into an ever-present emotional state, which triggers physical changes as the body responds in an attempt to adapt. The combination of these physical and emotional symptoms can result in such problems as panic disorder, phobias, obsessive-compulsive disorders, and posttraumatic stress disorder. Anxiety is also associated with the development of depression and substance abuse problems. It is important to recognize and treat anxiety in children as early as possible because long-standing problems with anxiety may become difficult to change.

Box 15-2 Signs and Symptoms of Depression in Adolescents

Moodiness characterized by irritable moods and acting-out behaviors
Decreased social activity
Decreased school performance
Difficulty in thinking
Inability to concentrate, make decisions, or solve problems
Somatic complaints: loss of energy, headache, stomachache, eating and sleeping problems

Adolescents with affective or mood disorders display a wide range of behaviors from profound depression to racing hyperactivity. One's mood is the ever-present emotional state that colors one's perception of the world. Because adolescents are struggling with issues of self-image and confidence, their moods change rapidly. Teens are expected to have short periods of "the blues," but when sad moods are prolonged or the teen's behavior alternates between extreme highs and lows, an emotional disorder is suspected. Refer to Box 15-2 for the primary signs and symptoms of depression in adolescents.

Other interpersonal difficulties are often present, such as problems with parents and siblings, the use of drugs, and fighting. Acting out one's depression through antisocial behaviors, such as theft, vandalism, and truancy, may result in involvement with the law and its criminal justice system. Sexual acting out is also common. Depression in adolescence is "characterized by irritable moods and acting-out behaviors, in contrast to the classic 'depressed mood' and 'loss of interest' characteristic of adults" (Hogarth, 1991). In short, depressed adults lose interest; depressed teens act out.

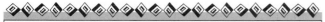

Modified from Serdula MK and others: *Annals of Internal Medicine* 119(7 pt 2):667, 1993.

Severe anxiety and depression are not average adolescent conditions. The majority of adolescents negotiate this developmental period without major problems, develop a positive personal identity, and manage adaptive peer relationships at the same time they maintain close family ties. The best prevention for emotional disorders in teens involves early recognition. Emotional problems left unrecognized and untreated in adolescence frequently develop into serious mental health disorders in adulthood.

Eating Disorders

Adolescents' eating patterns and food behaviors may follow the latest trend or change to reflect the preferences of the peer group, but as long as the teen is well nourished there is little cause for concern. Eating disorders are characterized by "severe disturbances in eating behavior" (American Psychiatric Association, 1994), which can result in a body that is far below or over its ideal weight.

The weight control practices of adolescents have been a cause for concern in today's society. The message of "slim equals attractive" bombards individuals throughout childhood; therefore weight control becomes an important concern for many teens. The Think About box describes a research study that demonstrates this concern.

Obesity is defined as a body weight that is 20% or more above the average weight for a person of the same height and build. Because the eating patterns of obese teens do not pose an immediate threat, chronic overeating is not considered a mental health disorder. However,

many people who become overweight as teens use food to help them through troubled times. In these cases, mental health interventions may help assist individuals in finding more effective ways of satisfying their needs. It has been estimated that between 5% and 10% of all female adolescents suffer from eating disorders. About 90% to 95% of teens with eating disorders are girls, but eating disorders do occur in male teenagers, usually athletes (Zerbe, 1995). The mortality rate for eating disorders is about 9%.

Common eating disorders in adolescence are anorexia nervosa and bulimia. **Anorexia nervosa** is a prolonged refusal to eat to keep body weight at a reasonable minimum. It is characterized by an intense fear of becoming fat and a relentless pursuit of thinness. **Bulimia** is the uncontrolled ingestion of large amounts of food (called *binge eating*) followed by inappropriate compensatory methods to prevent weight gain (called *purging*). In short, bulimia is a cycle of binge eating followed by purging. Anorexia is seen from about 12 years old, with peaks around 13 to 14 and again at 17 to 18. Bulimia often may not present until 17 or so. Both disorders also occur in adults, but the incidence decreases sharply after the midthirties.

The typical picture of an anorectic teen is one of an overly cooperative, achievement-oriented girl who sees herself as overweight and begins to diet. There may be a history of eating or mood disorders in the family. Over a period of months, her concern with dieting evolves into an obsessive need to be thin. All her behaviors soon center around remaining thin. She may restrict calories, exercise excessively, induce vomiting, or use pills (laxatives, diuretics, diet pills, or street drugs) to prevent even the smallest weight gain.

As the disorder progresses, the teen cuts back on her social activities and begins to avoid friends. She becomes increasingly anxious, irritable, and depressed. Now all her thoughts focus on food and weight loss to the exclusion of all else. Although it is glaringly apparent to everyone who sees her, the anorectic teen will deny that a problem even exists. Soon the physical and psychological effects of starvation begin to appear (Figure 15-1). Long-term, even life-threatening, complications can result unless medical and mental health interventions are undertaken.

Bulimia is more difficult to detect due to the secretive nature of the problem. However, it is estimated that as many as 20% of college-age women are bulimic. The road to bulimia begins with an intense interest in dieting. Struggles with food result in secret binge-eating episodes in which she consumes 5,000 to 20,000 calories of high-carbohydrate foods. Bingeing is followed by feelings of intense guilt or depression, and the teen then makes extreme attempts to control weight gain through vomiting, exercise, or the use of drugs. Self-imposed starvation may occur between binges. Some weight loss may occur,

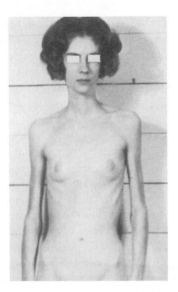

Figure 15-1 Woman with anorexia nervosa. (From Ezrin D and others: *Systematic endocrinology*, ed 2, New York, 1979, Harper & Row.)

but body weight usually remains within 20% of normal. The medical complications of bulimia include erosion of tooth enamel, gastric dilation, inflammation of the pancreas, and electrolyte abnormalities. Most people with bulimia are aware of their behavior, but they are ashamed and afraid to admit that they are out of control. Binge episodes frequently follow a stressful life event.

Treatment for eating disorders has three goals:
1. Manage the medical dangers, such as metabolic disturbances, cardiac problems, and dehydration
2. Restore normal nutrition and eating patterns
3. Meet the psychiatric treatment needs of the client and the family

Nursing (care team) diagnoses for eating disorders include activity intolerance, altered nutrition, altered thought processes, body image disturbance, chronic low self-esteem, defensive coping, denial, and ineffective family coping. Attempts are made to treat the teen within the family setting, but if the condition is severe, the teen is hospitalized. A plan to gradually improve the teen's nutritional intake (a refeeding program) is developed by the dietitian and other treatment team members. Therapeutic interventions are designed to stabilize the client's physical condition. Force feeding is discouraged because the goal is to get the teen to choose to eat.

As the teen begins to feel better, she is encouraged to express her feelings. With both types of eating disorders, the primary issue is one of control, not food. Psychotherapy is designed to help the teen recognize underlying depression that is often present and develop more effective coping skills.

Box 15-3 Stages of Chemical Dependency

1. Experimentation: Pleasant moods and social belonging associated with drugs are experienced; drugs are used for the first time within the comfort of the peer or other social group.
2. Actively seeking: Teen looks forward to and actively seeks out the mood changes brought about by the chemicals; becomes expert in the use of chemicals to regulate moods; schoolwork and relationships with family erode; friends become limited to other teens who "use."
3. Preoccupation: Teen believes that he or she cannot cope without chemicals; has lost control over the use of the drug; develops a tolerance and may begin to use other substances; chemical is now used to prevent withdrawal symptoms; psychosocial functioning begins to fail; friends are lost and may be replaced with antisocial, illegal, or violent behaviors.
4. Burnout: Focus of drug use now is to prevent negative feelings; if the teen attempts to stop using the chemical, withdrawal symptoms appear; those who progress to this level of addiction are usually no longer able to function productively in society; most are late adolescents or young adults.

Chemical Dependency

For adolescents, the temptation to "find out what it is like" is a strong motivator. Most teens who experiment with alcohol and drugs do not become dependent or addicted. However, for a growing number of teens, the use of chemicals is becoming a way of coping with the difficulties of life. The problems associated with substance abuse are many: accidents caused by lack of judgment, interpersonal violence, depression, and worsening relationships with others. Young adolescents who use chemical substances usually become sexually active at an earlier age. Perhaps the most critical fact is that the use of chemicals interferes with normal adolescent growth and development.

All adolescents are at risk for developing substance abuse problems, especially those who were abused as young children; teens from families who approve of, use, or promote the use of chemicals; and teens who suffer from other mental health problems. **Chemical dependency** is a state in which one's body physically and psychologically requires a drug. Identifying teens with substance abuse or chemical dependency problems is difficult. Many of the signs and symptoms of long-term abuse are absent.

Teens who become chemically dependent progress through four general stages: experimentation, active seeking, preoccupation, and burnout (Box 15-3).

Frequently the most important clues to substance abuse in teens are small ones. A change in habits, mood, or personality often hints of a problem. Sometimes a teen will suddenly become rebellious. More often, though, the adolescent will disappear with friends and take every necessary step to avoid contact with family members. The teen who becomes chemically dependent needs mental health intervention. Underneath a hardened exterior, there usually lies an individual who has few friends and little or no self-esteem.

Treatment is focused on helping replace their use of chemicals with more effective coping skills. Many of the treatment programs in the United States, Canada, and Great Britain are modeled on the principles of Alcoholics Anonymous, whose goal is a chemical-free lifestyle. Settings for treating teens range from outpatient counseling to residential treatment programs and therapeutic communities. Individual and group psychotherapy is often combined with behavioral and cognitive therapies. Therapeutic care is focused on providing a safe environment because many of these teens are suicidal.

Drug and alcohol abuse is a complex problem that affects all aspects of an adolescent's life. Few teens seek treatment, and the therapies for chemical dependency vary in their effectiveness. Prevention and early recognition remain the most effective tools for coping with adolescent substance abuse.

Personality Disorders

One's personality is an important part of identity. Personality is the combination of behavioral patterns that each of us develops to cope with living. Our personalities characterize us as unique individuals and allow us to function effectively within society. However, there are some adolescents who have long histories of inappropriate or maladaptive behaviors. These teens may be diagnosed as having a **personality disorder,** which is defined as "an enduring pattern of inner experience and behavior that:

1. deviates markedly from the expectations of the individual's culture,
2. is universal and inflexible,
3. has an onset in adolescence or early adulthood,
4. is stable over time, and
5. leads to distress or impairment" (American Psychiatric Association, 2000).

A major characteristic of the adolescent with a personality disorder is impulsivity—the temptation to engage in acts harmful to oneself or others. These spur-of-the-moment decisions lead to inappropriate actions, such as overeating, casual sexual practices, shoplifting, and thrill-seeking behaviors. Intense emotional changes lead to anger and depression. Self-esteem and self-confidence are low. The ability to look inward (introspection) is minimal. These teens tend to develop "all-or-nothing relationships," where others are either idealized or considered worthless. They flip between

distance and closeness within their relationships and harbor a deep fear of being abandoned. Some become suspicious, and many attempt suicide. Frequently a personality disorder will coexist with another mental health diagnosis.

Treatment for teens with personality disorders involves the use of psychotherapy and various medications. Recent studies have shown that personality disorders may be related to a problem with the neurotransmitter serotonin. Treatment with selective serotonin reuptake inhibitors, such as fluoxetine hydrochloride (Prozac), has been successful. Long-term individual therapy, in combination with selective medications, provides a promising outlook for teens who are suffering from personality disorders.

Sexual Disorders

One of the tasks during adolescence is to establish a sexual identity and role. To do this, many teens experiment with various sexual attitudes, outlooks, and behaviors. Attitudes about sexuality change as societies evolve, therefore the definition of a **sexual disorder** must be characterized by significant distress and impaired ability to function.

Adolescents with sexual disorders relating to gender identity are still struggling with conflicts that began in childhood. Individuals with gender identity disorders have a continual discomfort with their assigned sex. The child has a strong and persistent need to identify with the other sex and often insists on wearing clothing designed for the other sex. During play the child identifies with or role plays the opposite sex. Playmates and activities are limited to those associated with the desired sex. For example, a boy might like to wear dresses, play house acting as the mother, and choose only girls as friends.

As these teens grow older, they become preoccupied with ridding themselves of their sexual characteristics and assuming those of the desired sex. They may request hormonal therapy, surgery, or other procedures that may produce characteristics of the desired sex. Treatment consists of medical and mental health therapies that are designed to relieve distress and help teens solve their problems.

Sexually acting out is not uncommon for teens. However, if their behaviors result in discomfort or harm for themselves or others, society defines the behaviors as inappropriate. Many sexual problems faced by adolescents can be solved with good communication skills. Sometimes just replacing ignorance with accurate knowledge can assist a teen along the road toward healthy sexual maturity.

Psychosis

The defining feature of **schizophrenia** and other psychoses is a grossly impaired ability to function due to a loss of

---

Think About

Neurotic behaviors are recognized by the person as unacceptable, recurring, and persistent. Behaviors may be odd or unusual, but they are within socially acceptable limits. The individual is in contact with reality and able to carry out the activities of daily living.

Psychotic behaviors are characterized by personality disintegration, reduced awareness, and an inability to function within socially acceptable limits. The individual is not in contact with reality and is unable to carry out the activities of daily living.

◆ When do neurotic behaviors become psychotic?

Box 15-4   Warning Signs of Teen Suicide

Change in grades at school
Loss of interest, initiative
Rapidly changing emotional highs and lows
Defies rules, regulations, pushes limits
May become secretive
Withdraws from family interactions
Changes in personal hygiene
Isolates self from others
Discusses suicide with peers, close friends
Gives away prized possessions
Hints about intentions (e.g., "After I'm gone . . .")

---

being in touch with reality. Psychotic disorders are discussed in detail in a later chapter, but here it is important to know that the onset of schizophrenia usually takes place in adolescence. The adolescent who suffers from schizophrenia is typically a good child who begins to develop a whole new set of (sometimes bizarre) behaviors and activities. Psychosis can result from head injury, substance abuse, or extreme stress (see Think About box).

The major characteristic of adolescent psychosis is loss of contact with reality. The teen may have hallucinations, delusions, and feelings of paranoia. He or she lacks judgment, behaves impulsively, and shows little insight. Behaviors may become inappropriate, ritualistic, or repetitive. Disordered thought patterns lead to communication problems and difficulties with peer relationships. Because of the loss of contact with reality, personal hygiene (even eating and drinking) may be neglected. The teen usually requires hospitalization and close supervision.

Treatment for psychosis includes a combination of psychotherapy and medications. Antipsychotics, antidepressants, and lithium may be ordered. Care is focused on providing basic physical needs, including feeding, bathing, and exercise; providing a safe environment; and developing skills for successful living. As the adolescent begins to respond to treatment, education about the nature and control of the disorder is begun. Schizophrenia is lifelong, and the major problem in management is the poor compliance with taking the prescribed medications. Both adolescents and their families need ongoing support. Family members are often encouraged to join a support group for the emotional assistance required to cope with a teen who has a psychosis.

Suicide

The number of adolescents who take their own lives is growing at an alarming rate. From 1960 to 1998, the rate of **adolescent suicide** more than doubled (U.S. Bureau of the Census, 1998). Adolescent girls attempt suicide three

times more often than their male counterparts, but boys are more successful in their attempts because they choose more lethal methods.. Teens who have been hospitalized for injuries or motor vehicle (especially single-car) accidents may be actually attempting suicide.

A suicide attempt by an adolescent is a call for help. Today's society is complex and has many influences on a developing adolescent. Factors that may influence suicidal behavior include more competition for fewer resources, exposure to child abuse and neglect, instability within the family, the presence of depression or other illness, the availability of handguns and other weapons, and an increased use of alcohol and drugs. Box 15-4 lists the warning signs of suicide.

Teenagers who attempt suicide usually fall into one of three groups: the teen with depression, the teen who is trying to influence others, and the teen with a serious mental health problem. When a teen cannot keep up with school and social activities, withdraws from others, has problems eating or sleeping, and feels hopeless, then he or she is at risk for suicide resulting from depression.

The teen who uses a suicidal gesture as a way to get back at someone (usually parents or boyfriend or girlfriend) is attempting to influence someone. Often there is little or no depression and no real wish to die. The teen is angry, and the gesture is done with the goal of gaining attention or scaring another person. Teenage girls engage in this type of suicidal behavior much more commonly than boys.

The third group of adolescents who attempt suicide are seriously ill. They can see no other way out of their discomfort and actually welcome the relief they expect death to bring.

The highest risk group for suicide is the older white adolescent boy who has expressed his intention to die. Previous attempts, written plans, and available tools for committing suicide all heighten the risk for future attempts. Increases in suicidal attempts are often seen

Sample Client Care Plan   Suicidal Adolescent

Assessment

History: Rita is a 15-year-old girl admitted to the medical unit of the local hospital for suicidal attempts. About 4 hours ago, she consumed approximately 35 tablets of diazepam (Valium) and had her stomach pumped in the emergency room. Three earlier suicidal attempts have involved drug overdoses and slashed wrists.

Current Findings: A sleepy teenage girl in no acute distress. Answers questions with one-word statements. States she attempted suicide to "get everyone off my back." Skin on wrists and forearms has numerous jagged scars. Rita refused further physical assessment.

Multidisciplinary Diagnosis

Violence, self-directed related to family behaviors, developmental conflict

Planning/Goals

Rita will contract with staff for no suicidal attempts.
Rita will verbalize an awareness of her pattern of self-harm by May 7.

Therapeutic Interventions

Intervention	Rationale	Team Member
1. Assess potential for self-harm.	Helps prevent harm or injury; helps determine level of surveillance needed.	All
2. Ensure safety; place on suicidal precautions.	Prevents impulsive reactions to stressful situations.	Nsg
3. Monitor activities continually for first 24 hours.	Helps assess level of suicidal intention, effectiveness of behaviors.	Nsg
4. Establish a verbal or written contract not to harm self; renew every 24 hours.	Prevents suicidal behaviors, demonstrates respect.	Nsg
5. Establish rapport; offer support; be available to listen; ensure confidentiality.	Acceptance of Rita's feelings shows respect and encourages self-worth even though her behavior is unacceptable.	All
6. Encourage Rita to keep a diary and write in it daily.	Helps Rita identify her reactions and behaviors.	Psy

Evaluation

Rita willingly contracted each day for no self-harm. By May 1 Rita was seeking Mary P., a nurse, for interaction. By May 7 Rita was able to identify one area in which she was having problems.

A complete client care plan includes several other diagnoses and interventions.

after a schoolmate has committed suicide. Health care providers who work with adolescents must assess every teen for his or her suicidal risk. Chapter 27 takes a more in-depth look at this problem.

The goals of treatment for suicidal adolescents are to protect them from harm, build trusting therapeutic relationships, and assist them in developing self-awareness and alternate coping skills. The Sample Client Care Plan illustrates a nursing care plan designed for a suicidal adolescent.

THERAPEUTIC INTERVENTIONS

Adolescents require special care because they are developing and maturing at the same time they are experiencing mental health problems. Although each adolescent is unique, several therapeutic interventions can serve as strategies for working with all teens. The relationship between client and nurse serves as an instrument for understanding and helping each teen. Nurses use therapeutic communication skills to help adolescents define their problems and then develop new and more effective ways of solving them. Specific interventions for adolescents center around five basic strategies: surveillance, limit setting, building self-esteem and confidence, role modeling, and skill development (Box 15-5).

Surveillance and Limit Setting

Surveillance is defined as the process of watching over clients to determine if they are safe, are keeping their

> **Box 15-5** **Therapeutic (Nursing) Interventions for Suicidal Teens**
>
> Surveillance
> Limit setting
> Building self-esteem and confidence
> Role modeling
> Skill development

> **Box 15-6** **Interventions to Build Self-Esteem in Adolescents**
>
> Use *eye contact.*
> Address each individual by his or her *name.*
> *Actively listen* (use the therapeutic communications in Chapter 11).
> Convey *respect*—ask, don't order.
> Help teens to assume *responsibility* for their behaviors and their consequences.
> *Praise* each effort at changing behaviors and point out their progress and successes.
> Teach *problem solving* and help them apply it to their own behaviors and problems.
> *Enforce limits respectfully;* focus on the behaviors that need to be changed.
> The goal is to *encourage responsibility* for one's actions and self-development.

rules, are making good decisions, or need adult intervention. The amount of surveillance is determined by the degree of the problem. Some adolescents need only minimal supervision, whereas others may require 24-hour-a-day observation. The goal of surveillance is to assist teens in developing new skills and coping methods, as well as to protect them from harm. The alert nurse can turn a potential crisis situation into an opportunity for growth.

Setting limits is also essential for adolescents. Part of the process of growing up is to test the limits of authority. Teens are struggling with learning to control their emotions. Nurses work to change the focus of control from external to internal (self-control). Situations in which the teen attempts to exceed the limits are treated as learning experiences. When limits are set on an adolescent's behaviors, it is important that the teen understand the rules of acceptable behavior and the consequences of inappropriate behaviors.

Quite often, adolescents do well with the problem-solving approach. Here the nurse asks the teen what he or she is feeling and doing. Then the teen is asked if the behavior is helping him or her get what he or she wants. The teen then develops a plan for meeting the goal or coping with the feelings and follows it through. This process helps adolescents learn to solve problems and gain some control over their situations. Positive actions are praised and reinforced, and the teen is encouraged to apply the process to other situations.

Building Self-Esteem

Adolescents, even the most well-adjusted, experience the discomfort of low self-esteem at some time or another; but for the teen with mental health problems, these discomforts can be great. Teenagers are masters at reading nonverbal behaviors. Nurses who use eye contact, address each teen by name, and actively listen make adolescents feel accepted and valued. Do not lecture or give advice. Instead, direct teens toward problem solving and assuming responsibility for their own feelings. Convey respect by requesting rather than ordering and by thanking them for their help. Praise each small effort toward success, and point out the adolescent's progress. If limits must be enforced, do so without anger or embarrassment for the

teen. The goal of setting limits is to encourage responsibility (Box 15-6).

Self-esteem is also fostered through the use of role models. The impression caregivers present will have an impact on the effectiveness of therapeutic actions. Adolescents watch how their therapists and care providers interact with each other and solve the problems that arise among them. It is important to remember that caregivers are always being watched and evaluated. If teens feel that your behaviors are effective, they will often adopt them for use in similar situations. Acting as a role model for healthy behavior requires a lot of energy, but it is a highly effective way of helping an adolescent learn to cope.

Skill Development

One of the most important therapeutic interventions involves assisting adolescents in developing the skills that are essential for functional living. Caregivers help their teen clients with cognitive (intellectual) skills, such as applying the problem-solving process to actual problems. They help young clients practice appropriate social skills. Working cooperatively within a group, learning how to listen to others, and exploring new methods for controlling anger or aggression are other therapeutic actions designed to help adolescents develop effective living skills. Working with adolescent clients is demanding and rewarding. Effective mental health interventions at this stage of life are extremely important if we are to prevent future problems.

KEY CONCEPTS

◆ The passage from childhood to adulthood is a time of physical, sexual, and psychosocial growth.

◆ Many common problems of adolescence can be classified into two categories: internal sources and external sources.

◆ A mental health problem exists when an adolescent's problems impair performance or threaten physical well-being.

◆ The category of disruptive behavioral disorders is divided into two basic diagnoses: attention-deficit hyperactivity disorder and conduct disorders.

◆ Emotional ups and downs are a normal part of adolescence, and many teens suffer from anxiety and mood disorders.

◆ Anorexia nervosa and bulimia are eating disorders characterized by severe disturbances in eating behavior, which can result in a body that is far below its ideal weight.

◆ Teens who become chemically dependent or addicted progress through four general stages: experimentation, active seeking, preoccupation, and burnout.

◆ Adolescents with long histories of inappropriate or maladaptive behaviors may be diagnosed with a personality disorder.

◆ A sexual disorder is diagnosed when problems cause the teen significant distress and impair his or her ability to function.

◆ The major characteristic of adolescent psychosis, such as schizophrenia, is a loss of contact with reality.

◆ Teenagers who attempt suicide usually fall into one of three groups: the teen with depression, the teen who is trying to influence others, and the teen with a serious mental health problem.

◆ In addition to the use of therapeutic relationships and communications, interventions for adolescents center around five basic strategies: surveillance, limit setting, building self-esteem and confidence, role modeling, and skill development.

Suggestions for Further Reading

"Abstinence Is Not the Only Answer," by Monica Poliafico (*RN* 62[1]:58, 1999), argues for the knowledge necessary to make responsible choices about alcohol.

The website: http://itsa.ucsf.edu/-mww/ offers information relating to child advocacy.

References

American Psychiatric Association: *Diagnostic and statistical manual of mental disorders,* ed 4, text revision, Washington, DC, 2000, The Association.

Clark RB: Psychosocial aspects of pediatrics and psychiatric disorders. In Hay WW and others, editors: *Current pediatric diagnosis and treatment,* ed 3, Norwalk, Conn, 1996, Appleton & Lange.

Hogarth CR: *Adolescent psychiatric nursing,* St. Louis, 1991, Mosby.

Inmates' kids may fill cells themselves in future, *New York Times,* p 4, April 7, 1999.

Kadzin AE: Adolescent mental health: prevention and treatment programs, *American Psychologist* 48(2):127, 1993.

Kaplan DW, Mammel KA: Adolescence. In Hay WW and others, editors: *Current pediatric diagnosis and treatment,* ed 3, Norwalk, Conn, 1996, Appleton & Lange.

Serdula MK and others: Weight control practices of U.S. adolescents and adults, *Annals of Internal Medicine* 119(7 pt 2):667, 1993.

U.S. Bureau of the Census: *Statistical abstract of the United States: 1998,* ed 118, Washington, DC, 1998, U.S. Government Printing Office.

Wong DL: *Whaley and Wong's nursing care of infants and children,* ed 6, St. Louis, 1998, Mosby.

Zerbe KJ: Eating disordered men require diverse treatment, *Menninger Letter* 3(9):4, 1995.

Chapter 16

Problems of Adulthood

Learning Objectives

1. List two developmental tasks of young adults.
2. Explain the importance of having a strong sense of personal identity.
3. Identify three characteristics of a successful adult.
4. Discuss three developmental problems faced by most adults.
5. Name four stresses associated with parenting or guiding the next generation.
6. Describe how environmental problems can limit an adult's ability to function effectively.
7. Identify two effects of a lack of social support for adults.
8. Explain how the fear of human immunodeficiency virus (HIV) and acquired immunodeficiency syndrome (AIDS) is affecting young adults.
9. Name three therapeutic interventions to help the psychosocial functioning of adults with problems.

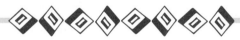

Key Terms

acquired immunodeficiency syndrome (AIDS)

adulthood

marriage

maturity

mortality

poverty

social isolation

For many years, adulthood was considered the end of growth and development. Once an adolescent reached the age of 21 years or so, he or she was viewed as an adult, completely matured and ready to assume a full place in society. **Maturity** is defined as the ability to accept responsibility for one's actions, delay gratification, and make priorities. Adulthood was once viewed as a time of stability with little or no change. Today, however, we see the period that follows adolescence as a dynamic one, filled with learning, struggle, rewards, and change. Adulthood is a time of personal, professional, and social development. It is the time to nurture and guide the next generation and for individuals to move beyond themselves and direct their energies for the benefit of others. The period of life labeled **adulthood** includes ages (approximately) 18 to 65 years. Remember, these divisions are for the sake of discussion. In reality, each adult is an individual who ages at his or her own particular pace.

Adulthood, like every other age, is filled with tasks, problems, and opportunities for learning. Refer back to Chapter 5 and review Erikson's developmental theory and Maslow's hierarchy of needs. All young adults are faced with the challenge of establishing their careers, their identities, and the relationships that will emotionally support them throughout their lives. As they age, adults must learn to cope with changes in families, careers, and relationships. All this is accomplished within a society so complex that no single person is able to understand its workings.

ADULT GROWTH AND DEVELOPMENT

Physical growth for men is complete by about 21 years of age. Women mature earlier, reaching their full growth around 17 years of age. Physical abilities are at their peak efficiency in young adulthood. Body systems have a remarkable ability to compensate, so the young adult is able to maintain a healthy state with little interruption, even during periods of illness (Edelman and Mandle, 1998). Because of this remarkable ability, young adults usually have few if any concerns about their health. Although many adults begin to show signs of aging after age 30, a healthy lifestyle and the absence of any chronic conditions usually allow then to enjoy good health well into later life.

Although physical growth may be complete, adults continue to develop in other dimensions. The emotional, intellectual, sociocultural, and spiritual dimensions of one's character begin to receive attention. Young adulthood is a time to establish oneself as fully functional and capable of living and thriving independently, whereas middle adulthood sees the growth and maturity of one's family and profession. Young adults must face the realities of choosing a career or vocation that provides them with the ability to secure the basic necessities of daily life, establishing long-term goals, and committing themselves to personal relationships with others. For many, adulthood is also a time of marriage, creation of a family, and parenting. As individuals encounter each life change, they rely on previously learned behaviors to help them cope. If one has learned to solve problems effectively as a child, then adulthood will pose fewer crises. However, problems of childhood, if not resolved, can follow one through life.

Emotional development of young adults is centered on learning to function within a stressful environment. Work and school offer many opportunities to cope with stress. When used positively, stress motivates young adults to achieve their goals, some of which are long term. When ignored, stress can lead to many problems. Young adults still have occasional emotional outbursts, but they attempt to find new ways of coping with the many feelings experienced during this time. Nurses who care for young adults must be willing to explore inappropriate or troublesome feelings with them. Assessments of the emotional status for all adults should include "the client's perception of how his emotions affect his ability to develop satisfactory relationships or achieve professional goals" (Rawlins, Williams, and Beck, 1993).

Later in adulthood, emotional development deals with the struggle of seeing oneself age. Individuals who have successfully coped with life's problems, gracefully accept and adapt to the fact that they are growing older. The anxiety generated by the prospect of a limited time on this earth motivates many middle adults to make the best of the benefits of middle age.

Fear of poor health, death, and loss of financial security causes anxiety in many adults, which can result in stress-related illness and behavioral problems. Feelings of anger can arise when interactions with work and family members are not as expected. Guilt can be experienced over parents, children, and the failure to meet personal goals. Health care providers should always assess their adult clients for signs of stress, anxiety, and depression. About 15% of adults in the United States experience a major depressive problem at some time, but fewer than one third receive treatment.

Intellectual development focuses on the young adult's ability to solve intellectual and abstract problems. Young adults must process large amounts of information and learn many new skills to become successful in education or employment. As young adults effectively cope with their situations, their horizons broaden and they develop flexibility—the ability to adapt to change. This flexibility, combined with the willingness to take risks, encourages them to respond to available personal and career opportunities.

Adults continue to grow intellectually if they use their abilities to think. People who exercise their intellects "have little, if any, loss of mental ability, whereas those who do not engage in productive mental activities may experience a decline in intellectual performance" (Rawlins, Williams, and Beck, 1993). The "use it or lose it principle" also applies to the use of intellectual abilities.

Social development for young adults focuses on interactions and relationships with others. If the sense of personal identity is strong and well established, individuals learn to form close personal relationships and become willing to make lasting commitments.

Habits learned in childhood are likely to become lifelong. Patterns of communicating and interacting with others establish young adults' interactional styles, which have a strong impact on employment, relationships, and choice of goals. For example, low self-esteem and withdrawal from social situations may result from an ineffective interactional style with inadequate social or communication skills.

Establishing intimacy is an important task for young adults. Those who have strong senses of personal identity are able to merge themselves with another in marriage or a long-term relationship. Individuals still struggling with their identities may seek relationships to fill their unmet psychosocial needs.

Parenting is a major challenge for most adults. The responsibilities of parenthood force an individual to shift energies from self to caring for others. Parenthood is a 24-hour-a-day career. Its demands may create anxiety, feelings of inadequacy, and a sense of isolation and helplessness. Women who manage both parenting and working outside the home are especially vulnerable. As the family unit gradually stabilizes and children begin to gain independence, parents often expand their focus beyond the immediate family or work situation and become involved in community activities.

The social tasks for adults also relate to the change from parent back to the role of partner. As children prepare for their careers and move out of the home, the middle-age couple has the opportunity to redefine their marriage relationship. With the responsibilities of parenting over, the couple begins to explore the 'communication, commitment, and compromise' aspects of their relationship (Box 16-1).

Marriages that have weathered the challenges of career and parenting are based on a solid foundation. Each partner recognizes the individuality of the other and his or her need to achieve personal growth. Couples who have effective *communications* are able to freely share their attitudes, opinions, and emotions. They reaffirm their *commitment* to each other and the relationship. Couples who find themselves unable to communicate are frequently faced with the possibility of divorce or separation.

Compromise involves the willingness to negotiate and to enter into interactions in which neither person wins nor loses. Conflicts are resolved by defining and solving the problem. The focus is kept on the issue. Couples who compromise communicate openly, listen carefully, and try to understand their partner's point of view. Their relationship is respected and cherished.

Development within the spiritual dimension focuses on defining one's value system and belief system. Young adults often challenge their current religious practices by changing churches or refusing to attend services. As individuals become established within the community and begin to raise families, they reexamine their values. Children offer many opportunities for parents to reflect on their values, beliefs, and ethics.

The spiritual tasks of adults are concerned with finding meaning in life. Religious and spiritual beliefs are reexamined in light of one's own **mortality** (eventually having to die). Religious, social, and community activities become important. Volunteering to help others enriches their lives and provides many opportunities for socialization. It is not uncommon for middle-age adults to dramatically change their lifestyles. The 40-year-old wealthy businessman who sells everything and volunteers at a homeless shelter and the mother who begins to study for a college degree are examples. Adults who do not or cannot find meaning in their lives become stagnant, self-absorbed, and isolated. The potential for serious mental health problems is greater for the unhappy, self-focused adult, no matter what the age.

To summarize, adults with good mental health are able to successfully adapt to life's changes. Once their personal identities have been established, they are capable of using each life experience as a lesson in personal growth. They develop the ability to solve problems and learn. Healthy

---

Box 16-1 **Social Tasks of Adults**

Commitment—to significant other, to career
Communications—with significant other, with children, with co-workers
Compromise—with significant other, with children, with co-workers

---

Box 16-2 **Characteristics of Successful Adults**

Accepts self
Adapts to changes, is flexible
Establishes priorities
Sets realistic goals and expectations
Learns from past experiences
Functions in stressful circumstances
Has achieved emotional control
Solves problems and thinks abstractly
Makes sound decisions
Establishes and maintains intimate and social relationships
Guides next generation
Finds meaning in life
Finds balance between give and take
Has inner strength to effectively adapt to new situations

---

adults are able to set priorities and reasonable expectations for themselves. They form bonds with other people and are willing to devote their energies to guiding the next generation or making the world a better place in which to live. They are able to give of themselves in both intimate and social situations, and their self-confidence remains unaffected by the opinions of others. There is a balance between give and take. In short, successful adults have developed the inner strength to carry them through the joys, sorrows, and everyday activities of daily living (Box 16-2).

COMMON PROBLEMS OF ADULTHOOD

Diagnosable mental health disorders that affect adults are described in detail in later chapters. (See Box 16-5 for the DSM-IV–TR classification of adult mental health problems.) Here we consider some of the risk factors and difficulties faced by many adults in today's society.

All adults are faced with situations that produce anxiety. The stresses that accompany everyday life are many, and stress-related problems can develop when individuals become too anxious. The common difficulties that challenge adults are divided into internal and external types of problems. One's personal outlook (internal) defines stressful or anxious situations, whereas the environment (external) plays an important role in determining the opportunities for jobs, education, and living conditions.

Internal (Developmental) Problems

Because life is a dynamic process, people must cope with change. As they do, they learn and (hopefully) develop more effective ways of living. As children, our developmental problems are clear. As adolescents, we discover that a unique individual lies within a seemingly ever-changing body.

Adults experience developmental problems too, but theirs are not so obvious. Choices made affect one's life. When adults feel they have made the right choices, they develop the inner strength to weather future storms. When they allow anxiety, anger, or other emotions to be the focus, effective adaptation does not occur as easily. Those who provide health care for adults should be aware of clients' problems and coping skills. Intervening early is a good form of preventive mental health care.

Personal Identity

Problems with establishing a strong personal identity begin in childhood. People who were not guided, nurtured, or unconditionally accepted in childhood find it more difficult to feel good about themselves as adults. Overcoming a childhood filled with negative examples is a difficult task for many adults. It requires the willingness to look at one's behaviors and learn new methods of handling difficult situations. With the support and examples of effectively functioning people, many adults are able to overcome the difficulties of their pasts and mature into capable individuals with strong senses of personal identity and self-worth.

Nurses have many opportunities to assist individuals by offering the emotional support and encouragement to problem solve. They can act as valued resources, directing their clients to support groups and other community resources. Helping a young adult develop a positive personal identity will lessen the possibility of future mental health problems. Box 16-3 lists several interventions designed to help young adults establish a positive personal identity.

Problems of personal identity can also be related to a person's intellectual abilities: how one solves problems, makes decisions, and interprets stress. When an individual's ability to solve problems in effective ways is limited, behavioral and personality difficulties are much more common.

Emotional problems plague all adults, but those who are able to put things into perspective are able to cope with fewer stress-related effects. Mentally healthy adults can identify and accept their emotions without acting inappropriately on them. Unfortunately, anger-control

---

Box 16-3 Therapeutic Interventions for a Positive Personal Identity

Assist the individual to:
Define a life dream
Develop occupational choices and goals
Differentiate self from the nuclear family by sorting through the beliefs and values of childhood to establish a belief system that is one's own
Decide about relationship choices and levels of commitment, such as marriage, cohabitation, remaining single
Assess how one's emotions influence the ability to achieve professional goals and develop healthy interpersonal relationships

Data from Haber J and others: *Comprehensive psychiatric nursing,* ed 5, St. Louis, 1997, Mosby.

---

problems plague many adults, especially those who were exposed to aggressive acts as children. Drug and alcohol abuse may also be the result of a person's need to deal with emotional problems, such as feelings of inadequacy, anxiety, or depression.

Interpersonal Relationships

Human beings are always changing and adapting. Young adults, who are still discovering their unique natures, are also searching for the relationships that will fulfill their needs and encourage their personal growth. Adulthood is a time for commitment to others, be it through marriage or career. The need for intimacy and belonging is great throughout life, and adults usually form many relationships. Young adults often seek relationships in an attempt to fill a personal void or escape an unhappy situation. Sometimes errors in judgment have enormous consequences for their future.

Many adults commit themselves solely to another with the vows of marriage. In this society, **marriage** is a legal state that bonds two people as a single family unit. Most often, children are produced, and the responsibilities of life focus on nurturing and providing for the offspring. As children mature and leave home, the marriage relationship is reevaluated, and decisions are made to continue or end the relationship. Other adults choose to cohabitate (live together) in opposite or same sex relationships. Homosexual families fill the same needs and engage in the same tasks as traditional families, but they are at greater risk for mental health problems because of the stigma and discrimination that still exists.

Many adults (especially women) are caught in the cycle of violence that comes with abusive relationships. Chapter 26 discusses this problem in depth.

Caring for one's aging parents is fast becoming a problem for many adults. Today members of the "sandwich generation" are faced with the dual responsibilities of caring for their children and their aging parents at the same time. Providing care for both adds many new stresses to the family as adults work to balance the requirements of career, children, and parents.

Conflict relating to gender roles and their stereotypes can arise when adults wish to engage in activities, behaviors, or career choices that traditionally belong to one sex. To illustrate, a woman who aspires to become a heavy equipment operator faces greater social resistance than a woman who works as a beautician.

Problems with interpersonal relationships can extend to work and social environments. Individuals who have little or no ability to see how their attitudes and behaviors affect other people often have difficulties with long-term relationships. They become superficial and unwilling to consider the feelings of others. Small problems with social relationships can balloon into serious mental health problems. Learning effective communication and interpersonal skills can spell the difference between a functional adult and an unhappy, unfulfilled adult. Nurses can play an important role in preventing mental illness by identifying those clients with interpersonal problems and offering them support, education, and resources.

Guiding the Next Generation

Most adults, married or not, have children, and children are not isolated events. They arrive as package deals, along with responsibility, fatigue, self-doubt, love, and joy. If pregnancies are planned, children are eagerly anticipated. Unplanned pregnancies, however, are stressful and sometimes unwanted. Choices about terminating the pregnancy, single parenting, or marrying for the sake of the child are decisions faced by unmarried adults that will have an impact on the rest of their lives.

The child-rearing practices of adults vary considerably. Most parents raise their offspring based on how they were treated as children. Parents who were strongly disciplined as children tend to use physical discipline when correcting their children. Likewise, adults who were disciplined in nonphysical ways, continue the practices with their offspring. Other factors, such as money, family relationships, safety, housing, health practices, and spiritual beliefs all affect the family, parenting practices, and the children. For example, relationships between individuals and with extended family members, as well as social interactions, can support or discourage certain child-rearing habits (Box 16-4).

The rise of single-parent families must be considered. Today it is estimated that more than 14% of all households in the United States are headed by women alone (U.S. Bureau of the Census, 1998). In these families, the single parent must function as father, mother, and provider. The joys of children can become overshadowed by the work and stress of providing for them. Without support and intervention, these families have a high potential for developing several mental health problems.

> **Box 16-4** **Factors That Influence Child-Rearing Practices**
>
> Family relationships
> Financial status
> Health practices
> Housing, living environment, safety
> Parenting styles
> Socialization with others
> Spiritual beliefs
> Type of discipline

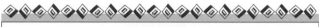

> **Think About**
>
> A single mother of two young children has lost her job and will soon be forced to leave her home.
> ◆ What resources in your community are available to help her?

Single parenthood can also be a positive experience. Not having to experience the conflict of different outlooks about child-rearing practices, providing the guidance that allows children to experience life in positive ways, and securing an environment free from adult conflicts are some of the rewards of single parenthood.

With remarriages (blended families) and adoptive families, children and adults who were once strangers instantly become relatives "without the shared experience of developing their parent-child relationship over time" (Stanhope and Lancaster, 1996). These families must establish new relationships, roles, and family boundaries. Sometimes they must cope with a natural parent living outside the family.

Childless adults contribute to the next generation through devotion to a career or volunteer activities. The need to share and leave one's mark increases by middle adulthood.

Economics

One of the greatest stressors for adults of all ages is financial security. Young adults must choose a vocation or profession that offers an opportunity to provide the necessities of life. Food, shelter, and clothing cost money—a fact that many young adults fail to learn until they leave the security of the family. Decisions about education and training, made young in life, will affect the quality of living far into the future.

Unemployment is a multisided problem. When a parent does not work, he or she becomes unable to financially provide for the children. Loss of self-esteem and self-worth accompany loss of employment. This absence of a regular income and its associated stresses

Case Study

Joan is a nurse in a center for homeless people located in a large U.S. city. She describes the qualifications necessary for her position: patience, persistence, and the ability to apply creative approaches to client care problems. Her role is one of facilitator and advocate who helps clients gain access to other services in the community. She ensures that each person is clean and presentable when requesting services. Although the shelter provides shower and laundry facilities, Joan makes sure everyone uses the toothbrushes, deodorant, soap, and razors.

She reschedules missed appointments for her homeless clients, providing for transportation if necessary. Clarifying instructions from other agencies and helping clients with job applications are also on her list of caregiving interventions. Every opportunity to provide client education is taken.

Joan instructs her homeless clients on the importance of good nutrition, safe sexual practices, communicable diseases, and other health-related subjects. She works with each individual to set and reach realistic goals. She sees every person as worthy of respect and dignity. Although her successes may be small, "hearing someone express that since he was able to get help for his problems, he now feels better about himself and is motivated to change his lifestyle provides this nurse's personal reward and professional satisfaction in working with the homeless" (Foster, 1992).

◆ According to Maslow, what needs is Joan helping her clients fulfill? (Refer to Chapter 5.)

◆ What resources are available for the homeless in your community?

---

begins the family on a downward spiral that may include poverty, physical illness, and psychosocial disorders. A stressful family environment with an unemployed head of household is associated with child neglect, maltreatment, and abuse. Nurses can play an important role in assisting families in finding support and retraining services (see Think About box).

Although adults experience many challenges, most learn to cope with each difficulty and apply lessons learned to the next problem. As time passes, the inner strength built through experience becomes a part of who they are. This inner strength provides encouragement to grow and expand beyond the limits of who they are today.

External (Environmental) Problems

The environment plays a strong role in the development of an individual during childhood. In adulthood, one's environment can either limit or encourage further development. Some of the major environmental problems affecting adults today include a lack of education, poverty, homelessness, substance abuse, HIV/AIDS, and lack of social support. Each of these problems can have a strong impact on the mental health of adults. Health care providers should be aware of these problems.

Education, Economics

An individual's training or education is closely associated with his or her economic status. Less educated people tend to be poorer, with few savings or financial reserves. Many families live "from paycheck to paycheck," where one small financial demand (e.g., the car breaking down or a sick child) can throw the family into turmoil. Adults who are vocationally trained or educated tend to have more financial and health care resources and are better able to cope with the problems of everyday life. Encourage your clients to seek further education or training by referring them to various community agencies that offer help or

training. A lack of education limits abilities and fosters disabilities.

The result of unemployment (or underemployment) is poverty. **Poverty** is the lack of resources necessary for reasonable and comfortable living. Poverty means unstable housing, poor educational opportunities, work problems, and an increased risk of becoming a victim. Adults who survive below the poverty line often have children who suffer as a result of their parents' misfortune. Poverty, homelessness, and a lack of education go hand in hand. Adults who must cope with this three-pronged dilemma usually need some kind of support and intervention.

The homeless are a diverse group. Many are single men, but almost a third are homeless women and children. Many chronically mentally ill people inhabit the streets because they are unable to use their resources wisely. Discouraged by their prospects, homeless individuals run a much greater risk for depression, drug abuse, and other mental health disorders.

Homeless people have special health care needs. Health care interventions must consider each individual situation and lifestyle. Therapeutic actions will be more effective when they are realistic and attainable (see Case Study box).

Lack of Social Support

Perhaps one of the most distressing problems for adults is **social isolation**—a lack of meaningful interactions with others. Before the time of rapid transportation, families tended to remain in one geographic area for generations. Small communities were often composed of relatives and extended family members who could provide strong emotional and social support during difficult times. People shared their anxieties, hopes, and difficulties with each other and received the emotional support and energy to cope with their problems.

Today, families live physically apart from each other—surviving as isolated, single units. The social interconnectedness that bonded people together is no longer intact. Adults must establish new connections, new relationships, and new support systems every time they move to a different community. This results in many people feeling socially isolated and disconnected from their fellow human beings.

Social support is the friendship from others that helps carry individuals through life's more difficult moments. With trusted friends, adults can share their problems, concerns, and stresses. These interactions—this social support given by friends—can make the difference between mental health and illness. Be sure to assess clients' social support systems (ask about friendships, and help them identify possible support people, such as neighbors or co-workers) and refer them to various support or community groups as needed. Remember that social isolation is not healthy for human beings. Acknowledging this fact can help prevent many future mental health difficulties.

Acquired Immunodeficiency Syndrome

Acquired immunodeficiency syndrome (AIDS) was first recognized in the United States in 1981. Since then, millions of people, especially adolescents and young adults, have been exposed to this devastating disease, which is caused by HIV. It is spread through sexual activities, the sharing of needles, or exposure to blood and body fluids. Acquired immunodeficiency syndrome prevents the body from fighting off infectious diseases, and its signs and symptoms are not recognized for many years in some cases.

People with AIDS often have vague physical complaints, such as night sweats, cough, weight loss, or fever. Other problems can include ear, nose, throat, or stomach complaints or skin changes. About one third suffer from anxiety, depression, or lapses in memory.

Acquired immunodeficiency syndrome has an impact on all members of society, but it is especially felt among sexually active young adults. People this age are more vulnerable to contracting the disease because they (1) lack the emotional maturity and judgment to make sound decisions and (2) feel the invulnerability of youth—the attitude that "it will never happen to me." It is only when a friend or loved one contracts the disease that its reality strikes home. Adults who can appreciate the seriousness of the disease have either made changes in their lifestyles or suffer the anxieties associated with high-risk behaviors.

Fear of AIDS has spread to persons whose lifestyles offer little likelihood of contracting the disease. The term AFRAIDS (Acute Fear Regarding AIDS) has been coined to describe an anxiety-related condition caused by a fear of AIDS. Individuals with poor or marginal coping skills may find it difficult to deal with the emotional aspects of this epidemic (Cook and others, 1994).

Every health care provider has a responsibility to educate clients about AIDS. The most important tool in the treatment of this devastating disease is education. Knowledge can be a powerful weapon if it leads adolescents and adults toward making health-promoting decisions. Knowledge can decrease the fear and anxiety felt by those who do not know the facts. Knowledge can help in detecting the need for diagnosis and treatment. It is true that AIDS has many physical consequences, but its psychosocial and emotional effects can be equally devastating.

There are many potential health problems, both physical and mental, in the adult world. Drug use is increasing as it becomes a way of coping with the difficulties of life. Decisions made regarding oneself and one's environment have greater consequences than they did during earlier years. Health care providers working with adult clients can find many opportunities to encourage and teach healthy living practices, which in turn can prevent future problems from developing.

MENTAL HEALTH PROBLEMS OF ADULTS

A great number of the mental health disorders suffered by adults have their roots in childhood. Adults who were diagnosed with attention-deficit hyperactivity disorder (ADHD), conduct disorders, or learning disorders in adolescence must now learn to cope with the responsibilities of adulthood. Many become substance abusers, others become members of the prison system, and a few progress toward successful adulthood. "It is striking to think that in a given year, 22% of the adult population in

---

Box 16-5 DSM-IV–TR Classification of Adult Mental Health Disorders

Adjustment disorders
Anxiety disorders
Cognitive disorders: delirium, dementia, amnesia
Dissociative disorders
Eating disorders
Factitious disorders
Impulse-control disorders
Mental disorders resulting from a general medical condition
Mood disorders
Personality disorders
Schizophrenia and other psychotic disorders
Sexual and gender identity disorders
Sleep disorders
Somatoform disorders
Substance-related disorders

Data from American Psychiatric Association: *Diagnostic and statistical manual of mental disorders*, ed 4, text revision, Washington, DC, 2000, The Association.

the United States have some diagnosable mental disorder or that 5 million people meet the criteria for severe mental illness" (Garritson, 1994). Millions of adults are struggling with depression or addictions (alcohol, gambling, or shopping). All must cope with the problems and crises of everyday living. One can understand why health care providers have many opportunities to provide the psychosocial care so needed by so many.

According to the *Diagnostic and Statistical Manual of Mental Disorders* (DSM-IV–TR) (see Appendix B), there are 15 categories of mental disorders. Box 16-5 lists each category. Remember, though, that beyond the diagnostic label lies an individual. If nurses are willing to put aside their biases and values, they will do much to encourage the higher levels of functioning in each client.

►►► Sample Client Care Plan — Ineffective Coping

Assessment

History: Jed is a 33-year-old man who has recently lost his job and his wife and is now being sued. Last night he had several drinks before driving home. His car ran off an embankment and rolled into an irrigation ditch. Jed was found uninjured, sleeping in the car early this morning. He has been referred to the clinic for evaluation.

Current Findings: In no acute distress; several bruises on arms and face; odor of alcohol. Jed states that 6 months ago his business as a roofer failed. After 4 months of trying to find employment, Jed began to drink. One evening he and his wife had an argument. When he returned later that night, she had moved her personal belongings out of the house and left a note saying that his drinking was becoming more than she could tolerate. For the past 2 months Jed has been spending his time "getting drunk."

Multidisciplinary Diagnosis

Ineffective individual coping related to loss of support systems

Planning/Goals

Jed will remain sober throughout treatment.

Jed will attend Alcoholic Anonymous meetings every evening.

Jed will recognize his maladaptive behaviors and take action to solve his identified problems.

Therapeutic Interventions

Intervention	Rationale	Team Member
1. Establish a trusting relationship with Jed.	Trust must be present if problems are to be solved.	All
2. Assess for degree of anxiety, depression, intent to do self-harm.	To determine interventions needed; to understand Jed's viewpoint	All
3. Help Jed identify each of his problems and current coping mechanisms.	Problems must be defined before they can be solved.	Psy, Nsg
4. Have Jed make a list of his available resources and support systems	Use of previously successful coping mechanism helps develop multiple skills.	Soc Svc
5. Replace the use of alcohol with crisis support person and phone number to call at any time.	Jed knows his drinking is an excuse to forget about his problems and is willing to call his support person when he wants a drink.	Nsg, Soc Svs
6. Help Jed devise new, more effective coping responses.	Builds on Jed's current abilities to solve problems.	All
7. Refer to Social Services for placement in the employment program.	Provides new resources for exploring job availability and opportunities.	

Evaluation

During the first 3 weeks of clinic visits, Jed had been drinking. By the fourth week, he had decided to quit drinking so that he could concentrate on "getting (his) life back together." By the sixth week, Jed was able to identify his most pressing problems.

A complete client care plan includes several other diagnoses and interventions.

Therapeutic Interventions

Although specific therapeutic interventions for each mental health disorder are described in later chapters, a look at the interventions available in every practice setting may be helpful. The focus of most therapeutic mental health interventions relates to prevention or assisting clients to cope.

Health Care Interventions

When working with adults, nurses can use their assessment skills to uncover clients' descriptions of their difficulties. Frequently the physician or nurse will actively intervene with a problem that is not as important to a client as it is to the health care provider. Make sure clients define their problems. Therapeutic actions will have greater results if the goals of care are as important to the client as they are to the health care provider. The Sample Client Care Plan for an adult with situational problems offers some suggestions for interventions.

Work within the client's reality. Learn about the client's living conditions. It does no good to instruct a client to take medication four times a day if he or she has no watch or means of telling the time. Too many therapeutic interventions fail because the client's total situation is not considered.

Give clients *written instructions* if you expect educational efforts to be effective. Everyone experiences anxiety when interacting with the health care system. People do not remember information when they are under stress. Written instructions allow them to refer back to the information when they are less anxious and more willing to follow instructions.

Preventing Mental Illness

Health care providers in every setting can do much to prevent mental-emotional disorders. Always remember that it is the whole person who receives our care. We may separate the human being into physical, mental, social, cultural, intellectual, and emotional parts, but we must consider and treat the entire person.

Each physical illness has emotional components, and each mental disorder is accompanied by physical changes. Therapeutic interventions need to include all aspects of the client's problems. A positive step toward preventing mental illness is to recognize the need for making mental health interventions available for all individuals, not just those people who are "diagnosed" with a mental disorder.

KEY CONCEPTS

◆ Adults continue to develop the emotional, intellectual, sociocultural, and spiritual dimensions of their characters.

◆ Parenting provides many challenges for most adults.

◆ The social tasks for middle-age adults include changes from being a parent back to the role of partner.

◆ Adults who are responsible for their behavior, use effective communications, are willing to make commitments, and cooperate with others successfully adapt to life's changes.

◆ Adults experience developmental problems, but they are not as obvious as those of children or adolescents.

◆ Problems of personal identity may be related to negative childhood experiences or a person's intellectual abilities.

◆ Anger-control problems plague many adults, especially those who were exposed to aggressive acts as children.

◆ Factors such as money, family relationships, safety, housing, health practices, and spiritual beliefs affect the family, parenting practices, and children.

◆ Some of the major environmental problems affecting adults today include a lack of education, poverty, homelessness, substance abuse, and minimal social support.

◆ The term AFRAIDS (acute fear regarding AIDS) has been coined to describe an anxiety-related condition caused by fear of AIDS.

◆ Each physical illness has emotional components, and each mental disorder is accompanied by physical changes.

◆ Health care providers must recognize the need for making mental health interventions available for all clients.

Suggestions for Further Reading

The *Fact Sheet on Mental Illness* (http://mentalhelp.net/may/facts.htm) is filled with interesting data about mental health problems.

References

Cook JA and others: HIV-risk for psychiatric rehabilitation clientele: implications for community-based services, *Psychosocial Rehabilitation Journal* 17(4):105, 1994.

Edelman CL, Mandle CL: *Health promotion throughout the lifespan,* ed 3, St. Louis, 1998, Mosby.

Foster J: The nurse in a center for the homeless, *Nursing Management* 23(4):38, 1992.

Garritson SH: Comments on health care reform for Americans with severe mental illness: report of the National Advisory Mental Health Council, *Community Psychiatric Nursing* 1(1):31, 1994.

Haber J and others: *Comprehensive psychiatric nursing,* ed 5, St. Louis, 1997, Mosby.

Rawlins RP, Williams SR, Beck CK: *Mental health-psychiatric nursing: a holistic life-cycle approach,* ed 3, St. Louis, 1993, Mosby.

Stanhope M, Lancaster J: *Community health nursing,* ed 4, St. Louis, 1996, Mosby.

U.S. Bureau of the Census: Statistical abstract of the United States: 1998, ed 118, Washington, DC, 1998, U.S. Government Printing Office.

Chapter 17

Problems of Late Adulthood

Learning Objectives

1. Name six physical changes associated with older adults.
2. Identify three mental changes seen in older adults.
3. Explain how a lack of finances or access to health care affects the mental health of older adults.
4. Describe the drug misuse (abuse) patterns of older adults.
5. Define the term elder abuse and describe a typical victim.
6. Explain how depression can affect older adults' abilities to function.
7. Describe the signs and symptoms seen during the progression of Alzheimer's disease.
8. List three mental health care goals for clients with Alzheimer's disease, dementia, or confusion.
9. Discuss how the standards of geriatric nursing care are used in other health care practices and vocations.
10. Identify three therapeutic interventions that promote mental health in older adults.

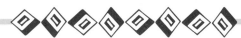

Key Terms

adaptation
affective losses
aging
Alzheimer's disease (AD)
catastrophic reactions
conative loss

delirium
dementia
elder abuse
functional assessment
gerontophobia
hoarding

integrity
maturity
memory loss
sundown syndrome

Aging is the process of growing older. Older adulthood, or **maturity**, is defined as the period in life from 65 years of age until death. Until recently, people older than 65 were considered "old," but our ideas of aging have changed and are no longer based on the number of years an individual has been alive. There are several theories or ideas about the aging process. Biological theories attempt to explain why we age physically, whereas psychosocial theories focus on the mental health aspects of aging. This chapter focuses on the psychosocial adaptations made by older adults and the mental health disorders that affect this age group.

OVERVIEW OF AGING

The **aging** process begins at birth, but few signs are noticed until well into middle age. With the passage of time, however, changes become apparent, and physical maturity begins to be replaced by the aging process. These are the senior citizen, geriatric, or elderly years—a time where outlooks can range from deep satisfaction and happiness to despair and sadness (Figure 17-1).

The number of people 65 years of age and older is growing dramatically. Today, because of scientific, medical, and technological advances, people are living

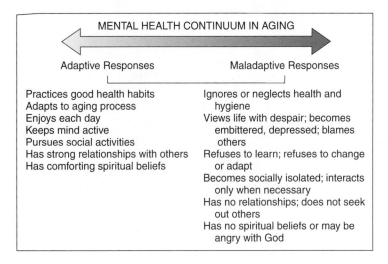

Figure 17-1 Mental health continuum in aging.

Box 17-1 Statistics Are Changing for Older Adults

The number of older Americans has increased by almost four times since the early 1900s.

In 1980 there were about 24 million adults over the age of 65 in the United States.

In 1998 there were more than 34 million older Americans.

Nearly one of every eight adults in the United States is 65 or older.

 Cultural Aspects

In traditional Korean families, elders hold a high place of honor. The responsibility of caring for them in old age falls to the first-born son, who inherits the family leadership and most of the property.

The Japanese have close ties between the generations. Care of the elderly traditionally falls to the oldest son or an unmarried adult in the family. Until recently there were few long-term care facilities for the aged in Japan.

Native Americans value the wisdom of their older adults. Historically most of their tribal leaders had attained much experience and knowledge before assuming leadership positions. Native American families are large, extended groups, and the care of the elderly is shared by every family member.

The Chinese value the family and consider it their responsibility to care for their elders. Older Chinese family members are respected and obeyed. Decisions are made through agreement of family members.

African-Americans have large support groups that offer help and comfort for their elderly.

Hispanic-American elderly live with their married children when they are no longer self-sufficient. Cultural and folk medicine beliefs are passed down by older family members.

longer and enjoying better health than their ancestors (Box 17-1).

Older adults are an important segment of the population. Many continue to remain active members of their communities. Such organizations as the Grey Panthers and AARP have strong economic and political influences in the United States today. In 1990 more than 11% of people over age 65 were still employed. By 2005 estimates place that number at 18% (U.S. Bureau of the Census, 1998).

Facts and Myths of Aging

Many people carry mental pictures or myths of older adults as people who are wearing out, biding their time until the inescapable end arrives. This is a myth—a belief based on little or no fact. In reality, the majority of older adults are dynamic individuals, living within their homes and functioning successfully within their communities (Edelman and Mandle, 1998).

Another myth of aging is that elders live in nursing homes. The facts show that over 95% of seniors live outside institutions, "except in the 85-year-and-older age group, in which approximately 20% are in institutions" (Hogstel, 1995). More than half the adults older than 65 are still living at home with a spouse, and many maintain their households alone.

"The majority of the elderly are poor" and "the majority of the elderly are rich" are two myths that explode on further examination. In reality, the economic status of older adults is as varied as that of any other age group. Incomes for the majority of people older than 65 fall somewhere between the 500,000 millionaires and 12% of older adults who are living in poverty.

Perhaps the cruelest myth, though, is that young and attractive is "good," whereas old and imperfect is "bad." Today's modern society places little value on its elders. Other cultures hold older adults in high esteem and value their wisdom and experience (Giger and Davidhizar, 1999) (see Cultural Aspects box).

It is difficult for young people to imagine growing old. As they mature, adults and children alike are repeatedly exposed to the negative aspects of aging. Over a period of years a fear of growing old develops, and anything associated with aging is avoided. "This fear of aging and refusal to accept the elderly into the mainstream of society is known as **gerontophobia**" (Wold, 1998). This attitude leads to stereotyping older adults. It is important for health care providers who work with older adults to look at their attitudes and values about aging. The journey through life is, for the most part, taken as an adult, living in the currents of change.

Physical Health Changes

As an individual ages, so does every body system. The physical changes of aging are not noticeable until the late 30s. By the 50s, one cannot deny the effects of time. Signs of aging continue to show themselves until around 85. After that, people appear to age little until their deaths.

The physical aging process varies greatly. It is affected by genetics, early physical and mental health care, current lifestyle practices, and attitude. Refer to a basic text for a discussion of the physical changes that are associated with normal aging. Figure 17-2 shows one effect of decreasing sensory abilities in an elderly woman.

Mental Health Changes

Older adulthood is a time for adjusting to change, or **adaptation.** Developmental tasks at this stage are challenging. According to the theorist Erikson, older adults who have developed a sense of personal **integrity** (state of wholeness) accept the worth and uniqueness of their lifestyles. They are able to find order and meaning in their lives. A sense of the flow of time (past, present, future) allows them to face life's challenges with grace and inner strength. They know they will survive because they have so many times in the past. If relationships with their children have been positive, they experience love and respect from their offspring. In short, the elder is able to accept his or her life (as it actually was and is) and value the contributions that he or she has made.

For older adults who have not reached a sense of wholeness, life is viewed with despair. Individuals become unhappy, feel that life has been a waste, and focus on "what might have been." They blame others for life's misfortunes. A sense of loss and contempt for other people leads these individuals to a sad and lonely lifestyle.

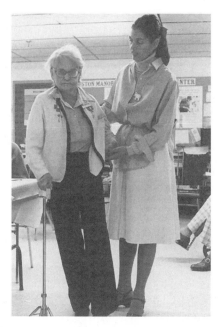

Figure 17-2 Decreased sensory abilities and function. (From Edelman CL, Mandle CL: *Health promotion throughout the lifespan*, ed 4, St. Louis, 1998, Mosby.)

Recently, mental health changes in older adults have been the subject of much study. The popular belief was that mental abilities decrease slowly with advancing age. The truth, we are learning, is not so simple. Some mental functions peak in childhood, others in adolescence. Although short-term memory and speed begin to decline in the 40s, mental capabilities, such as judgment and wisdom, continue to improve as one grows older (Table 17-1). Research over the past decades shows that the mind constantly adjusts its way of doing things and compensates nicely for the many losses in efficiency.

COMMON PROBLEMS OF OLDER ADULTS

Older adults must cope with many changes. They are required to adjust to physical changes that accompany the passage of time. Older adults are faced with loss through the death of spouse, family, and friends. Retirement brings a loss of income and opportunities for socialization. Living arrangements may need to be changed, and relationships with adult children are often redefined. Sometimes, several losses occur at the same time. For example, the individual who has just suffered a stroke (CVA) faces the loss of function, physical health, mobility, body image, and independence at the same time. Losses that occur at the same time seriously decrease the older person's ability to cope effectively. Older adults "must also learn to acquire new activities and interests to maintain the quality of life" (Potter and Perry, 1998). For some older adults, adaptation to change comes easily and

Table 17-1	Normal Mental Changes of Aging
Area of function	**Changes associated with aging**
Attention: Alertness, maintaining focus, noticing	Attention is fully developed by college age; declines slowly after age 70; easy to distract
Cognitive style: Ability to adapt, to roll with punches of life	Mental decline is more rapid in people who are rigid; flexibility in midlife reduces risk of mental decline
Crystallized intelligence: Specialized accumulated knowledge (nursing, engineering, technical skills)	Remains intact until 75 or older; may possibly remain intact until death
Episodic memory: Ability to register and store memories of events in time and space, to retrieve memories	Retains memories of recent events when able to anchor them to own experiences, knowledge base
Information processing: Ability to relate to, store, and retrieve information	Processing speed decreases with age; may take longer to retrieve information
Learning new tasks	Learning enhances many mental functions; people who do not continue to learn experience slowing and decline in many areas (which is reversible when one resumes learning)
Memory: Names and faces	Decreases fairly rapidly in middle age; often considered worse than truly is; like people of all ages, older adults must process information by associating it to related data
Metamemory: Judgment of one's ability to monitor and control one's own mental processes	After 40, older adults make conscious efforts to learn, manage, store, and remember new information; metamemory remains active in older adults who use their intelligence and lead active lives
Mood: Emotions, feelings	People with frequent negative emotions have higher incidence of depression; depression is common in older adults
Perceptual speed: Ability to become alert and respond	Perceptual speed slows after age 50 but may not be noticed; elderly score lower on timed tests but better on others
Personality: Behavioral traits that make one a unique individual	Personality is established in childhood and remains stable throughout life; if one was happy child, one is usually happy older adult
Reasoning: Ability to solve problems and make choices, comparisons, and judgments	Great individual differences between 60 and 80; after 80, some loss noticed; people with active mental lives decline more slowly
Retrieval of information: Ability to bring stored information into active consciousness	Takes longer after 50; more errors in retrieving; as persons age, there are more data to match up; slower information retrieval is sign of rich, well-stocked memory
Working memory: Random access memory; memory to which one refers	Increases through childhood and peaks during early adulthood; strengthens with use through connecting of neurons that occurs with learning

Modified from White K: *Psychology Today* 26(6):38, 1993. Reprinted with permission from *Psychology Today* magazine, Copyright © 1993 Sussex Publishers, Inc.

without discomfort. For others, however, each life change is stormy and produces major stresses.

Health care providers, especially those in the nursing profession, play a major role in caring for older adults. The problems of elderly clients challenge and test our resources. As the population ages, health care providers will be called on to assist many clients in coping with the changes of growing older.

Physical Adaptations

Because of normal changes associated with aging, many people believe that an inability to perform physical activity is the natural result of growing older. However, much research has pointed to the importance of remain-

ing physically active throughout life. Aerobic and muscle-strengthening exercises can prevent many of the physical problems associated with aging. Although the 70-year-old man cannot perform the same amount of physical labor in the same time a 30-year-old man does, he can perform the same amount if given extra time. The task will be done—it just takes longer. It is important to encourage daily physical activity in every client. A sound physical body has a better chance of housing a sound psychosocial "body."

Besides changes in endurance and the ability to do physical work, older adults must cope with a body that wants to adjust itself to a new routine. Changes in eating and sleeping patterns take place as one ages. Once, one was able to sleep through the night. Now some need or another often awakens the older adult. One used to be able to eat anything, and now antacids are placed at strategic locations throughout the house. The volume on the television creeps up; lights are adjusted to decrease the glare, and the odors drifting from the kitchen while awaiting dinner seem to be less inviting. Even without the problems of a chronic illness, older adults must adjust to the small, everyday physical changes of aging.

Older adults face many alterations in their lifestyles that may affect them physically. Older individuals who live alone, for example, tend to neglect their nutritional needs. They may eat too much or not enough or use their limited finances to buy less costly, empty-calorie foods. Many elders are not physically able to prepare their meals. Others suffer from sensory, dental, or digestive problems. Over time, the lack of adequate food intake results in chronic malnutrition. Resistance to the effects of stress and disease drops, and the risk for serious health problems increases. The Case Study box presents a typical experience.

Sexuality remains important for many older adults. The focus shifts from having children to an expression of caring, intimate communication, and sharing. Adaptations may be needed in the expression of sexuality because of physical limits or the presence of chronic health problems. A decrease in hormone levels leads to physical changes in the reproductive systems of older adults, but both men and women are capable of remaining sexually active well into their 90s.

Physical adaptations to aging include the loss of ability to move about freely. Losing a driver's license has a strong impact on one's independence and ability to provide for the necessities of living. Without private or public transportation, many of our elderly are severely restricted in their abilities to move freely about the community.

Adapting to the physical changes of aging can pose many problems that place an individual at higher risk for mental health disorders. Physical problems can lead to changes in mental status. Older adults commonly have vague, generally nonspecific physical signs and symptoms that may mask a mental health disorder. Drug-drug interactions, food-drug interactions, or drug side effects can cause both physical and psychological problems. Every health care provider who works with older adults must be alert for the existence of physical problems. Early assessment and intervention are the key for keeping older adults' minor physical problems from becoming major ones.

Health Care

The availability of health care is an important factor in maintaining the health of older adults. In the United States people older than 65 are covered by a national health program called Medicare, whereas Canadian and British citizens have national health insurance for people of all

---

◈ Case Study

Ned was 70 years of age when he lost his beloved Molly, his wife of 52 years. They met while they were still in high school, married soon after the war, and vowed never to be apart again. Four children filled the years with joy and hard work, and retirement was packed with new friends and experiences. But once Molly was gone, life for Ned became filled with gloom. He no longer sought out his long-time friends and stopped playing golf or horseshoes. He sold the motor home and retired into his darkened living room. Well-meaning friends often stopped by, but by the time they departed, they had taken on Ned's gloom instead of cheering him.

Soon Ned stopped eating. Molly had always prepared his meals, and he felt lost and unhappy every time he walked into the kitchen where Molly had spent so many hours. By the time his daughter visited Ned, he was confused and unable to care for himself. Assuming he had suffered a stroke, Ned's children admitted him to a long-term care facility.

◆ Describe early interventions that could have prevented Ned from being removed from his home.
◆ Discuss the advantages and disadvantages of care in the home compared with institutional care.

---

ages. Medicaid programs are state-administered programs that are designed to help "defray expenses for those who could not meet the cost of Medicare contributions or who exhausted their Medicare benefits" (Ebersole and Hess, 1998). Most older Americans receive benefits from Medicare or Medicaid.

Older adults in the United States must pay premiums for their medical insurance. In addition, they are required to cover other out-of-pocket expenses, such as medication costs and associated deductible and coinsurance costs. Do not assume that older clients are receiving medical care because they are covered by Medicare. Many elderly place their health care needs in the background when they are unable to afford the costs.

Health services may be available and affordable, but without transportation, visits to health care providers are few. Older adults who live alone or have sensory problems often find it difficult to obtain health services because of the obstacles they must overcome. Periods of confusion and forgetfulness may cloud an elder's ability to follow therapeutic instructions, and many confused people attempt to disguise or cover up the problem by being very cooperative and voicing understanding.

Psychosocial Adaptations

Before the 1920s it was not uncommon for individuals to grow up, marry, raise a family, and grow old within one community or group of people. People were cared for in their homes as they aged, with relatives or friends attending to their well-being. If they became confused or forgetful, friends and surroundings were a source of comfort and familiarity.

Today growing old has become more impersonal. The comforts of family and friends may lay miles away. Older adults may have problems relating to money, adequate food and housing, or health care. The loss of loved ones, social status, and earning power withers social support systems, and decreasing sensory abilities leave many elders questioning the soundness of their judgments.

The majority of older adults benefit from health care interventions. Nurses, because of their focus on the activities of daily living, are able to help the elderly fill many of their needs. Health care providers who work with older adults also help to fill the gap for missing family members by providing emotional and social support. The following section discusses a few of the most important problems faced by the elderly and some basic therapeutic interventions.

Economics

The outlook of older adults concerning money and financial security differs greatly from that of young adults. People in their 80s were born before the Great Depression of the 1930s. They were old enough to feel the pangs of hunger that arrive when food is scarce. They remember men selling apples on the street corners and have experienced the uncertainty of wondering how they were going to survive tomorrow. Many of these people even raised children during the Depression, sacrificing food from their own mouths to feed their offspring. The Depression years of the 1930s forged an indelible memory on our older adults. Many of their seemingly strange behaviors, such as **hoarding,** (the act of collecting and saving assorted, seemingly useless items) are the result of attitudes learned during those difficult years. The 90-year-old who takes doggie bags from the restaurant to wither in the refrigerator remembers the Great Depression and cannot bear to waste food. The collections of newspaper, clothing, string, old magazines, and other assorted odds and ends, are protection for leaner days that may lie ahead.

Because of inflation, the value of a country's currency (e.g., dollar, pound, or mark) changes, sometimes dramatically. Older adults in the United States have seen the price of a loaf of bread go from five cents to $2. During this time, many elderly people have followed savings plans or invested for their later years. Some are now financially comfortable, whereas others, not having realized the change in the actual value of a dollar, are coping with fewer resources than they had expected. People who made no preparations for later life often find themselves at the mercy of an impersonal system, living on meager resources with little quality in their lives.

The elderly are also faced with the problem of being

financially vulnerable. Older people were taught to trust other people and to take them "at their word." This background, combined with diminishing senses or understanding, leaves older adults vulnerable to the scams, deceptions, and threats of con men and criminals. Many older adults have lost their life's savings because they could not understand the language on a contract or allowed themselves to be charmed or intimidated out of their money.

Interventions relating to money are most often provided by social workers, whereas other caregivers can assess for indications of financial problems and refer clients to the appropriate resource. Remember to monitor elderly clients, because worry about money can lead to mental health problems such as depression, anxiety, or paranoia (Box 17-2).

Housing

Problems with housing for older adults range from having "too much house" to having none at all. In the United States, the majority of adults older than 65 live in their own homes with their spouses. About a third live alone, and about 15% live with someone else (U.S. Bureau of the Census, 1998). These statistics, of course, do not account for the number of elderly who have no homes because homeless people are difficult to count.

The problems of "too much house" usually arise when one spouse passes away and the remaining person is unable to care for the property. Because women tend to outlive men, the most common scenario is that of a newly widowed woman who is faced with the care of a house about whose maintenance she knows nothing. She may live there for many years of widowhood, but eventually she will be forced to move to a safer environment that requires less responsibility and upkeep.

The problems of "too little house" (inadequate housing) include homelessness and despair. Many of the elderly who experience homelessness are mentally ill. and are "usually sicker and have more needs for health services than the younger homeless" (Hogstel, 1995).

Box 17-2 Financial Assessment for Older Adults

Demonstrate respect during questioning, but ask about:
Sources of income
Housing and food costs
If they have money left for health costs
How they obtain their medications, do they share medications?
Money remaining (after paying expenses) for clothing and recreation

Others have been forced out of their homes because they were unable to afford the expenses associated with them.

As the population of older adults increases, new arrangements in housing are being developed. Today inventive new plans and living arrangements are evolving for older adults. Independent living centers, life contract facilities, foster homes, subsidized housing, and assisted living situations are all being explored as options for housing the elderly.

Loss and Death

We tend to travel life's paths with companions, friends, relatives, and people who have become important in our lives. With the passage of time, many older adults lose the individuals who are important for their emotional support and well-being. When a spouse of many years is lost, the remaining partner is left to cope alone. Depression often becomes one's companion after the death of a spouse or significant other. Not infrequently, couples who have been together for many years will die within months of each other. It seems the will to carry on without the loved one is lost, and death becomes an opportunity to be reunited.

Losses during the older years also arrive in various other forms. The loss of physical stamina and endurance and the loss of sharp senses with which to enjoy the world present problems and challenges for older adults. Although the concept of loss is described in a later chapter, it is important to remember that coping with loss is one of the most difficult problems of older adults. Compassion, understanding, and support help them reestablish the psychosocial connections that bind us together (see Think About box).

Substance Abuse

The misuse or abuse of chemicals is a complex issue for older adults. The elderly receive a great number of prescription drugs to treat multiple and chronic health problems (Box 17-3).

Older adults also metabolize and excrete drugs more slowly. Their decreased tolerance for most drugs can result in overdoses and severe interactions with other medications and foods. Problems with sight and memory also contribute to the misuse of medications by older adults.

Elders with several health problems may visit many specialists, with each one prescribing a different medication. The purchase of over-the-counter drugs compounds the situation by increasing the potential for adverse reactions. In addition, many of the elderly use several pharmacies, share their prescriptions with friends, and follow the recommendations of those offering relief from their discomfort. Hoarding drugs is common because of the expense and the possible need for them in the future. Many individuals will underdose themselves to save money and make medications last longer. Outdated medications are seldom thrown away.

Nurses have a special responsibility to assure that their older clients are using their medications correctly. Other caregivers can use this tool to gather vital information about clients' drug use. This responsibility includes a thorough assessment of a client's drug history, current drug use (prescribed, over-the-counter, and recreational), and an understanding of the medications currently being taken (see Drug Alert box).

Although the use of recreational or street drugs decreases with age, some drugs, especially alcohol, still cause problems for many older adults. Alcohol use helps to provide a substitute for social interactions, and many of the elderly drink to dull the discomforts associated with isolation. Older adults who were heavy drinkers in the past often show the results of long-term alcohol abuse.

The use of opiates (heroin, opium) is even more invisible than the use of alcohol. Older Asian-Americans with opium addictions or retired white-collar workers addicted to cocaine seldom reach the attention of health care providers because their habits do not usually result in the serious medical complications usually associated with alcohol.

All health care providers need to assess older adults for signs of substance abuse, especially when an unusual accident or event occurs. Often a history of minor accidents and injuries signals a problem with drugs. If problems with drug or alcohol use are suspected, the

---

Think About

◆ How do you picture yourself at 80 years of age?
◆ How physically active do you expect to be?
◆ Have you thought about or made any plans for retirement?
◆ At what age do you feel a person should think about retirement?

Box 17-3 Prescription Drug Use by the Elderly

Persons over age 65:
75% use some kind of medication
More than 30% of those medications are over-the-counter drugs
25% of all prescriptions are written for persons over age 65
Many older adults share medications or skip their medications to help keep costs down
Few of the elderly have knowledge of side effects or drug interactions.

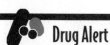

Drug Alert

Nursing Process

Assessment

1. Obtain a complete drug history: name of drug, reason prescribed, amount taken, how often taken. Is drug taken with other medications, on an empty or full stomach, at a certain time? What is your client's knowledge about the drug's side effects, drug-food interactions?
2. Instruct the client to put every medication he or she has into a paper bag and bring them to you. Check each medication for its expiration date. Be alert for several bottles of the same medication. Do not forget to include all over-the-counter products, vitamins, and herbal or natural remedies.
3. Assess client's ability to follow verbal and written instructions and willingness to learn about each medication.

Planning

1. Based on the client's abilities to understand and cooperate, develop a plan for teaching and monitoring the client's use of each drug.
2. Arrange for the client to show you the steps in identifying and taking the medication if necessary. Include family members in the teaching process when possible.

Nursing Diagnoses

Possible nursing diagnoses include:
Knowledge deficit relating to use, administration, and monitoring of prescribed medications

Ineffective management of therapeutic regimen because of sensory loss
Noncompliance related to altered thought processes

Therapeutic Interventions

1. Teach the client and significant others about the proper use and dosage of each medication, side effects and what to do about them, and expected therapeutic actions.
2. Devise a system for taking daily medications. Pill dispensers are available at most pharmacies. These multiboxed units can hold up to 1 week's medications. They usually consist of a series of small compartments, which are filled with all the drugs that must be taken at a certain time. The client opens the compartment at the prescribed time and takes every medication in the box. Having the client return weekly with his or her medications and pill dispenser allows the nurse and other caregivers to monitor the medications taken.

Evaluation

1. Assess the client's therapeutic response to the medications. What is the blood pressure? Has the pain been relieved? Did the drug do what it was intended to do?
2. Evaluate the client's willingness and ability to cooperate. Has there been any change in the client's alertness, level of understanding, or memory?

---

client is first referred to a physician for a medical assessment.

MENTAL HEALTH PROBLEMS OF OLDER ADULTS

People over age 65 suffer from the same mental health disorders as adolescents and younger adults, but they are also faced with the problems of vulnerability, abuse, memory loss, dementia, and Alzheimer's disease. Mental health difficulties can result from physical or biochemical disorders, such as diabetes or medication imbalances. Many mental health threats arise from loneliness and social isolation. Psychological problems with which individuals have struggled throughout their lives follow them into old age. Although all major mental health disorders can occur in older adults, by far the most common disorders relate to loss, depression, abuse, and dementia.

Elder Abuse

Older adults view the world from a different point of view than younger people. Many are lonely and easily trust someone who is kind or interested in them. Older adults

without adequate support are a vulnerable population—those people who are open to assault or attack by others. They are the abused elderly.

Elder abuse is defined as any action that takes advantage of an older person, his or her emotional well-being, or property. The three basic categories of elder abuse are domestic abuse, where the abuser has a special relationship with the elder; institutional abuse, where caregivers who are legally obligated to provide protective care fail to do so; and self-neglect or self-abuse. Acts of elder abuse appear in various forms, ranging from physical neglect to stealing money and exploiting the older person's resources. Table 17-2 lists several ways in which elder abuse occurs.

The victims of elder abuse are divided into those in which the elder has physical or mental impairment and depends on the family for daily care needs and those whose care needs are minimal or overshadowed by the abusive behavior of the caregiver. The typical abused elder is a woman at least 75 years of age with physical or mental problems who is living with a relative. Often the responsibilities of care can lead even well-intentioned family members or caregivers to lose

Table 17-2 Forms of Elder Abuse

Type of abuse	Description and examples
Exploitation	Improper use of a person for one's own profit. *Examples:* theft of objects, diversion of elder's money into own pocket, use of legal power assigned by the older adult for own gain. An estimated 10% of the elderly are exploited.
Neglect	Refusing to meet basic physical and mental health needs. *Examples:* depriving food, drink, clothing, shelter, hygiene, corrective and remedial devices (e.g., glasses, hearing aids); refusal to seek medical care, even when urgently needed; refusing to interact, to provide for love, belonging, social needs. About 65% of abused elderly are neglected.
Physical abuse	Physical harm caused by the actions of another person. *Examples:* beating, whipping, scalding, cigarette burns, bruises, fractures.
Psychological abuse	Threats to mental health caused by another person. *Examples:* poor personal hygiene, grooming, environmental conditions; threats of nursing home placement; being humiliated, threatened, or socially isolated; verbal assaults, name calling; being treated like a child; being placed in seclusion.
Violation of rights	The refusal to allow another the exercise of individual rights. These rights include the right to consent for medical treatment or surgery, refuse treatment, live in a safe environment of choice, privacy, and the right to use personal financial resources as desired.

Modified from Hogstel MO: *Geropsychiatric nursing,* ed 2, St. Louis, 1995, Mosby.

their tempers when they are stressed or feel pressured. However, losing control assists neither the victim nor the caregiver.

Abuse of the elderly is not new, but it has just begun to receive public attention. The actual numbers of abused elderly are unknown, but experts agree that current statistics show only the tip of the iceberg and the actual numbers of abused elderly are far greater (National Commission on Elder Abuse, 1999). Nurses must be aware of and alert for the indications of abuse in every older client. Chapter 26 focuses on the recognition, prevention, and treatment of this problem.

Depression

Along with the losses experienced through death, retirement, and relocation, many older adults are faced with losing their social supports. As stresses mount and resources are lost, many older individuals become saddened. This emotional state continues, and unless it is interrupted by the attentions of others, their outlook is bleak and hopeless. The mood becomes overpowering and reaches into every aspect of one's life. Individuals feel hopelessness and powerless to do anything about it. The future holds no joy, only the possibility of suffering more tomorrow than today. This is the face of depression in older adults (see Chapter 21).

Depression is probably the most common mental health disorder of late adulthood. It is estimated that more than 15% of older adults in the community have depressive signs and symptoms. Elders in long-term care institutions or hospitals have even higher rates. Depression is commonly underdiagnosed and undertreated. Sometimes vague complaints are the only clue. Other times, depression will mask itself as a physical illness. Knowing clients' lifestyles, preferences, social habits, and attitudes toward life is important. With this knowledge, nurses can assess for the behaviors that signal the onset of depression. Box 17-4 lists several signs and symptoms of elder depression.

Frequently the signs and symptoms of depression can mimic dementia. Careful assessments are required to distinguish the difference. Many medications, such as cardiovascular, anticancer, and psychotropic drugs, hormones, and antiinflammatory agents are associated with the development of elder depression.

Depression is treated with individual and group therapy and medications. Reminiscence therapy has proved effective in improving spirits. Antidepressant drugs have mixed effects because clients may experience unwanted reactions or toxic accumulations. Nortriptyline (Pamelor) and selective serotonin reuptake inhibitor (SSRI) antidepressants have fewer side effects in the elderly than other medications. Clients must be monitored for orthostatic hypotension (rapid drop in blood pressure on arising) and gastrointestinal (GI) symptoms. Offering emotional support and interest helps prevent depression by reestablishing the human connection that elders so often need. Remember that one person can make a difference in the quality of an elderly individual's life.

Dementia and Alzheimer's Disease

Dementia describes mental health problems caused by a medical condition or substance (e.g., abused drug, medication, toxin). Problems of this nature were referred to as organic brain syndromes in the past. The cognitive (intellectual) changes of older adults may range from mild lapses in memory to multiple, severe behavioral changes. **Memory loss** is the inability to recall a certain detail or event. It is a natural part of the aging process and affects most people older than 70. **Delirium** is a change of consciousness that occurs over a short period of time. It can be caused by various medical conditions, a variety of drugs and their interactions, or other problems.

Dementia is a loss of multiple abilities, including short-term and long-term memory, language, and the ability to think and understand. It is a broad term that describes a group of symptoms relating to a severe loss of intellectual functions (Hamdy and others, 1998). The condition may be reversible if the cause is discovered and treated early. There are more than 60 causes associated with dementia, including metabolic problems; hormonal abnormalities; infections; cardiovascular disorders; brain traumas, infections, or tumors; pain; sensory deprivations; toxic alcoholic reactions; anemia; chemical intoxication; drug interactions; and nutritional deficiencies such as vitamin B_{12}, folic acid, or niacin. Refer to Box 17-5 for an easy way to remember the causes of dementia.

Remember to assess older clients thoroughly and completely. The minor observations of one nurse can prevent a client from suffering the consequences of dementia. The label *dementia* should never be applied until the client's abilities have been thoroughly investigated.

Sundown syndrome describes a group of behaviors characterized by confusion, agitation, and disruptive actions that occur in the late afternoon or evening. The cause is unknown but sundowning is associated with dementia, loss of cognitive functions, and physical or social stressors. As visual cues and social interactions decrease with the onset of nighttime, individuals become more confused, irritable, and agitated. Box 17-6 lists assessments and interventions for sundown syndrome.

Dementia of the Alzheimer's type presents special challenges. As many as 4 million Americans are affected by Alzheimer's disease, and by the year 2050, approximately 14 million Americans will be affected (Hamdy and others, 1998). **Alzheimer's disease (AD)** is a progressive, degenerative disorder that affects brain cells and results in impaired memory, thinking, and behavior.

The unique characteristics of this condition were first described by a German psychiatrist, Alois Alzheimer, in 1907. He related the case of a 51-year-old woman who had a severely impaired ability to encode information, compromised language functions, and delusions. When she died from this severe form of progressive dementia, an autopsy of her brain revealed that it was shrunken, contained abnormal tangles of nerve fibers, and had clusters of degenerated nerve endings throughout the cortex. Since this first description, the pathological findings of AD have been the subject of intense study and research.

Box 17-4 Signs and Symptoms of Depression in Older Adults

Physical

Muscle aches
Abdominal pain, nausea/vomiting
Dry mouth
Headache

Cognitive (Intellectual)

Decreased or slowed memory
Slowing intellectual functions
Agitation
Paranoia
Focus on the past
Thoughts of death and suicide

Emotional

Fatigue
Lack of interest
Increased anxiety or dependence
Inability to experience pleasure or laughter
Feels useless, hopeless, helpless

Behavioral

Activities of daily living become difficult
Changes in appetite
Changes in sleeping patterns
Lowered energy levels
Poor grooming
Withdrawal from people and activities

Box 17-5 Possible Causes of Dementia

Remember: MEND A MIND

Metabolic disorders	Arterial disease	Mechanical disorders
Electrical disorders		Infectious disease
Neoplastic disease (cancer)		Nutritional disorders
Degenerative disease		Drug toxicity

The number of older adults with dementia increases with age. More than 50% of these people suffer from AD. Each year more than 250,000 new cases of AD are diagnosed. Because people with AD can live more than 20 years after diagnosis, many elderly people need extensive care. Caregivers need to be knowledgeable about the effects of AD and other dementias.

The diagnosis of AD is not clear-cut. Therefore a diagnosis is usually made by exclusion—that is, by exploring and ruling out all other causes of dementia. Many times a client's confusion or dementia may be the result of a drug interaction or reaction. Other times, dementia occurs as the result of a medical condition. Careful and thorough history, physical examination, and mental status examinations are performed, and the diagnosis of AD is made after all the findings are considered. Today researchers are working intensively to develop a diagnostic test for AD. Promising results have been seen with a type of skin testing, brain imaging techniques, and genetic studies (Fackelmann, 1995).

Alzheimer's disease involves a gradual, progressive death of one's brain and its functions. It is found in people as young as 40, but the incidence increases with advancing age. Alzheimer's disease progresses slowly and involves a loss in every area of functioning. In normal aging, cognitive (intellectual) and psychomotor (physical) changes are to be expected. Reaction times slow, and lapses of memory commonly occur. Learning new skills requires more time and practice, but intelligence and understanding (cognitive functions) remain intact.

Box 17-6 Care for Clients With Sundown Syndrome

Assess for:
Hunger, thirst, pain, the need to eliminate,
Feelings of fear, insecurity
Isolation, little contact with other people
Recent move or change in routine

Therapeutic (Nursing) Interventions

Maintain comfort, toilet as necessary, keep dry.
Control pain with nondrug interventions (back rub, massage, touch, distraction).
Reduce environmental stimulation during late afternoon and evening.
Maintain daily routine.
Provide environmental cues, turn on lights before dusk, provide night-light.
Provide soothing music.
Provide reassurance and companionship during evening hours.

People with AD, however, lose their cognitive abilities and suffer many intellectual losses. They cannot recall any recent events or process new information, become increasingly forgetful, and may display personality changes. Slowly other changes take place. As the disease progresses, individuals usually develop one or more of the following:

Aphasia: A loss of language
Apraxia: Loss of ability to perform everyday actions, activities
Visual agnosia: Loss of recognition of previously known or familiar people and objects

Soon individuals with AD become unable to make even the simplest decisions or choices. Following a conversation becomes impossible as speech becomes disjointed, simplified, and empty. As the disease continues, many people develop mutism (inability to speak) or speak in grunts.

The intellectual losses of AD are accompanied by the slow drain of one's own personality (**affective losses**). Emotional control declines as the individual fades into childlike, antisocial, or emotionally labile behaviors. As the disease progresses and the ability to process information is lost, people with AD become lost and absorbed in themselves. Some may even experience delusions, hallucinations, and feelings of paranoia.

Another loss for people with AD relates to the ability to make and carry out plans (**conative loss**) even for the simplest activities. The everyday tasks of living, such as dressing, grooming, and bathing, become overwhelming challenges. The harder they concentrate on the activity, the more difficult the activity becomes to perform. Stress, anger, and frustration increase fatigue levels because everything requires so much energy. Short-term memory fades, and everything seems to be happening for the first time.

Finally, there is the loss of the ability to withstand stress. People with AD become less and less able to cope with stress as the disease progresses. What once were minor anxieties cascade into full **catastrophic reactions,** in which the person becomes increasingly confused, agitated, and fearful. They may wander, become noisy, act compulsively, or behave violently. Because of the lowered stress threshold, it takes fewer and fewer stimuli to produce these overwhelming behavioral reactions. For this reason, care for clients with AD centers around providing a low-stimuli environment with as few as possible stress-provoking situations.

Treatments for AD are presently limited to providing physical and emotional support. Drug therapy is beginning to show promise with medications such as tacrine (Cognex), donepezil (Aricept), and calcium channel blockers (Schweiger and Huey, 1999). Certain antiinflammatory drugs may slow the rate of decline. Care of

---

Box 17-7　Tips for Managing Confusion

Determine physical, social, and psychological history of client before confusion.

Identify potential dangers to client in environment.

Place identification bracelet on client.

Touch client to convey acceptance if appropriate.

Identify strategies used by home caregiver to provide comfort.

Monitor cognitive functioning using an appropriate screening tool.

Avoid unfamiliar situations when possible.

Identify usual patterns of behavior for such activities as sleep, medication use, elimination, food intake, and hygiene.

Allow client to eat alone if appropriate.

Provide finger foods to maintain nutrition for client who will not sit and eat.

Provide client a general orientation to season of year by using holiday decorations.

Decrease noise levels.

Select one-to-one activities geared to client's cognitive abilities and interests.

Label familiar photos with names of individuals.

Limit visitors to one or two people at a time.

Give one simple direction at a time.

Address client by name.

Provide visual boundaries, such as red or yellow tape on the floor.

Place client's name in large block letters in his or her room, and on his or her clothing.

Use pictures to assist client to locate room, bathroom, or other equipment.

Refrain from using physical restraints.

Monitor carefully for physiological causes for increased confusion.

Modified from McCloskey JC, Bulechek GM: *Nursing interventions classification (NIC)*, ed 3, St. Louis, 2000, Mosby.

---

people suffering from AD is focused on providing the highest quality of life possible during the slow progression of the disease.

Most people with AD are cared for in the home by family members. Some day care facilities are available to care for AD clients while family members work or attend to other obligations. When the demands of care become too great or the individual's safety is threatened (e.g., wandering or smoking), most are admitted to long-term care facilities. Others arrive earlier if family support is unavailable because people with AD cannot be left alone for any time. Once the client adjusts to his or her new surroundings, the quality of life often improves. Family members are frequently relieved as the tremendous responsibility of constantly providing for every need of their loved one (without recognition or thanks) is lifted off their shoulders.

Care providers should first perform a **functional assessment**—an analysis of each client's abilities to perform the activities of daily living. How does the client eat, bathe, move, and provide for his or her hygiene? This information helps to establish an important baseline for comparisons later as the client deteriorates. Therapeutic care for clients with AD has three major goals:

1. Provide for clients' safety and well-being
2. Manage client behaviors therapeutically
3. Provide support for family, relatives, and caregivers

People with AD are unable to care for themselves, even in the most basic ways. Bathing, grooming, eating, and physical activity for persons with AD all require interventions tailored to the individual.

Elders with AD have no sense of safety or idea of danger. When they wander, they may walk in the street, step out in front of moving vehicles, or sit on the railroad tracks. Because of this absent sense, many facilities that care for AD clients have restricted or locked environments. Here clients are safe from both the threats of physical harm and overstimulation. When clients behave inappropriately, they are gently redirected in less stressful activities. Box 17-7 offers a few tips for managing confusion in the elderly.

Family members and friends who visit often are included in planning care, and many therapeutic actions are directed at providing support and understanding for them. It has often been said that AD is worse on the caregivers, who must stand by helplessly as they watch the person they love fade into a vague, unconscious existence. Never forget that clients' loved ones need your attention as much as the client. Alzheimer's disease and other dementias are serious problems, but with continued research and good care, we may someday be able to lessen the sad effects of these devastating conditions.

THERAPEUTIC INTERVENTIONS

Therapeutic care for older adults cannot effectively be accomplished unless a special ingredient is present. That special ingredient is *respect*: the courtesy, consideration, and esteem due each individual who has reached this stage of life. Every older adult, alert or not, cooperative or not, deserves respect, which is demonstrated by

Box 17-8 Standards of Geriatric Nursing Practice

I. Organization of Geriatric Nursing Services
Services are directed by a baccalaureate- or masters-prepared nurse with geriatric experience.

II. Theory
Nurses participate in developing new theories and use concepts to guide their practice.

III. Data Collection
Clients are routinely assessed, and the results are shared with clients, family, and multidisciplinary team members.

IV. Nursing Diagnosis
Nurses use assessments to develop nursing diagnoses (nursing process).

V. Planning and Continuity of Care
Nurses collaborate to develop a plan of care to help clients achieve the highest level of health, well-being, and quality of life possible, including a peaceful death.

VI. Intervention
Nurses provide care to maintain or restore abilities and prevent complications.

VII. Evaluation
Nurses continually evaluate client and family responses to determine progress toward goals and care plan revisions.

VIII. Interdisciplinary Collaboration
Nurses plan and meet regularly with other members of the health care team to evaluate and adjust the plan of care.

IX. Research
Nurses participate in, share, and use research knowledge.

X. Ethics
Nurses use the ANA code of ethics to guide decision making in practice.

XI. Professional Development
Nurses assume responsibility for professional growth through peer review and evaluations of the quality of nursing practice. Nurses contribute to the professional growth of other health care team members.

---

each action and each interaction we perform. Treat clients as you would like to be treated if you were in their situation.

Standards of Geriatric Care

The American Nurses Association (ANA) has developed guidelines (standards) for nurses who work with older adults. These standards offer nurses a means for providing and measuring the nursing care they deliver to older adults. Every nurse who works with older adults is responsible for following the standards of geriatric nursing practice. Other caregivers have the responsibility to care for older adults with respect, kindness, and sensitivity. Box 17-8 lists each standard.

Mental Health Promotion and Prevention

Many problems of older adults can be prevented or minimized if they are discovered early. Health care providers must work together to grasp every opportunity to promote healthful practices in their older clients. They should assess clients for changes in social, emotional, behavioral, and physical functioning and intervene early. Caregivers should not hesitate to help satisfy clients' needs, even though it may take some creative planning. Newer interventions, such as using dolls and stuffed animals to provide comfort (doll therapy) and life review (reminiscence therapy), are proving effective with many older adults. The Sample Client Care Plan focuses on an older adult who is having trouble recovering from a significant loss.

Caregivers play a major role in the care of the elderly. Interventions often require the services of several specialists, such as nurses, physical therapists, social workers, and homemakers. Sharing information and coordinating cares promotes quality in the lives of older adults. Health care providers also have the opportunity to make a significant difference in the direction of public policies regarding older adults, as well as in the lives of all the persons they touch.

KEY CONCEPTS

- Older adulthood, or maturity, is defined as the period of life from 65 years of age until death.
- According to the theorist Erikson, older adults with a well-developed sense of personal integrity accept the worth and uniqueness of their own lifestyles.
- Although short-term memory and speed begin to decline in the 40s, such mental capabilities as judgment and wisdom continue to improve as one grows older.
- Physical problems can lead to changes in mental status.
- Older adults experience several physical and social losses.
- Problems with housing for older adults range from having too much house to having none at all.
- The availability of health care for the elderly is an important factor in maintaining both physical and mental health.

> ### Sample Client Care Plan   Dysfunctional Grieving

Assessment

History: Moe and Mary had been married for more than 40 years when Mary died last month. Since her death, Moe has refused to leave his home. His days are spent in front of the television, eating snack food. Friends no longer visit because Moe refuses to turn off the TV, and it is too difficult to converse above the noise. For the past week, Moe has not bathed or changed his clothes. **Current Findings:** A sad-looking man, untidy, with a strong body odor. Speech is slow, answers with one word. When asked, states that "life is no longer worth living without Mary."

Multidisciplinary Diagnosis

Dysfunctional grieving related to loss of long-time spouse

Planning/Goals

Moe will acknowledge his loss and express emotions appropriate to the grief process.

Therapeutic Interventions

Intervention	Rationale	Team Member
1. Identify which task of mourning must be accomplished (acknowledge loss, work with pain, adjustment to loss).	Helps client begin grief work and reintegration into life.	Psy, Nsg
2. Help Moe express his feelings about Mary's death.	To prevent unexpressed emotions from bein directed inward.	All
3. Assure Moe that his emotions are normal expressions of grief.	Provides reassurance, acceptance of feelings.	All
4. Encourage Moe to talk about both positive and negative sides of their relationship.	Realistic appraisal of loss gives clearer perspective and promotes acceptance of current situation.	All
5. Engage Moe in social activities and refer to senior support group.	Decreases isolation and withdrawal; helps regain trust that "life will go on."	Soc Svc

Evaluation

After 3 weeks, Moe was able to discuss his feelings of loss, anger, and hopelessness associated with Mary's death.

A complete client care plan includes several other diagnoses and interventions.

◆ One of the greatest mental health challenges is coping with the loss of loved ones and friends.
◆ The misuse or abuse of drugs and alcohol is a complex issue for older adults who receive a great number of prescription drugs to treat multiple and chronic health problems.
◆ Elder abuse is defined as any action on the part of a caregiver to take advantage of an older person, his or her emotional well-being, or property.
◆ Depression is one of the most common mental health disorders of late adulthood.
◆ Alzheimer's disease and other dementias are behavioral or mental health problems caused by a medical condition.
◆ Dementia is a loss of multiple abilities, including short-term and long-term memory, language, and the ability to understand.

◆ Care for older adults cannot be effective without respect, courtesy, consideration, and the esteem due each individual who has reached this stage of life.

Suggestions for Further Reading

"Alzheimer's Disease: Your Role in the Caregiving Equation," by Joyce Schweiger and Ruth Huey (*Nursing 99* 29[6]:35, 1999), describes assessment methods, new treatments, and behavioral techniques for working with AD clients.
The website address www3.healthgate.com/aginghealth offers a wealth of information relating to older adults and the aging process.

References

Ebersole P, Hess P: *Towards healthy aging; human needs and nursing response*, ed 5, St. Louis, 1998, Mosby
Edelman CL, Mandle CL: *Health promotion throughout the lifespan*, ed 4, St. Louis, 1998, Mosby.
Fackelmann K: Brain changes may foretell Alzheimer's, *Science News* 147(12):180, 1995.

Giger JM, Davidhizar RE: *Transcultural nursing: assessment and intervention,* ed 3, St. Louis, 1999, Mosby.

Hamdy RC and others: *Alzheimer's disease: a handbook for caregivers,* ed 3, St. Louis, 1998, Mosby.

Hogstel MO: *Geropsychiatric nursing,* ed 2, St. Louis, 1995, Mosby.

McCloskey JC, Bulechek GM: *Nursing interventions classification,* ed 3, St. Louis, 2000, Mosby.

National Commission on Elder Abuse: *The basics: what is elder abuse,* pamphlet, 1999, The Commission.

Potter PA, Perry AG: *Basic nursing: theory and practice,* ed 4, St. Louis, 1998, Mosby.

Schweiger JL, Huey RA: Alzheimer's disease: your role in the caregiving equation, *Nursing 99* 29(6):35, 1999.

U.S. Bureau of the Census: Statistical abstracts of the United States: 1998, ed 118, Washington, DC, 1998, U.S. Government Printing Office.

White K: How the mind ages, *Psychology Today* 26(6):38, 1993.

Wold G: *Basic geriatric nursing,* ed 2, St. Louis, 1998, Mosby.

Chapter 18

Illness and Hospitalization

Learning Objectives

1. Explain the difference between health and illness.
2. Outline the five stages of illness.
3. Identify how denial is used as a protective mechanism during illness.
4. Explain why hospitalization is considered a situational crisis.
5. Describe the three stages of the hospitalization experience.
6. Compare hospitalization for psychiatric problems with hospitalization for physical problems.
7. Discuss how emotional support of significant others affects the outcome of a client's illness.
8. Identify three nondrug methods for managing pain.
9. Examine the importance of discharge planning for hospitalized persons.

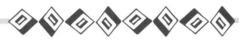

Key Terms

body image
denial
discharge planning
health

homeostasis
hospitalization
illness
pain management

sick role
situational crisis

Remember the first time you visited a hospital? Perhaps you were a visitor or even a patient. Can you recall how you felt? First, the hospital appeared to be huge. Even small hospitals are confusing, with mazes of hallways and mysterious little rooms everywhere. The odors were extra clean, antiseptic smells, like no other odors. The people who worked there were all dressed in ceremonial garb and paraded through the hallway mazes with business-like efficiency. Then there is the equipment—the machines and equipment that do one thing or another. It seemed that every piece came with a bell, whistle, or other annoying tone to periodically remind us of its presence. Generally, a health care facility can be a scary, intimidating place, not one in which most people choose to spend time.

For those of us in the health care professions, however,

the hospital (or nursing home or clinic) is a known environment, filled with the familiar. We often forget that the thought of "going to the hospital" brings immediate anxiety to the hearts of many. For these people, hospitalization can be an overwhelming and threatening experience (see Case Study box).

This chapter explores the mental health aspects of illness and the situational crisis of hospitalization. It describes the process of illness and its psychosocial adaptations, and it offers several therapeutic interventions for decreasing or eliminating the anxieties that accompany the illness and hospitalization experiences. Most importantly, it reminds us of the discomforts shared by the individuals who must cope with and adapt to the inpatient environment—a world we health care providers take for granted.

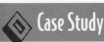

Case Study

Bob was an 82-year-old retired printer, living in a small retirement village with his wife, who had diabetes mellitus. He has enjoyed excellent health throughout his life. Other than periodic visits to his physician, he has had no contact with the medical community.

One evening, Bob noticed that he was bleeding when he urinated. After referral to a specialist, he was scheduled for a simple operative procedure to remove the extra tissue blocking the flow of urine and causing the bleeding. They were instructed to arrive at the hospital early the following morning.

On admission, nurses, noting Bob's age, assumed that he had some experience in a hospital—after all, he was older than 80. He was quickly admitted and prepared for surgery.

The surgical procedure was completed without problems. Bob was taken to the recovery room in good condition with a Foley catheter to straight drainage and an intravenous line in his right forearm. The first hour following the procedure was uneventful; however, the minute Bob regained consciousness, he insisted on going home. Nurses reassured

him that he would be discharged as soon as the physician saw him. He nodded and then dozed off. Seeing him sleeping, they turned their attention to other clients.

Bob hopped off the gurney and went on to detach himself from the intravenous line and Foley catheter. He was last seen walking out the door to his car in his hospital gown and bleeding from the urethra. As a result of the mishap, Bob was chased down, "captured" against his will, and hospitalized for 3 days to control the bleeding from the traumatic catheter removal. You can imagine what a challenging time that was for Bob and his wife, not to mention his health care providers.

Regretfully, not one health care provider assessed this man's previous experiences relating to hospitalization or medical treatment. Bob was under the false assumption that once the task was completed, he was free to return home.

◆ What actions could have prevented this situation from occurring?

◆ How could the lessons from this study be applied to your practice?

THE NATURE OF ILLNESS

Health is a dynamic state of physical, mental, and social well-being, as well as the absence of disease or abnormal conditions (Potter and Perry, 1998). Our state of health constantly changes as we respond and adapt to the challenges of life. This constant change process is called **homeostasis,** and it serves us well throughout our lives. When individuals become unable to adapt or regain the balance of homeostasis, they become ill and must mobilize critical energies to return to a state of health.

Illness is a state of imbalance. It is an "abnormal process in which aspects of the social, physical, emotional, or intellectual condition and function of a person are diminished or impaired, compared with that person's previous condition" (Anderson, Anderson, and Glanze, 1998). When you are ill or sick, you feel poorly. The body is not working correctly, energy is sapped, and spirits are low. Activities performed without a thought yesterday now loom as obstacles. Getting dressed for work becomes such a challenge that you seriously wonder how you will make it through the day. You need some rest, but your will is reminding you of your commitments and obligations. Sound familiar?

Illness is the body's way of communicating its need for attention. It will adjust to the demands placed on it until it is no longer capable of compensating. Eventually the individual becomes too exhausted to carry on without some attention. The example of the person with hallucinations who collapses from malnutrition because his visions told him he should not accept food from

others reminds us of the complexity of the mind-body interaction.

Stages of the Illness Experience

The subjective experiences associated with illness and disability are very personal. Some individuals consider being ill a minor annoyance, whereas others analyze their sickness for hidden evidence of certain doom. The illness experience is roughly divided into five stages. Each stage is associated with certain perceptions, decisions, and behaviors (Table 18-1).

Because nurses and other health care providers support clients throughout their institutional stays, it is important to be familiar with the emotional and behavioral reactions during each phase of the illness experience, be it physical or mental.

Stage 1: Symptoms

The illness experience begins when a person becomes aware that something is not right. It may be a physical or emotional discomfort, but something is perceived as wrong. During this stage, an individual becomes aware of an undesirable change, analyzes and evaluates the change, makes a decision that the change indicates an illness, and acts to remedy the situation based on the decision and the accompanying emotional response.

Many factors, such as the nature of the symptoms, the knowledge of the individual, and the availability of treatment resources, enter into determining if an illness exists. Emotional responses often govern behavior during this stage. If signs and symptoms are mild, one may

Table 18-1	Stages of the Illness Experience		
Stage	**Decision**	**Behavior**
1. Symptom experience	Aware that something is wrong	Symptom control, folk medicine, self-medicates
2. Assumes sick role	Gives up normal roles	Seeks support for sick role
3. Medical care contact	Seeks professional advice	Seeks sick role approval from an authority, negotiates treatments and procedures
4. Dependent patient role	Accepts health care treatment	Receives treatment, follows regimen
5. Recovery and rehabilitation	Gives up sick role	Resumes normal roles and responsibilities

self-medicate with various over-the-counter drugs, visit a local cultural folk healer, pray or meditate, or ignore the situation. For more serious symptoms, the individual may seek medical care or continue to deny a problem exists. When an individual recognizes the presence of a health problem, he or she begins to move into the second stage.

Stage 2: The Sick Role

Once a person acknowledges the presence of an illness, he or she seeks to confirm it by talking with other people. Family members, fellow workers, and friends are consulted for their opinions. The social group supports the presence of an illness, and the individual either assumes the **sick role** (actions and behaviors of a person who is ill) or continues to deny the illness.

Assuming the sick role serves several purposes. First, the person is excused from everyday duties and responsibilities. Other people "take up the slack" by assuming the ill person's duties. Second, permission is given for the individual to rest and conserve energy for healing. Third, the social responsibilities of interacting with others are relieved during the illness. In short, permission is given to focus on restoring the balance between health and illness.

Stage 3: Medical Care

If symptoms of the illness persist and home remedies fail, the person usually becomes motivated to seek professional intervention. The authoritative advice of a health professional confirms the presence of an illness, provides treatment, and informs the individual about the causes, course, and future implications of the illness. At this time, the individual can either accept the diagnosis and follow the plan of treatment or continue to deny the problem. Many people consult several different health care professionals (shop around) in an attempt to receive a diagnosis more to their liking or until they finally accept the professionals' opinions.

Stage 4: Dependency

In the dependency stage, the ill individual accepts the attentions of other people. A dependent role is assumed in which one must rely on the kindness and energies of others. "Care, sympathy, and protection from the demands and stresses of life" (Potter and Perry, 1998) are provided by family, friends, or health care providers. The individual is relieved of obligation, allowed to be passive and dependent, but expected to get well. The sick person may feel ambivalent: grateful for the help but resentful of the limitations. People in this stage have a particular need to be informed and emotionally supported.

Stage 5: Recovery and Rehabilitation

Movement into the recovery and rehabilitation stage can occur suddenly (e.g., a response to drug therapy or the breaking of a fever) or more slowly (e.g., recovery from a stroke or mental disorder). If recovery is rapid and complete, the individual gradually gives up the sick role and resumes his or her normal obligations and duties. For those whose recoveries are prolonged, arrangements for long-term care are made. Whenever possible, arrangements are made for individuals to recover in their homes. When this is not an option, the individual is usually transferred to another institution for further rehabilitation or care.

Not all people pass through every stage of the illness experience, and progression through the stages occurs at a very individual rate. However, nurses who understand the emotional aspects of the illness experience are better able to plan and implement effective client care.

Impacts of Illness

Illness is not an isolated event. It affects the activities of the individual and those who come in contact with the sick person. When illness occurs, it challenges the resources and changes the activities of all those involved. Illness has an impact on the individual. Short-term acute illnesses, such as the flu or a cold, have little effect on behavior, but a serious health problem (physical or mental) can lead to major emotional and behavioral changes. Individuals may react to illness with anxiety, anger, denial, shock, or withdrawal (Box 18-1).

If the illness involves a change in physical appearance it will have a strong impact on the individual's **body image**

Box 18-1 **Behavioral and Emotional Changes Associated With Illness**

Anxiety: Stress, feelings of apprehension, uncertainty about the illness. Responses to anxiety vary with the individual and the stage of the illness.
Anger: A response to feeling mistreated, injured, or opposed; may be directed inward or outward, may be irrational (has no basis in fact), and may affect the person's social functioning.
Denial: Refusal to acknowledge painful facts. Short-term denial helps mobilize resources, but long-standing denial results in maladaptive behaviors.
Shock: An overwhelming emotional state; individual is unable to process the information within the environment; may trigger both effective and maladaptive behaviors. (Refer to the stages of crisis discussed in Chapter 6.)
Withdrawal: The removal of self from others; individual refuses to interact; is often a sign of depression. Family members and/or the ill person may withdraw from each other.

Modified from Potter PA, Perry AG: *Basic nursing: theory and practice,* ed 4, St. Louis, 1998, Mosby.

(one's concept of his or her body). Threats to body image occur with surgery, extensive diagnostic procedures, and acute and chronic illness. One's self-concept also becomes threatened if the illness progresses beyond the expected time. Tension and conflict with other family members can further erode the ill person's confidence, and a depressed mood may begin to take hold.

Psychosocially, illness has an impact on the family. Changes in routine add more pressure to an already threatened family. Because the obligations and responsibilities of the ill individual cannot be met, family members often take on heavier work loads during times of illness. If the illness is prolonged, family members may experience situational stress, leading to an imbalance in family stability (Edelman and Mandle, 1998) until new roles and habits are established.

Illness has many faces. Remember, when assessing the physical signs and symptoms of illness, we are touching only the tip of the iceberg. Underneath lie other emotions, reactions, and behaviors that arrive with the package called "illness."

Illness Behaviors

During each stage of the illness experience, people are faced with several emotional choices. Some emotions serve to protect the individual from further stresses or mobilize resources to be devoted to healing, but other emotions can be destructive if they block efforts toward resolving health problems. For example, the emotion of denial can be useful or paralyzing.

Denial is a psychological defense mechanism (see Table 5-1, Chapter 5) used to ward off the painful feelings associated with problems. Denial can be helpful when it allows the time to collect and reorganize thoughts and plans, but it can be deadly when it clouds judgments and prevents individuals from taking the needed steps to restore themselves to health. Clients in denial require patience and understanding. They are struggling with the emotional aspects of illness and attempting to restore themselves to a more comfortable state of functioning.

Fortunately most people experience illness, recover to previous levels of functioning, and move on with their lives. They have actively or passively taken part in returning themselves to a state of homeostasis. Becoming ill and experiencing disability is not a comfortable experience, and nurses should remember that illness is the most important priority for the individual who is suffering from it.

THE HOSPITALIZATION EXPERIENCE

The great majority of illnesses are treated successfully in the home. However, some individuals are placed in an inpatient setting for treatment. **Hospitalization** is the placing of an ill or injured person into an inpatient health care facility that provides continuous nursing care and an organized medical staff.

People have vastly different experiences relating to stays in a hospital. Attitudes are also affected by what one hears. The relative who drags out minor historic facts about the hospital experiences of every family member and the horror stories from tabloid newspapers adds to one's concerns about receiving care in a hospital.

People who are hospitalized experience several emotional threats to their well-being and progress through different stages throughout their hospital stays (Robinson, 1984). During each stage, certain anxieties and emotional issues surface and challenge the client's coping abilities. Nurses should be aware of these issues and include them in the client's plan of care. Persons who are hospitalized are faced with physical, emotional, and environmental problems all at the same time. For most individuals, being hospitalized is seen as a crisis, an event with which they are unable to cope.

Situational Crisis

People are generally hospitalized in one of two ways: either the admission is planned in advance or an emergency requires special health care resources. In the case of the planned admission, one has time to experience the anxieties and work with the complications that occur as a result of the individual's absence. Although emotional reactions may be intense and the event may be viewed as a crisis, persons who elect to be hospitalized have the luxury of time to prepare themselves and their loved ones, both physically and emotionally. For those individuals brought to the hospital through the emergency department, no time is allowed for preparation. Their lives have suddenly been disrupted. If the health problems require complicated or long-term treatment, major adjustments in lifestyles must be made quickly.

Review the principles of crisis intervention discussed in Chapter 6 and apply them to the crisis of being hospitalized. Remember, a **situational crisis** is one that relates to outside or environmental problems. In the case of the client who has been coping with an illness or dysfunction for a time before admission, the precrisis behaviors consist of efforts to deal with the health problem. For the individual whose admission was an emergency, the precrisis behaviors were a healthy person's usual activities of daily living with no thought of illness or injury.

The actual crisis in both cases though is about being removed from one's familiar home environment to be cared for by strangers in an impersonal, uncomfortable setting (Aguilera, 1998). All hospitalized clients have one thing in common—the feeling of being out of control and dependent on the mercy, knowledge, and expertise of unknown health care providers. If nurses are sensitive to the fact that their clients are experiencing a crisis, therapeutic interventions will meet with greater success.

The Person Becomes a Patient

The process of becoming a patient is peppered with problems. The dilemma becomes more anxiety provoking as the admission process transforms an individual into a "patient or client." The name band around the wrist provides a means of identity that removes the requirement of a vocal inquiry because now caregivers can identify individuals by their arm bands. The demand for the paperwork diminishes a person into an account number and saps what little energy is present. "Next, an institutional gown helps the sick person to exchange his role as a functioning adult for that of a patient" (Robinson, 1984) (Figure 18-1). The individual goes to bed and becomes surrounded by caregiving people. In this vulnerable position, a person is expected to passively submit to scrutiny of body and behavior. All this is expected to be done gracefully and cooperatively, denying the fear, anger, and humiliation that are actually being experienced. The sick individual has made an agreement, a deal of sorts, whereby privacy is offered in exchange for treatments and interventions that will return him or her to wellness. The focus of treatment may be on the physical body, but care providers must stay aware of the psychosocial aspects of clients' health problems and hospitalization experiences.

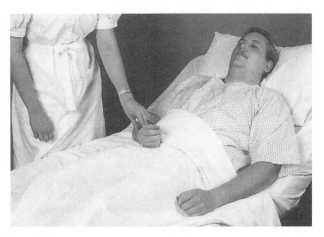

Figure 18-1 Becoming a patient. (From Potter PA, Perry AG: *Basic nursing: a critical thinking approach,* ed 4, St. Louis, 1998, Mosby.)

Individuals who are experiencing hospitalization progress through three steps. The first stage is the sense of being *overwhelmed.* The intensity of being separated from loved ones and left alone in an unfamiliar environment leaves many individuals exhausted. Energies needed to cope with the illness were diverted to surviving the admission process, separating from loved ones, and tolerating various diagnostic procedures. As a result, many clients withdraw into themselves and interact only when necessary. They must focus their attention inward in an effort to replace the energies that have been drained by the experiences of illness, crisis, and hospitalization.

During the second stage, *stabilization,* the hospitalized person gradually gains the strength to reestablish some personal identity. Individuals can become self-centered in this phase. The intellectual understanding that one is not the only person requiring care exists, but the emotional needs for reassurance and personal interest frequently must be asserted.

Adaptation marks the third stage. In this stage, the individual has regained enough of a personal identity to adapt. He or she often becomes interested and willing to learn about health problems, coping techniques, or preventive measures. Energies are replenished, the body feels better, and emotional responses are stable. Reorganization has taken place, and most people are again able to function effectively. For those persons who are transferred to another institution, the crisis begins again.

Common Reactions to Hospitalization

The rule of thumb for clients' reactions is "every person will react in his or her way." The manner in which individuals respond to the stresses of being hospitalized is determined by how they react to every other threat or crisis. The executive who controls a large company commonly reacts by attempting to gain control over his or her hospital environment. The woman dominated by her spouse makes few decisions without his opinion; and the helpless individual often becomes more so in the hospital. Please remember that even though some of your clients' behaviors may be distasteful, they are coping with their situations to the best of their abilities.

Hospitalization may also hold some symbolic meaning. For some persons, hospitalization confirms the fear that this is no ordinary illness, that there may be something seriously amiss. For others, especially the elderly, the hospital is the place where one goes to die, and for some, it is a place of respite where one is removed from the stresses of daily living. Attitudes and meanings concerning inpatient treatment for mental health problems differ from those relating to institutional stays for physical problems.

Psychiatric Hospitalization

The experience of entering a psychiatric treatment facility differs from hospitalization for physical reasons in several ways. Individual and family must cope with the stigma of mental illness. Friends may be reluctant to discuss the illness or feel awkward about offering their support. Employers may question the individual's fitness for the job, and insurance companies may deny payment for treatment.

The ill person has received a diagnostic label that will follow him or her for years to come. They are also affected by the numerous stories about life in psychiatric hospitals. Admission may be seen as confirmation that he or she is truly crazy.

If clients are alert and aware, they may fear other client's behaviors. Odd or inappropriate behaviors may create anxiety and feelings of the need to protect oneself. Frequent contact and support from the health care staff during the admission and adjustment period help clients cope with the anxieties of psychiatric hospitalization.

THERAPEUTIC INTERVENTIONS

Nurses play a vital role in the care of the sick within the hospital setting. Clients remember the people who provided their care. The caregiver who went that extra mile for a personal favor, the therapist who made certain a client's pet was fed, and the nurse who sat at the bedside when a client was too anxious to sleep are remembered clearly. Unfortunately the opposite is also true. Clients remember the short temper, the cutting words, and negative nonverbal messages more easily than acts of kindness and concern. All health care providers need to remember that psychosocial attention is just as important as good physical care and need to be willing to meet both the physical and nonphysical needs of all clients. Box 18-2 lists several nursing diagnoses (problem statements) that apply to the experience of illness and hospitalization.

Psychosocial Care

"Good physical care is always the first place to start in meeting the emotional needs of persons who have physical illness" (Taylor, 1994). Therapeutic care communicates a willingness to focus attention on the client, offers opportunities for interaction, and allows nurses to assess the client's adaptation to the changes resulting from treatment. Good psychosocial care begins with an assessment of the client's coping status (Ferszt, 1995). Perform a crisis assessment using criteria listed in Table 18-2. This allows you to identify problems before a crisis develops and plan preventive interventions.

Next, get to know your clients as individuals and real persons. Use active listening skills to encourage clients to discuss their anxieties and concerns. Clarify the clients' perception of the problems and their roles in treatment (Campbell and Anderson, 1999). Listen more than you talk because most clients need to share their emotions about the illness experience. No matter what your personal opinions are, do not pass judgment on clients' emotions and behaviors. Creating an accepting environment gives clients permission to share themselves, thereby beginning to establish trust in the therapeutic relationship.

Assist clients to cope with the fight-or-flight response brought about by the illness or hospitalization. According to Lazarus, stress is defined by the individual's

---

Box 18-2 NANDA Nursing Diagnoses Relating to Illness and Hospitalization

Activity intolerance
Adjustment, impaired
Anxiety
Body image disturbance
Communication, impaired verbal
Coping, ineffective, individual, family
Decisional conflict
Denial, ineffective
Diversional activity deficit
Family processes, altered
Fear
Grieving, anticipatory
Growth and development, altered
Hopelessness
Self-esteem disturbance
Sexual patterns, altered
Sleep pattern disturbance
Social interaction, impaired
Spiritual distress

From North American Nursing Diagnosis Association: *NANDA nursing diagnoses: definitions and classification 1999-2000,* Philadelphia, 1999, The Association.

cognitive evaluation of the situation and the importance or significance he or she attaches to it (Haber and others, 1997). Some individuals interpret the hospitalization experience as comforting and healing, whereas others may feel it is the first step toward dying. Teach and encourage clients to practice muscle relaxation techniques, imagery, and conscious sedation techniques to help ease their stresses. If the client practices a certain spiritual belief, notify the appropriate priest, minister, or spiritual practitioner. Also, be alert for any cultural practices that bring emotional support and comfort. Box 18-3 illustrates the use of the therapeutic (nursing) process as applied to the hospitalized client.

Support clients throughout each stage of the illness experience. Be aware of the behaviors associated with each stage of illness and hospitalization. Assist clients with the emotional discomforts of illness, whether physical or psychological. The Sample Client Care Plan addresses some of these factors.

Supporting Significant Others

An individual's family is an important group in one's life. The family of the traditional mother, father, siblings, and relatives is being replaced by newer forms, such as the single-parent family, the same-sex couple family, and the blended family in which the children of previous

Table 18-2 Crisis Assessment

Assessment steps	Description
Assess client's history of loss	What types of losses (physical, psychological, social, or spiritual) has client experienced in past?
	Who or what has helped client through crises in past?
	Older and younger persons have more difficulty coping with crisis.
Assess what illness means to client	What is client's understanding of current situation?
	What has client been told about condition, treatment, chances for recovery?
	How have client and family been affected?
Assess for other risk factors	Assess client's level of support from supportive significant others and friends.
	How easily does client adapt to new situations?
	Assess for other crises. Other problems can exist in addition to the crisis.
	Older adults and children have more trouble cooperating and following therapeutic plans.

Modified from Ferszt GG: *Nursing 95* 25(5): 88, 1995.

Box 18-3 Nursing Process Related to Hospitalized Clients

Assessment

1. Perform a complete physical and psychosocial assessment, including previous hospitalizations. Have client describe each hospitalization and his or her reactions to and opinions of the experience.
2. Ask client to describe any particular concerns or fears about being hospitalized.
3. Ask if there is a special routine or ritual that is important to the client.

Planning

1. Based on the data obtained in the interview, develop a plan to decrease the client's concerns and anxieties related to hospitalization.
2. Involve client and significant others in the planning process.

Nursing Diagnoses

See Box 18-2 for a list of possible diagnoses.

Interventions

1. Convey respect and politeness when interacting with clients.
2. Maintain a pleasant environment. Pay attention to noise levels, lighting, staff interactions.
3. Encourage client to cooperate and participate in his or her care.
4. Use therapeutic communications and offer emotional support. Listen to what the client is saying.

Evaluation

1. Evaluate the client's responses to the therapeutic interventions. Does the client demonstrate a decrease in his or her level of anxiety? Have the clients' concerns been addressed?
2. Ask the client to evaluate his or her hospital experience.

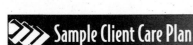 **Sample Client Care Plan**   # Hospitalization

Assessment

History: Mac is a 72-year-old man who has enjoyed excellent health until approximately 6 weeks ago, when he noticed a lump in the right abdominal area. Because of the possibility of extensive surgery, the physician would prefer to perform the biopsy at the hospital. Mac is being admitted the evening before surgery for preparation.

Current Findings: A nervous, pale man, appearing his stated age. Appearance, speech, and motor activity are all within normal limits. Mac states he is "a little concerned" about the surgery. Although alert, oriented, and cooperative, he has difficulty following instructions.

Multidisciplinary Diagnosis

Anxiety related to situational crisis of hospitalization and outcome of surgery

Planning/Goals

Mac will verbalize his concerns over his illness, outcome, and management of care.
Mac will understand and cooperate with his care.

Therapeutic Interventions

Intervention	Rationale	Team Member
1. Address client by his preferred name.	Demonstrates respect and insures that dignity will be maintained.	All
2. Obtain history of previous hospitalizations.	Helps plan care based on individual needs and experiences.	Nsg
3. Actively listen to and accept Mac's feelings of anxiety and the threat it poses to his self-esteem.	Conveys respect, self-worth; assures him that his concerns will be addressed.	All
4. Explain each procedure and gain cooperation before beginning.	Helps decrease anxiety and fear of unknown.	All
5. Assist Mac to identify and build on past successful coping mechanisms.	When added to newly learned ones, past successful coping mechanisms equip Mac with more skills.	All
6. Help Mac identify new ways to cope with his anxiety.	To help him manage anxiety.	Psy
7. Inform Mac frequently of his status and progress made during hospitalization.	Knowledge of one's condition decreases anxieties associated with the lack of control during hospitalization.	All

Evaluation

By the morning of surgery, Mac was able to discuss his concerns with the nurse. Recovery from anesthesia was uneventful.

A complete client care plan includes several other diagnoses and interventions.

relationships are blended into a new family group. Clients' families can have a significant impact on the outcome of their illnesses.

In many societies, the man is a symbol of strength and stability. When men from these societies are ill or hospitalized, their roles as providers change and they become receivers. Because they are unable to fulfill their roles, they feel inadequate and humiliated. This change of roles leaves family members bewildered and uncertain. If the condition is serious or chronic, loved ones are also faced with the issues of long-term care placement or death. In addition, each family member is trying to cope with all the internal emotional problems associated with the illness of a loved one.

Care providers should be alert to how the family's interactions affect their clients. Family members should be included and consulted for details about the client's care. All family members should be kept informed about the client's progress.

Also, remember that family members are people in crisis themselves, and gentle interventions provide some much-needed emotional support. When family members are satisfied that their loved one is receiving good care, the decrease in anxiety can help promote clients' recoveries.

Pain Management

An important component of any illness, hospitalization, or surgery relates to the concept of pain—that unpleasant sensation of nerve endings being unkindly stimulated. Pain is associated with many illnesses and hospital stays. It is a subjective experience and can be felt only by the individual experiencing it. People view pain individually based on their own experiences, attitudes, and anxieties.

To manage clients' pain effectively, nurses must discover their clients' expectations of pain, what they think may happen to them, and how much they expect it will hurt. Many clients believe that, if they complain, the physicians and nurses will be distracted from their real job—helping them to heal. Taking the time to learn about the clients' viewpoints will help you plan and implement more effective pain relief measures.

An essential step in helping clients control their pain (**pain management**) is mutual goal setting. Using a pain scale of 1 to 10, the client is asked to pick a target, a "pain score." The objective is to keep pain at or below the pain score level throughout the illness or hospital stay. This concrete goal helps both nurses and clients set realistic, attainable goals for pain management. For diagnostic procedures associated with pain, conscious sedation may be ordered (Messinger and others, 1999).

Assess your client's pain frequently. Try natural remedies to decrease the discomforts before resorting to pain medications. Massage, visualization, distraction, and therapeutic touch have all been found helpful in relieving pain. Pain has an emotional component attached to it. If nurses can decrease the anxiety associated with pain, the chances of a speedy recovery are much greater, because energy that was once used to control pain can now be used to focus on healing.

Discharge Planning

To help clients cope with the hurdles of illness or dysfunction, early identification and intervention of their problems following hospitalization are essential. This process is called **discharge planning**. After the initial admission assessment, possible home care needs are identified. Then referrals are made to appropriate resources. For example, home health nursing is arranged for the client who must recover from a fracture at home, or the social worker is notified of a client's need for psychiatric day care or housing. For clients who are living with others, discharge planning helps discover educational needs relating to the care of the recovering individual.

Illness affects the entire family group. New anxieties about the individual returning home must be addressed before release from the hospital. During the client's hospitalization, make an effort to discuss home care requirements with the family. Note and correct any misleading or inaccurate information. Use time with family members to teach health care practices related to client care. Most loved ones are more than willing to learn about good home care.

For people living alone, especially older adults, discharge planning is vital if individuals are to return to their homes after leaving the health care institution. Basic needs are a high priority for persons living alone. When those needs are met, anxieties are diminished, and people can get on with the business of living. Discharge planning is an important component of every client's care plan and a valuable tool for assessing and meeting clients' after-hospitalization needs.

Illness and hospitalization are stressful. Although many thousands of people are treated in hospitals yearly, every admission is a crisis. Do not become so comfortable in your work environment that you cannot appreciate your clients' emotional reactions to their situations.

KEY CONCEPTS

◆ Health is a dynamic state of physical, mental, and social well-being.

◆ Illness is an abnormal process in which aspects of the social, physical, emotional, or intellectual condition and function of a person are diminished or impaired.

◆ The illness experience is roughly divided into five stages, with each stage associated with certain perceptions, decisions, and behaviors.

◆ During each stage of the illness experience, people are faced with several emotional choices and with reactions frequently involving feelings of denial, anger, frustration, shame, and helplessness.

◆ Hospitalization is the placing of an ill or injured person into an inpatient health care facility that provides continuous care by nurses, allied health care providers, and an organized medical staff.

◆ The situational crisis of inpatient treatment is about being removed from one's familiar home environment to be cared for by strangers in an impersonal, uncomfortable building.

◆ It is important for clients to be emotionally supported through the psychiatric hospitalization experience because of the associated stigma and anxiety.

◆ Health care providers must remember that psychosocial attention is just as important as good physical care.

◆ Pain has an emotional component. Decreasing the anxiety associated with pain, increases chances of a speedy recovery because the energy used to control the pain can be focused on healing.

◆ Psychosocial care for hospitalized clients focuses on supporting clients and their families throughout the illness experience.

Suggestions for Further Reading

"Healing Touch: An Energetic Approach," by Cynthia Hutchison (*American Journal of Nursing* 99[4]:43, 1999), states that the images we focus on can evoke physical changes throughout the body and offers us a powerful technique for guiding our clients' images and energies in a positive, healing direction.

Nursing Net (www.nursingnet.org) offers interesting suggestions for client care.

References

Aguilera DC: *Crisis intervention: theory and methodology,* ed 8, St. Louis, 1998, Mosby.

Anderson KN, Anderson LE, Glanze WD: *Mosby's medical, nursing, and allied health dictionary,* ed 5, St. Louis, 1998, Mosby.

Campbell DB, Anderson BJ: Setting behavioral limits, *American Journal of Nursing* 99(12):40, 1999.

Edelman CL, Mandle CL: *Health promotion through the lifespan,* ed 4, St. Louis, 1998, Mosby.

Ferszt GG: Performing a crisis assessment, *Nursing 95* 25(5):88, 1995.

Haber J and others: *Comprehensive psychiatric nursing,* ed 5, St. Louis, 1997, Mosby.

Messinger JA and others: Getting conscious sedation right, *American Journal of Nursing* 99(12):44, 1999.

North American Nursing Diagnosis Association: *NANDA nursing diagnoses: definitions and classification 1999-2000,* Philadelphia, 1999, The Association.

Potter PA, Perry AG: *Basic nursing: theory and practice,* ed 4, St. Louis, 1998, Mosby.

Robinson L: *Psychological aspects of the care of hospitalized patients,* ed 4, Baltimore, 1984, FA Davis.

Taylor CM: *Essentials of psychiatric nursing,* ed 14, St. Louis, 1994, Mosby.

Chapter 19

Loss and Grief

Learning Objectives

1. Describe two characteristics of loss.
2. Illustrate four behaviors associated with loss.
3. Explain the differences between anticipatory, healthy, and unresolved grief.
4. State three techniques that help health care providers cope with their own feelings of grief.
5. Compare the reactions of being diagnosed with a potentially fatal illness to those of having a terminal diagnosis.
6. Describe how cultural factors can influence attitudes about death, grief, and mourning.
7. Outline each stage of the dying process.
8. Explain the meaning of a "good death."
9. Describe the support provided by nurses who provide hospice care for terminally ill persons.

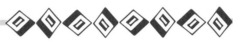

Key Terms

anticipatory grief

bereavement

bereavement-related depression

complicated grief

dying process

external losses

grief

grieving process

hospice

internal losses

loss

mourning

terminal illness

ife is a series of situations, challenges, joys, and losses—a dynamic process that requires continual adaptation and adjustment for survival. Life is filled with gains and losses on every level of functioning. Although change is an interwoven part of every individual's life, reactions to change and the accompanying losses vary according to our sociocultural perceptions. We each tend to react to our worlds as we were taught. Culture influences attitudes about proper living, relationships with others, and what is considered important in life. It also has a strong influence on a society's attitudes and practices relating to loss, the expression of a loss, and the dying process (Koenig and Gates-Williams, 1995) (see Cultural Aspects box).

This chapter explores the human reactions to loss. It offers several suggestions for assisting clients and their loved ones through the emotions associated with loss, and it encourages you to consider a "client-centered and peaceful death" as an appropriate therapeutic goal.

THE NATURE OF LOSS

The word **loss** has several meanings. It is a form of the verb "to lose," which means to bring about the destruction of; to become unable to find, to misplace; a failure to keep, win, or gain; and to have taken from one by accident, separation, or death. Add to this the emotional perceptions attached to loss, and one can see how loss becomes a very individual and personal experience.

Because losses are an unavoidable part of life, everyone must cope with them. Emotional reactions and their resultant behaviors were learned from childhood observations and experiences. How individuals cope with problems, successes, and losses is influenced by the success or failure of past experiences and present attitudes. How people react and behave during times of loss is highly individual. Responses to loss can range from quiet withdrawal to angry rampages, depending on how the loss is perceived, valued, and supported by others.

Losses can be classified as external or internal (self) losses. **External losses** include those losses outside the individual that relate to objects, possessions, the environment, loved ones, and support. **Internal losses** are more personal and include the losses that involve some part of oneself: the loss of physical, emotional, sociocultural, or spiritual self. An understanding of the characteristics of loss is important if nurses and other health care providers are to provide the psychosocial interventions that are so important in helping clients (and themselves) cope effectively with the emotional times associated with loss.

Characteristics of Loss

In the health care professions, loss is defined as "an actual or potential state in which a valued object, person, or body part that was formerly present is lost or changed and can no longer be seen, felt, heard, known, or experienced" (Rawlins, Williams, and Beck, 1993). This broad statement requires some analysis.

First, loss is an actual or potential state. A loss can be real—an actual threat or a situation based in reality. For example, the family whose home burns in flames is experiencing an actual loss. Potential losses are defined by the individual experiencing them. The industrial worker who is facing a layoff is coping with the possibility of losing his means of providing for his family. A college student who loses her confidence is faced with a less overt, but still important, potential loss. Losses can also be imagined—perceived as a loss. The case of a newlywed who loses her breast to cancer and imagines that her husband will reject her (even though that is not actually the case) illustrates an imagined loss that resulted from an actual loss.

Consider the next portion of the definition—"in which a valued object, person, or body part . . . is lost or changed." How a loss is defined depends on the value, importance, and significance of the item to the individual. Often the significance of a loss will be different for the client and the care provider. For example, the young mother who has just experienced her fourth miscarriage may define her loss differently than the nurse who has never been pregnant. Remember to assess the meaning of loss for each client.

The last portion of the definition, "and can no longer be seen, felt, heard, known, or experienced," explains the state of loss. When the valued person, object, or concept is gone, something is changed. This change leads to certain emotional reactions and responses that we call grief.

Losses may also be temporary or permanent, expected or unexpected. They may occur suddenly or gradually. Illness, for example, results in the temporary loss of roles and obligations, but the loss of a limb is definitely a permanent loss. Expected losses arrive with many situations. For example, a chronically ill 70-year-old does not expect to compete in the Senior Olympics because he knows he has gradually lost physical abilities. The individual diagnosed with a terminal illness is coping with an expected loss. Unexpected losses are just that. They are the unknown occurrences that arrive suddenly and without warning. The automobile accident, the diagnosis of human immunodeficiency virus (HIV), and the suicide of a cherished friend illustrate unexpected losses.

Losses can also be maturational, in which an individual must give up something to gain a higher level of development. The 18-year-old who is moving into her own apartment loses the comfort and security of family to establish herself as an independent adult. The loss here is ideally offset by the gains in self-development and maturity.

Situational losses occur in response to external events. In a situational loss, the individual has no control over the event leading to the loss. The death of a loved one, a natural disaster, and the divorce of family members are typical situational losses.

Behaviors Associated With Loss

Each person reacts to loss based on his or her level of development, past experiences, and current support systems. To support clients in coping with their losses, it is important to understand how people at various developmental stages react to loss.

Children's understanding of and reactions to loss change as they grow and develop (Wong, 1998). Newborns and infants feel the loss of their caregivers but show little emotional reaction to the loss as long as their basic needs are being met. Toddlers are concerned with themselves. Although they may repeat phrases such as "Daddy is gone," they have no grasp of the real meaning of loss. Because of their sense of time, preschoolers cannot understand a permanent loss such as death. Preschoolers use magical thinking (they believe that their thoughts can control events) to explain their losses. This can result in a child carrying the burdens of shame, doubt, and guilt when his or her thinking is associated with the loss. To illustrate, Jerry, a 3-year old, believes that if he were not such a bad boy, his mother would not have gone away. Younger children may react to the same loss more intensely than older children or adults because they have fewer coping mechanisms.

School-age children have some idea about cause and effect, but they still associate bad thoughts or misdeeds with losses. At this age, children experience great feelings of grief over the loss of a body part or function. They may feel overwhelming responsibility and guilt about an event, but they respond well to simple, logical explanations. Children around 6 or 7 often apply a broad definition to loss, especially death, by giving responsibility for the loss to the devil, God, or the bogeyman. By 9 or 10 years of age, most children have an adult concept of loss and death. They realize that some losses such as death are permanent, whereas others are only temporary. Their attitudes, reactions, and responses to their losses are now firmly established.

Adolescents can react to loss with adult thinking and childlike emotions. Although they can understand the concepts of loss and death, they are the age group least likely to accept the situation. Adolescents grieve acutely over the loss of a body part or function and fear rejection from their peers. Death is particularly difficult to accept at this age because the developmental task of adolescence is to define who they are and to establish an identity. Threats of loss at this age may make a person stand out from the peer group, so many adolescents ignore or minimize the loss or deny their own mortality.

Adults facing loss are able to perceive events more abstractly than younger persons. They can tell the difference between temporary and permanent losses. Most are able to accept their losses and grow from the experiences. As they continue to encounter and cope with various losses, most adults develop a "hardiness," a sense of self-confidence and motivation about life and death. This strength helps stave off the depression so common in older adults who have experienced significant losses. Hardy people are able to problem solve. They are in control of their emotions, their lives, and their reactions to loss. By the time most individuals have reached old age, their emotional hardiness has carried them through many of life's losses.

THE NATURE OF GRIEF AND MOURNING

Although the terms grief, mourning, and bereavement are used interchangeably, each has a separate meaning. **Grief** is the set of emotional reactions that accompany a loss. **Mourning** is the process of working through or resolving grief, and **bereavement** is the emotional and behavioral state of thoughts, feelings, and activities that follow a loss. The period of grief and mourning after a loss can be intense and painful. It may last for a short period or remain as a deep emotional scar. Feelings of loss, grief, and mourning are deeply personal, and each of us has our own way of coping with these emotions. There is no right or wrong way to grieve.

The Grieving Process

To work through the emotional responses to loss, one must experience the **grieving process**—a method for resolving losses and a way of healing or recovering. Grieving, mourning, and bereavement are normal, healthy responses to loss. Working through the grieving process allows people to "piece themselves back together," to reintegrate their lives, to find meaning in new relationships, and to reestablish a positive picture of themselves. It is a healing process that encourages people to continue even after the loss. The nurse's role during the grieving process is to provide an atmosphere for clients and support them in accomplishing the painful work of grieving (Lueckenotte, 2000).

The grieving process was first studied by Sigmund Freud in the early 1900s. Since then, many theories have been developed to explain the work of grieving. Although various theories consider different aspects of grieving, all include stages that individuals experience while resolving their grief.

The first step in the process of grieving is to say "NO." It begins with a feeling of shock. One wants to deny the loss, to say "no," and to refuse to give up the cherished object and accept the loss. Individuals may refuse to acknowledge that a loss has even occurred. They may behave as if nothing has happened or pretend that the loved object is still present. *Denial* at this stage provides an emotional buffer that gives grieving persons time to mobilize their resources for the work ahead.

As the realization that the loss can no longer be ignored sets in, denial turns to *yearning*. During this stage, the reality of the loss begins to sink in and the griever becomes overwhelmed. Crying, self-blame, and anger are common, and some may even strike out at self or others. The griever "falls apart"—becomes disorganized, depressed, and unable to complete daily living activities. He or she may try to postpone coping with the loss by ignoring it. They may feel that life is not worth living and consider or attempt suicide (Box 19-1). This is an

Box 19-1 | **Suicide Alert**

Individuals experiencing acute emotions of grief and loss often feel that life is not worth continuing. Any medications, over-the-counter drugs, or other chemicals in the environment have the potential of being used for a suicide attempt. Grieving persons have been known to ingest medications prescribed for the deceased with the purpose of committing suicide during the grieving process.

Sometimes grief is so intense that they will resort to slitting their wrists or using a weapon on themselves. Health care providers should be alert to the signs and symptoms of possible suicidal actions. See Chapter 27 for a more thorough discussion of suicide.

---

extremely difficult time for people. They need the emotional support and caring of friends and family to remind them of all that still remains, even after loss and suffering.

As the impact of the loss is felt in daily living, *depression and identification* with the lost object settle over the grieving individual. The work of mourning begins as the full impact of the loss is realized. Feelings of guilt and remorse are frequent as attempts are made to cope with the painful void left by the loss. The grieving individual may withdraw from social interactions, engage in unhealthy behaviors, or experience overwhelming loneliness. As time passes, however, most people become willing to share their memories and rely on the emotional support of others.

Acceptance and recovery begin when grieving individuals begin to focus their energies toward the living. The loss is a reality, but life continues, so they begin to reinvest their feelings in others and nurture their remaining relationships. Steps are taken to reorganize their lives by filling the void created by the loss. Eventually, a new self-awareness and inner strength evolve from the grieving experience. The good times start to outweigh the bad, and life once again slowly stabilizes.

The grieving process is dynamic, and most individuals do not move through the process step-by-step. They may "backslide" or regress into earlier stages or make multiple adjustments at one time. The actual length of time required for the work of grieving varies considerably, depending on the severity of the loss and coping resources available. Some theorists state that the intense reactions of grief gradually decrease within 6 to 12 months, but active mourning may continue for 5 years or longer.

Because resolving an important loss occurs slowly, time is allowed for people to mourn, to sort through their emotions, then cope with them. When the grieving process and its accompanying mourning behaviors are experienced successfully, people emerge with hope and a new

sense of involvement with life. The loss has been recognized, accepted, and placed in memory. Although life may never be the same, a new appreciation and interest in current activities gradually replaces the grief. One becomes healed and able to continue.

If an individual becomes aware of an impending loss, such as a diagnosis involving the loss of a body part or a terminal condition, he or she may experience **anticipatory grief**—the process of grieving before the actual event occurs. During divorce proceedings, for example, many persons grieve for the part of life that has been lost and what they know will be lost in the future. Anticipatory grieving allows individuals time to prepare for the loss.

Unresolved Grief

When the grieving process is prolonged or impairs functioning over time, mental health problems can result. Unresolved grief, also termed *dysfunctional grief* or *complicated bereavement,* describes unhealthy or ineffective grief reactions. People who suffer from unresolved grief are unable to shift their attention from their loss to the realities of everyday life and become so preoccupied with the loss that they are unable to function effectively. There are two types of unresolved grief: bereavement-related depression and complicated grief. Both are associated with expressions of distress about the loss, changes in eating or sleeping patterns, and changes in activity levels.

With **bereavement-related depression**, the griever feels the loss so intensely that feelings of despair and worthlessness overwhelm everything in life. Every day is a gray fog with no light as one looks toward the future. Life becomes a burden, and each new day is faced with remorse. This attitude overshadows all else, and the griever experiences changes in eating, sleeping, and activity levels; angry or hostile moods; and an inability to concentrate or complete work tasks. To complicate matters, individuals often become more and more socially isolated, and react with hostility or anger when friends express concern. This type of grief commonly leads to suicide but responds well to treatment when it is recognized and interventions are begun early. A combination of psychotherapy and drug therapy has been effective, but emotional and social support are always important factors.

Complicated grief is a persistent yearning for a deceased person that often occurs without signs of depression. Although the symptoms appear to be those of normal grieving, they are associated with impaired psychological functioning and disturbances of mood, sleep, and self-esteem. The griever becomes preoccupied with the loss and may idealize and search for the lost person or object or relive past experiences. Because life in the present is not as desirable as past memories, the individual may become intolerant of others and socially

Think About

Your client displays all the signs and symptoms of complicated grief. It is recommend that she start attending a support group for widows, but she refuses. With gentle questioning, she confides that she has no money for transportation to the meetings and is too proud to ask for help.

◆ What therapeutic interventions would help this client meet the goal of regularly attending the support group meetings?

 ## Cultural Aspects

In the Navaho culture of North America, it is a taboo to touch a dead or dying person or articles associated with the dying individual.

Filipino clients view death as a spiritual event and will surround themselves with objects of spiritual or religious significance. Often the family will pray at the bedside and wash the body after death has occurred.

Haitians may relate to death with guilt and anger. As part of the grieving process, they may take on the symptoms of the lost person's last illness.

From Giger JM, Davidhizar RE: *Transcultural nursing: assessment and intervention,* ed 3, St. Louis, 1999, Mosby.

isolated. Treatment for unresolved grief depends on the presence of depressive symptoms. A psychotherapeutic and psychopharmacological approach treats depression, whereas grief is helped by emotional support and someone to listen. Support groups and opportunities for social interactions add to the effectiveness of treatment in most cases (see Think About box).

The therapeutic interventions for both types of unresolved grief involve listening, providing emotional support, and referring to appropriate resources. Nurses and direct caregivers are often the first to identify the signs and symptoms of unresolved grieving because of their focus on clients' activities of daily living. Therapeutic listening helps in understanding the needs of the grieving individual. It also offers an opportunity to provide emotional support and comfort. Sometimes when grievers are encouraged to verbalize their feelings, the real healing begins. Health care providers are instrumental in referring their clients to the therapists, support groups, and educational opportunities that may help them work through the grieving process.

Caregivers' Grief

Caregivers experience the same grief as others when faced with loss. Many nurses work with dying clients, some on a daily basis. Relationships are formed between caregivers and clients that develop into understanding and rapport. The focus is on the client, and the caregiver acts therapeutically, but the bond between individuals grows with the relationship. When that relationship is lost, even if it was an expected loss, caregivers grieve, and that is a necessary process for health.

However, the caregiver's role in offering support and comfort to grieving loved ones can become complicated if one's personal feelings of grief overshadow one's effectiveness. Caregivers should share in the grief experience, but they need to remember that the primary goal is to provide support for the remaining loved ones. Many health care facilities offer support groups for nurses and other caregivers who work with dying clients in an effort to assist them with their own grief experiences. Learn to

appreciate the experiences of dying and grieving clients. Understand the steps of the grieving process and how you cope with losses. Finally, do not forget to find a way to renew your energies. When we know and accept our own attitudes and feelings about loss and grieving, we are better able to provide the therapeutic interventions so needed by others.

THE DYING PROCESS

Dying is the last stage of growth and development. Like birth, it is an intensely personal process. Unlike birth, however, an individual is often aware and consciously takes part in the process. Death means different things to each of us. For some, it is a welcome relief from suffering. For others, it is the ultimate fear. The process of dying remains unchanged, but attitudes, beliefs, and behaviors surrounding death are as variable as the individuals who practice them (see Cultural Aspects box).

Death may occur suddenly or gradually. It may be expected or arrive as a total surprise. One may be fortunate enough to die in familiar surroundings, attended to by loved ones and friends, or be faced with the fate of dying alone and unloved. During earlier days in American history, most families cared for their elders and ill at home. Children witnessed the births of their siblings and the deaths of their grandparents. It was all accepted as a part of living. Today children know little about dying because older adults no longer live in the family home. More than two thirds of all deaths now occur in health care facilities, hospitals, and nursing homes (Ebersole and Hess, 1998).

Age Differences and Dying

The impact of death is only as strong as one's understanding of it. Before the age of 8, most children do not understand the permanency of death, but they do experience a sense of doom and danger associated with dying. By age 12, children are aware that death is irreversible, but they do not relate to their own deaths. Adolescents and young adults do not relate to death unless forced. As people grow older they begin to lose family and friends and must begin to face their own mortality.

A special word about the dying child is needed here. Children are remarkably observant and have an intuitive ability to understand the seriousness of their illness and its outcomes. However, their immediate concerns focus on how the illness affects the activities of daily living and limits their abilities. Children are also very aware of the family's reactions and hesitate to discuss issues they think may be upsetting to the family. Whenever possible, parents should be encouraged to communicate with the dying child. Open discussions of the illness and its outcome help children cope with the feelings of isolation, anxiety, and guilt over causing distress in the family. Sharing feelings and insecurities helps to bond family members together and gain strength from each other. Children who are able to share their emotions have fewer behavioral problems, less depression, and higher self-esteem than those who suppress their feelings (Calandra, 1993). They adapt to the difficulties of their disease and its treatment better than those who must cope with the isolation of dying emotionally alone. Siblings of the dying child also need extra attention during this time because feelings of jealousy, anger, and guilt are often present.

Terminal Illness

A **terminal illness** is a condition in which the outcome is death. The diagnosis of a terminal illness is perhaps one of the most difficult challenges an individual must face in his or her lifetime. In today's world the diagnosis of HIV/acquired immunodeficiency virus (AIDS) is especially devastating for young adults. The course of the disease is long and marked by periods of physical improvement and hope alternating with times of illness and suffering. Grieving occurs throughout the course of the illness.

How a person responds to and prepares for death depends on two factors: the meaning of death and the coping mechanisms used throughout life to deal with problems. If the individual is comfortable and satisfied with life, death is usually accepted without fear; but if the person lived struggling and fighting, the experience of dying will be much the same. People tend to cope with dying in the same ways in which they coped with living.

The diagnosis of a fatal illness or condition is usually received with disbelief and shock—true crisis. This is a time of great uncertainty because client and family are struggling to cope with the illness, its effects, and its final outcome. Crisis interventions can be very effective at this stage.

As the condition progresses, denial and hope allow the client and family to slowly adjust to the reality of the situation. Hope is future oriented and helps individuals

endure the suffering of the present because it offers the possibility that soon things will be better. Denial offers a way of coping with each little loss until the reality of the situation is finally accepted. During this time, the individual is encouraged to continue with daily activities until he or she is no longer able. As time goes by, both the family and individual either accept the final outcome and prepare for death or continue to deny the reality of the situation, sometimes until it is no longer possible.

Receiving the diagnosis of a potentially fatal illness, along with the possibility of death, can bring forth a variety of reactions. Individuals who are young and feel healthy may refuse to accept that a problem exists. For others, the diagnosis of a potentially terminal condition acts as a wake-up call and a motivator to make major lifestyle changes. The Case Study illustrates such a situation.

Case Study

Brittany was just 35 years of age when she received the diagnosis of severe coronary artery disease. She became short of breath one day while doing household chores and decided that she must be hanging on to the cold received from her 8-year old a few weeks ago. She decided to schedule an appointment with her family physician.

Dr. Dunn had worked with Brittany's family for many years. He knew about her smoking, eating, and exercise habits. He had encouraged her to consider weight loss and had referred her to a smoking cessation program several times in the past few years, but to no avail. After a thorough physical examination and an electrocardiogram, Dr. Dunn scheduled Brittany for a cardiac catheterization at the local hospital the following day. Brittany left the office in shock, stunned by the realization that she may actually not live long enough to see her children grow into adults. She knew inside her heart that this was the warning call to take her life and health more seriously. She only hoped that she had the strength to make the changes she knew would be required if she wanted to live a while longer.

The results of Brittany's cardiac catheterization showed that three of her coronary arteries were seriously blocked and the blood supply to the heart was inadequate. Her physician recommended surgery to restore the blood supply to the heart but firmly stated that this was only a temporary measure. Without major lifestyle changes, the problem would reappear. At this point Brittany had to make some life-and-death decisions. As she saw it, she had two options: to continue with her easy-going, comfortable lifestyle and run the risk of dropping over with a heart attack at an early age or to change her diet, stop her unhealthy habits, begin to exercise, and learn to defuse her stress.

◆ What therapeutic interventions would help Brittany make a sound decision?

Many people often make the major changes necessary to prevent the condition from becoming fatal. Others value their present ways of living too much or feel that the work is not worth the extra time gained. The decisions about one's remaining time belong to and should be made by the individual. Caregivers should accept and support clients' decisions about terminal illness and structure the goals of care to provide the best possible interventions within the realities of each situation.

Cultural Factors, Dying, and Mourning

Although death is a personal experience, it occurs within a cultural and social context. Cultural practices regarding dying, grief, and mourning have a strong influence on behaviors. To illustrate, many modern North Americans see death as the final loss in life. East Indian Hindus, however, believe that all creatures are in a process of spiritual evolution that extends through the boundaries of time and space. They view death as a passage from one existence to another (Giger and Davidhizar, 1999).

Culture also dictates many funeral, burial, and mourning practices. The length of time for mourning and public displays of grief are culturally determined. Special clothing is often worn during the grieving process to symbolize the loss. To illustrate, traditional Chinese wear white as a sign of mourning, whereas black is the required color for mourning in North America and Russia.

The beliefs, rituals, and practices of one's culture may be very important to one individual and barely matter to another member of that same culture. Nurses must be careful to assess and understand the meaning of each client's cultural, religious, and social practices (Geissler, 1998). Many variations exist in every group of people, no matter which culture. Do not assume how a client feels about his or her cultural beliefs and practices. Find out what is important and, if at all possible, incorporate it into the client's plan of care. Never take a person's cultural background for granted.

Stages of Dying

Unless death arrives suddenly, both individuals and family members progress through several psychological stages. These stages or phases, called the **dying process,** allow people to cope with the overwhelming emotional reactions associated with dying and losing loved ones. Several theories about the process of dying have been developed during the past decades. The most well known is Elizabeth Kübler-Ross's five stages of dying: denial, anger, bargaining, depression, and acceptance (Kübler-Ross, 1969). Later theorists simplified Ross's five stages into three basic phases of resistance, working, and acceptance.

During the *resistance* stage, the individual fights the issue through denial, avoidance, anger, and bargaining. The *working* or review stage broadens consciousness as one's life is reviewed: "the struggle or resistance disappears and the individual begins to deal with unfinished

business and reclaims a part of the self, becoming more in tune to the self of the present rather than of the past" (Hess, 1998). In the last stage, called *acceptance,* the individual is comfortable and accepting of death. He or she can discuss death with peace and calm. Increasingly greater amounts of time are spent focusing inward, moving one's energies away from reality. Some individuals have near-death experiences that they describe as a passage into another realm of consciousness or a "vivid personal journey . . . when they were on the brink of death" (Hayes and others, 1998). Eventually, the dying person fades from this life, leaving only a body behind.

A broader perspective of the dying process is offered by Glaser and Strauss (1963), whose models of awareness of dying can be applied to family, friends, and health professionals who care for the dying individual. They describe the *closed awareness* model as one in which medical personnel know that the condition is fatal but still "keep the secret" or withhold the information from the client. Once the dying individual becomes suspicious of the truth, a battle for control of information ensues. This type of closed awareness was commonly practiced by health care providers in the past. Frequently clients were not told of the seriousness of their illness because it was believed that the news was too upsetting. Most terminally ill persons know that they are dying. Many still experience death locked into a denial supported by health care providers.

The *mutual pretense* model is a "let's pretend" kind of awareness. Both caregivers and the dying individual are aware of the impending death, but nobody talks about it. Although no one really expects the client to recover, it is easier to pretend that things will get better. Unfortunately the true feelings of everyone remain hidden, unspoken, and unresolved.

In the *open awareness* model, the approaching death is openly acknowledged and accepted. The client is resigned to dying and accepts each day as it can be lived. Family members, health care providers, and the dying have permission to discuss their fears, concerns, and experiences. The open awareness method of coping allows mutual support and comfort to be given and received. It also encourages loved ones to grieve *with,* rather than for, the dying.

THERAPEUTIC INTERVENTIONS

One of the most rewarding experiences in health care is assisting an individual to experience a "good death," one in which the dying and the living participate fully and completely. In a good death, individuals control their own destiny. Clients decide when to stop aggressive treatments, refuse the one last surgical procedure, or end the discomfort of a painful therapy. Peace, serenity, and acceptance replace denial, fighting, and anger. Individuals value and cherish each day but look forward to the day when their suffering will end. They are not afraid of death—rather, it is the last step of the growth process, which draws a productive and fruitful life to a close.

Nurses and other health care providers bring their own sets of attitudes, values, beliefs, and biases to the care of the dying. The way caregivers perceive "the act of dying, as painful, upsetting, indifferent, or a blessing, influences the treatment the dying patient will receive in the last days, whether in the hospital or nursing home" (Ebersole and Hess, 1998). Explore your own attitudes about death; the quality of your clients' care depends on it.

Never limit your clients by placing labels on them. It is easy for nurses to focus on the dying person's biological or physical needs. It is nonthreatening to help relieve the physical symptoms associated with dying, but it is another thing to become involved in a meaningful therapeutic relationship that supports the dying individual. Box 19-2 lists nursing diagnoses (problem statements) that relate to dying clients.

Hospice Care

In the past most of the dying were cared for in the home by family and friends. As society gradually became more mobile, families became separated from relatives when they moved to different locations. Dying at home was no longer an alternative for many people, so they were sent to hospitals and long-term care facilities. For many years health care providers assisted their clients through the dying process, providing comfort where they could, but

realizing that there must be better ways to meet life's final challenge.

Finally, during the 1960s, a model for humane care of the dying was developed and tested at Saint Christopher's Hospice in London, England. Since then the number of hospices has grown tremendously. In the United States today, almost 600,000 clients are receiving hospice care. (U.S. Bureau of the Census, 1998). The term **hospice** symbolizes a philosophy of care for people with terminal illnesses or conditions and their loved ones. Guidelines for hospice care have been developed by the National Hospice Organization (NHO), which is dedicated to promoting the principles and standards of high-quality hospice care.

The goal of hospice care is to make the remainder of an individual's life as meaningful and comfortable as humanly possible. Hospice care differs from institutional care in several ways. The focus of health care reorients from the institution to the home, where hospice services are available 24 hours a day. Hospice care redefines family relationships because care of the dying individual requires the energies of loved ones and friends. Hospice care helps the family retain control for the dying individual, and it allows individuals to experience death with the dignity

---

Box 19-2 NANDA Nursing Diagnoses Related to Dying

Adjustment, impaired
Anxiety
Caregiver role strain
Coping, ineffective
Decisional conflict
Denial, ineffective
Grieving, anticipatory
Grieving, dysfunctional
Hopelessness
Knowledge deficit
Nutrition, altered: more or less than body requirements
Powerlessness
Self-esteem disturbance
Sleep pattern disturbance
Social interaction, impaired
Social isolation
Spiritual distress
Violence, risk for: self-directed

From North American Nursing Diagnosis Association: *NANDA nursing diagnoses: definitions and classification 1999-2000*, Philadelphia, 1999, The Association.

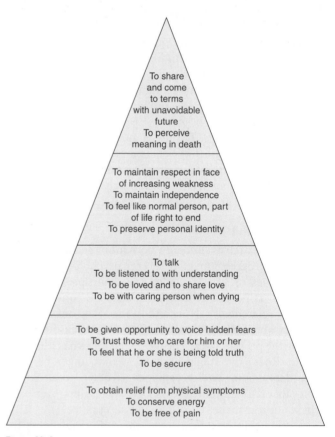

Figure 19-1 Hierarchy of the dying person's needs. (Redrawn from Ebersole P, Hess P: *Toward healthy aging: human needs and nursing response*, ed 5, St. Louis, 1998, Mosby.)

they deserve. Many care providers are choosing to specialize in hospice care today because it is such a rewarding area of practice.

Meeting the Needs of Dying Clients

Dying clients have special needs during their final days (Figure 19-1). One of the most urgent needs is to be free from pain and discomfort. This can usually be accomplished by around-the-clock administration of pain-relieving medications. Addiction is not an issue in caring for the terminally ill.

Freedom from loneliness is not always so easily accomplished. Many dying individuals have already suffered numerous losses, both physical and emotional. The strange surroundings of an institution and unfamiliar caregivers can add to a person's sense of isolation and loneliness. Dying clients need to know that someone who really cares for their welfare is there to help. Health care providers should assess for loneliness in clients and offer personal attention.

Individuals with terminal illnesses also need to preserve their self-esteem. The pride of a lifetime of work

and struggle can be easily shattered by the thoughtless words or actions of a caregiver. Respect is always an important factor in caring for clients, especially older adults. One of the most important principles to remember when working with terminally ill clients is that a dying person lives with the same needs as the rest of us. Life and its needs for love, friendship, and self-esteem continue, even when an individual is in the process of dying.

As death approaches, many physical and emotional changes begin to take place (Tables 19-1 and 19-2). This is a time to provide comfort and solace and meet the physical needs of care, but most important, it is a time to support those who must say goodbye and those who are left behind.

Loss, Grief, and Mental Health

Loss is a part of living. The behaviors associated with grief and mourning allow us to heal after suffering a loss. For many people, death represents the ultimate loss. How effectively individuals cope with their losses has a large effect on their mental and emotional health. The Sample

Table 19-1 Physical Signs/Symptoms Associated With the Final Stages of Dying: Rationale and Interventions

Symptoms	Rationale	Interventions
Coolness, color and temperature change in hands, arms, feet, and legs	Peripheral circulation diminishes to facilitate increased circulation to vital organs	Place socks on feet. Cover with light cotton blanket.
Increased sleeping	Conservation of energy	Spend time with the client; hold client's hand; speak normally to the client even though there may be a lack of verbal response or consciousness.
Disorientation, confusion of time, place, or person	Metabolic changes	Identify self by name before speaking to client; speak softly, clearly, and truthfully.
Incontinence of urine and feces	Increased muscle relaxation and decreased consciousness	Maintain vigilance and change bedding as appropriate.
Congestion	Poor circulation of body fluids, immobilization, and inability to expectorate secretions causing gurgling, rattles, bubbling	Elevate the head and gently turn the head to the side to drain secretions.
Restlessness	Metabolic changes and a decrease in oxygen to the brain	Calm the client by speech and action. Reduce light; gently rub back, stroke arms, or read aloud, play soothing music. DO NOT USE RESTRAINTS.
Decreased intake of food and liquids	Body conservation of energy for function	Do not force client to eat or drink. Give ice chips, soft drinks, juice, and popsicles as appropriate. Apply petroleum jelly to dry lips. If client is a mouth breather, apply protective jelly more frequently as needed.
Decreased urine output	Decreased fluid intake and decreased circulation to kidney	None
Altered breathing pattern	Metabolic and oxygen changes to respiratory centers	Elevate the head of bed; hold hand, speak gently.

Modified from Beare PG, Meyers J, editors: *Principles and practice of adult health nursing*, ed 3, St. Louis, 1998, Mosby.

Table 19-2 Emotional/Spiritual Symptoms of Approaching Death: Rationale and Interventions

Symptoms	Rationale	Interventions
Withdrawal	Prepares the client for release and detachment and letting go of relationships and surroundings	Continue communicating in a normal manner using a normal voice tone. Identify self by name: hold hand, say what you want person to hear from you.
Visionlike experiences (dead friends or family, religious vision)	Preparation for transition	Do not contradict or argue regarding whether this is or is not a real experience. If the client is frightened, reassure that he or she is not crazy, but that these aberrations do occur.
Restlessness	Tension, fear, unfinished business	Listen to client express fears, sadness, and anger associated with dying. Give permission to go.
Decreased socialization	As energy diminishes, the client withdraws and begins to make the transition	Express support; give permission to die.
Unusual communication: out of character statements, gestures, requests	Signals readiness to let go	Say what needs to be said to the dying client; kiss, hug, or cry with him or her.

Modified from McCracken AL, Gerdsen L: *Journal of Gerontological Nursing* 17(12), 1991.

Client Care Plan offers an example of a care plan for an individual who is coping with grief.

Many of the behaviors associated with the grieving process could be diagnosed as mental health disorders except for the fact that they are short lived. Mental health problems arise only when a person is stuck or immobilized during a stage of the grief reaction. Clinically, the *Diagnostic and Statistical Manual of Mental Disorders* (DSM-IV–TR) diagnoses of bereavement and bereavement-related depression are applied only to those grievers who are significantly impaired in their abilities to accomplish the activities of daily living for more than 2 months.

For persons who currently suffer from a mental health disorder, the stresses of loss and grief can overwhelm delicate coping mechanisms and lead to further problems. For example, the 23-year-old with schizophrenia who has lived with her family all her life will have great difficulties in grieving for the loss of her mother. Caregivers must remember that people with existing mental health problems require much emotional support during periods of loss or grieving.

How each human being copes with loss is unique and individual. Coping mechanisms may be effective and result in growth and healing. They may also be inadequate or dysfunctional, resulting in distress, depression, or other mental health problems. Nurses need to assess their clients' abilities and resources to cope with their losses. By encouraging effective coping skills and providing physical and emotional support, health care providers become able to help their clients (and themselves) in successfully working through life's losses and grief.

KEY CONCEPTS

◆ Life is filled with gains and losses on every level of functioning.

◆ Grief is the set of emotional reactions accompanying loss, whereas mourning is the process of working through or resolving one's grief.

◆ Bereavement is the emotional and behavioral state of thoughts, feelings, and activities that follow a loss.

◆ The steps of the grieving process are shock, disbelief, and denial; anger, bargaining, reviewing; depression; and acceptance.

◆ Two types of dysfunctional (unresolved) grief are known as bereavement-related depression and complicated grief.

◆ The nurse's role in offering support and comfort to grieving loved ones can become complicated if one's personal grief overshadows his or her effectiveness.

◆ Dying is the last stage in the development of an individual.

◆ How an individual responds to and prepares for death depends on what death means and the coping mechanisms used throughout life.

◆ Terminally ill children who are able to share their feelings have fewer problems and adapt better than those who must cope with emotional isolation.

◆ One of the most rewarding experiences in health care is assisting an individual in experiencing a client-

Sample Client Care Plan — Grieving

Assessment

History: Jerry was 14 when he lost his leg in an automobile accident 8 weeks ago. His attitude toward the loss of his leg was casual at first, but soon he became angry and withdrawn. Complaints of chronic fatigue, poor appetite, and an inability to concentrate have prompted his mother to seek health care.

Current Findings: An alert adolescent boy who complains that he is unable to sleep. Speech is slow with delayed responses. Left leg is amputated above the knee. Uses crutches for mobility.

Multidisciplinary Diagnosis

Dysfunctional grieving related to loss of body part and physiological functioning

Planning/Goals

Jerry will attend each counseling session.
Jerry will identify his feelings of loss and anger by February 21.

Therapeutic Interventions

Intervention	Rationale	Team Member
1. Establish trust and open communication.	Adolescents must trust in the relationship before they commit themselves.	All
2. Assure Jerry that his feelings are important and give permission to discuss them.	Shows interest and respect; helps maintain self-worth and dignity.	All
3. Assist Jerry in acknowledging his feelings associated with losing his leg.	Helps Jerry to connect his anger with the loss and begin the work of grieving.	All
4. Help Jerry and family understand that anger is a normal response to loss.	Assures him that his emotions are a normal part of the grieving response.	All
5. Assist Jerry in finding appropriate outlets for his anger rather than projecting it onto others.	Provides structure, gives a sense of control, and helps him focus on more effective ways of emotional expression.	Psy, Soc Svc
6. Encourage Jerry to make plans for the future and set goals.	Goals help change the focus from the past to the future.	Psy, Nsg

Evaluation

Jerry missed the first two appointments but has kept every appointment for the past month. Jerry is able to identify three reasons why he feels angry and frustrated. Jerry was unwilling to make any plans for the future at time of evaluation.

A complete client care plan includes several other diagnoses and interventions.

centered, peaceful death, one in which the dying and the living participate fully and completely.

◆ The term *hospice* has come to mean a philosophy of care for people with terminal illnesses or conditions and their loved ones.

◆ Dying clients have special needs during their final days, including the need to be free from pain and discomfort, freedom from loneliness, and preservation of self-esteem.

◆ One of the most important principles to remember is that a dying person lives with the same needs as the rest of us.

Suggestions for Further Reading

On Death and Dying, by Elizabeth Kübler-Ross (New York, 1969, MacMillian), is the classical work on the dying and grief processes.

Crisis, Grief, and Healing (www.webhealing.com) offers information and resources for grieving individuals and families.

References

American Psychiatric Association: *Diagnostic and statistical manual of mental disorders,* ed 4, text revision, Washington, DC, 2000, The Association.

Beare P, Meyers J, editors: *Principles and practices of adult care nursing,* ed 3, St. Louis, 1998, Mosby.

Calandra B: A death in the family: helping children cope, *Advances in Nursing Practice* 1(3):17, 1993.

Ebersole P, Hess P: *Toward healthy aging: human needs and nursing response,* ed 5, St. Louis, 1998, Mosby.

Geissler EM: *Pocket guide to cultural assessment,* ed 2, St. Louis, 1998, Mosby.

Giger JM, Davidhizar RE: *Transcultural nursing: assessment and intervention,* ed 3, St. Louis, 1999, Mosby.

Glaser B, Strauss A: *Awareness of dying,* Chicago, 1963, AVC.

Hayes ER and others: Near death: back from beyond, *RN* 61(12):54, 1998.

Hess PA: Loss, grief, and dying. In Beare P, Meyers J, editors: *Principles and practices of adult care nursing,* ed 3, St. Louis, 1998, Mosby.

Koenig BA, Gates-Williams J: Understanding cultural differences in caring for dying patients, *Western Journal of Medicine* 163(3):244, 1995.

Kübler-Ross: *On death and dying,* New York, 1969, MacMillian.

Luekenotte AG: *Gerontologic nursing,* ed 2, St. Louis, 2000, Mosby.

North American Nursing Diagnosis Association: *NANDA nursing diagnoses: definitions and classification 1999-2000,* Philadelphia, 1999, The Association.

Rawlins PR, Williams SR, Beck CK: *Mental health-psychiatric nursing: a holistic life-cycle approach,* ed 3, St. Louis, 1993, Mosby.

U.S. Bureau of the Census: *Statistical abstract of the United States: 1998,* ed 118, Washington, DC, 1998, U.S. Government Printing Office.

Wong DL: *Whaley and Wong's nursing care of infants and children,* ed 6, St. Louis, 1998, Mosby.

Chapter 20

Anxiety Disorders

Learning Objectives

1. Describe the continuum of responses to anxiety.
2. Identify three types of coping mechanisms used to decrease anxiety.
3. Explain how anxiety is experienced through each life cycle.
4. Compare the difference between normal anxiety and an anxiety disorder.
5. Discuss the difference between phobic and obsessive-compulsive behaviors.
6. Examine three features of posttraumatic stress disorder.
7. List two therapeutic interventions for the client with rape-trauma syndrome.
8. Explain the importance of monitoring medication use for clients with high levels of anxiety.
9. Examine three methods for recognizing and preventing anxiety.

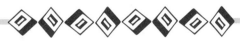

Key Terms

addictive behaviors

agoraphobia

anxiety

anxiety disorder

anxiety state

anxiety trait

avoidance behaviors

compulsion

coping mechanisms

fear

flashbacks

obsession

panic attack

phobia

signal anxiety

traumatic stress reaction

Anxiety is a feeling of uneasiness, uncertainty, and helplessness—a state of tension sometimes associated with feelings of dread or doom. Anxiety is the normal emotional response to a threat or stressor, whereas **fear** is an intellectual appraisal of a dangerous stressor.

Anxiety occurs as the result of a perceived threat to one's physical or psychological self. The threat itself may be real or a response to what one thinks is happening. The actual object of one's anxiety often cannot be identified, but the feelings associated with the experience are all too real.

For the sake of discussion, anxiety has been described by type. **Signal anxiety** is a learned response to an anticipated event. The usually calm student who becomes nauseated during examinations is an example of signal anxiety. An **anxiety state** occurs when an individual's coping abilities are overwhelmed and emotional control is lost. Many emergencies, accidents, and traumas are associated with anxiety states. Last is an **anxiety trait** which is a learned component of the personality. Persons with anxiety traits react to relatively nonstressful situations with anxiety. The teen who is always giving reasons for his or her behavior, even when they are not requested, is an example of trait anxiety.

Anxiety serves several purposes. It is a warning of impending danger. Mild anxiety can increase learning by helping with concentration and focus, and anxiety can serve to motivate an individual. However, uncontrolled anxiety can often lead to ineffective and maladaptive behaviors. Anxiety is a part of survival and growth. How individuals use and control anxiety is one of the measures of mental health or mental illness.

CONTINUUM OF ANXIETY RESPONSES

Reactions to anxiety occur along a continuum of behavioral responses (Stuart and Laraia, 2001) (Figure 20-1). Adaptive responses to anxiety result in positive outcomes, new learning, and greater self-esteem. When anxiety is focused positively, the individual adapts, learns, and grows. However, maladaptive responses to anxiety are ineffective attempts to cope; they do nothing to resolve the problem or eliminate feelings of anxiety.

Most individuals deal with anxiety by using a number of behaviors or **coping mechanisms** to help decrease discomfort. Coping mechanisms in the physical realm of functioning include efforts to directly face and handle the problem. The woman who fights the thief who is attempting to snatch her purse, for example, is directly dealing with the source of her anxiety. Intellectual coping mecha-

Table 20-1	Levels of Anxiety		
Anxiety level	**Physiological**	**Cognitive/Perceptual**	**Emotional/Behavioral**
Mild	Vital signs normal. Minimal muscle tension. Pupils normal, constricted.	Perceptual field is broad. Awareness of multiple environmental and internal stimuli. Thoughts may be random, but controlled.	Feelings of relative comfort and safety. Relaxed, calm appearance and voice. Performance is automatic; habitual behaviors occur here.
Moderate	Vital signs normal or slightly elevated. Tension experienced; may be uncomfortable or pleasurable (labeled as "tense" or "excited").	Alert; perception narrowed, focused. Optimum state for problem solving and learning. Attentive.	Feelings of readiness and challenge, energized. Engage in competitive activity and learn new skills. Voice, facial expression interested or concerned.
Severe	Fight-or-flight response. Autonomic nervous system excessively stimulated (vital signs increased, diaphoresis increased, urinary urgency and frequency, diarrhea, dry mouth, appetite decreased, pupils dilated). Muscles rigid, tense. Senses affected; hearing decreased, pain sensation decreased.	Perceptual field greatly narrowed. Problem solving difficult. Selective attention (focus on one detail). Selective inattention (block out threatening stimuli). Distortion of time (things seem faster or slower than actual). Dissociative tendencies; vigilambulism (automatic behavior).	Feels threatened; startles with new stimuli; feels on "overload." Activity may increase or decrease (may pace, run away, wring hands, moan, shake, stutter, become very disorganized or withdrawn, freeze in position/unable to move). May seem and feel depressed. Demonstrates denial; may complain of aches or pains; may be agitated or irritable. Need for space increased. Eyes may dart around room or gaze may be fixed. May close eyes to shut out environment.
Panic	Above symptoms escalate until sympathetic nervous system release occurs. Person may become pale, blood pressure decreases, hypotension. Muscle coordination poor. Pain, hearing sensations minimal.	Perception totally scattered or closed. Unable to take in stimuli. Problem solving and logical thinking highly improbable. Perception of unreality about self, environment, or event. Dissociation may occur.	Feels helpless with total loss of control. May be angry, terrified; may become combative or totally withdrawn, cry, run. Completely disorganized. Behavior is usually extremely active or inactive.

From Fortinash KM: *Psychiatric nursing care plans,* ed 3, St. Louis, 1999, Mosby.

nisms are aimed at making the threat less meaningful by changing the definition of the threat, whereas emotional responses use ego defense mechanisms to reduce anxiety.

Responses to anxiety occur on four levels, ranging from mild to panic (Table 20-1). During periods of anxiety, many physical, intellectual, emotional, and behavioral responses are called on to help an individual cope. In periods of severe anxiety, the autonomic nervous system stimulates the fight-or-flight response, which triggers many physical changes.

Self-Awareness and Anxiety

A basic characteristic of anxiety is that it is contagious. Like a cold or influenza virus, anxiety is easily transmitted to others. Clients have an uncanny ability to focus on the anxiety levels of their health care providers. Sometimes the client can become the therapeutic agent for an anxious caregiver. The therapeutic relationship is built on trust.

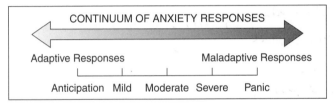

Figure 20-1 Continuum of anxiety responses. (Redrawn from Stuart GW, Laraia MT: *Principles and practice of psychiatric nursing*, ed 7, St. Louis, 2001, Mosby.)

Case Study

Cathy's appointment with her doctor was for 10 AM. By the time she had waited for more than 2 hours, Cathy was feeling frustrated. After a 2½-hour wait, she was downright anxious. Just as she began to leave, her name was called, and she was ushered into a rather impersonal examination room, where she changed into the paper gown and waited, shivering, for her physician.

After what seemed another hour, the door finally opened. Her physician, a woman of many words, began the interaction with "My gads, what a day! One thing goes wrong in the morning, and I spend the rest of the day chasing myself to catch up."

Noting her doctor's tension and rapid speech, Cathy responded, "You certainly look tired. Sounds like you have been working too hard." Her physician countered with, "That's not the half of it," and then proceeded to share each of her day's frustrations.

◆ Who was the therapeutic one in this situation?

◆ How did the physician's behavior affect therapeutic interactions with this client?

Inherent in that trust is the caregiver's responsibility to listen and communicate effectively. High levels of anxiety can impair one's ability to therapeutically interact with the client. For this reason, it is important for caregivers to recognize and cope effectively with their own anxieties. Remember, we may not choose our anxieties, but we do choose *how* we deal with them. The Case Study box provides an example of how a health care provider's anxiety can affect the therapeutic relationship.

THEORIES RELATING TO ANXIETY

A number of theories have been developed since Sigmund Freud first listed anxiety as a defense mechanism. Today the causes of anxiety are still uncertain, but research indicates that a combination of biological, psychosocial, and environmental factors are involved. A few of the more well-known theories of anxiety are discussed here.

Biological Models

The group of theories receiving the most recent attention attempts to find a biological or physical basis for anxiety. The work of Charles Darwin first posed the possibility of a link between emotions and the ability to adapt. Later Hans Selye demonstrated a connection between the perception of stress and physical changes in the body with his fight-or-flight response. During the 1990s, called "the decade of the brain," many advances in the understanding of emotions and mental illness have been made. Today we are beginning to gain an understanding of the role emotions play in health and illness as researchers unveil new information.

One of the most popular current theories of anxiety relates to the role of neurochemicals. Research into the role of these body chemicals, called neurotransmitters, has resulted in evidence that emotions may be linked to changes in brain development and biochemistry (Hyman, 1998). Anxiety is thought to result from the dysfunction of two or more neurotransmitters. Some studies have demonstrated inappropriately activated norepinephrine and imbalances between this and other neurotransmitters. Further research is being done to investigate specific medications designed to alter neurotransmitter activity. Other ongoing studies are investigating the role of the autonomic nervous system in the development of anxiety. Many medical disorders, hormonal imbalances, problems with substance use, even fatigue, are related to the development of anxiety.

Psychodynamic Model

According to Freud's psychoanalytical point of view, anxiety results from a conflict between two opposing forces within the personality—the ego and the id. Neurotic or maladaptive behaviors are the result of attempts to defend oneself against anxiety, just as adaptive behaviors do. Today many psychotherapists have broadened the psychoanalytical theory to define anxiety as the result of a conflict between two opposing forces within an individual.

Interpersonal Model

With the interpersonal model, anxiety is explained in terms of interactions with others. Anxiety develops when early childhood interactions with significant others result in negative outcomes, such as disapproval. Over a period of time, an individual's experience of and responses to anxiety form the basis for low self-esteem and poor self-concept.

Interpersonal theorists work with a broad definition of anxiety. Its most famous theorist, Harry Stack Sullivan, believed that children acquire the values of their parents because they are dependent on others for approval or disapproval. In adulthood, individuals cope with anxiety based on their perceptions and on how they were taught to cope with conflict as children. Using this interpersonal model, one can see the importance of early assessment and intervention for children who are anxious.

Behavioral Model

The behavioral theories consider anxiety a learned response. Children who experienced anxiety in one situation link those feelings to more general situations. Anxiety results when individuals encounter a signal that reminds them of earlier anxious times. Thus individuals learn to react with anxiety by linking anxious experiences.

Other Models

Other theories explain anxiety as the result of a loss of life's meaning (existential theory). Environmental models tie anxiety with uncontrollable events or situations. Fires, floods, or other natural disasters, along with assaults and human-induced traumas, all serve as stressors for the individual.

Many health care providers have chosen to view anxiety from a holistic mode. Anxiety is viewed as having an impact on every realm of human functioning. Physical reactions, such as the fight-or-flight reaction, result from anxiety. Strong emotional responses occur when one is anxious. Social areas of functioning can become impaired as a result of anxiety, and even one's spirituality comes into question during times of great or prolonged anxiety. By considering each area of functioning, nurses are better able to plan and implement effective therapeutic interventions for relieving anxiety.

ANXIETY THROUGHOUT THE LIFE CYCLE

Anxiety is a universal experience that begins early in life, as soon as an individual is capable of realizing that something could go wrong. Responses to anxiety grow and evolve with the individual. Behavioral reactions to anxiety change as effective (anxiety-reducing) actions are added to current coping mechanisms. Responses or behaviors that are ineffective or serve no purpose are discarded. An understanding of how individuals at various developmental stages perceive and cope with anxiety helps nurses plan and implement individualized care for all clients experiencing anxiety.

Anxiety in Childhood

Children learn to cope with anxiety by watching and imitating others. Most children are happy, active individuals with few anxieties; but if their needs for nurturing are not met, high levels of anxiety can result. Children's needs for love and belonging are so great that later-life emotional problems are often related to unmet needs in childhood. "Although children are not strangers to stress, some children appear to be more vulnerable than others" (Wong, 1998). Recognizing signs of childhood stress and intervening early prevents anxiety from becoming overwhelming and helps teach children how to cope successfully.

Anxiety is experienced in relation to a child's developmental level. Infants feel a sense of discomfort if their basic needs are not met immediately. Toddlers become anxious when they perceive something that is larger or more ferocious than themselves and capable of harming them. Their anxiety relates to power and lasts until their balance of power can be restored. Anxiety in preschool children revolves around the experience of separating from the security of parents. As children learn that the separations are not permanent, anxieties lessen and coping abilities improve. School-age children learn to cope with the anxieties of becoming members of a group outside the family.

The development of certain behavioral habits early in childhood appears to help children relieve anxiety. Thumb sucking, nail biting, hair pulling, and rhythmic body movements are examples of behaviors that seem to soothe and lessen anxiety for young children. Excessive anxiety appears to develop when children resist their feelings of anxiety and focus them elsewhere. Problems associated with anxiety in childhood include compulsions, phobias, separation anxiety disorder, overanxious disorder, and avoidant disorders.

Separation anxiety disorder is diagnosed when children are unable to be without their parents for any length of time. By about 6 months of age, infants are able to recognize their mother's absence from the room and protest. They soon become very aware of mother's activities and learn to identify the behaviors indicating mother is leaving the area. By 11 months, most children learn to protest before their mother leaves. During the next 4 years, children learn to tolerate varying degrees of separation from parents. By school age, most children separate from parents easily, and the focus of their anxieties changes to coping with school life.

Children with separation anxiety disorder, however, experience severe anxiety that may even develop into panic when separated from their parents or significant others. Physical complaints such as headaches, nausea, or vomiting are common when children anticipate separation. Nightmares occur frequently. Associated fears of death, animals, monsters, and harmful situations are seen in children with separation anxiety disorder.

Overanxious disorder appears during childhood with unrealistic levels of anxiety lasting longer than 6 months—a long time in the life of a child. These children worry about everything, from past events to future expectations. Overanxious disorder is often seen in children whose parents focus on overachievement and downplay their children's actual accomplishments.

Children can also experience severe anxiety during times of great change in the family. Reactions to divorce, death, or separation often lead to situational anxiety or **avoidance behaviors** in which the child refuses to cope with the anxiety-producing situation by ignoring it.

Sadly, children are not immune to the effects of unresolved anxiety. Occurrences of posttraumatic stress disorder, depression, and suicide are on the rise in children. Children with behavioral problems often have underlying anxieties. If children are to be given opportunities to grow and mature into effective, adaptable individuals, we must learn to recognize and treat the signs of anxiety early. The old proverb "A stitch in time saves nine" is worth remembering when working with children.

Anxiety in Adolescence

Coping skills learned in childhood continue to be refined throughout adolescence. If teens have successfully handled anxieties in childhood, the distresses of becoming adults offer opportunities for personal growth and maturation. Adolescents who ineffectively cope with anxiety often express themselves by running away from home; becoming angry, defiant, aggressive, or manipulative; experimenting with drugs; and engaging in high-risk behaviors. They frequently use denial to cope with their stresses and resist attempts to explore the anxiety-producing aspects that lead to understanding. When anxieties are extreme, adolescents may engage in self-mutilating behaviors or develop the characteristics of anorexia nervosa or bulimia.

Many beginning symptoms of schizophrenia and other psychoses begin in adolescence. Signs of maladaptive behaviors, such as flights from reality, strict ritualistic behaviors, or withdrawal from others, may actually be symptoms of serious mental health problems.

Unfortunately adolescents are a forgotten population when it comes to mental health care. "According to recent studies, large numbers of children and adolescents with serious emotional or behavioral disorders receive either no mental health treatment or treatment inappropriate to their needs" (Collins and Collins, 1994). Health care providers who work with adolescents must learn to recognize clients' anxiety levels and offer interventions and education early, before anxiety becomes the fuel for more serious mental health problems.

Anxiety in Adulthood

By young adulthood, coping behaviors are well established. Adults are more likely to encounter situations that provoke anxiety as they move through their worlds of work, family, and community. Some adults appear to lead a "charmed life" with few stresses and anxieties. Others seem to continually struggle, only to rebound from one misfortune after another. Like their younger counterparts, adults handle anxiety using earlier, established coping mechanisms.

Adults must cope with many anxiety-producing situations. Developmental tasks, such as establishing a career and family, present numerous stressors. The loss of income, spouse, or physical ability can lead to severe anxiety. Uncontrollable situations, such as fires, floods, earthquakes, or wars, often result in long-lasting anxiety, which, unless resolved, can evolve into posttraumatic stress syndrome. When adult anxieties are not focused or controlled, a number of mental health problems may result. Generalized or situational anxiety disorders are diagnosed when individuals become overwhelmed and nonfunctional as a result of their anxieties. Other maladaptive responses to anxiety in adults include panic disorders, phobias, behavioral addictions, obsessions, and compulsive activities.

Anxiety in Older Adulthood

Older adults face a combination of unique, anxiety-producing life hazards. They tend to express anxieties in less overt ways than younger persons. "Older people tend to deny or somatize (express physically) feelings of depression, anxiety, and tension, either because of social desirability factors such as 'looking good' to others and projecting an image of self-reliance, or a lack of self-awareness as to what they really are experiencing" (Hogstel, 1995).

Although few actual statistics are available, anxiety appears to be a common problem for many older adults. Elders face an uncertain future and must cope with a number of problems in the present. Issues about loss of self-determination and control can cause much anxiety in the elderly.

Many of today's elders have experienced difficult times, when work and food were scarce. Socially they were taught that it is inappropriate to share one's fears and anxieties. Because older adults are less likely to directly share feelings, it becomes more difficult for nurses to recognize the signs of anxiety in elderly clients. Behaviors indicating the presence of anxiety include apathy; changes in eating, sleeping, and ability to concentrate; impatience; and fatigue. Stating observations of behaviors that indicate anxiety promotes an atmosphere that allows expression of what is being experienced. One of the most effective methods for assessing anxiety in older adults is to simply ask the client to explain his or her anxious feelings, because the elderly appreciate the interest of concerned nurses.

ANXIETY DISORDERS

If anxiety is a normal human response, when does its expression become a disorder? An **anxiety disorder** exists when anxiety is expressed in ineffective or maladaptive ways and one's coping mechanisms (behaviors) do not successfully relieve the distress. People cope with or handle anxiety using every area of functioning. In the physical realm, one attempts to cope directly with the source of the anxiety. Intellectual efforts are directed at analyzing the situation, problem solving, or changing the meaning of the problem. When efforts in these areas fail, ego defense mechanisms attempt to reduce the emotional distress associated with anxiety. Many individuals call on their spiritual resources in an effort to cope with anxiety-producing problems.

The diagnosis of an anxiety disorder is based on a description of the behaviors used to express distress. The *Diagnostic and Statistical Manual of Mental Disorders* (DSM-IV–TR) classifies anxiety disorders as generalized, panic, phobic, obsessive-compulsive, behavioral, and posttraumatic. Because these disorders are commonly encountered in every culture, society, and health care setting (see Cultural Aspects box), it is important for nurses to understand their nature.

Generalized Anxiety Disorder

Anxiety disorders are usually seen in adolescence or early adulthood. A generalized anxiety disorder is diagnosed when an individual's anxiety is broad, long-lasting, and excessive. It is primarily a disturbance in the emotional area of functioning that eventually affects every other aspect of one's world. People with generalized anxiety disorder are worried and anxious more often than not. They tend to fret about numerous things and find it difficult to control their worries. Often they are so anxious they find it difficult to concentrate on a task long enough to complete it. Responses are far out of proportion with the actual situation. Physical signs and symptoms usually accompany the anxiety and can range from muscle tension to full fight-or-flight responses. Generalized anxiety disorder is often seen in persons with irritable bowel syndrome, headaches, sleep disturbances, and substance abuse.

When generalized anxiety is seen in children, it is diagnosed as overanxious disorder of childhood. These children tend to worry about their school performance and social interactions, whereas adults with generalized anxiety concentrate on worrying about the everyday events.

Panic Disorders

Panic disorders offer a challenge to health care providers because their signs and symptoms are difficult to distinguish from actual physical dysfunctions. A **panic attack** is a brief period of intense fear or discomfort. It is always accompanied by various physical and emotional reactions (Box 20-1). The duration of the actual attack is short (1 to 15 minutes), with a peak in anxiety after about 10 minutes.

Panic disorders are more common than once thought. Research has shown that many clients seen in primary

---

Cultural Aspects

Anxiety appears to occur in most, if not every, culture. Expressions of anxiety, however, differ greatly:

Japanese people tend to somatize or handle anxiety by becoming physically ill.

Mothers in the Dominican Republic cope with the anxiety of the "evil eye" by wearing red and saving the infant's umbilical cord.

Greek men consider body hair a sign of manhood. Shaving their hair in preparation for a surgical procedure can result in great anxiety.

Box 20-1 Panic Attack Criteria

A panic attack is a period of intense fear or discomfort in which at least four of the following symptoms develop abruptly and reach a peak within 10 minutes:

1. Palpitations, pounding heart, or accelerated heart rate
2. Sweating
3. Trembling or shaking
4. Feelings of shortness of breath, smothering
5. Feeling of choking
6. Chest pain or discomfort
7. Nausea or abdominal distress
8. Feeling dizzy, unsteady, light-headed, or faint
9. Derealization (feelings of unreality) or depersonalization (being detached from oneself)
10. Fear of losing control or going crazy
11. Fear of dying
12. Paresthesias (numbness, tingling sensations)
13. Chills or hot flushes

From Stuart GW, Laraia MT: *Stuart and Sundeen's pocket guide to psychiatric nursing,* ed 4, St. Louis, 1998, Mosby.

care settings suffer from panic disorders. Often these disorders are either misdiagnosed or inadequately treated. Panic disorders are more common in women (70%), people who are separated or divorced, and persons of both sexes between ages 24 and 44 (American Psychiatric Association, 2000). Typically, an individual with a panic attack presents with physical complaints that may indicate a life-threatening situation.

There are two kinds of panic disorders: those associated with agoraphobia and those that are not. **Agoraphobia** is anxiety about possible situations in which a panic attack may occur. People with agoraphobia avoid people, places, or events from which escape would be difficult or embarrassing. Fear accompanies a sense of helplessness and embarrassment with the thought of a panic attack occurring. Typically, agoraphobia is associated with public situations, such being in a crowd, standing in line, traveling on a bus or plane, standing on a bridge, or being afraid to leave the house alone. The presence of chronic stressors complicates the picture for treatment and improvement.

Treatment for panic disorders focuses on educating clients about the nature of the disorder, blocking the panic attacks pharmacologically, and assisting clients in developing more adaptive ways of coping with their anxieties. Cognitive therapy helps individuals identify their emotions and behaviors, whereas psychotherapy allows them to explore social or personal difficulties. Education and emotional support are important therapeutic measures for clients who suffer with panic disorders.

Phobic Disorders

A **phobia** is an unnatural fear. Phobias may be expressed as a fear of people, animals, objects, situations, or occurrences. For example, a social phobia is characterized by an unrealistic and persistent fear of any situation in which other people could be judging. Individuals with social phobias are constantly worried about looking foolish. They fear their hands will tremble if they try to write, their voice will quaver if they attempt to talk, or they will vomit if they start to eat. Some are especially anxious in the presence of authority figures or persons with high social contacts. Even eye contact (or the lack of it) from others can be misunderstood as scrutiny and rejection. When the anxieties associated with the social phobia are intense, a full-blown panic attack often results. Persons with severe social phobias often avoid contact with anyone outside their immediate family. Life for many socially phobic individuals can be a lonely and isolated existence.

Phobias differ from common fears. First, phobias are obsessive in nature. Individuals with phobias tend to dwell on their object of fear almost to the point of fascination. Thinking may take the form of fantasies about the fear, such as the person with thanatophobia (fear of dying) rehearsing his or her funeral.

People with phobias handle their anxieties differently. "A phobia typically produces so high a level of anxiety that it is immobilizing, preventing the person from acting in a way that could prove effective in alleviating the anxiety" (Corsini, 1994). The experience of great anxiety or fear that normally protects a person immobilizes the individual with a phobia.

The characteristics of phobias vary with the culture. In some cultures, fears of hexes, spells, magical spirits, and unseen forces result in phobic reactions. Health professionals should remember cultural backgrounds when assessing clients for phobic responses to anxiety (see Think About box).

Obsessive-Compulsive Disorder

An **obsession** is a distressing persistent thought. A **compulsion** is a distressing recurring behavior. An obsession must be persistent, recurring, inappropriate, and distressing. Compulsions are not just habits. They are specific behaviors that *must* be performed to reduce anxiety. Although all of us have repeated worries or routines that we recognize as not entirely sensible, persons with obsessive-compulsive disorder (OCD) are consumed by self-destructive, anxiety-reducing thoughts and actions. Obsessive-compulsive disorders were once thought to be relatively rare, but recent studies have demonstrated that OCD occurs in many more individuals than previously thought.

Symptoms of OCD can occur as early as 3 years of age, but usually they begin in adolescence. Men and women appear to be equally affected, although symptoms frequently appear an average of 5 years earlier in men. A high rate of OCD occurs in persons with other mental health problems, especially

Think About

The client believes that his abdominal abscess is caused by a hex placed on him by his neighbor with whom he has an ongoing dispute over the placement of the shared fence. Last week a particularly angry interaction took place. His neighbor shouted curses and threatened to have a hex placed on him. Less than 24 hours later, the client began to experience abdominal pain, which he endured for 3 days before seeking treatment.

At this time, you are preparing the client for surgery to drain the abscess. Noting his anxious expression, you ask what is bothering him. He replies by telling you that the surgery will not cure his condition until the hex is removed, and the only way to do that is to appease his neighbor.

◆ How would you react to your client's anxiety associated with the hex?

◆ Which therapeutic interventions would you choose if you were this client's care provider?

depression and schizophrenia. The most common obsessions relate to cleanliness, dirt, and germs; aggressive and sexual impulses; health concerns; safety concerns; and order and symmetry. Obsessions can take the form of thoughts, doubts, fears, images, or impulses. People with OCD use the ego defense mechanisms of repression to cope with distressing obsessions. They focus anxieties into compulsive actions (displacement) and engage in undoing behaviors to relieve stress. They know, intellectually, that their attempts to relieve anxiety are maladaptive but feel emotionally compelled to yield to their distressing obsessions. Many people with OCD are unable to maintain social relationships because their compulsions are too time-consuming or inappropriate.

OCD is seen in families, and many studies are exploring possible genetic and hormonal causes. Treatment for OCD consists of a combination of drug and behavioral therapy. A number of antidepressants and selective serotonin reuptake inhibitor (SSRI)–antidepressant medications have been successfully used to treat OCD.

For behaviors to be called obsessions and compulsions, they must meet the criteria in Box 20-2.

Box 20-2 Obsessions and Compulsions Criteria

Obsessions

1. Recurrent and persistent thoughts, impulses, or images that are experienced as intrusive or inappropriate and cause marked anxiety or distress. The thoughts, impulses, or images are not simply excessive worries about real-life problems.
2. The person attempts to ignore, suppress or neutralize such thoughts.
3. The person recognizes that the thoughts, impulses, or images are a product of his or her own mind

Compulsions

1. Repetitive behaviors (e.g., hand washing, ordering, checking) or mental acts (e.g., praying, counting, repeating words silently) that the person feels driven to perform in response to an obsession or according to rules that must be applied rigidly.
2. The behaviors or mental acts are aimed at reducing distress or preventing some dreaded event or situation; however, these behaviors or mental acts either are not connected in a realistic way with what they are designed to neutralize or they are clearly excessive.

From Stuart GW, Laria MT: *Stuart and Sundeen's pocket guide to psychiatric nursing*, ed 4, St. Louis, 1998, Mosby.

Behavioral Addictions

Obsessive-compulsive activities may also take the form of certain **addictive behaviors,** such as gambling, shopping, working, or engaging in excessive sexual activity. Compulsive gambling or wagering is a problem for many people as more and more states legalize gambling and open casinos. Estimates put the number of compulsive gamblers in the United States at more than 9 million people (Simon, 1995). If left unchecked, obsessive-compulsive activities can destroy personal, professional, and financial relationships. Compulsive sexual activity has the added factor of increased risk of contracting and spreading sexually transmitted diseases.

Traumatic Stress Reaction

A **traumatic stress reaction** is a series of behavioral and emotional responses following an overwhelmingly stressful event. People at high risk for being exposed to traumatic stress are persons with current mental health problems, victims or observers of violence, victims of sexual assault (especially as a child), victims of spouse abuse, and homeless persons. Traumatic stress reactions are always considered with people who have been sexually assaulted. Reactions to traumas, specifically rape-trauma syndrome, follow a predictable clinical course: fear and anguish, recovery and repair, and adaptation.

Following a traumatic event, "the initial response generally consists of an outcry of *anguish* or fear. Then the patient tries to *recover* from the traumatic event and repair the immediate damage" (Forster and King, 1994). During the repair and recovery stage, most individuals make reasonably adaptive responses, but some will react ineffectively and develop chronic stress reactions or posttraumatic stress disorder. The *adaptation* phase is heralded by a return to real-world situations and appropriate coping behaviors. Providing psychological stability, emotional support, and advocacy are the most important therapeutic interventions for clients with rape-trauma and other traumatic stress reactions.

Posttraumatic Stress Disorder

Individuals with posttraumatic stress disorder (PTSD) have at some time in their lives been exposed to a traumatic experience outside the realm of normal life experiences in which intense fear, horror, or helplessness was experienced. Posttraumatic stress disorder is the reliving of the traumatic events or situations. Symptoms of PTSD include **flashbacks,** which are vivid recollections of the event, in which the individual relives the frightening experience. Flashbacks can last from a few seconds to longer than a half an hour. During a flashback the experience is vividly real and life-threatening to the individual. Health care providers must remember this fact when coping with a client who is experiencing a flashback. Interventions are to assure everyone's safety and reorient the client to his or her present surroundings.

Anxiety, depression, and nightmares can complicate the picture, and individuals may reduce their involvement with others as their responsiveness to life numbs. Frequently people with severe PTSD isolate themselves from society by living in sparsely populated rural areas. Children with PTSD express themselves through disorganized or agitated behaviors. Long-term interventions include pharmacological and psychological therapy and emotional support.

THERAPEUTIC INTERVENTIONS

The most effective way to cope with anxiety is to prevent it. Learn to recognize the signs and symptoms of anxiety and include an anxiety level assessment for every client. Be especially alert to the signs of anxiety in children. Teaching children to appropriately cope with their anxieties can prevent or minimize a number of mental health problems later in life.

Therapeutic interventions for individuals with maladaptive responses to anxiety involve a combination of mental health therapies and medications. Psychotherapy helps clients to discover the basis for their anxiety. Two behavioral therapies that are successful in treating phobias are systematic desensitization and flooding.

With systematic desensitization, clients learn to cope with one anxiety-provoking stimulus at a time until the stressor is no longer associated with anxiety. This step-by-step method gradually removes the anxiety from the distress-causing event and allows clients to develop more effective ways of perceiving their anxiety.

Flooding is just the opposite. This method for treating phobias rapidly and repeatedly exposes clients to the feared object or situation until anxiety levels diminish.

Table 20-2	Side Effects of Benzodiazepines and Nursing Care
Side effects*	**Nursing (therapeutic) interventions**
Central Nervous System	
Dizziness, drowsiness, sedation, headache, tremors, depression, insomnia, hallucinations	Ensure safety, prevent falls, assist with ambulation, use side rails. Reassure that symptoms are common when first beginning the medication. Assess mental status routinely.
Gastrointestinal	
Dry mouth, anorexia, nausea, vomiting, constipation, diarrhea	Give with food or milk. Ensure frequent oral care. Offer hard candy, gum, sips of water frequently.
Cardiovascular	
Electrocardiogram changes, *orthostatic hypotension, tachycardia*	Monitor intake and output if anorexia, vomiting, diarrhea. Assess blood pressure, pulse (lying and standing); if systolic pressure drops 20 mm Hg, hold drug, notify physician. Monitor complete blood count and other laboratory studies during long-term therapy.
Eyes, Ears, Nose, Throat	
Blurred vision, ringing in ears	Provide reassurance. Ensure safety.
Integument (skin)	
Itching, rash, dermatitis	Encourage use of tepid baths without soap. Assess rash and report to physician.
Emotional	
Feelings of detachment, irritability, increased hostility	Encourage social interactions. Assess for loss of control over emotions and aggression.
Long-Term Effects	
Increased drug tolerance, physical and psychological dependency, rebound anxiety and insomnia	Drug dose is tapered slowly after 4 months of treatment. Help client identify difference between symptoms of drug withdrawal and original feelings of anxiety.

*The most common side effects are in italics.

Box 20-3 NANDA Nursing Diagnoses Related to Anxiety Responses

Adjustment, impaired
Anxiety*
Breathing pattern, ineffective
Communication, impaired verbal
Coping, ineffective individual*
Diarrhea
Energy field disturbance
Fear*
Health maintenance, altered
Incontinence, stress
Injury, risk for
Nutrition, altered
Posttrauma syndrome
Powerlessness
Self-esteem disturbance
Sensory/perceptual alterations (specify)
Sleep pattern disturbance
Social interaction, impaired
Social isolation
Thought processes, altered
Urinary elimination, altered

From North American Nursing Diagnosis Association: *NANDA nursing diagnoses: definitions and classification 1999-2000,* Philadelphia, 1999, The Association.
*Primary nursing diagnosis for anxiety.

Other treatments, such as rational-emotive therapy, are designed to help clients learn how their illogical thinking leads to maladaptive behaviors. Anxiety is also treated with various medications, including benzodiazepines, antidepressants, antihistamines, propranolol, and the anxiolytic drug called buspirone (BuSpar). Because each type of drug is associated with possibly severe side effects, nurses must monitor their clients' responses to drug therapy. Table 20-2 lists the side effects of the most commonly used antianxiety agents, benzodiazepines, and suggested therapeutic interventions.

After a complete nursing history and thorough physical examination, the most appropriate nursing diagnoses, which can be used as problem statements by the health care team, are selected (McCloskey and Bulechek, 1999) (Box 20-3).

This information is then brought to the health care team, where overall client goals are established and interventions are chosen.

One of the first priorities of care is to protect the client from possible injury to self and others. Establishing a trusting therapeutic relationship helps clients to explore their distresses and learn to link their behaviors to the sources of their anxiety. Problem-solving techniques assist clients in developing more

effective coping mechanisms. Relaxation techniques, such as meditation, and stress-reducing exercises help clients counter the anxieties being experienced. The Sample Client Care Plan provides an example of a care plan for anxiety responses. Health care providers are in an excellent position to help clients cope effectively with the effects of stress and anxiety. Handling small, everyday distresses successfully is key to preventing complicated mental health problems that arise as maladaptive expressions of anxiety.

KEY CONCEPTS

- Anxiety is a diffuse feeling of uneasiness, uncertainty, and helplessness; it is a normal emotional response to a threat or stressor.
- Adaptive responses to anxiety result in positive outcomes, new learning, and greater self-esteem.
- Maladaptive responses to anxiety are ineffective attempts to cope that do nothing to eliminate feelings of anxiety.
- An understanding of how individuals at various developmental stages perceive and cope with anxiety is important for health care providers.
- The specific causes of anxiety are still uncertain, but research indicates that a combination of physical, psychosocial, and environmental factors are involved.
- An anxiety disorder exists when one's coping mechanisms or behaviors do not relieve anxiety's distress.
- A generalized anxiety disorder is diagnosed when anxiety is broad, long-lasting, and excessive.
- A panic attack is a brief period of intense fear or discomfort accompanied by physical and emotional reactions.
- A phobia is an unnatural fear of people, animals, objects, situations, or occurrences.
- An obsession is a distressing, recurring, persistent thought.
- A compulsion is a distressing recurring behavior.
- Posttraumatic stress disorder (PTSD) is the reexperiencing of previously experienced traumatic events or situations.
- One of the first priorities of care is to protect the client from possible injury to self and others.
- Medications for treating anxiety include the benzodiazepines, antihistamines, propranolol, buspirone, and antidepressants.
- Establishing a trusting therapeutic relationship is a therapeutic intervention that helps clients to explore their distresses and learn to connect behaviors with the sources of their anxiety.
- Problem-solving techniques assist clients in developing new, more effective coping mechanisms.
- Relaxation techniques help clients counter the anxieties currently being experienced.

Sample Client Care Plan — Anxiety

Assessment

History: Joe is a 44-year-old man who lost his wife, job, and car within the past 3 months. Last night, after Joe and his buddies "had a few drinks," Joe became suspicious and accused his friends of trying to steal "what little I have left. I just know something awful is going to happen." Today Joe is seeking treatment for his upset stomach and inability to sleep.

Current Findings: An untidy man who appears older than his stated age. There is an odor of alcohol. Vital signs are increased, with a pulse rate of 116 beats/min. He complains of shortness of breath, upset stomach, frequent urination, and lack of sleep. When questioned about the recent changes in his lifestyle, he replies, "It's no big deal. I'll get by."

Multidisciplinary Diagnosis

Anxiety related to loss of wife and job

Planning/Goals

Joe will identify the causes of his anxiety and make two attempts to decrease the level of anxiety he is experiencing.

Therapeutic Interventions

Intervention	Rationale	Team Member
1. Establish trust with Joe.	Trust helps client to explore new ways of coping.	All
2. Contract with him to refrain from hurting himself and others for the duration of therapy.	To ensure safety of Joe and others during expressions of anxiety.	Nsg
3. Use active listening to encourage Joe to link his anxiety with recent experiences.	Allows time to assess Joe's perspective; helps Joe to connect his emotions with his feelings of anxiety.	All
4. Assess Joe's statements of self-worth and reinforce personal strengths that he has identified.	Helps determine Joe's perception of himself, energy flows where it is focused.	All
5. Help Joe identify areas of his life over which he has control.	Learning to direct one's energies decreases anxiety, promotes relaxation, and increases sense of control.	All
6. Give positive feedback for attempts to reduce anxiety.	One small success builds on another when recognized.	All
7. Encourage Joe to continue already established relationships.	Established relationships can be source of comfort and support.	All
8. Help identify areas of strength and limitations in social interactions.	Positive reinforcement encourages appropriate actions, the first step in changing behaviors in identifying them.	Soc Svc, Nsg
9. Job skill and employment testing.	A source of income helps satisfy basic needs.	Soc Svc, OT
10. Monitor for therapeutic response, side effects of Buspar.	Drug has several side effects that can be disturbing for client.	Nsg

Evaluation

Joe attended four counseling sessions before he recognized that he was anxious. By the seventh session, he was able to reduce his anxiety about 15% of the time.

A complete client care plan includes several other diagnoses and interventions.

Suggestions for Further Reading

An article that discusses the latest research findings on anxiety is "A New Image for Fear and Emotion" by Steven E. Hyman (*Nature* 393(6684):417, 1998).

The American Psychiatric Association (www.psych.org) provides updated information about anxiety disorders.

References

American Psychiatric Association: *Diagnostic and statistical manual of mental disorders,* ed 4, text revision, Washington DC, 2000, The Association.

Collins BG, Collins TM: Child and adolescent mental health: building a system of care, *Journal of Counseling and Development* 72(3):239, 1994.

Corsini RJ, editor: *Encyclopedia of psychology,* ed 2, New York, 1994, John Wiley.

Forster P, King J: Traumatic stress reactions and the psychiatric emergency, *Psychiatric Annals* 24:603, 1994.

Fortinash KM: *Psychiatric nursing care plans,* ed 3, St. Louis, 1999, Mosby.

Hogstel MO: *Geropsychiatric nursing,* ed 2, St. Louis, 1995, Mosby.

Hyman SE: A new image for fear and emotion, *Nature* 393(6684):417, 1998.

McCloskey JC, Bulechek GM: *Nursing interventions classification,* ed 3, St. Louis, 1999, Mosby.

North American Nursing Diagnosis Association: *NANDA nursing diagnoses: definitions and classification 1999-2000,* Philadelphia, 1999, The Association.

Simon P: Gambling addiction, Congressional Record for 104th Congress 141:10912, July 31, 1995.

Stuart GW, Laraia MT: *Principles and practice of psychiatric nursing,* ed 7, St. Louis, 2001, Mosby.

Stuart GW, Laraia MT: *Stuart and Sundeen's pocket guide to psychiatric nursing,* ed 4, St. Louis, 1998, Mosby.

Wong DL: *Whaley and Wong's nursing care of infants and children,* ed 6, St. Louis, 1998, Mosby.

Chapter 21

Depression and Other Mood Disorders

Learning Objectives

1. Describe the continuum of emotional responses.
2. Compare four theories relating to emotions and their disorders.
3. Explain how emotions affect individuals throughout the life cycle.
4. Compare the differences between a depressive episode and a depressive disorder.
5. List the diagnostic criteria for bipolar disorders.
6. Discuss behaviors associated with postpartum depression.
7. Explain seasonal affective disorder.
8. Identify three drug classes used for the treatment of depression and other mood disorders.
9. Apply four nursing (therapeutic) interventions for clients with mood disorders.

Key Terms

affect

bipolar disorder

cyclothymic disorder

depression

dysthymia

emotion

hypomania

mania

manic depression

mood

mood disorder

postpartum depression

religiosity

seasonal affective disorder

situational depression

The emotional realm of human functioning affects all areas of behavior. Emotions can lead to physical changes, new intellectual perspectives, and altered social roles. It is safe to say that emotions play an important role in the lives of human beings. An **emotion** is a feeling—a nonintellectual response. Emotions are reactions to various stimuli based on individual points of view. The Think About box presents an example of how perceptions affect emotional reactions.

CONTINUUM OF EMOTIONAL RESPONSES

The spectrum of human emotion ranges from elation to despair. Emotional responses can be growth promoting and adaptive, or they can lead to ineffective behaviors that could soon become maladaptive. Figure 21-1 illustrates the continuum of emotional responses. As individuals repeatedly react to their own behaviors, interactions with others, society, and the environment, they establish

Think About

Ted and Fred, two neighborhood teens, are working on building a model airplane in Fred's backyard.

A piece of the model breaks and they begin to argue over each other's clumsiness. The emotions grow, and soon scuffling, swearing, and fighting ensue.

The commotion brings both fathers to the scene. Fred's father shakes his fist and shouts, "That's a boy! Punch him good. No son of mine is going to let someone get the best of him!"

Ted's father, also seeing the scene, reacts with, "Boys! Stop fighting! There are better ways to solve your problems than beating each other up."

◆ How did each father's perception of the situation differ?

◆ What do you think caused the difference in their reactions?

◆ What do you think Fred and Ted learned from observing each father's response?

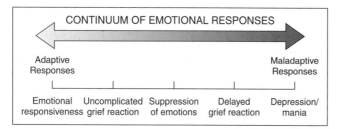

Figure 21-1 Continuum of emotional responses. (Redrawn from Stuart GW, Laraia MT: *Principles and practice of psychiatric nursing,* ed 7, St. Louis, 2001, Mosby.)

patterns of emotional responses that become moods, and moods evolve into an overall point of view or outlook on life. From this outlook, people interpret and react to the world about them. Some of the reactions are emotional, and the cycle continues.

THEORIES RELATING TO EMOTIONS AND THEIR DISORDERS

A **mood** is described as a "prolonged emotional state that influences one's whole personality and life functioning" (Rollant and Deppoliti, 1996). Mood disorders were once considered simple, correctable imbalances in behavior. Today evidence suggests that a combination of physical, psychological, and environmental factors are involved in the development of mood disorders. Many theories about the cause of mood disorders have been presented throughout the years, but none fully explains the complexities of these conditions.

Box 21-1　Factors Related to Causes of Mood Disorders

Genetic susceptibility
Biochemical imbalances (neurotransmitters, hormones)
Childhood and adult experiences
Social circumstances

Biological Evidence

Over the past decade much has been learned about the physical nature of mood disorders. The causes of these disorders are complex. When sad moods deepen and persist, the individual is unable to restore emotional equilibrium or balance because of unusual stress or poor internal regulation. Box 21-1 lists the possible causes of the faulty regulatory mechanism or excessive stress.

Defects in the immune system have been implicated in depression. Genetics may be a factor in mood disorders because high rates of depression and bipolar illness are seen in individuals who have relatives with mood disorders.

Studies of the effects of neurochemical messengers (neurotransmitters) and hormones on behavior have revealed that behaviors and body chemistries are interrelated. The major neurotransmitters, the monoamines norepinephrine and serotonin, excite or inhibit the brain circuits involved in mood regulation. Monoamines are longer acting and actually modify the sensitivity of the neurons. When an imbalance in this complex system occurs, depression occurs.

One of the ways the pituitary gland controls the secretions of hormones in the body is by balancing thyroid and adrenal hormones. This balance is often poorly regulated in those with mood disorders. Serotonin, estrogen, and progesterone imbalances may help explain the fact that women are more than twice as likely to develop depression (Scott, 1998).

Investigators have also found that the biological rhythms of depressed persons are different from those of nondepressed persons. Depression is also related to physical illness. Many individuals who are being treated for a physical condition show signs of depression or other mood disorder. As research efforts continue, new information about the biology of mood disorders will be uncovered.

Other Theories

Psychoanalytical theories see mood disorders as anger turned inward. Behaviorists view depression as a group of learned responses, whereas social theorists consider depression the result of faulty social interactions. Beck's cognitive theory focuses on restructuring faulty beliefs and assumptions. A holistic viewpoint is usually used by health care providers because it considers all areas (realms) of human functioning and provides a framework from which to work with the whole person.

Many social factors have an influence on the development of mood disorders. Family relationships are important. Adults who were not nurtured as children are at higher risk for depression. Losses, role changes, and physical illnesses have an impact on the development of emotional problems. Poor social support, such as few friends and no significant others, heightens the loneliness of individuals, and repeated reactions to stress and crises wear down one's emotional resistance. Although the exact cause of depression and other mood disorders remains unclear, we do know that early recognition and treatment greatly improve the lives of people who suffer from severe and prolonged emotional problems.

EMOTIONS THROUGHOUT THE LIFE CYCLE

Because emotional responses are one of the realms of human functioning, they grow and develop as the individual does. When we are young, emotions are often experienced but seldom controlled. With growth and maturity, emotional control is slowly gained as individuals test and learn about the appropriateness of their emotionally expressive behaviors. By adulthood, most societies expect people to control their emotions and express them in appropriate ways. (See Chapter 16, Box 16-2 for the characteristics of successful adults.)

Emotions in Childhood

When infants' basic needs are met, they usually feel a sense of contentment. Any delay in meeting those needs, however, is often announced by verbal expressions of frustration or even anger. Toddlers struggle to cope with many newly experienced emotions, such as fear, helplessness, and anxiety. Many of these feelings are acted out rather than identified because young children are often unable to express themselves verbally. School-age children learn to identify, express, and control their emotions. The emotional intensity of adolescence offers new challenges for learning emotional control.

Most depressive responses in children are tied to a specific event or situation. This type of depression is called acute depression or **situational depression** because it can be traced to a recognizable cause. Once the stressors are removed or decreased, the depression is relieved. Situational depression occurs in all age groups.

Children who are depressed have a distinct way of thinking that involves feelings of hopelessness, low self-esteem, and a tendency to take the blame for every negative event (Wong, 1998). They often respond with

irritability, tearfulness, and sadness. Schoolwork and friendships suffer as more and more time is spent alone, especially watching television. Some children become clinging and dependent, whereas others engage in aggressive or disruptive behaviors. Many show changes in eating and sleeping behaviors. Fortunately, most acute episodes of childhood depression fade with family and social support.

During childhood, individuals begin to establish their self-esteem, coping mechanisms, and problem-solving abilities. If they have been successful in developing these skills, they are well prepared to handle the emotional distresses of later life. If self-esteem fails to grow or coping mechanisms and problem-solving abilities fail to develop, a mood disorder or other mental health problem may arise. The incidence of depression in childhood is increasing, and health care providers should include an assessment of mood for all young clients.

Emotions in Adolescence

During the teen years, individuals struggle to identify, gain control over, and express emotions. The moods of adolescents commonly swing from feeling vulnerable and dependent to knowing that they are smarter than everyone else in the family. Most adolescents establish their personal and social identities without significant psychological problems or emotional disorders, but a growing number of teens are showing evidence of depression.

Depression in adolescence appears to be related to four factors: self-esteem, loneliness, family strengths, and parent-adolescent communications. Age and gender are lesser factors, but women with depression outnumber men by two to one. Many individuals tend to react with a sense of helplessness and feelings of depression when self-esteem is low. They perceive the world as bleak and themselves as small and insignificant. Feelings of low self-esteem feed other negative emotions, and a cycle of depression and low self-esteem is established. Grades drop as interest in school activities fades.

Loneliness is an aspect of depression in all age groups, but especially in adolescence. People need other people; as loneliness increases, so does depression. The emotionally isolated teen may be surrounded by others, yet still feel like an outcast.

Family relationships also have an influence on adolescent depression. Studies of mothers of depressed adolescents revealed that higher standards of achievement were expected, but the children were seldom rewarded. Often adolescents rebel against what they feel are impossible standards by withdrawing into depression. Parent-adolescent communication patterns also have an impact on the teen's ability or willingness to discuss problems. Teens who can discuss their concerns with understanding parents have lower rates of depression.

Data from Keltner NL, Schwecke LH, Bostrom CE: *Psychiatric nursing,* ed 3, St. Louis, 1998, Mosby.

The occurrence of depression and other mood disorders in adolescence reaches across gender and cultural lines.

Depression in adolescence must be recognized as serious. Depressions arising during adolescence tend to last, have a high rate of recurrence, and are associated with long-standing interpersonal problems. Teaching adolescents to cope effectively is essential if we are to protect the mental health of our greatest "natural resource," our children.

Emotions in Adulthood

During adulthood, society expects people to practice emotional control. Unfortunately, many adults have difficulties with emotional control, and mood disorders are among the most common serious mental health problems today (Box 21-2).

Adults must cope with a wide range of situations, events, developmental tasks, and responsibilities, as well as the emotional reactions that accompany each. Family interactions have a strong influence on adults. Many are also challenged with the problems of physical illness or dysfunction. Sometimes the practice of certain behaviors, such as drug use, dieting, or refusal to seek help for distressing symptoms, can result in the development of a mood disorder. Unfortunately, mood disorders are stigmatized by the public (and clients themselves) and seen as being caused by a lack of will power or a character flaw. Thus adults who suffer from depression or bipolar disorder must endure the additional burden of being stigmatized and stereotyped as "mentally ill." A sensitivity to this issue assists health care providers in providing support for adults with emotional difficulties.

Emotions in Older Adulthood

Depression is very common in the elderly. Major depression affects as many as 40% of older Americans. The highest rates are found in elderly women, the medically ill, and individuals who receive long-term care.

Depression is not a normal consequence of aging. Most older adults live full, active, and rewarding lives.

When depression or other mood disturbance occurs suddenly in an older adult, it is most likely linked to a physical cause. Depression can be treated, but failure to recognize its symptoms prevents many elders from receiving therapy.

Older adults often express their feelings of depression in more subtle ways than younger persons. Most do not complain or volunteer to share their feelings. Signals of depression in the elderly include changes in daily routine, eating, sleeping, or activity patterns; decreased concentration, communications, and motivation; feelings of envy, failure, indecision, guilt, and hopelessness; loss of interest, self-confidence, and self-esteem; and worry or talk about death. Active listening, gentle questioning, and alert assessments help nurses detect signs of depression.

CHARACTERISTICS OF MOOD DISORDERS

Affect is the outward expression of one's emotions. Affects can be described as blunted (restricted), flat, inappropriate, and labile (rapidly changing). A **mood disorder** is defined as a disturbance in the emotional dimension of human functioning. Mood disorders have also been called affective disorders. Problems with emotions occur when one is extremely happy or sad. We all experience emotional extremes; but when feelings interfere with effective living, they become maladaptive.

Problems with emotions range from mania to depression. **Mania** refers to an emotional state in which a person has an elevated, expansive, and irritable mood accompanied by a loss of identity, increased activity, and grandiose thoughts and actions. **Depression,** the opposite of mania, is characterized by feelings of sadness, disappointment, and despair. It is an illness that affects about 20% of the U.S. population (Mood disorders, 1997). More than 19 million people in the United States will suffer from a depressive illness each year (National Institute of Mental Health, 1999). Depression is found in all races, ethnic groups, age groups, and socioeconomic levels. It commonly affects twice as many women as men. It is easy to see that emotional problems are a large part of the distresses suffered by people.

MOOD DISORDERS

According to the *Diagnostic and Statistical Manual of Mental Disorders* (DSM-IV–TR), mood disorders are divided into two basic categories: depression and mania (Figure 21-2). Depression is further classified into depressive episodes and depressive disorders, based on time and recurring patterns of the behaviors. Mania is seen in **bipolar disorders,** which are divided into bipolar I, bipolar II, and cyclothymic disorders.

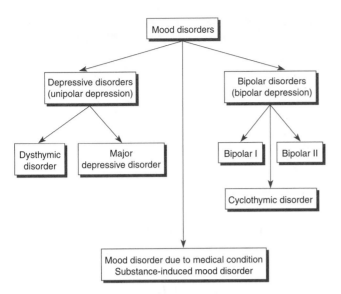

Figure 21-2 Classification of mood disorders.

Depression is a "whole body" illness that involves emotional, physical, intellectual, social, and spiritual problems. It can be transitory (lasting only a few days), or it can plague an individual for many years. It is one of the most common and treatable mental disorders (Isaacs, 1998). Table 21-1 lists many of the behaviors associated with depression. Study it carefully, because a client's nonverbal messages may be the only clues to the presence of this mood disorder.

Depression can occur on several levels. *Mild depression* is short-lived and usually triggered by life events or situations outside the individual. For example, mild depression is common after suffering an important loss. With mild depression, individuals frequently complain of feeling lost, let down, or disappointed. Drug or alcohol use may increase during this time. Mild depression is usually self-limiting and subsides as interest in life returns to normal.

In contrast, *moderate depression* (**dysthymia**) persists over time. Feelings of depression begin to seriously interfere with activities of living, because individuals lack the energy to make it through the day. Physically, they are fatigued (anergia) and drag themselves around. Eating and sleeping difficulties and changes in sexual functioning and menstrual cycles begin to surface (Perry, 1999). Emotionally, these individuals are also drained of energy. They feel despondent, dejected, and gloomy and unable to find joy in life (anhedonia). Feelings of helplessness, low self-esteem, ineffectiveness, and worthlessness reinforce their negative outlooks. Judgment and decision making are clouded by gloom. With moderate depression, the intellectual realm is focused on proving how really bad they are. Slowed thoughts and impaired concentration add to the picture of ineptness. Problem-solving skills fail, hopelessness sets in, and escape from emotional turmoil

seems impossible. Persons with moderate levels of depression are at higher risk of suicide as their depression increases.

Major Depressive Episode

When depression is severe and lasts more than 2 weeks, it is called a major depressive episode. Severe depression encompasses one's whole being—every realm of human functioning. "The zest for life has vanished. It left without notice. Hours, days drag into weeks, months, even years. The simplest tasks loom over us like impossible demands. Energy is gone. Hope and joy are only meaningless words. Truly, darkness rules" (National Depressive and Manic-Depressive Association, 1993).

Behaviors associated with severe depression range from paralysis to agitation. Feelings of worthlessness, guilt, and despair are expressed in every thought, every movement, and every activity. Physical appearance declines as eating and sleeping become distasteful chores. Poor concentration and an inability to follow through on tasks lead to feelings of powerlessness and helplessness. Suicidal thoughts are entertained, and suicide is seen as the only way to cope with the misery. Individuals suffering a major depressive episode practically drag through the day, unable to function, caring about nothing, and interested only in their suffering. As truly distressed human beings, they are caught in a downward emotional cycle. Major depressive episodes can occur in response to situations, events, and developmental tasks. They are frequently seen in combination with other mental health problems.

Major Depressive Disorder

When major depressive episodes routinely repeat themselves (for more than 2 years), a depressive disorder is diagnosed. Persons with major depressive disorders have a high mortality rate. "Up to 15% of individuals with severe major depressive disorder die by suicide. Statistical evidence also suggests that there is a fourfold increase in death rates in individuals with major depressive disorder who are over age 55 years" (American Psychiatric Association, 2000). Major depressive disorder occurs twice as often in adolescent girls and adult women than in men. Symptoms may begin at any age, but the average age of symptom onset is in the early 20s. The course of the disorder is variable. Some individuals experience depressive episodes separated by many years, whereas others suffer more frequent episodes as they grow older. Families with one depressed member are at an increased risk of other members developing the disorder. Some families appear to be genetically vulnerable to depression.

Severe, prolonged depression results in many physical changes and increases one's risk for illness. Studies have demonstrated an association between depression and low immune system functions. Researchers who follow depressed individuals over time have found that depressed

Table 21-1 Behaviors Associated With Depression

Emotional	Physical	Intellectual	Behavioral
Anger	Abdominal pain	Ambivalence	Aggressiveness
Anxiety	Anorexia or overeating	Confusion	Agitation
Apathy	Backache	Inability to concentrate	Alcoholism
Bitterness	Chest pain	Indecisiveness	Altered activity level
Dejection	Constipation	Loss of interest and motivation	Drug addiction
Denial of feelings	Dizziness	Pessimism	Intolerance
Despondency	Fatigue	Self-blame	Irritability
Guilt	Headache	Self-depreciation	Lack of spontaneity
Helplessness	Impotence	Self-destructive thoughts	Overdependency
Hopelessness	Indigestion or nausea	Uncertainty	Poor personal hygiene
Loneliness	Insomnia		Psychomotor retardation
Low self-esteem	Lassitude		Social isolation
Sadness	Menstrual changes		Tearfulness
Sense of personal worthlessness	Sexual nonresponsiveness		Underachievement
	Sleep disturbances		Withdrawal
	Vomiting		
	Weight change		

Handwritten notes: suicide & elopement; milieu therapy; Seclusion; restraint

Modified from Stuart GW, Laraia MT: *Principles and practice of psychiatric nursing*, ed 7, St. Louis, 2001, Mosby.

Handwritten note: Somatic Therapy

persons face more physical and mental impairments than individuals with chronic illnesses. Major depressive disorders are truly debilitating.

Dysthymic Disorder

A dysthymic disorder is daily moderate depression that lasts for more than 2 years. People with dysthymic disorder are chronically sad and self-critical. They see themselves as incapable and uninteresting. Usually they experience many symptoms of moderate depression, such as low energy levels, poor decision-making skills, and eating or sleeping difficulties. Because the feelings of depression have lasted so long, they become a part of everyday experiences. Individuals with dysthymia have learned to see the world from a negative point of view and will often tell you that they have "always" been this way. During periods of intense stress, these persons may experience major depressive episodes along with the existing dysthymia.

Dysthymic disorders can begin in childhood or as late as early adulthood. Because they develop slowly, dysthymic disorders are often difficult to recognize and diagnose. Persons with dysthymia can often carry out their daily living activities, but they are unable to enjoy them.

Bipolar Disorders

The hallmark of a **bipolar disorder** is sudden and dramatic shifts in emotional extremes. Persons with bipolar disorders live in a world that seesaws in cycles between the emotional extremes of mania and depression. Thoughts, moods, and behaviors swing from normal to grandiose to depressed. Then a return to normal functioning follows, the "in-between time," before the cycle begins

again. Time intervals between manic episodes vary, and individuals who cycle rapidly have a poorer prognosis.

Mania is defined as "an abnormally and persistently elevated, expansive, or irritable mood" (American Psychiatric Association, 2000). During periods of mania, behaviors build in intensity as the individual moves through three stages or levels of mania (Table 21-2). **Hypomania,** an exaggerated sense of cheerfulness, begins the cycle. Soon cheerfulness progresses to the unstable "high" of mania. If allowed to continue, the extreme excitement of delirium may result.

During the manic phase, the individual's behaviors become more and more impaired. If not treated, the manic phase of bipolar illness can last for as long as 3 months. Eventually the depressive phase begins again. Hospitalization is often required to break the cycle of mania and to protect the person from the negative consequences of poor judgments and actions. An episode of mania is presented in the Case Study box.

Bipolar disorders (also called **manic depression**) exist in two forms. Bipolar I disorder is characterized by episodes of depression alternating with episodes of mania. It is the more severe and incapacitating form of bipolar illness. Delusions are common during periods of mania, and hallucinations can occur. With bipolar II disorder, individuals suffer major episodes of depression alternating with periods of hypomania. Bipolar II disorder often results in 1 to 2 weeks of severe lethargy, withdrawal, and melancholy, followed by several days of elevated or irritable mood, constant activity, and risky decision making. Although the depths of depression and mania may not be as severe as with bipolar I disorder, the effects of bipolar II disorder are just as devastating.

Table 21-2	Levels of Manic Behavior
Level of mania	**Description of behaviors**
Hypomania	Outgoing, happy-go-lucky, free of worry; catchy euphoria (observers feel euphoric), confident, uninhibited; unconcerned about feelings of others; increased motor activity, sexual drives, distractibility, sense of importance; decreased ability to concentrate; moves quickly from one topic to another (flight of ideas); becomes easily irritated
Mania	"High," expansive, unstable affect; angers quickly; pressured speech, flight of ideas, delusions of persecution and grandiosity; dresses inappropriately (layers of clothing, bizarre outfits, excessive makeup and jewelry); inappropriate behaviors (meddles in other's affairs, spends money recklessly, engages in risky activities); sexually driven; little food or sleep but still hyperactive
Delirium	Period of extreme excitement, anger, elation; has grandiose or religious delusions; becomes disoriented, incoherent, agitated; may injure self or others; poor hygiene, disheveled, physically drained; death from exhaustion may occur if mania goes untreated

Modified from Rollant PD, Deppoliti DB: *Mosby's review series: mental health nursing*, St. Louis, 1996, Mosby.

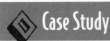

Case Study

Kevin was ordinarily a quiet and reserved person, but today he felt extraordinarily good—full of confidence and vigor. He even convinced himself that this would be his lucky day. By the time he started dressing, he had already decided to "skip" work. He was going to the casino because he could do no wrong today. Too impatient to eat or finish dressing, he bolted from the house and jogged the 4 miles to the casino.

By noon Kevin had lost his pocket money and had consumed four scotch and sodas. He became angry with the cashier when she refused to cash a check without identification. "She should certainly know who I am. Why should I need identification? Everyone in town knows who I am! How dare they demand to see my identification!" Kevin screamed as he paced agitatedly.

After being forcibly removed from the casino, Kevin began a tour of every business in town. He demanded to see the owners and then offered them a contract to share a portion of his winnings if they financed his gambling now. By the time he visited the fourth establishment, the police were waiting. Kevin made his offer to both police officers and was promptly admitted to the local hospital for mental health care. After 3 days of hospitalization, Kevin traded his extraordinarily good feelings for depressive ones.

◆ What clues (signs/symptoms) in Kevin's behavior indicate that he was in the manic phase of bipolar illness?

Cyclothymic Disorder

The extreme emotional swings of bipolar disorders are less intense in persons with cyclothymic problems. As the name implies, a **cyclothymic disorder** is a pattern that involves repeated mood swings alternating between hypomania and depressive symptoms. With cyclothymia, there are no periods of "normal" functioning. No day is free of symptoms because individuals bounce from "too high" to "too low." Many persons with cyclothymic problems eventually progress to full-blown (clinically definable) bipolar disorders.

Other Problems With Affect

Many other emotional problems exist in society today. **Seasonal affective disorder** (also known as winter depression) occurs in many individuals from October to April. Levels of mild and moderate depression are experienced during long winter days, and the symptoms begin to lift with the coming of spring. Daily exposure to full-spectrum light (phototherapy) lessens the symptoms of sadness and social withdrawal in persons with seasonal affective disorder.

Phototherapy or light therapy has also been found to be useful in treating women with late luteal phase dysphoric disorder—the depression associated with the onset of menses. Every month, these women experience the melancholy and sadness of depression. In these cases the cause, however, lies within the rhythms of their hormone cycles.

A connection between hormonal balance and emotions is implicated as a possible cause of **postpartum depression.** Symptoms of tearfulness, irritability, hypochondria, sleeplessness, impairment of concentration, and headache in the days and weeks following childbirth are characteristic (Perry, 1999). Mild postpartum depression often clears within days, but symptoms lasting longer than 2 weeks should be investigated. Women who have experienced complicated pregnancies or difficult deliveries and women who are not emotionally prepared for motherhood are at higher risk for postpartum depression.

A substance-induced mood disorder is defined as a persistent emotional disturbance that can be directly traced to the physiological effects of a chemical. Many illegal chemicals (street drugs), such as amphetamines, cocaine, marijuana, and heroin, as well as alcohol, are associated with changes in mood. Also, many therapeutic

Table 21-3	**Phases of Treatment for Depression**	
Phase	Time period	Goal of treatment
Acute treatment	6 to 12 weeks	To reduce symptoms and inappropriate behaviors
Continuation	4 to 9 months	To prevent relapses into distressing emotional states
Maintenance	Indefinite	To prevent recurrences

medications are related to the development of mood disorders. The Drug Alert box lists common medications that have depressive effects.

Medical Problems and Mood Disorders

Depression is a common condition among hospitalized persons, and most physically ill people are depressed to some degree. Because the whole person is involved, a physical illness always has emotional consequences. Many physical problems and medical conditions are associated with mood disorders. It is common for people to feel depressed when ill or feeling poorly. Depression is a response to chronic illness or lingering disability because people anticipate their losses and lifestyle changes. Because it is often encountered within health care settings, an important responsibility of each health care provider is to assess for signs and symptoms of mood disorders in every client, from the youngest to the oldest.

THERAPEUTIC INTERVENTIONS

Mood disorders present many treatment challenges. Perhaps the greatest is that fewer than half of the people with mood disorders receive treatment. Feelings of hopelessness and the stigma of having a mental illness prevent many people from seeking treatment. Others are misdiagnosed or treated for a medical illness because their symptoms are mainly physical. Also, men are less likely to receive treatment because they often hide their emotions behind alcohol, drugs, or aggression. Depression responds well to treatment, especially if begun early. Serious disturbances of severe depression and bipolar disorders may involve years of therapy.

Treatment and Therapy

The therapeutic plan for clients with mood disorders is often arranged into three phases. The *acute treatment phase* lasts 6 to 12 weeks. The goal during this phase is to reduce symptoms and inappropriate behaviors. Inpatient hospitalization may be required when clients are too impaired to continue with the activities of daily living or too suicidal to be left alone.

The goal of the *continuation phase* is to prevent relapses into distressing emotional states. This period usually lasts from 4 to 9 months and is carried out on an outpatient basis. Medications and psychotherapy are continued. Clients are educated about the nature of their conditions and their medications and encouraged to try new coping behaviors.

The *maintenance treatment phase* concentrates on preventing recurrences in clients with prior episodes of depression and/or mania. Maintenance psychotherapy and medications help prevent new episodes or recurrences (Table 21-3).

Current standard treatments for mood disorders include psychotherapy, pharmacological therapy, and electroconvulsive therapy. During each phase of treatment, nurses and other health care providers play important roles because they are the ones who help teach, encourage, and guide clients toward living effectively with their disorders.

Psychotherapies

Various psychotherapies are effective in treating mild and moderate depression. Cognitive-behavioral therapy is used to help clients identify and correct self-defeating thoughts and actions that keep self-esteem low. Interpersonal therapy assists clients with relationships and interactions, and psychodynamic therapy encourages the growth of personal insight. Support groups and organizations have also been found to be very helpful for clients and families coping with mood disorders.

Electroconvulsive Therapy

Electroconvulsive therapy (ECT) is the introduction of a controlled grand mal seizure by passing an electrical current through the brain. Electroconvulsive therapy appears to work by raising the levels of the neurotransmitter norepinephrine, which are low in many people with depression. Electroconvulsive therapy is used only after attempts to stabilize the depression with various medications have failed.

Each ECT treatment requires about 15 minutes, but the actual shock lasts for only a few seconds. Generally, 6 to 12 treatments are administered over a course of several weeks, and most individuals receive ECT two to three times a week.

Electroconvulsive therapy is not prescribed for clients with a recent myocardial infarction (MI) (heart attack), heart disease, high or low blood pressure, stroke, or congestive heart failure because the treatment slows heart rate and lowers blood pressure followed by a reflex rise in heart rate and blood pressure. It is contraindicated in people with increased intracranial pressure and tumors of the nervous system. Each client is evaluated for ECT on an individual basis, and the benefits must outweigh the risks before treatment is prescribed.

Electroconvulsive therapy may be administered on an outpatient or inpatient basis. The preparation of the client includes physical and emotional care, as well as education about the expected side effects of ECT. Consent for treatment forms are signed, and the client is reminded that confusion and memory loss are common after treatment. Clients treated on an outpatient basis must be accompanied by someone who can care for them following treatment.

Clients must eat nothing by mouth for at least 8 hours before treatment. Baseline vital signs are obtained, and the client is attached to cardiac, blood pressure, and oxygen monitors. Short-acting muscle relaxants, sedatives, and an anesthetic agent are administered intravenously.

Eelectroencephalogram (EEG) monitors and electrodes are positioned at certain points on the head by the physician. An airway is established, and an electrical shock, resulting in a controlled seizure of about 30 to 60 seconds, is delivered. Often the only evidence of a seizure is a flexing of the client's big toes. Brain waves are monitored throughout the procedure, and the client sleeps for about an hour following the treatment.

Common side effects of ECT include headache, confusion on awakening from the treatment, and short-term amnesia, but the client's mood improves rapidly. Many individuals can be managed on an outpatient basis with good postprocedure nursing management and appropriate client teaching. The responsibilities of the nurse when working with clients undergoing ECT include initiating intravenous therapy, administering ordered medications, and monitoring the client's responses before, during, and after treatment.

Drug Therapies

Medications are a mainstay in the treatment of mood disorders. However, their use must be carefully assessed, monitored, and evaluated because of the possibility of side effects and drug misuse. The most commonly used drug classes for treating mood disorders are four classes of antidepressants and several mood-stabilizing drugs All work to increase neurotransmitter levels in the body, which leads to improvement of depression.

Based on their chemical composition, antidepressants are divided into five categories: tricyclics, monoamine oxidase inhibitors (MAOIs), selective serotonin reuptake inhibitors (SSRIs), and atypical antidepressants. Each type alters a part of the brain's neurochemical balance or function. Many antidepressants require from 2 to 4 weeks before their effects are noticed and the client's well-being improves. For this reason some clients believe that antidepressants are ineffective. They require education and reminders that these drugs require time to take effect and encouragement to continue taking their medications.

Tricyclic antidepressants were once the first choice for the treatment for depression The SSRIs are now more often prescribed because of their low incidence of side effects. Last choice for use are the MAOIs because of their severe and potentially fatal side effects. New antidepressants, which are chemically unrelated to the other classes, are currently being introduced into the market. Nurses who administer these chemicals are responsible for maintaining current knowledge about their uses and effects.

Tricyclic antidepressants can produce severe central nervous system (CNS) depression when they interact with the barbiturates, certain anticonvulsants, drugs, and alcohol. Selective serotonin reuptake inhibitors act specifically to prevent the uptake of the neurochemical serotonin. They have fewer side effects than the tricyclics. Headache, nausea, nervousness, and insomnia are the most common side effects.

When MAOI antidepressants are combined with certain substances and foods containing the enzyme tyramine, the nervous system can become overexcited. This can lead to severely elevated blood pressure levels and hypertensive crisis. Refer back to Chapter 7 for a review of antidepressants, diet restrictions, and education for clients who are receiving MAOIs. Profound CNS depression or severe anticholinergic effects can occur. Elderly male clients receiving antidepressants should be observed for urinary retention, which can develop quickly. Side effects, such as blurred vision and dry mouth, can cause problems with compliance because individuals stop taking their medications as a result of these bothersome effects. Atypical and other antidepressants achieve the same effect as other antidepressants using different mechanisms of action. Box 21-3 lists various antidepressant and mood-stabilizing drugs.

Basically antidepressants exert their unwelcome side effects on both the central and peripheral nervous systems. Therapeutic interventions are often needed to

Box 21-3 Antidepressants and Mood-Stabilizing Drugs

Tricyclic Antidepressants

Amitriptyline (Elavil)   Clomipramine (Anafranil)
Doxepin (Adapin, Sinequan)   Imipramine (Tofranil)
Trimipramine (Surmontil)   Desipramine (Norpramin)
Nortriptyline (Pamelor)   Protriptyline (Vivactil)

Monoamine Oxidase Inhibitors (MAOIs)

Isocarboxazid (Marplan)   Phenelzine (Nardil)
Tranylcypromine (Parnate)

Selective Serotonin Reuptake Inhibitors (SSRIs)

Fluoxetine (Prozac)   Fluvoxamine (Luvox)
Paroxetine (Paxil)   Sertraline (Zoloft)

Other Antidepressants

Amoxapine (Asendin)   Bupropion (Wellbutrin)
Trazodone (Desyrel)   Venlafaxine (Effexor)

Mood-Stabilizing

Lithium (Lithobid, Lithonate)
Carbamazepine (Tegretol)   Clonazepam (Klonopin)

From Stuart GW, Laraia MT: *Principles and practice of psychiatric nursing*, ed 7, St. Louis, 2001, Mosby.

help clients adjust to their medications. Table 21-4 lists common side effects and therapeutic actions.

Because antidepressants may alter liver and kidney functions, hepatic and renal studies should be obtained monthly. Nurses should review all laboratory results for each client. Often blood levels of certain drugs are measured to determine the amount of drug still in the system. Toxic antidepressant levels can result if clients are not carefully monitored. Headaches, palpitations, changes in levels of consciousness, and stiffness in the neck should be reported to the physician immediately.

Lithium is a naturally occurring salt that helps to control the exaggerated thoughts and behaviors associated with mania. Because lithium does not bind to body proteins (as many other drugs do), it does not need to be metabolized by the liver. Lithium is distributed throughout the body fluids, where it competes with sodium. It is excreted by the kidneys more rapidly than sodium; therefore an important interaction between the level of lithium in the blood and common table salt exists.

When clients who are taking lithium ingest large amounts of salt, lithium levels usually drop because of rapid kidney excretion of lithium. The opposite is also true. When clients decrease their salt intake or lose salt through sweating, diarrhea, or altered kidney function, lithium levels in the blood are likely to increase. Because

the range between therapeutic response and toxic effects is very narrow, clients must be instructed not to change their diet or activity habits abruptly. The narrow therapeutic index of lithium requires close observation of client responses. If blood levels of the drug are too low, manic behavior returns; if levels are too high, an uncomfortable and possibly life-threatening toxicity may result. Most side effects of lithium are directly related to dosage and blood serum levels (Table 21-5). Polyuria (large urinary output) and polydipsia (increased thirst) are frequently seen in people beginning lithium therapy. Common unwanted gastrointestinal tract reactions include a metallic taste, dry mouth, thirst, nausea, diarrhea, a bloated feeling, and weight gain. Sleepiness, light-headedness, drowsiness, and a mild hand tremor are common during the first weeks of therapy.

Because the signs and symptoms of lithium toxicity are the same as the side effects during the first weeks of therapy, all caregivers should be aware of clients' responses to their lithium therapy. Most side effects disappear or decrease to a tolerable level by the sixth week of treatment. If they continue, be alert for the possibility of early lithium toxicity.

Blood tests for thyroid and kidney function, in addition to lithium levels, are routinely performed. Therapeutic blood levels of lithium range from 0.6 to 1.2 mEq/L. Toxic reactions occur when lithium levels in the blood are greater than 1.5 mEq/L (Table 21-6). Lithium toxicity can be life-threatening, and no specific antidote exists. Therefore it is one of the nurse's most important responsibilities to frequently assess each client's response during treatment with lithium or any other antimanic medication and monitor for signs and symptoms of toxicity. Review Chapter 7 for more information about client care and education for persons taking lithium. Study the procedure for a prelithium workup and be alert to the special educational needs of clients who require lithium.

Once the client is no longer manic, the need for lithium drops dramatically. Toxicity may set in rapidly unless the dose is reduced. Clients must be carefully monitored during the first weeks of lithium therapy. If little response is seen by the sixth week of treatment, the physician usually considers other therapies.

Nursing Process

Therapeutic care for clients with disturbances in mood relates to the whole person. Clients are first assessed for level of depression or mania. Next, a thorough history and physical examination help to establish the database. Nursing diagnoses are then chosen based on the individual's most distressing problems (Box 21-4).

Therapeutic interventions for the physical realm focus on helping clients with personal hygiene, maintaining adequate nutrition, and encouraging physical

Table 21-4 Side Effects of Antidepressants and Nursing Care

Side effects	Nursing care
Tricyclic Antidepressants	
Fatigue, sedation, slow psychomotor reactions, poor concentration, tremors, ataxia	Give at bedtime (h.s.); increase dose slowly; teach caution when using machinery; write instructions; document behaviors.
Suicidal gestures	Institute suicide precautions; drug increases energy for suicide.
Anticholinergic effects: dry mouth, decreased tearing, blurred vision (common)	Encourage frequent oral care, water, gum; use artificial tears; ensure that vision clears in 2 weeks; report eye pain immediately.
Constipation, urinary hesitancy or retention, excessive sweating	Monitor food and fluid intake; promote high-fiber diet (more than 30 mg/day); encourage water intake of at least 2500 ml/day; teach importance of adequate fluids, clothing, and sensible exercise; avoid hot showers, baths, dehydration; monitor urinary output, especially in older men.
Nontricyclic Antidepressants	
Dizziness, drowsiness, anxiety, confusion, tremors, weakness, dry mouth, nausea, diarrhea, increased appetite, paralytic ileus, urinary retention	Ensure safety; monitor mental status, moods, affect, level of consciousness, increased symptoms; weigh weekly; monitor for weight gain; encourage fluids to 2500 ml/day; monitor intake and output.
Orthostatic hypotension, tachycardia, palpitations	Teach client to rise slowly; monitor and report vital signs.
Monoamine Oxidase Inhibitors (MAOIs)	
Increased CNS stimulation	Reassure client; monitor for psychosis, seizures, hypoactivity.
Postural hypotension	Teach client to rise slowly; assure client that symptoms will decrease.
Muscle twitching	Vitamin B$_6$ (300 mg/day) is helpful.
Fluid retention, urinary hesitancy	Monitor intake and output; administer thiazide diuretics as ordered.
Insomnia	Give last dose as early as possible; encourage relaxation in evening.
Food-drug interaction with tyramine (common amino acid)	Avoid tyramine-rich foods; avoid drugs with epinephrine or stimulants.
Selective Serotonin Reuptake Inhibitors	
Dry mouth	Encourage fluids, good oral care.
Nausea, diarrhea	Give drug with meals; maintain bland diet; encourage good hydration; administer lower dose.
Drowsiness, dizziness, nervousness	Give h.s.; keep active during day; institute safety precautions; instruct client to avoid machinery.
Sweating	Maintain good hygiene; wear cotton clothing; encourage fluids.
Headaches	Teach relaxation techniques; administer mild analgesic for headache.
Insomnia	Give medications early; encourage good sleep habits and relaxation.
Nonselective Reuptake Inhibitors (Venlafaxine)	
Increased blood pressure	Monitor vital signs; report to physician if blood pressure stays high; may reduce dose.
Weakness, sweating, sleepiness, dry mouth, nausea, vomiting, constipation, anorexia, blurred vision, anxiety, tremors	Refer to nursing care for other drug classes of antidepressants.

activity. If clients are suicidal, special precautions and observations are implemented. In the emotional realm, care revolves around the therapeutic relationship. Acceptance and support are powerful tools in this area. Once trust is established, clients feel the encouragement to cope with their problems. In the intellectual realm, extreme emotional responses alter one's ability to think logically long enough to complete anything. Nurses should remember that these clients need extra patience and nonjudgmental guidance when attempting to follow

Table 21-5 Side Effects of Lithium and Nursing Care

Side effects	Nursing care
Abdominal discomfort, nausea, soft stools, diarrhea	Give lithium with food or milk; reassure that signs/symptoms are temporary and should subside.
Edema, especially feet	Reassure that signs/symptoms are temporary; check with physician about salt restriction.
Hair loss, hypothyroidism	Obtain thyroid function tests; reassure that condition is temporary; if continues, notify physician, who may discontinue drug.
Muscle weakness, fatigue	Provide reassurance; give more frequent divided doses per physician order.
Polyuria (can progress to diabetes insipidus)	Provide reassurance; increased output is expected; monitor intake and output; report if output greater than 3000 ml/24 hr.
Thirst	Encourage client to quench thirst but maintain stable fluid intake.
Tremors	Provide reassurance; eliminate caffeine; give slow-release form per physician order.
Weight gain	Provide reassurance that weight gain is common; moderately restrict calories; advise client against restricting fluids or salt.

Table 21-6 Signs/Symptoms of Lithium Toxicity

Level of toxicity	Signs/Symptoms
Mild Toxicity Blood serum levels 1.5 mEq/L	Apathy, sluggishness, drowsiness, and lethargy; diminished concentration; mild incoordination, muscle weakness, muscle twitches, coarse hand tremors
Moderate Toxicity Blood serum levels 1.5 to 2.5 mEq/L	Nausea, vomiting, severe diarrhea; slurred speech, blurred vision, ringing in the ears; apathy, drowsiness, lethargy, moderate sluggishness; muscle weakness, irregular tremors, ataxia, frank muscle twitching, increased tonicity
Severe Toxicity Blood serum levels above 2.5 mEq/L	Nystagmus; irregular muscle tremors, fasciculations (twitches of single muscle groups), hyperactive deep tendon reflexes; oliguria, decreased urine output, severe changes in level of consciousness, hallucinations; grand mal seizures, coma, death

Box 21-4 NANDA Nursing Diagnoses Related to Emotional Responses

Anxiety	Powerlessness*
Communication, impaired verbal	Self-care deficit
Community coping, ineffective	Self-esteem disturbance
Coping, ineffective individual	Sexual dysfunction
Grieving, anticipatory	Sleep pattern disturbance
Grieving, dysfunctional*	Social isolation
Hopelessness*	Spiritual distress*
Injury, risk for	Thought processes, altered
Loneliness, risk for	Violence, risk for: self-directed
Nutrition, altered	

From North American Nursing Diagnosis Association: *NANDA nursing diagnoses: definitions and classification 1999-2000*, Philadelphia, 1999, The Association.
*Primary nursing diagnosis for disturbances in mood.

Sample Client Care Plan   Major Depressive Episode

Assessment

History: Leanne is a 22-year-old woman with a diagnosis of major depressive episode following the loss of her infant son. Her childhood was uneventful except for a domineering father. She reports no abuse during childhood but admits being intimidated by her father's loud voice and gruff manner.

During her first year in college, she met and married Mark, a senior majoring in marketing. The first 10 months of the marriage went well, until Leanne discovered she was pregnant. The news of her pregnancy infuriated Mark, who insisted that she "do something." Leanne insisted on keeping the baby but was plagued by the guilt of adding an extra burden to Mark's load throughout the pregnancy. On May 10, she delivered a son.

Leanne's postpartum course was difficult. She was trying to care for her son, attend school, and appease her husband, who had become somewhat more interested in the baby. One morning she noticed that her son was too quiet. Attempts to revive him were unsuccessful, and the diagnosis of sudden infant death syndrome was made on autopsy. Three weeks later, Mark filed for divorce, stating that Leanne was not a "good mother."

Current Findings: A disheveled-appearing young woman with uncombed hair and wrinkled clothes. Speech is soft, almost inaudible. Does not maintain eye contact. Eyes red and swollen. Offers no information but when questioned admits to "being a complete failure," and "not worth the space I'm taking up." She describes her history as "filled with failures."

Multidisciplinary Diagnosis

Hopelessness related to loss of significant others as evidenced by an inability to perform activities of daily living

Planning/Goals

Leanne will use effective coping methods to counteract her feelings of hopelessness by November 29.

Leanne will express hopeful thoughts by December 15.

Therapeutic Interventions

Intervention	Rationale	Team Member
1. Assess risk for suicidal behaviors.	Suicide rates are high in depressed persons.	Nsg, All
2. Establish a no-self-harm contract with Leanne.	Demonstrates caring and helps to prevent suicidal gestures.	Psy, Nsg
3. Assist with activities of daily living as needed.	Supports Leanne until she is able to care for herself.	Nsg
4. Monitor fluid and food intake.	Depressed persons often do not eat or drink.	Nsg, Diet
5. Use active listening to encourage her to identify and express fellings.	Gives her an opportunity to explore and vent her emotions realistically.	All
6. Assess progress through the grief reaction and offer appropriate support.	Unresolved grief can cause depression; Leanne may not have grieved for the loss of her child yet.	Psy, Nsg
7. Help her to focus on the positive aspects and support systems in her life.	When energies are positively focused, success is encouraged.	All

Evaluation

After 5 days on the unit, Leanne assumed self-care activities and appeared well groomed throughout the remainder of her stay. By December 1, Leanne was able to discuss her feelings with two staff members. On December 14, Leanne joined a support group for mothers who have lost children.

A complete client care plan includes several other diagnoses and interventions

through on tasks. Give instructions slowly and clearly. Repeat them as needed, but do not become impatient. Remember, it is difficult to cope when one cannot think straight. Socially, most persons with mood disorders are lonely and afraid of associating with others. Once medications have begun to stabilize the client's moods, gentle encouragement to begin interacting with others may be needed.

Mood disorders involve the spiritual realm too. Many individuals with depression often question their spiritual beliefs. Manic clients commonly have delusions of **religiosity,** believing they have powers to communicate with God or become a spirit. Therapeutic listening is a helpful intervention, but do not hesitate to contact a cleric if the client so requests. The Sample Client Care Plan offers a plan for clients with a mood disorder. Remember, each actual plan will be unique according to the needs of the individual client.

Emotions, both positive and negative, add texture and meaning to the tapestry of our lives. Although we may not understand the exact connections between mind and body, we do know that our emotions are determined in large part by the way we think, the way we perceive the world, and our "self-talk." So powerful is this optimistic or pessimistic view that it determines not only our emotions, but the very condition of our physical and mental health. Stay healthy by thinking positively. You and your clients will both benefit.

KEY CONCEPTS

- An emotion is a nonintellectual response in the affective realm of human functioning.
- A mood disorder is defined as a disturbance in the emotional dimension of human functioning.
- Emotional responses grow and develop with the individual.
- Current evidence suggests that a combination of physical, psychological, and environmental factors are involved in the development of mood disorders.
- Depression is a "whole body" illness that involves emotional, physical, intellectual, social, and spiritual problems.
- Depression can be experienced as mild, moderate, or severe.
- When depression is severe and lasts more than 2 weeks, it is called a major depressive episode.
- When major depressive episodes routinely repeat themselves (for more than 2 years), a depressive disorder is diagnosed.
- A dysthymic disorder is daily moderate depression that lasts for longer than 2 years.

- The hallmark of bipolar disorders is sudden and dramatic shifts in emotional extremes.
- Bipolar I disorder is characterized by episodes of depression alternating with episodes of mania.
- With bipolar II disorder, individuals suffer major episodes of depression, alternating with periods of hypomania.
- Other problems with depression include seasonal affective disorder, postpartum depression, and depression associated with menses, medical conditions, or substance use.
- The therapeutic plan for clients with mood disorders is arranged into three phases: acute treatment phase, continuation phase, and maintenance phase.
- Various psychotherapies are effective in treating mild and moderate depression.
- The most commonly used drug classes for treating mood disorders are antidepressants and mood-stabilizing drugs.
- Electroconvulsive therapy (ECT) is used to relieve depression by inducing a controlled grand mal seizure by passing an electrical current through the brain.
- Therapeutic care for clients with disturbances in mood relates to each realm of functioning.

Suggestions for Further Reading

"Spotting Depression in Asian Patients," by Phyllis J. Estin (*RN* 62(4):39, 1999), is an excellent reminder of how cultural differences influence the signs and symptoms of depression.

General information about several mood disorders is available at www.psych.helsinki.fi

References

American Psychiatric Association: *Diagnostic and statistical manual of mental disorders,* ed 4, text revision, Washington, DC, 2000, The Association.

Issacs A: Depression and your patient, *American Journal of Nursing* 98(7):26, 1998.

Keltner NL, Schwecke LH, Bostrom CE: *Psychiatric nursing,* ed 3, St. Louis, 1998, Mosby.

Mood disorders: an overview, part I, *Harvard Mental Health Letter* 14(6):6, 1997.

National Depressive and Manic-Depressive Association: *Depression and bipolar illness,* Chicago, 1993, The Association.

National Institute of Mental Health: *The numbers count,* Boston, Mass, June 1, 1999, The Institute.

North American Nursing Diagnosis Association: *NANDA nursing diagnoses: definitions and classification 1999-2000,* Philadelphia, 1999, The Association.

Perry BL: A 45-year old woman with premenstrual dysphoric disorder, *Journal of the American Medical Association* 281(4):368, 1999.

Rollant PD, Deppoliti DB: *Mosby's review series: mental health nursing,* St. Louis, 1996, Mosby.

Scott S: Biology and mental health: why do women suffer more depression and anxiety? *Maclean's* 111(2):62, 1998.

Stuart GW, Laraia MT: *Principles and practice of psychiatric nursing,* ed 7, St. Louis, 2001, Mosby.

Wong DL: *Whaley and Wong's nursing care of infants and children,* ed 6, St. Louis, 1998, Mosby.

Chapter 22

Physical Problems, Psychological Sources

Learning Objectives

1. Explain the purpose of the physiological stress response.
2. Illustrate how stress can affect immune system functions.
3. Describe five conditions related to the physiological stress response.
4. Examine three theories that attempt to explain the role of emotions in the development of illnesses.
5. Compare three culturally related somatization disorders.
6. Explain the differences between conversion disorders and somatization disorders.
7. Describe the most essential feature of hypochondriasis.
8. Compare the difference between hypochondriasis and malingering.
9. Plan three therapeutic goals when caring for clients with psychophysiological disorders.

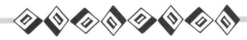

Key Terms

body dysmorphic disorder
conversion disorder
factitious disorder
health
hypochondriasis

la belle indifference
malingering
physiological stress response
primary gain
psychophysical disorders

psychosomatic illnesses
secondary gains
somatization
somatoform disorder

For centuries, mankind has questioned the interactions of mind and body and the roles emotions play in health. In ancient China, around the year 2000 BC, the emperor Huang Ti recorded his keen observations of the physical illnesses arising from emotional causes in his book titled *Classic of Internal Medicine*. Hippocrates instructed people to care for the spirit as well as the body. Throughout the Middle Ages, magical and symbolic thinking kept body and mind inseparably linked. People whose behavior or physical appearance differed were condemned as witches and workers of the devil.

Toward the end of the nineteenth century, scientific advances were made in biology, chemistry, and microbiology that shifted the focus of research to the cause and treatment of physical disease. By the time Freud's theories were introduced, the study of human beings had evolved into two distinct divisions: the biological (or physical) and all other aspects of human functioning (or the psychological). Complex human beings were now officially categorized into convenient sections for study, discussion, research, and treatment.

Today, however, researchers and practitioners alike are remembering that no such divisions between the mind and body exist. Human beings are dynamic, complicated physical organisms that are affected by many nonphysical events. Each of us is a unique individual—a combination of genetics, culture, and experience. Each of us has psychological aspects to our being, and our own way of coping with the stresses of life.

This chapter explores the connection between the physical and psychological aspects of people. It is an important chapter because clients with psychologically based physical problems are encountered in every practice setting. Health care providers who understand the role emotions play in the development of health problems are better able to assess client needs and plan more effective care.

ROLE OF EMOTIONS IN HEALTH

Health is a concept embodying the whole person. It is a state of well-being in which the psychological is in balance with the physical in a state of homeostasis. All animals, including humans, must live with and adapt to stress. The antelope on the African savanna must deal with the stress of becoming some carnivore's lunch every day of its life. To do this, the antelope is equipped with a delicate internal mechanism of biochemicals, all wired to the appropriate organs. When the animal is stressed, a response is activated and the antelope can run faster, jump higher, and endure the chase longer. In short, animals have evolved a stress response mechanism that protects them during times of threat or illness. It is called the *fight-or-flight response,* and it is an essential part of every animal's survival mechanisms.

Anxiety and Stress

Human beings are also equipped with a **physiological stress response** mechanism. This biochemical fight-or-flight system is a biological survival tool designed to provide the energy for fighting opponents or running to save one's skin. The physical stress response served early man effectively, but as people became civilized and adopted rules for behavior, fighting and running were replaced by more socially acceptable (but biochemically stifling) behaviors. Today the stressors of modern life are many, but outlets for the stress response are few.

In his book *Stress of Life,* Hans Selye "proposed that all humans show the same general bodily response to stress" (Corsini, 1994). Selye studied the biochemical reactions of the stress response and their effects on various body systems and called these reactions the general adaptation syndrome. Today, it is known that stress activates primitive regions in the brain that also control eating, aggression, and immune responses. These responses to the stresses of modern life are biochemically identical to the responses that early humans experienced

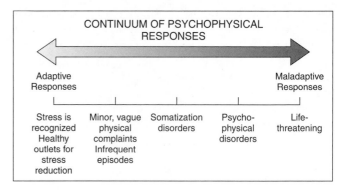

Figure 22-1 Continuum of psychophysical responses.

when fighting to stay alive. The problem today is that the fight-or-flight response occurs in non–life-threatening situations, stimulating the body for actions that never occur. The stress response mechanism can even work overtime when individuals are routinely exposed to stressors.

When an individual perceives stress, tension, or anxiety, the body initiates a cascade of biochemicals. The body's central command post, the hypothalamus, communicates to the pituitary gland, which in turn notifies the adrenal glands. The adrenal glands manufacture and release the body's four major stress hormones—dopamine, epinephrine, norepinephrine, and cortisol. The basic functions of the body are so responsive to these chemicals that even small changes in their levels can have a significant impact on one's state of health. Responses to stress exist along a continuum, ranging from high-level adaptive responses to life-threatening disorders (Figure 22-1).

Scientific investigation is beginning to show that the immune system is affected by one's level of stress. Several studies have demonstrated that significant immune function and blood pressure changes occur in people who displayed hostile or negative behaviors during periods of conflict. One study revealed that married couples who frequently argued had less effective immune systems. Other studies have demonstrated the importance of a positive attitude in physical healing.

The psychological side of an individual has a strong impact on the ability to identify and successfully cope with stress. People who are able to recognize and defuse their stressors early seldom experience the physical effects of stress. Others struggle with stressors and the body's response to them. Some individuals focus their stress into bodily activities and functions, thus developing physical problems that arise from psychological sources. These problems are called *somatoform, psychosomatic,* or *psychophysical disorders.*

Childhood Sources

How an individual perceives and responds to stress is established in childhood. The link between mind and body is made early in infancy because infants require the routine attentions of a consistent caregiver—someone who feeds, cuddles, and protects them. As children learn to cope with stresses, the brain becomes patterned. Biochemical reactions to stress alter the physical patterns of the brain and sensitize children to future stressors. This patterning sets up automatic chemical responses to stress—every time one is exposed to stress, the body responds with its biochemical program, even though the individual may not consciously feel stressed. Children who have experienced an unstable home environment, for example, may react to stress with exaggerated hormonal mechanisms as adults.

People experience stress related to their levels of development. In infancy mechanisms for coping with stress are limited. The only means of expression is through the body, so infants create physical signs and symptoms to help cope with their stresses. Problems such as colic, atopic dermatitis, allergic reactions, and obesity may all arise from the effects of stress. Older children can express their stresses by developing allergic skin reactions, asthma, gastrointestinal tract complaints, or joint aches and pains.

Families who emotionally support and encouraged their children to effectively cope with their stresses, have few physical complaints. Families filled with conflict and uncertainty often live with numerous physical problems, as well as psychological distresses. Most psychosomatic problems and somatoform disorders (physical problems with emotional sources) start in childhood and become established during adolescence. By adulthood, individuals can be significantly impaired in their daily living activities because of their reactions to stress.

COMMON PSYCHOPHYSICAL PROBLEMS

The physical signs and symptoms of emotional distress are very real to the individual who is suffering from them. The discomfort of an upset stomach is the same, whether it is caused by too much pizza or a disturbing piece of news. The effects of emotionally caused illnesses are the same as those arising from physical sources.

When the body is under continual or repeated stress, it responds by overactivating its stress response mechanism, which can result in many of the physical signs and symptoms of an illness, disease, or disability. (Refer to the stress adaptation theory in Chapter 6.) In the past these symptoms were often referred to as **psychosomatic illnesses,** meaning emotionally (psycho) related physical (somatic) disorders. Unfortunately, this term has come to mean an imaginary illness in popular vocabulary. The more recent term, **psychophysical disorders,** was coined to refer to the stress-related physical problems. The physiological stress response affects many body systems (Box 22-1).

Box 22-1 Physical Conditions Affected by Psychological Factors

Cardiovascular

Migraine headaches
Tension headaches
Hypertension (high blood pressure)
Angina (chest pain)

Musculoskeletal

Rheumatoid arthritis
Low back pain

Respiratory

Hyperventilation
Asthma

Gastrointestinal

Anorexia nervosa
Obesity
Peptic ulcer
Irritable bowel syndrome
Colitis

Skin

Neurodermatitis
Eczema
Psoriasis
Pruritus (itching)

Genitourinary

Impotence
Frigidity
Premenstrual syndrome

Endocrine System

Hyperthyroidism
Diabetes

From Stuart GW, Laraia MT: *Stuart and Sundeen's pocket guide to psychiatric nursing,* ed 4, St. Louis, 1998, Mosby.

One of the systems that receives much of the stress response is the gastrointestinal tract. Common stress-related problems include indigestion, vomiting, constipation, and diarrhea. Ulcerative colitis and gastric, peptic, and duodenal ulcers can also occur when the gastrointestinal tract is the focus of one's stress. The respiratory system can develop asthma, and the cardiac system can raise blood pressure when subjected to prolonged stress. Many mental health conditions, such as anxiety, are expressions of stress.

Theories of Psychophysical Disorders

Although it is known that emotions play an important role in the development or prevention of illness, just how this connection works is uncertain. Several theories attempt to explain this relationship.

The stress response theory states that individuals are biochemically patterned to react to stress. During times of stress, the autonomic nervous system prepares the body for fight or flight. Because the threat is not external, no physical outlet for the biochemical response is usually possible. Consequently, nothing is done to relieve the conflict, and soon a cycle of biochemical stimulus-response is established. This pattern eventually results in physical disturbances within the body.

A second theory focuses on the symbolism attached to a symptom or illness. For example, the angry young executive who needs to vent his rage, but feels that displays of anger are inappropriate, may develop ulcerative colitis or high blood pressure as a way of coping with his anger.

Another theory states that certain personality types are prone to developing certain illnesses. The hard-working, independent, overly ambitious businessman is considered at high risk for the development of cardiac problems because of his aggressive personality. The quiet, uncomplaining, overburdened clerk may suffer from ulcers, joint problems, or skin rashes.

Last is the theory of organic weakness, which states that every individual has one body system that is more sensitive than other systems. When a person has underlying emotional problems that affect functioning he or she may develop a physical illness as a means of coping with the unconscious problem.

Although these theories may appear unrelated, all of them have several concepts in common:

1. Unconscious emotional conflict that increases anxiety and interferes with activities is the basis for many psychophysical problems.
2. The development of physical symptoms is the result of attempts to lower anxieties associated with conflict.
3. The illness is real to the person, regardless of whether organic changes exist. In some cases, physical changes can be life-threatening, so never treat a client's complaints casually.
4. Most often, the onset of the illness or problem is related to a stressful event.

The physical signs and symptoms of an illness often relieve an individual's anxieties by masking their inner emotional turmoil. This anxiety-reducing benefit is called **primary gain** because the symptoms reduce anxiety. There are other benefits, called **secondary gains,** to assuming the sick role. These include being relieved of responsibilities, receiving the special attentions of others, and having dependency needs met. Frequently these gains tend to reinforce the pattern of psychophysical symptoms and encourage illness behaviors to continue.

SOMATOFORM DISORDERS

Somatization is term for feeling physical symptoms in the absence of disease or out of proportion to an ailment (Corr, 1992). It is a common stress-reducing mechanism that may or may not result in pathological functioning. Persons suffering from a somatoform disorder demonstrate no objective causes or physical dysfunctions for their signs and symptoms. The diagnosis of a **somatoform disorder** is made by first excluding any possible physical dysfunctions, the presence of drugs or other toxic substances, or other mental health problems that may be related to the symptoms. Finally, if investigations reveal no diagnosable medical condition that accounts for the client's physical condition, a diagnosis of one of the somatoform disorders is made.

Somatization is common in the United States. Almost 80% of basically healthy people have somatic symptoms in any given week. Many health care dollars (about one in five) are spent treating nonphysically based complaints, and "nearly half of the patients seen in physicians' offices are the 'worried well' " (Corr, 1992). Somatization costs more than just money. Often individuals with somatoform disorders will subject themselves to painful or dangerous diagnostic procedures and treatments. Cardiac pain, for example, must be investigated to determine whether its origin is emotional or physical.

The signs and symptoms of illness may be the client's way of coping with emotional distress. Emotional distress depletes the body's energies and results in decreased immune functions, which can make the person more susceptible to actual illness and disease. Remember, people with somatoform disorders also fall ill to the same maladies as everyone else, so do not dismiss any clients' complaints as trivial.

Cultural Influences

Cultural differences are associated with certain illnesses, both physical and mental. Many somatization disorders are culturally related, and their treatment depends on understanding the problem within the client's cultural context or framework (Table 22-1).

Health care providers who work with clients from different cultures must be aware of the meaning or importance that the problem holds for the person (Giger and Davidhizar, 1999). Many somatic illnesses are based in cultural or spiritual beliefs. Assessments and treatment plans must not threaten or challenge these beliefs if therapeutic interventions are to be effective. Culturally appropriate nursing interventions are based on knowledge of and respect for another's way of living (Geissler, 1998). The effective health care provider does not hesitate to learn as much as possible about other cultures.

Criteria for Diagnosis

Expressing emotions through the body (somatization) is a common coping mechanism for many people. It fulfills needs and relieves anxiety. Because every physical sign or symptom may have a biological cause, each complaint must be investigated thoroughly before it is labeled as emotionally based. Therefore, the first criteria for diagnosis is that *no organic medical condition to explain the symptoms can be found.*

The second condition for diagnosis is that *the disorder significantly disrupts or impairs one's level of functioning.* Because of the somatoform problem, the person is unable to engage in the activities of daily living, perform work, or engage in social activities. This adds significant distress to an already emotionally charged situation.

The third criteria for diagnosis is that *the client is unaware of or unable to express his or her emotional*

Table 22-1 | Culturally Related Somatic Disorders

Cultural group	Description
Japanese	*Gaman* means to internally suppress emotions, especially anger. Emotional distresses are expressed through physical signs or symptoms. Illness is a socially acceptable way of receiving care. Body functions are of concern, especially blood pressure. Headaches are related to depression.
Southeast Asians	Mental distress is not discussed but expressed via various physical ailments. *Koro* is fear of penis shrinking into abdomen, which results in death.
Hispanics	*Mal ojo* (the evil eye) is associated with fever, headaches, diarrhea, restlessness, irritability, and weight loss.
East Indians (India)	*Dhat* syndrome consists of male reproductive signs/symptoms caused by fear and concern about losing semen.
Koreans	The body is the property of the ancestors. Mental and emotional illnesses are expressed as physical (somatic) complaints.

distress. Acknowledging emotional distress may be seen as a weakness, especially for men. Experiencing physical problems, however, enables individuals to accept the attention and the sympathy that anxiety or emotional expression would not elicit. Somatization is a common way for many emotional problems to make themselves known.

The *Diagnostic and Statistical Manual of Mental Disorders* (DSM-IV–TR) lists six types of somatoform disorders: somatization disorder, undifferentiated somatoform disorder, conversion disorder, pain disorder, hypochondriasis, and body dysmorphic disorder. Most eating and sleeping disorders arise from emotional sources, and they are considered in the next chapter. Individuals with **factitious disorder** intentionally produce signs and symptoms of illness or disability in order to assume the sick role. Because most of these clients are seen in general medical settings, such as clinics and physicians' offices, it is important for all caregivers to be familiar with somatoform disorders.

Somatization Disorder

Somatization disorder has been historically referred to as *Briquet's syndrome* or *hysteria.* As a polysymptomatic disorder, the condition is associated with many signs and symptoms. It begins before age 30, sometimes as early as adolescence or childhood, and can persist for many years. Somatization disorder occurs more frequently in women and appears to occur in a family pattern. It is seen in 10% to 20% of the daughters of women diagnosed with the disorder. The male relatives of these women show an increased risk of antisocial personality disorders and substance-abuse problems (American Psychiatric Association, 2000). Both genetic and environmental factors contribute to the risk of developing a somatization disorder.

 Drug Alert

Nurses need to ask all clients if they are currently seeing any other health care providers, natural healers, or any other practitioners.

Obtain a full drug history from each client, including the use of over-the-counter drugs, home remedies, and herbs.

Individuals with somatization disorder often possess a long history of vague complaints. Their complaints are usually described in colorful and exaggerated terms but offer few facts. Although the descriptions of their illnesses may be vivid, they actually give a poor history of their medical problems. In addition, it is not uncommon for individuals with somatization disorder to seek treatment from several physicians at the same time. This dangerous practice can lead to hazardous events for these clients if the combined drugs and therapies are not compatible (see Drug Alert box).

The most common client complaints are a combination of gastrointestinal tract and sexual problems, with pain and false neurological symptoms. The Case Study box explains a typical case.

For a diagnosis of somatization disorder to be made, the client must meet the criteria listed in Box 22-2.

Signs of anxiety and depression are very common in people with somatization disorders. They may also behave in impulsive, antisocial, or suicidal manners. Frequently their lives are associated with chaos, marital discord, and social problems with lifestyles as complicated as their medical histories.

Three features may help health care providers to differentiate a somatization disorder from a medical

Case Study

Sarah was a single 31-year-old woman who came to the clinic with complaints of diarrhea, nausea, pain, and weight loss over a period of 5 years. During the health history Sarah revealed that she was the only one of five children still living at home with her mother. Sarah described younger years as always being "sickly," but she could not identify any specific health problems.

Her father, whom Sarah described as "silent and cold," died when she was 15. She remembers feeling little loss at her father's death. Sarah's relationship with her mother became very important after the death of her father. Sarah and her mother did everything together, even to the point of sharing the same bed. Upon graduation from high school, Sarah worked in a candy shop for a few years but found the work too demanding and quit. She has not been employed in over 7 years.

It seems that just before the symptoms of her illness began, Sarah's mother's sister became widowed and decided to move in with Sarah and her mother. Aunt Sally arrived with much of her furniture, including a pair of twin beds. Soon thereafter, the mother sold the large double bed and substituted the twin beds, forcing Sarah to sleep alone. Although she did not protest, Sarah felt angry and deserted. A few weeks later she developed abdominal pain, diarrhea, and nausea.

◆ How do you think the onset of Sarah's symptoms relates to her family situation?

◆ Consider which therapeutic (nursing) interventions would be most effective with Sarah.

Box 22-2 Criteria for Diagnosis of Somatization Disorder

1. A history of pain related to at least four different sites (e.g., headache, backache, or joint, extremity, chest, or abdominal pain) or functions (e.g., menstrual, sexual, or urinary dysfunctions).
2. A history of at least two gastrointestinal tract symptoms (other than pain), such as nausea, abdominal bloating, vomiting, diarrhea, and food intolerance.
3. A history of one sexual or reproductive problem other than pain. For women, these include irregular or difficult menses, heavy menstrual bleeding, or vomiting throughout pregnancy. For men there may be erectile or ejaculatory problems. Both men and women are often sexually indifferent.
4. A history of at least one symptom that suggests a neurological disorder, such as impaired coordination, localized weakness, and double vision.

problem (Kirmayer, Robbins, and Paris, 1994). First, the involvement of multiple organ systems suggests somatization disorder. Second, the disorder is characterized by an early onset and chronic condition in which no physical changes occur over time. Third, the absence of any significant laboratory values indicates that the underlying problems may be emotionally based. It is important to remember that the onset of multiple complaints in an older person is almost always caused by a medical condition, not somatization. Also, having a somatization disorder does not protect individuals from developing a physical problem.

Clients with somatization disorder are difficult to diagnose and even more challenging to effectively treat.

"Conflict between patients' experience of illness and physicians' diagnostic categories, and fear of blaming the patient, complicate naming and characterizing the illness" (Epstein, Quill, and McWhinney, 1999). These individuals are not consciously aware of the conflicts related to their difficulties. Long-term therapy is usually indicated when clients are willing to recognize and work with the emotional conflicts that are at the basis of their physical problems.

Conversion Disorder

The term *conversion* is derived from Freud's theory of conversion hysteria, which stated that a psychosexual conflict is focused or converted into a physical disturbance. Today this relatively uncommon condition, called a **conversion disorder,** is considered to be a somatoform disorder in which the individual presents problems related to the sensory or motor functions (Table 22-2).

Conversion disorders appear more commonly in persons of lower socioeconomic status, those living in rural areas, and people with little health care knowledge. Approximately 1% to 3% of referrals to mental health clinics involve clients with conversion reactions (Kirmayer, Robbins, and Paris, 1994). When clients with conversion disorders are assessed, it is important to consider their social and cultural backgrounds.

Men and women differ in relation to conversion disorder, and the disorder is much more common in women. As many as 10 women for every 1 man are diagnosed with conversion disorders. In men, conversion disorders are often associated with military service, industrial accidents, and antisocial personalities. The onset of problems is usually during late childhood through early adulthood, but almost always after 10 and before 35 years of age. There have been reports, however, of conversion reactions in persons in their 90s. Children

Table 22-2 DSM–IV–TR Medical Diagnoses for Somatoform Disorders

DSM–IV–TR diagnosis	Essential features
Somatization disorder	A history of many physical complaints beginning before the age of 30, occurring over a period of several years, and resulting in treatment being sought or significant impairment in social or occupational functioning. The patient must display at least four pain symptoms, two gastrointestinal symptoms, one sexual symptom, and one symptom suggesting a neurological disorder.
Conversion disorder	One or more symptoms or deficits affecting voluntary motor or sensory function suggesting a neurological or general medical condition. Psychological factors are judged to be associated with the symptom or deficit because the initiation or exacerbation of the symptom or deficit is preceded by conflicts or other stressors. The symptom or deficit cannot be fully explained by a neurological or general medical condition and is not a culturally sanctioned behavior or experience.
Hypochondriasis	Preoccupation with fears of having, or ideas that one has, a serious disease based on the person's misinterpretation of bodily symptoms. The preoccupation persists despite appropriate medical evaluation and reassurance and has existed for at least 6 months. It causes clinically significant distress or impairment in functioning.

Modified from American Psychiatric Association: *Diagnostic and statistical manual of mental disorders*, ed 4, text revision, Washington, DC, 2000, The Association.

usually present with gait problems or seizures. In older individuals, the signs and symptoms usually appear as sensory or motor disturbances. Symptoms often appear suddenly, but they can also begin slowly and increase over time and typically last only a short time. In hospitalized clients, symptoms often disappear within 2 weeks. However, recurring episodes are common, and as many as 25% of clients have a return of symptoms within 1 year.

✔ Conversion disorders are thought to be the result of an emotional (psychic) conflict. Situational factors, such as environmental stressors or interpersonal conflicts, can frequently trigger the appearance of conversion reactions. For a conversion disorder to be diagnosed, the client must meet four criteria (Box 22-3).

Conversion signs and symptoms tend to be more in keeping with the individual's ideas of what the problems should be. For example, a "paralyzed" arm that is raised over the head by the nurse remains suspended for a moment and then falls to the side rather than on its owner's head, or an extremity that is "paralyzed" moves automatically when the client is not paying attention to it. Individuals with conversion "seizures" vary in their seizure activity, and few if any changes are noted on an electroencephalogram (EEG). In short, the course of the signs and symptoms is not in keeping with physically-based disease processes but rather the client's ideas.

An interesting feature of conversion disorders is **la belle indifference,** which is a lack of concern or indifference about the signs or symptoms. Some individuals with conversion disorders appear totally indifferent to their symptoms, whereas others present their complaints in dramatic or hysterical manners. Symptoms are more

Box 22-3 Criteria for Diagnosis of a Conversion Disorder

1. At least one of the signs or symptoms involves the voluntary motor or sensory system and suggests the presence of a neurological problem.
2. The signs and symptoms are brought on or worsened by the presence of a conflict or other stressor.
3. The signs and symptoms are not intentionally produced.
4. The signs and symptoms cause significant distress and impairment in daily functions.
5. After extensive investigation, the signs and symptoms cannot be explained by a pathological condition, the effects of a substance, or a culturally appropriate behavior.

apparent during times of extreme psychological stress, such as the loss of a loved one or change in fortune. People with conversion disorders are often very suggestible, and their symptoms can be modified or intensified by the reactions of others in their environments. Laboratory and other diagnostic examinations show no specific abnormalities. In fact, it is the absence of diagnostic findings that helps to establish the diagnosis.

Treatment goals focus on eliminating the possibility of any physical causes and then assisting clients in identifying the conflicts responsible for their signs and symptoms. Individuals and their families are frequently referred for psychotherapy, wherein antidepressants and antianxiety agents are often prescribed. Behavior modification techniques are successful in some cases.

Hypochondriasis

Hypochondriasis is a somatoform disorder in which one has an intense fear of or preoccupation with having a serious disease or medical condition based on a misinterpretation of body signs and symptoms. Hypochondriasis is a persistent fear that something is physically wrong, even when all diagnostic test results are negative and reassurances have been given by various physicians. Although the individual can acknowledge the possibility that the symptoms are being exaggerated or blown out of proportion, he or she continues to hold onto the belief that something is physically wrong.

Symptoms commonly relate to minor abnormalities (a sore on the skin, a cough), body functions (heartbeat, sweating), or vague physical sensations, such as "tired blood" or "aching veins." The meaning, source, and nature of the symptoms cause great concern to the client despite repeated negative test results and reassurances from health care providers. These people commonly "doctor shop," seeing several physicians at the same time. Often their relationships with health care providers become strained because clients with hypochondriasis feel they never receive the proper medical care and usually resist referral to mental health care settings.

Hypochondriasis can begin at any age, but the symptoms most commonly occur in early adulthood. It is more frequent in persons who were exposed to a serious illness or life-threatening condition in childhood. The course of the disorder follows a seesaw pattern and tends to become chronic. In some cases the disorder is first diagnosed following a severe stressor, such as the death of a loved one. Although exact statistics are not available, it is estimated that from 4% to 9% of the clients seen in a general medical practice are suffering from hypochondriasis.

People with hypochondriasis often have strained interpersonal relationships. Because they are so focused on themselves, many expect special consideration and treatment. Family and social lives can become quite disturbed because they center around clients' pictures of their health. Individuals may be able to remain employed if the appearance of symptoms is limited to nonwork time; time is frequently missed from work. In the most severe cases, people become complete invalids. The client must meet five criteria (Box 22-4) before a diagnosis of hypochondriasis is made.

Anxiety, depression, and compulsive personality traits are often present along with hypochondriasis. These clients are frequently demanding and a challenge to treat because they can be critical and suspicious of all offered health care. Patience, therapeutic communication skills, and alert observations are needed when caring for individuals with hypochondriasis.

Because of the chronic nature of the disorder and the fact that these clients are "doctor shoppers," hypochondriasis is difficult to treat. Often clients show poor insight or little concern about the source of their preoccupations. Psychotherapy and emotional support assist some clients in identifying the sources of their problems. Antianxiety and antidepressive medications may be prescribed. Because of the chronic and interfering nature of the disorder, long-term therapy and support are indicated.

Other Somatoform Disorders

Table 22-2 presents a summary of the essential features of the three most common somatoform disorders. Two less common but important somatoform disorders relate to the perceptions of pain and disfigurement. Somatoform pain disorder may be diagnosed when pain or discomfort is the major focus of distress *and* no other cause of the pain can be identified. Many times these individuals benefit from attending pain clinics.

Body dysmorphic disorder is characterized by a preoccupation with a physical difference or defect in one's body. The most common site of concern is the face or head. Clients may be concerned about their ears, noses, thinning hair, drooping chin, crooked teeth, or numerous other imperfections. They describe their distress as tormenting, devastating, or intensely painful. Because of their concern and embarrassment over their perceived defect, these individuals often describe themselves as "ugly" or "unacceptable" and often avoid work, social, or public gatherings. Their distress can lead to repeated hospitalizations for treatment of the perceived defect, as well as suicide attempts.

FACTITIOUS DISORDERS AND MALINGERING

Factitious disorders and malingering differ from somatoform disorders in that signs and symptoms are *intentionally* produced. People who are malingering or engaging in factitious behaviors are purposefully and willfully pro-

---

Box 22-4 **Criteria for Diagnosis of Hypochondriasis**

1. A preoccupation with fears of having a serious disease based on a misunderstanding of body messages.
2. The preoccupation is not delusional (clients can admit that they have an unreasonable concern).
3. The preoccupation persists despite negative diagnostic testing results.
4. The preoccupation causes significant distress or impairment in the client's activities of daily living.
5. The preoccupation has been present for at least 6 months.

ducing the signs or symptoms of illness for some form of gain. Both psychological and physical signs and symptoms can be expressed. Clients are rarely diagnosed with factitious disorder because they tend to move from physician to physician and undergo various operative procedures in different facilities. Some spend the major focus of their lives seeking admission or staying in health care facilities.

Factitious disorder by proxy, also called *Munchausen's syndrome*, is the deliberate production of signs and symptoms in another person. Situations most often involve a caregiver (mother, baby-sitter) who induces signs of illness in a child and then presents the child for medical care. The type and severity of signs and symptoms vary with the medical knowledge of the offender. Diagnosis is difficult because offenders commonly remove their victims as soon as the disorder is suspected.

Clinical Presentations

The difference between a factitious disorder and malingering lies with the *intent* of the individual.

The most important feature of a **factitious disorder** is that symptoms are purposefully produced to assume the sick role. Presenting complaints include psychological signs and symptoms, self-inflicted illnesses or injuries, and exaggerated symptoms of actual physical problems. Examples include complaining of acute abdominal pain, producing abscesses by injecting saliva under the skin, ingesting medications to produce dramatic side effects, or pretending to have a seizure with no actual history of epilepsy. The motivation for the client's behaviors is to assume the sick role.

The medical history of individuals with factitious disorders may be dramatic and colorful, but clients are vague and inconsistent when questioned. Often they lie

---

Box 22-5 NANDA Nursing Diagnoses Related to Psychophysiological Responses

Adjustment, impaired*
Anxiety
Body image disturbance
Constipation
Coping, ineffective individual
Denial, ineffective
Diarrhea
Diversional activity deficit
Family processes, altered
Fear
Gas exchange, impaired
Health maintenance, altered
Hopelessness
Nutrition, altered: less than body requirements
Pain, chronic*
Physical mobility, impaired
Powerlessness
Self-care deficit
Self-esteem, chronic low
Self-esteem, situational low
Self-esteem, disturbance
Skin integrity, impaired
Sleep pattern disturbance*
Social interaction, impaired
Social isolation
Spiritual distress

From North American Nursing Diagnosis Association: *NANDA nursing diagnoses: definitions and classification 1999-2000,* Philadelphia, 1999, The Association.
*Primary nursing diagnosis for maladaptive psychophysiological responses.

Think About

Clients who have been diagnosed with somatoform disorders receive more than just a name for their symptoms. They are also the recipients of health care provider's attitudes.

Caring for individuals with somatoform problems is often demanding and difficult, testing the patience and goodwill of health care providers As a result, caregivers sometimes engage in forced politeness and interact with these clients as little as possible. These people soon become labeled as "uncooperative," and this label follows them through all areas of the health care system.
◆ How would you feel about caring for these clients?
◆ How do you think the negative labeling affects the health care received by this type of client?

Box 22-6 Key Interventions for Clients With Psychophysical Problems

Convey an attitude of acceptance and understanding.
Meet all physical needs of the client during acute feelings of illness.
Minimize secondary gains once the acute phase of the illness is resolved.
Use the client's level of anxiety as a gauge to determine the amount and type of health teaching.
Acknowledge the client as a responsible adult while indirectly addressing dependency needs.
Encourage the client to talk about his or her feelings.
Assist the client and family to enlarge their social network.

From Taylor CM: *Essentials of psychiatric nursing,* ed 14, St. Louis, 1994, Mosby.

>>> Sample Client Care Plan Psychophysiological Responses

Assessment

History: Jasmine is a 20-year-old college student. Last year, during final examination week, she developed frequent bouts of nausea followed by vomiting. Once final examinations were over, her symptoms subsided until about 3 days ago.

Current Findings: A tense, young woman, sitting stiffly in the chair and wringing her hands. On questioning, Jasmine reveals that she has "never had problems with her stomach." She believes that her nausea and vomiting are related to the "institutional food" she eats while on campus. She is here at the clinic to "get some of those nausea pills." Final examinations for her four classes are scheduled for next week. Jasmine states school stresses "really have nothing to do with my stomach problems. It's the food that's the real problem here."

Multidisciplinary Diagnosis

Impaired adjustment related to anxiety about examinations

Planning/Goals

Jasmine will express her feelings verbally rather than through nausea and vomiting.

Therapeutic Interventions

Intervention	Rationale	Team Member
1. Assist Jasmine to identify stressful situations by reviewing the events surrounding the development of nausea and vomiting.	Identifying events relating to internal conflicts helps reduce the anxiety that results in nausea and vomiting.	Psy, Nsg
2. Help her see the association between thoughts, feelings, and behaviors.	Helps Jasmine to gain control over her expressions of emotions.	All
3. Explore more effective ways of coping with her anxieties.	Preserves dignity and self-respect; encourages effective coping behaviors.	Psy, All
4. Help her choose two new coping mechanisms for dealing with the stress of examinations.	Equips Jasmine with multiple ways to manage her anxieties and demonstrates the use of more effective behaviors.	Psy, Nsg
5. Actively encourage Jasmine to test the new coping mechanisms and provide feedback.	Change requires time, emotional support, and positive reinforcement from others.	All
6. Encourage physical activity and relaxation exercises.	Wellness requires a balance between physical and psychosocial needs.	Nsg
7. Assess eating and sleeping habits and encourage her to follow a routine schedule.	A healthy, well-cared-for body functions more effectively during stress.	Ns

Evaluation

During final examination week, Jasmine had two episodes of nausea but no vomiting. By the next final examination period, Jasmine had replaced nausea and vomiting with a 1-mile walk and 10 minutes of relaxation exercise during each examination day.

A complete client care plan includes several other diagnoses and interventions.

entertainingly about any aspect of their condition. Some may have extensive knowledge of hospital routines, diagnostic testing, and medical terminology. When the cause of the original symptoms is ruled out, individuals often develop new complaints and eagerly undergo invasive procedures. If they are confronted with evidence of their behaviors, they strongly deny it and discharge themselves from the institution or change health care providers.

On the other hand, the **malingering** individual produces symptoms to meet a recognizable goal. The student who fakes a stomachache to be excused from school for the day is a common example of malingering. Producing symptoms to avoid military service, the police, jury duty, or social obligations are examples. Not infrequently clients will produce symptoms with the goal of receiving compensation, food, or shelter for the night. However, once the motive becomes apparent to others, the symptoms usually disappear because they no longer serve a purpose.

IMPLICATIONS FOR CARE PROVIDERS

Caring for clients with somatoform disorders is both challenging and rewarding. The first goal of care in every case is to rule out the presence of any physical disease or dysfunction. As physicians order and interpret diagnostic tests, nurses and other caregivers observe and assess clients and their activities. Data are gathered and analyzed, physical dysfunctions are ruled out, and a health care team and nursing diagnoses are established (Box 22-5).

The development of trust is an important goal in the treatment of clients with somatoform disorders. Clients' sufferings are very real to them, and health care providers must be aware of how their behaviors and attitudes affect the clients for whom they care (see Think About box).

Nurses should attempt to understand the purposes served by clients' symptoms and work to encourage a trusting relationship with clients. Encourage the expression of feelings and emotional states rather than physical complaints. Also, teach the importance of good nutritional, exercise, and sleep habits using the client's anxiety level as a guide for teaching. Meet physical needs when necessary but encourage independence. Help clients fill their social needs and encourage them to explore more adaptive ways of handling their stresses. Box 22-6 summarizes key interventions for clients with somatoform disorders. The Sample Client Care Plan illustrates the care for a client. Finally, acknowledge clients as individuals and responsible adults who are capable of changing and developing more effective coping mechanisms.

KEY CONCEPTS

- No real divisions between mind and body exist because human beings are dynamic, complex organisms who are affected by many nonphysical events.
- The physical signs and symptoms of psychic (emotional) distress are very real to the individual who is suffering from them at the time.
- When the body is under continual stress, it activates its stress response mechanism.
- Theories about stress include the stress response, symbolism, personality, and organic weakness theories.

- Somatization is the term for feeling physical symptoms in the absence of disease or out of proportion to a given ailment.
- Many somatization disorders are culturally related.
- A somatoform disorder is diagnosed when no diagnosable organic medical condition can be found, the disorder significantly impairs one's level of functioning, and the client is unaware of or unable to express his or her emotional distress.
- Clients with a conversion disorder present with problems related to sensory or motor functions.
- Hypochondriasis is an intense fear of or preoccupation with having a serious disease or medical condition based on a misinterpretation of body signs or symptoms.
- The most important feature of factitious disorder is that symptoms are purposefully produced so that the individual can assume the sick role.
- The malingering individual produces symptoms to meet a recognizable external goal.
- The goals of care for every client with a somatoform disorder are to rule out the presence of any physical disease or dysfunction and to develop trust in the therapeutic relationship.

Suggestions for Further Reading

"Illness Without Disease, parts I and II, by Lester Grinspoon (*Harvard Mental Health Letter* 16(3):1, 1999), offers an excellent description of somatoform disorders and is written for the general public.

Patient information handouts on somatoform disorders are available at http://home.aafp/patientinfo.

References

American Psychiatric Association: *Diagnostic and statistical manual of mental disorders*, ed 4, text revision, Washington, DC, 2000, The Association.

Corr JM: Somatization: mind over matter, *Harvard Mental Health Letter* 17(6):4, 1992.

Corsini RJ, editor: *Encyclopedia of psychology*, ed 2, New York, 1994, John Wiley.

Epstein RM, Quill TE, McWhinney IR: Somatization reconsidered: incorporating the patient's experience of illness, *Archives of Internal Medicine* 159(3):215, 1999.

Geissler EM: *Pocket guide to cultural assessment*, ed 2, St. Louis, 1998, Mosby.

Giger JN, Davidhizar RE: *Transcultural nursing: assessment and intervention*, ed 3, St. Louis, 1999, Mosby.

Kirmayer LJ, Robbins JM, Paris J: Somatoform disorders: personality and the social matrix of somatic distress, *Journal of Abnormal Psychology* 103(1):125, 1994.

North American Nursing Diagnosis Association: *NANDA nursing diagnoses: definitions and classification 1999-2000*, Philadelphia, 1999, The Association.

Stuart GW, Laraia MT: *Stuart and Sundeen's pocket guide to psychiatric nursing*, ed 4, St. Louis, 1998, Mosby.

Taylor CM: *Essentials of psychiatric nursing*, ed 14, St. Louis, 1994, Mosby.

Chapter 23

Eating and Sleeping Disorders

Learning Objectives

1. List three criteria for the diagnosis of an eating disorder.
2. Compare the difference between anorexia nervosa and bulimia.
3. Forecast the prognosis (outcome) for a client with an untreated eating disorder.
4. Explain why obesity can be considered an eating disorder.
5. Examine the main therapeutic goal for treating clients with eating disorders.
6. Develop four therapeutic interventions for clients with eating disorders.
7. Describe three functions of sleep.
8. Discuss the signs and symptoms of a client suffering from insomnia.
9. Plan four therapeutic (nursing) interventions to assist clients with sleeping problems.

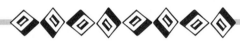

Key Terms

anorexia nervosa

binge eating

body image

bulimia

cataplexy

compulsive overeating

dyssomnias

eating disorder

insomnia

narcolepsy

obesity

parasomnias

pica

polysomnogram

purging

rumination disorder

sleep disorder

Every person has his or her own **body image**—the collection of perceptions, thoughts, feelings, and behaviors that relate to one's body size and appearance. Body image is an important part of self-concept. Positive body images lead to behaviors that express confidence and self-assurance. Negative body images can often lead to such problems as shyness and social isolation. Anxiety, depression, anorexia nervosa, bulimia, obesity, and other mental health problems are all interwoven with body image.

In the privacy of our thoughts, we all carry on dialogues or conversations with ourselves. Our internal dialogue that focuses on the body and appearance is our "private body talk." It is the content of our private body talk that helps to determine how we feel about our bodies.

Body image is also historically defined. Throughout European history, a large, fleshy body was considered a sign of wealth and prosperity. Only the wealthy could afford rich foods and extra pounds of body fat. Poor people were thin because they never got enough to eat. The same ideals followed our ancestors to the Americas. The wealthy remained well fed and overweight, while the remainder of the population worked hard and carried little extra weight.

By the early 1900s, things began to change. Economic situations became more secure, and people ate better. The style and attitude evolved from "fat's where it's at" to "thin is in," and the day of the dieter began. Since the early

262

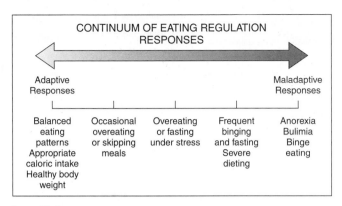

CONTINUUM OF EATING REGULATION RESPONSES

Adaptive Responses				Maladaptive Responses
Balanced eating patterns Appropriate caloric intake Healthy body weight	Occasional overeating or skipping meals	Overeating or fasting under stress	Frequent binging and fasting Severe dieting	Anorexia Bulimia Binge eating

Figure 23-1 Continuum of eating regulation responses. (Redrawn from Stuart GW, Laraia MT: *Principles and practice of psychiatric nursing,* ed 7, St. Louis, 2001, Mosby.)

part of this century, the emphasis on bodily appearance has centered around one's weight as a definition of beauty.

In most modern Western societies, a high value is placed on the thin body. Little tolerance is shown for individuals whose bodies are outside the range of "normal." Today anorexia nervosa is much more common in modern industrialized societies in which there is an abundance of food and a focus on being thin as a measure of attractiveness. A fear of obesity leads many persons to engage in unhealthy or destructive lifestyles. It seems that few people in modern Western societies are content with how their bodies look. Almost one third of Americans are dissatisfied with their weight. People who see themselves as too thin try to gain weight. People whose body images portray them as too fat try to lose weight.

Children learn early about which body images are desirable. It is not unusual to see boys imitating some popular, muscular hero or young girls dieting so that they may look like the latest underfed model. Because late childhood and early adolescence is a time for defining oneself, body image plays an important role (Wong, 1998). The desire for the perfect body can push young individuals toward many unsound physical and emotional habits.

This chapter focuses on the eating and sleeping problems considered mental health disorders. As with everything in life, an occasional skipped meal or night of lost sleep is not a problem (Figure 23-1), but when behaviors associated with eating or sleeping interfere with an individual's quality of daily life, they become mental health disorders.

EATING DISORDERS

An **eating disorder** is an ongoing disturbance in behaviors associated with the ingestion of food. The most common eating disorders are anorexia nervosa and bulimia.

Although obesity is not officially classified as an eating disorder, it presents problems for many individuals. According to the *Statistical Abstract of the United States* (U.S. Bureau of the Census, 1998), almost 30% of all adults consider that their actual weight is more than their desirable weight.

For adolescents the statistics relating to weight loss behaviors are alarming. Attempts to lose weight are very common among adolescents and adults. Girls as young as 8 years old are dieting, and the number of teens with serious eating disorders is increasing. Weight control methods practiced by adolescents include exercise, skipping meals, taking diet pills, and vomiting. The desire for thinness leads many young people into unhealthy behaviors that can eventually lead to severe mental health problems and life-threatening situations. Eating disorders are therefore one result of the quest for the perfect body.

Although the cause remains unknown, several theories and much research have attempted to explain the nature of eating disorders (Table 23-1).

Anorexia Nervosa

One of the most serious eating disorders is **anorexia nervosa,** a condition in which an individual does not maintain a normal body weight because of an intense fear of becoming fat. Actually the term *anorexia* (which in Greek means "want of appetite") is inaccurate because there is seldom an actual appetite loss associated with the disorder. The refusal to gain weight is a part of a strategy to solve a deep psychological problem and maintain some form of control. Because of the secrecy and social stigma associated with eating disorders, the exact number of persons with eating disorders is unknown.

Anorexia nervosa was first described more than 100 years ago as a mania to be thin. Since then the number of persons with this once-rare disorder has steadily grown to about 1 in 250 persons. Today approximately 90% to 95% of people with anorexia nervosa are female, but men are not immune to the disorder. Anorexia nervosa is seldom seen before puberty and rarely appears after 40 years of age. The average age of onset is about 17, but it is not uncommon to see anorectic behaviors in 12-year-olds. People who are concerned with their appearances for professional reasons, such as models, athletes, or flight attendants, are at a higher risk for developing anorexia nervosa. Early signs and symptoms of anorexia nervosa may be found in children with depressive symptoms and obsessive behaviors. Children from dysfunctional or abusive families are at a greater risk for developing the disorder.

Certain personality factors appear to be associated with anorexia nervosa. The classic description of a person with anorexia nervosa is a tense, alert, hyperactive, rigid woman who thinks, talks, and walks rapidly. She is very ambitious and drives herself to perfection. She is sensitive,

Table 23-1	Theories About the Nature of Eating Disorders

Theory	Description
Psychological	
Behavioral	Eating-disordered behaviors are attempts to reduce anxiety; discomfort with body image creates more anxiety, feelings of guilt and disgust, and loss of self-protecting boundaries.
Cognitive	Eating disorders are the result of deficits in attention, concentration, and vigilance related to underlying anxiety and depression.
Developmental	Individual fails to develop an appropriate sense of self and body; has problems with autonomy and self-identity; disorder is often brought about by a significant loss or crisis.
Sociocultural	Eating disorders are a response to a daily social emphasis on a stereotypical ideal of thinness; social stereotypes serve as stressors that drive women and girls to harmful dieting behaviors; anorexia nervosa is a way of mastering some control over the pressure on women to be successful in all areas of life.
Neurobiological	The causes for eating disorders involve complex relationships among the body's neurotransmitters; there is evidence of altered serotonin function; many of the same neuroendocrine findings are found in persons with depressive, and bipolar disorders; cortisol levels are altered in depression and eating disorders; anorexia nervosa decreases levels of luteinizing hormone and follicle-stimulating hormone, which results in menstrual irregularities.

Modified from Irwin EG: A focused overview of anorexia nervosa and bulimia: part 1, etiological issues, *Archives of Psychiatric Nursing* 7(6): 342, 1993.

insecure, and serious with a conscience that works overtime. Her neatness, self-will, and stubbornness make her difficult to treat, and her lack of warmth and friendliness allows her to make few friends. As she struggles to gain a self-respecting identity, she engages in "a relentless and successful pursuit of thinness that results in psychological and physiological disturbances" (Walsh, 1998).

The main issue is one of control, and the individual with anorexia nervosa becomes constricted, conforming, and obsessed with the need to control body weight. Some teenagers have a fear of growing up and sexually maturing. Anorexia nervosa allows them to prevent the onset of adulthood by delaying menses and the development of secondary sexual characteristics.

Clinical Presentation

Weight concerns put adolescents (especially girls) at a high risk for developing anorexia nervosa. Dieting, body dissatisfaction, current body weight below body weight ideals, and unusual eating patterns do not necessarily indicate an eating disorder, but when the quest for thinness results in the refusal to maintain a normal body weight, anorexia nervosa may be diagnosed.

To be diagnosed with anorexia nervosa, the individual must meet the four criteria listed in Box 23-1.

Figure 23-2 shows a typical anorectic woman before and after treatment.

People with anorexia nervosa have a self-esteem that is highly dependent on body size and shape. They often go to great measures to monitor their bodies, such as weighing three or four times a day, measuring body parts, and frequently looking in the mirror to check for areas of fat. The ability to lose weight is considered a sign of control and extraordinary self-discipline. Conversely, even the smallest gain in weight is seen as a threat and a failure of self-control. Some individuals may actually acknowledge their extreme thinness, but they typically deny the seriousness of their condition.

Anorexia nervosa is a *life-threatening disorder.* One study demonstrated that the mortality rate for anorexia "due to complications of starvation or suicide, is substantial, approximately 5% per decade of follow-up" (Walsh, 1998). This death rate is far higher than for any other mental illness. Death usually results from dehydration, loss of critical muscle mass, electrolyte imbalances, or suicide. Often clients are not seen by health professionals until the disorder has resulted in some physical problem.

Behaviorally, many anorectic persons have a preoccupation with food. They may save recipes or prepare elaborate meals and then cut their own food into small pieces and push it around the plate without eating. New evidence suggests that anorexia nervosa may stem from a food phobia (Travis, 1998). Obsessive behavior with food often extends into other obsessive-compulsive activities, such as a preoccupation with studying, exercising, or cleaning. Often individuals have poor sexual adjustment, with delayed sexual development or little interest in sex.

An inability to effectively cope or solve problems commonly exists. The history frequently is positive for anxiety, depression, or substance abuse. People with anorexia nervosa need intervention, but they often deny the seriousness of their problems until extensive physical

Criteria for Diagnosis of Anorexia Nervosa

1. A refusal to maintain body weight that is more than 15% below normal.
2. Even though the individual is underweight, an intense fear of becoming fat exists.
3. A distorted (inaccurate) significance placed on body weight and shape (person "feels fat" and perceives self as fat despite being underweight).
4. An absence of at least three menstrual cycles in a female who has previously menstruated.

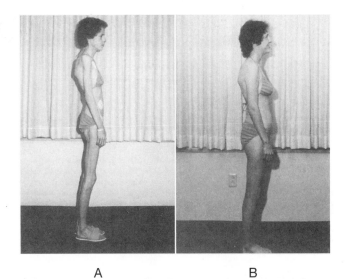

A   B

Figure 23-2 **A,** Anoretic woman before treatment. **B,** Same woman after gradual refeeding, nutritional management, and psychological therapy. (From Williams SR: *Basic nutrition and diet therapy,* ed 10, St. Louis, 1995, Mosby.)

damage has taken place. Nurses in every setting must be alert for the clues of anorexia nervosa because early intervention will often save a life that otherwise may literally waste away.

Bulimia

Bulimia is a disorder of binge eating and the use of inappropriate methods to prevent weight gain. Although anorexia nervosa may be a more dramatic problem, bulimia occurs more commonly. "The estimated incidence of anorexia nervosa in women is approximately 1%. Bulimia incidence rates vary among 4%, 8%, and 10.3%, depending on the population, method, and criteria used" (Carley and Rooda, 1995). Estimates of the incidence of bulimia in college-age women are as high as 19%.

Bulimia is most commonly found in young, white, middle-class and upper-class women. Men account for about one out of nine cases. There is an increased frequency of anxiety, depression, and drug abuse among individuals with bulimia. About one third to one half also meet the diagnostic criteria for a personality disorder. Because it is difficult to detect, many individuals with bulimia go untreated. Like anorexia nervosa, bulimia appears to be more of a problem in modern industrialized countries.

Binge eating is defined as consuming (within a certain period of time) an amount of food that is definitely larger than most individuals would eat in similar circumstances. During a binge, an individual often consumes large amounts of certain foods, usually carbohydrates. It is not unusual for the bingeing person to eat as much as 5000 calories in donuts, cakes, or other sweets. The binge lasts about 1 to 2 hours and then is followed by feelings of guilt and attempts to rid the body of the food just consumed.

Two subtypes of bulimia are classified according to the presence or absence of purging behaviors. **Purging** is an attempt to rid the gastrointestinal tract and body of unwanted food. The most common purging behaviors are vomiting and the use of diuretics and laxatives. Less commonly, some people use syrup of ipecac or enemas to purge.

The individual with "nonpurging type" of bulimia does not purge after a binge but uses other inappropriate methods to prevent weight gain, such as fasting between binges and exercising excessively.

The personality traits of persons with bulimia differ from those with anorexia nervosa. The average individual with bulimia is a woman who is slightly older and more outgoing than her anorectic counterpart. She is socially and sexually active and actually experiences hunger and feels distressed about her abnormal eating behaviors. Often her body weight is normal or even slightly above average. It is not uncommon for other mental health problems, such as substance abuse, self-mutilation, or hysteria, to be present at the same time. Refer to Table 23-2 for a comparison of the key features of anorexia nervosa and bulimia.

When it comes to body image, people with bulimia typically view themselves as fat or thin. Being in the middle, or average, is not considered. Not infrequently a woman with bulimia fears that she must follow a diet for the rest of her life if she gives up binge eating.

Perfectionism is often seen with bulimia and contributes to maintaining bulimic behaviors. Bulimic women frequently have unrealistic expectations about themselves and how their lives should run. They become frustrated by their own inabilities to reach unrealistic goals. If they experience failure, they conclude that they were unable to reach the goal because they were weak, not trying hard enough, inadequate, or unlovable or had some other negative failing. In short, these are the "I should have . . ."

Table 23-2	Key Features of Anorexia and Bulimia	
Anorexia nervosa	**Bulimia**
Rare use of vomiting, diuretics, laxatives	Vomiting or diuretics, laxative abuse
More severe weight loss	Less weight loss
Slightly younger	Slightly older
More introverted	More extroverted, social
Hunger denied	Hunger experienced
Eating behavior may be considered normal and source of esteem	Eating behavior considered foreign and a source of distress
Sexually inactive	More sexually active
May be obsessive or compulsive	May have hysterical or borderline, as well as obsessive, behaviors
Death from starvation or suicide	Death from hypokalemia or suicide
Amenorrhea	Menses irregular or absent
Fewer behavioral abnormalities	Stealing, drug and alcohol abuse, self-mutilation, and other behavioral abnormalities

Modified from Physicians of the Geisinger Health System: *Help for anorexia nervosa*, 1997.

Box 23-2 Criteria for Diagnosis of Bulimia

1. Recurring episodes of binge eating
2. Bingeing followed by recurring inappropriate behaviors to prevent weight gain
3. Eating binges occur at least twice a week for at least 3 months
4. Excessive emphasis is placed on body shape and weight in determining self-esteem

---

types who are never satisfied at their own efforts. Even when successful, they seldom can enjoy their accomplishments because they tell themselves that they should have done it better, sooner, or more efficiently. The desire to become the perfect person commonly leads to feelings of failure and uselessness. When life is based on the all-or-nothing principle, anything short of perfect is considered to be a failure. Unfortunately this means most of their time is spent in feeling that they are truly "nothing." Perfection, in reality, is not attainable.

Clinical Presentation

To receive the diagnosis of bulimia, a person must meet four basic criteria:

1. The most essential feature is recurring episodes of binge eating. Individuals are usually ashamed of their binges and often eat in secret. Episodes of binge eating may or may not be planned in advance. During the bingeing episodes, the individual feels out of control and often attacks eating in a frenzied state.
2. Bingeing is followed by recurring inappropriate behaviors to prevent weight gain. The most popular method of purging is to induce vomiting (80% to 90%), which

relieves the physical discomfort of a full stomach and the emotional fear of gaining weight. "In some cases vomiting becomes a goal in itself, and the person will binge in order to vomit or will vomit after eating a small amount of food" (American Psychiatric Association, 2000). Other methods of purging include the misuse of laxatives, diuretics, enemas, and syrup of ipecac. Some people use a combination of methods to purge, engage in strenuous exercise at inappropriate times, or follow semistarvation diets after a bingeing episode.

3. The eating binges must occur at least twice a week for at least 3 months. Patterns of binge eating range from several episodes a day to a regular and persistent pattern. Often episodes are triggered by a stressful event or experience.
4. Individuals place excessive emphasis on body shape and weight in determining their self-esteem. They are dissatisfied with their imperfect bodies, have a fear of gaining weight, and often restrict their caloric intake or choose low-calorie foods between binge-eating episodes (Box 23-2).

When purging behaviors are frequent, fluid and electrolyte abnormalities can result. The few persons who use syrup of ipecac are at risk for developing serious cardiac and skeletal muscle wasting. Although death from bulimia is rare, the underlying psychiatric problems are often more severe than those seen with anorectic persons.

Many times, the signs and of anorexia and bulimia occur together in the same individual. Both disorders are complex and often interrelated with other mental health problems.

Obesity

According to the *Diagnostic and Statistical Manual of Mental Disorders* (DSM-IV–TR), obesity is not listed as a mental health disorder because it has not been established that obesity is consistently associated with mental health or behavioral problems. However, obesity is linked to many physical and psychological problems that cause distress for most overweight individuals.

Obesity is defined as an excess of body weight. Clients are classified as mildly obese (20% to 40% above normal weight), moderately obese (41% to 100% above normal weight), and severely (morbidly) obese (over 100% above normal weight). Concern with being overweight is common in modern industrialized societies in which the luxury of chronic overeating and underexercising is available. Obesity is a relatively rare condition in less-developed societies. In some cultures it is seen as a sign of wealth and prosperity (see Cultural Aspects box).

Obesity is the result of too many calories consumed or not enough calories burned (Figure 23-3). As with the person with bulimia or alcoholism, many overweight individuals lose control over their eating. Although the eating patterns of obese individuals do not pose an immediate threat, being chronically overweight can eventually result in severe physical and emotional problems. Today much money and time are spent in the pursuit of losing weight throughout the industrialized world.

The causes of obesity are several. In addition to overeating, other factors have been discovered that may help explain obesity. Complicated neurochemical mechanisms that help to control appetite and eating behaviors are being studied. Heredity also appears to play a role in the development of obesity. The children of obese parents tend to be overweight themselves. Obese persons have larger fat cells in their bodies. Finally, a lack of sufficient exercise also contributes greatly to obesity.

Faulty eating behaviors appear to begin in childhood. Many overweight persons once relied on food to numb the discomforts of growing up. Throughout childhood, eating helped to relieve the emotional distresses of life. This pattern of lessening emotional pain by eating is called **compulsive overeating**. In time, food becomes like a drug, with a "fix" that temporarily lessens psychological discomforts of an ever-growing desire for more food.

As the individual continues to find comfort in food, he or she grows physically more obese and less attractive to others. (Remember our cultural stigmas against obesity.) This behavior serves only to increase feelings of worthlessness, and the person again eats to relieve the pain. A vicious circle soon becomes established, and the person begins to replace social relationships with the comforts of food. Compulsive overeating can become a lonely way of life.

Clinical Presentation

The first signs of obesity are seen early in life. An estimate may be made by comparing one's height and weight to a standardized chart. "Children who are 20% over normal

Cultural Aspects

The island nation of Nauru lies south of the equator in the western Pacific Ocean. Most Nauruans lead an inactive lifestyle because the island's phosphate mines are worked by immigrant miners. Almost all food and water is imported from Australia.

Eating processed foods is considered a sign of wealth. Obesity is seen as attractive, and overweight women are sought as wives. Nauru has the highest rate of diabetes in the world.

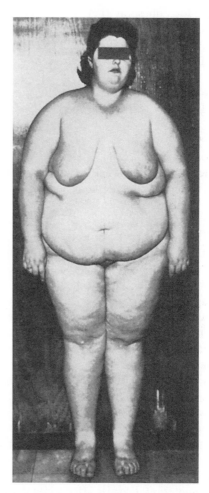

Figure 23-3 Obesity. (From Seidel HM and others: *Mosby's guide to physical examination,* ed 4, St. Louis, 1999, Mosby.)

for their height and weight should undergo further evaluation, including a height and weight history of the child, parents, and siblings, as well as eating habits, appetite, and hunger patterns, and physical activity" (Wong, 1998).

As overweight children grow and mature, they begin to sense society's disapproval of their obesity. Youngsters may begin to diet and exercise or react by continuing to find comfort in food. Dieting and other weight-loss methods soon become a way of life for many overweight people at a young age. During adolescence weight becomes an important part of a newly forming body image. Teens may rebel against parental nagging to lose weight or become unwilling to control their caloric intake. They may resort to unhealthy methods, such as prolonged fasting or purging, to gain some control over their weight. Not infrequently they will ignore their obesity and eat as though a problem does not exist.

The cycle of "I'm not attractive, so I'll eat because it makes me feel better" becomes ingrained as a way of coping in childhood. Many overweight individuals become even more obese as they grow older. Eventually, the numerous chronic health problems associated with moderate or severe obesity begin to appear. These problems increase anxiety and further encourage the individual to seek the comfort that food has so frequently brought in the past. The cycle continues, and problems grow.

Other Eating Disorders

Two less common eating disorders are pica and rumination. **Pica** is the persistent eating of nonnutritive substances (nonfood items) that lasts for more than 1 month. Substances, such as clay, laundry starch, insects, leaves, or pebbles are chosen for ingestion. The person with pica still eats and enjoys food. He or she just has an overwhelming need to eat the nonfood item. Many times the cause of pica can be traced to a vitamin, mineral, or calorie deficiency. The Case Study presents an interesting case history of pica. Treatment for pica is to rule out the presence of any physical problem or deficiency and then to assist clients in establishing more healthful eating habits.

Rumination disorder is an uncommon problem most often seen in childhood. It is defined as the regurgitation and rechewing of food. According to the DSM-IV–TR, "partially digested food is brought up into the mouth without apparent nausea, retching, disgust, or associated gastrointestinal disorder. The food is then either ejected from the mouth or, more frequently, chewed and reswallowed."

When rumination disorder affects infants, death from malnutrition can result. In older children and adults, malnutrition is less of a problem. This disorder can occur continuously or appear at intervals. Psychosocial problems, such as lack of attention, neglect, or a stressful environment, may be risk factors. Other feeding disorders of early childhood are discussed in Chapter 14.

Guidelines for Intervention

The main therapeutic goal for all eating disorders is to establish behaviors that promote health for the individual.

Although it sounds simple, this is a lofty goal. People with eating disorders have learned to cope with their stresses by focusing on food in one way or another. Those with anorexia nervosa attempt to cope by controlling, and the highest form of control is the ability to rule over one's body size. Individuals with bulimia learn to numb emotional pain by eating large amounts of food, and then they suffer through overwhelming guilt. Many persons who experience the discomforts of obesity have developed compulsive overeating habits to fill their needs for love and belonging.

Treatments and Therapies

The treatment for anorexia nervosa and bulimia requires medical and mental health interventions. There are three immediate (short-term) goals of treatment:
1. To stabilize existing medical problems
2. To reestablish normal nutritional and eating patterns
3. To help the client resolve the psychological or emotional issues that underlie the disordered eating behaviors

Medical care centers around nutritional management of the client. Individuals with severe weight loss may receive total parenteral nutrition (hyperalimentation), in which all the necessary nutrients are administered through an intravenous line placed in a large blood vessel. For less severely malnourished clients, intravenous therapy or tube feedings may be ordered, but the main focus is to encourage the client to voluntarily consume food.

Clients are weighed daily, and supplemental vitamins are usually prescribed. Clients are closely observed for secret anorectic or bulimic behaviors. The long-term goals of medical treatment (for both underweight and overweight clients) focus on teaching clients about good nutrition and assisting them in developing appropriate eating habits.

The goals of mental health care focus on helping clients improve their self-esteem and develop more effective coping skills. Once clients are physically stable, they are encouraged to adopt proper eating habits. Behavior modification techniques may help to reinforce healthful eating behaviors. Signs of depression are diagnosed and treated. Often family therapy is helpful. Individual or group therapy helps clients to focus on the psychological conflicts that underlie their inappropriate eating behaviors. Drug therapy can be quite effective, but only if it is combined with some form of psychotherapy. Amphetamines have been successfully used to treat obesity. However, their potential for addiction is high, and they are not frequently prescribed. Antidepressants or lithium has been used with success in the treatment of bulimia (see Drug Alert box).

Nurses and other health care providers play an important role in caring for individuals with altered eating patterns in both the hospital and community setting. The main goals are to assist clients in identifying and coping with the problems that led them to their inappropriate eating behaviors. Possible nursing diagnoses relating to eating disorders are listed in Box 23-3.

To accomplish the goals of care, nurses first work to establish rapport and trust with clients. Then they assist their clients in identifying how food is used to provide comfort and reduce anxiety. During the working phase of the therapeutic relationship, clients are helped to replace distorted ideas about their body images with thoughts and behaviors that build self-esteem. Problem-solving skills are taught, and clients are encouraged to identify the social support systems that encourage healthful practices. Refer to the Sample Client Care Plan for clients with eating disorders. Every individual with an eating disorder needs the understanding and compassion of health care providers. Hopefully, health care providers can help make the struggles of clients with eating disorders a little less difficult by nurturing and supporting more effective coping behaviors.

Case Study

Loren was assigned to rounds with the mobile clinic nurse, whose responsibility was to provide prenatal services for a group of poor women from a rural farming region. As he rode through the countryside, he was surprised to see how many pregnant women and children were working in the fields. He asked the clinic nurse how long field workers were expected to work during their pregnancies and was surprised to find that they were expected to be in the fields until the onset of labor. "How do they get enough to eat when they are working in the fields?" he wondered.

The mobile clinic nurse, sensing Loren's curiosity, assigned him to obtain dietary histories from as many of the farm workers as he could. By the time Loren had completed four histories, he was amazed. Not only were the workers' daily diets poor, but many of the pregnant clients made it a habit to carry laundry starch into the fields with them. During the day, as they became hungry, they would eat a handful of laundry starch and drink a few sips of water.

When Loren finally mustered enough courage to ask one of the women why she ate laundry starch, she told him that it "takes the edge off my hunger and lets me work a little longer. Some of the ladies even eat clay, if it's a good kind."

It seemed that eating the laundry starch provided these women with a substitute for more expensive calories. The need to eat clay may have indicated the presence of a mineral deficiency.

◆ How do you think the infants will be affected by their mothers' dietary habits?

SLEEP DISORDERS

Sleeping patterns and routines change as we grow older The 16 hours of nightly sleep required by the infant dwindles to less than 8 hours by adulthood. The afternoon naps of childhood are soon replaced by the all-day demands of school and work, whereas the ritual of the bedtime hour disappears altogether. By the time many persons reach adulthood, their sleeping habits may have changed dramatically. Most young adults have few difficulties with sleeping. However, sleep disorders begin to occur more frequently as adults grow older. By older adulthood, it is unusual to have a full night of uninterrupted sleep.

Although no one knows exactly why we must sleep every night, researchers have found that sleep serves several purposes. During sleep, bodily functions and

Drug Alert

Administering antidepressants to clients with anorexia nervosa before they regain weight may be hazardous if the individual has a history of cardiac problems or presently has a low serum potassium level. For this reason, the physician may order a trial dose of the antidepressants.

Be sure to check the laboratory results of clients with eating disorders. Withhold the medication and notify the physician if the potassium level drops below normal limits.

Box 23-3 NANDA Nursing Diagnoses Related to Eating Disorders

Activity intolerance
Adjustment, impaired
Body image disturbance*
Coping, ineffective individual*
Denial, ineffective
Failure to thrive, adult
Fluid volume deficit, risk for
Health maintenance, altered
Noncompliance
Nutrition, altered: less than body requirements*
Personal identity disturbance
Self-esteem disturbance*
Sexuality patterns, altered
Social isolation
Thought processes, altered, risk for
Violence, risk for: self-directed

From North American Nursing Diagnosis Association: *NANDA nursing diagnoses: definitions and classification 1999-2000,* Philadelphia, 1999, The Association.
*Primary nursing diagnosis for eating disorders.

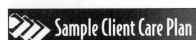 **Sample Client Care Plan**   Eating Disorder

Assessment

History: Erica is a 15-year-old who is 20 pounds under her usual body weight. She has always been a "chubby child" who had no problems eating until the beginning of this school year. Three months ago Erica told her mother to stop fixing "all those fattening foods" and began refusing her meals.

Current Findings: A thin, tired-appearing adolescent girl who appears older than her stated age. Face is hollow, eyes sunken, and skin is dry. Hair is fine and brittle. Skin is covered with lanugo (fine hair). Skin turgor is poor. Vital signs are low for age and size.

When questioned, Erica states that she "feels fine" and does not "know what all the fuss is about." "Just because I choose to lose a few pounds everybody gets upset. Sounds like this is their problem more than mine. I'm really still too fat."

Multidisciplinary Diagnosis

Alteration in nutrition: less than body requirements related to distorted self-image

Planning/Goals

Erica will voluntarily consume 2000 calories a day by July 4.

Erica will gain 1 pound of body weight per week.

Therapeutic Interventions

Intervention	Rationale	Team Member
1. Establish trust and gain Erica's cooperation.	Erica must first agree to work with the staff if other interventions are to achieve therapeutic results.	All
2. Perform a complete nutritional assessment.	Establishes a baseline from which to judge progress.	Diet, Nsg
3. Help Erica identify the consequences of her eating behaviors.	Helps her acknowledge the problem and its effects on her life.	Psy, Nsg
4. Monitor physical status daily for signs of malnutrition.	To prevent further physical problems and decline.	Nsg, MD
5. Explore other ways to achieve control over the parts of Erica's life that are causing distress.	When control is achieved in one area, it tends to spread to other areas; control builds self-image and confidence.	All
6. Involve family members in therapy if possible.	Erica may benefit from supportive family members; offers an opportunity to assess family interactions.	Psy, Nsg

Evaluation

During the first week Erica consumed an average of 1000 calories per day with much encouragement. By July 3, Erica was voluntarily consuming about 1800 calories per day. Weight gain averaged 1/2 pound per week.

A complete client care plan includes several other diagnoses and interventions.

---

metabolic rate slow, decreasing the workload on the heart. Muscles relax and the body conserves energy during sleep. One theory states that sleep is important for the renewal and repair of body cells and tissues. Sleep also "appears to be a critical cycle of brain activity important for learning, memory, and behavioral adaptation" (Potter and Perry, 1998).

The dreaming that takes place during sleep is also important for health. Dreaming allows us to gain insights, solve problems, work through emotional reactions, and prepare for the future. Many cultures place great meaning in dreams and use them to cope with the problems of everyday reality (see Think About box).

Sleep occurs in cycles of about 24 hours, depending on each individual's personal body rhythms. There are two phases to sleep: nonrapid eye movement (NREM sleep) and rapid eye movement (REM sleep). NREM sleep is divided into four stages.

The average adult's sleep pattern begins with a presleep period, lasting from about 10 to 30 minutes.

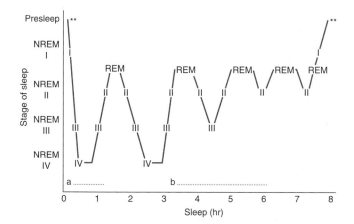

Figure 23-4 Normal adult sleep cycle and the stages of sleep. (Modified from Biddle C, Oaster TRF: Adult sleep cycles, *Journal of the American Association of Nurse Anesthetists* 58(1): 36, 1990.)

During this time, a gradual drowsiness develops until the individual "drops off to sleep" or enters stage 1 of NREM sleep. As the sleeper moves through each stage of NREM, the quality of sleep becomes deeper. During stage 4, the sleeper is most difficult to arouse. After reaching stage 4, the sleep pattern reverses, and the sleeper moves back through stages 3 and 2, where REM sleep takes place. Figure 23-4 illustrates the normal adult sleep cycle and its stages. If the sleeper is interrupted or awakened at any time during the cycle, he or she must return to stage 1 and begin the process again. If the disturbances occur frequently enough, the individual will experience the signs and symptoms of sleep deprivation. Everyone has the occasional poor night's sleep. For people with sleeping disorders, however, this experience becomes an unwelcome and unwanted way of life.

A **sleep disorder** is a condition or problem that repeatedly disrupts an individual's pattern of sleep. Problems with sleep are very common in modern societies in which the pace of life is fast and demanding. Sleep disorders occur more frequently in the elderly, but all age groups can be affected.

The diagnosis of a sleep disorder is based on a thorough history, physical examination, and the results of several tests. A **polysomnogram** monitors the client's electrophysical responses during sleep. It includes such measurements as brain wave activity (electroencephalo-gram), muscle movement (electromyogram), and extraocular eye movements (electrooculogram). Many medical centers have specially designed sleep laboratories where clients can be monitored for the quantity, quality, and characteristics of their sleep.

Sleep disorders are divided into two basic types: primary sleep disorders and those related to other conditions (secondary sleep disorders) (Figure 23-5). Primary sleep disorders are thought to be related to abnormal functioning of the sleep-wake or timing mechanisms of the body. The two subdivisions of primary sleep disorders are called the *dyssomnias* and the *parasomnias*.

Dyssomnias

Dyssomnias are characterized "by abnormalities in the amount, quality, or timing of sleep" (American Psychiatric Association, 2000) and include such problems as insomnia, hypersomnia, narcolepsy, breathing-related and circadian rhythm sleep disorders. Insomnia occurs most frequently.

Insomnia is a disorder of falling asleep or maintaining a sound sleep (Insomnia, 1998). It is often associated with increased physical and mental alertness at nighttime and sleepiness during the day. The individual who cannot regularly fall asleep often becomes preoccupied and distressed. This contributes to the development of more anxiety about sleep and sets up a vicious cycle in which the harder they "try" to fall asleep, the more difficult it becomes. Often, people are worried, anxious, or concerned about something when they prepare for sleep.

As nights of interrupted sleep continue, individuals become negatively conditioned toward sleep and begin to expect a poor night's sleep. Eventually, *chronic insomnia* develops and persists long after the problem that caused the initial sleep loss is solved. Chronic insomnia often leads to decreased feelings of well-being during waking hours, along with a lack of energy or motivation; decreased attention span, energy, and concentration; or a general worsening of moods and emotional reactions.

Insomnia is relatively rare in childhood and adolescence. Approximately 30% to 40% of adults have problems with insomnia, and the incidence increases with age. It is seen more often in women and usually begins in young adulthood or middle age with an initial period of poor sleep that progressively worsens over a period of months. Some people experience periodic episodes of insomnia, whereas others develop a chronic ineffective sleep pattern that may last for years. Many individuals with insomnia have a history of being "light sleepers" who are easily disturbed by environmental noises or other distractions.

Primary hypersomnia is an excessive sleepiness that usually begins between 15 and 30 years of age, slowly progresses over a period of weeks or months, and then becomes chronic and stable. Hypersomnia is character-

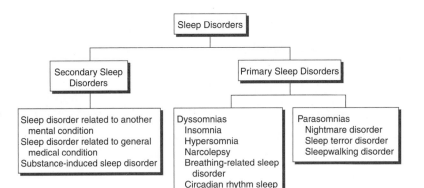

Figure 23-5 Classification of sleep disorders.

ized by prolonged sleep episodes or daytime sleeping that occurs daily for at least 1 month; excessive sleepiness severe enough to cause significant distress or impairment in the activities of daily living; and excessive sleepiness that is not caused by any other physical or mental health disorder.

In persons with hypersomnia, nighttime sleep may last from 8 to 12 hours, but it is often followed by difficulty awakening in the morning and excessive sleepiness during normal waking hours. During the day, these people may take long naps, which commonly last for more than an hour. After awakening, individuals do not feel more refreshed or alert.

Hypersomnia can lead to significant distress in a person's functioning. The long sleep and difficult morning awakenings make it nearly impossible to meet morning business or social obligations. Low levels of alertness result in decreased concentration, poor efficiency, and few memories of the day's events. Unplanned episodes of sleep can lead to embarrassing and even dangerous situations, such as falling asleep while driving a car. Daytime sleepiness can result in automatic behavior in which tasks are carried out with little or no memory of having done them. Sadly, people with excessive sleepiness are often thought of as lazy or indifferent.

Narcolepsy is an uncommon condition in which an individual has repeated attacks of sleep. Symptoms usually become apparent during adolescence, but a careful history often reveals a pattern of sleepiness dating back to preschool years. The onset of the disorder often follows a change in the person's sleep-wake schedule or a very stressful event.

The periods of sleepiness in narcolepsy are described as irresistible. Individuals fall asleep for about 10 to 20 minutes in any situation, whether it is appropriate to sleep or not. Episodes occur from two to six times a day. Some people with narcolepsy can "fight off" their sleep attacks, whereas others plan naps throughout the day to manage the condition.

Two other distressing features of narcolepsy are cataplexy and inappropriate rapid eye movement. Cata-

plexy is a sudden episode of muscle weakness and loss of muscle tone that lasts for seconds to minutes. These episodes are often brought about by an intense emotion. Inappropriate rapid eye movement occurs during the transition between sleep and wakefulness during which dreamlike hallucinations or paralysis of voluntary muscles occurs.

Breathing-related sleep disorders are more common than once thought. They are defined as sleep disruptions caused by abnormal ventilation during sleep. The most common form is called *obstructive sleep apnea* syndrome. During sleep a partially obstructed upper airway causes periods of apnea that repeatedly awaken the individual. Sleeping patterns are characterized by periods of loud snoring, followed by periods of apnea lasting as long as 90 seconds. The apneic event is ended when the individual gasps, moans, mumbles, or shakes with loud air-gulping snores. Although the person may not fully awaken during these events, sleep is disrupted enough to result in excessive sleepiness during the day. People who are extremely overweight are at risk for this disorder. The term *pickwickian syndrome* was coined to describe this disorder based on an obese character in a Charles Dickens novel.

Another dyssomnia is called *circadian rhythm sleep disorder,* a persistent pattern of sleep disruption that results from a mismatch between personal body rhythms and the demands of the environment. This disorder is most often seen in persons who do shift work or must travel frequently.

Disruptions in sleep can also be caused by environmental factors, restless leg syndrome, or nocturnal myoclonus. *Restless legs syndrome* is described as disagreeable sensations, such as pricking, tingling, itching, or crawling, that occur while falling asleep or during sleep. The sensations are relieved by moving the legs or walking and return when the legs are still. *Nocturnal myoclonus* is also called idiopathic periodic limb movements. These repeated, brief jerks occur mostly in the legs at the beginning of sleep and decrease during stage 4 NREM sleep. Because the movements take place every 20 to 60 seconds, they disturb normal sleep patterns.

Parasomnias

Sleep disorders characterized by abnormal behavioral or physical events during sleep are called **parasomnias.** It is believed that parasomnia sleep disorders are caused by the inappropriate activation of certain brain centers that govern physical and emotional functions (Hobson and Silvestri, 1999). People with parasomnias most often complain of unusual behaviors during sleep instead of daytime sleepiness. The most common parasomnias are nightmare disorder, sleep terror disorder, and sleepwalking disorder.

The most important feature of *nightmare disorder* is repeated frightening dreams that lead to abrupt awakenings. The individual is fully alert on awakening and significantly distressed from the experience. Awakenings may be accompanied by fight-flight responses, such as sweating, rapid respirations, and rapid heartbeat. Often a sense of anxiety lingers after the individual is awake, and he or she finds it difficult to return to sleep. The nightmares produce images that are often remembered in detail after awakening.

Sleep terror disorder is repeated nightmares and abrupt awakenings accompanied by a panicky cry or scream and intense fear. During the episode the person cannot be comforted or awakened without difficulty. Usually the individual does not awaken but returns to sleep. There is no memory of the event on morning awakening. Sleep terrors usually occur only once a night during stages 3 and 4 of NREM sleep. They are often accompanied by the physical signs of intense stress, such as increased heart rate, respirations, and muscle tone.

Sleepwalking disorder is characterized by episodes of complex motor movement during sleep. Individuals who sleepwalk rise from their beds and begin to walk around. They often have a blank stare and are not responsive to communication or efforts to awaken them. If awakened during or after an episode, they remember little about the event and may have a brief period of confusion until they become oriented. Sleepwalking is first seen between the ages of 4 and 8. It peaks by about age 12 and usually disappears by adolescence. First-time episodes of sleepwalking rarely occur in adults.

Other Sleep Disorders

Other sleep disorders can be traced to specific causes. They include sleep disorders related to a general medical condition, a mental health condition, and the use of chemical substances. Sleep disorders can result from many physical problems. The presence of a neurological, cardiovascular, or respiratory disorder or an infection has a significant effect on sleep. Pain from musculoskeletal disease and anxiety related to coughing or difficult breathing can lead to prolonged periods of inadequate sleep.

Many mental disorders are associated with sleep-related problems. Insomnia or hypersomnia is often seen in clients with major depressive, mood, anxiety, adjustment, somatoform, panic, and personality disorders. During flare-ups of schizophrenia, people have significant periods of insomnia.

Sleeping problems can occur during substance use (intoxication) or periods of withdrawal from the substance. Many prescription medications are associated with sleep disorders, including drugs that treat hypertension, cardiac problems, inflammatory processes, neurological conditions, and respiratory diseases. Chemicals such as alcohol, cocaine, and various street drugs affect sleep. Even the medications prescribed to induce sleep (hypnotics and sedatives) produce unwanted effects on the sleep cycle. Nurses and other caregivers must be aware of how various medications and chemicals affect each client's sleep.

Guidelines for Interventions

The first step in the treatment of sleep disorders is to teach prevention. Because many people do not regularly receive a good night's sleep, the need for good sleep hygiene habits is great. One of the best treatments for insomnia is to establish and maintain a regular sleeping routine by preparing both body and mind for the night's upcoming rest. Health care providers are in ideal positions to educate clients about the importance of receiving enough quality sleep. Box 23-4 offers several suggestions for effective sleep practices.

The main goal of care is to assist the client in obtaining a restful night's sleep. Short-term goals focus on helping clients establish a regular and healthy sleep pattern. Nursing diagnoses for sleep disorders include sleep pattern disturbance, high risk for injury, fatigue, altered thought processes, ineffective (individual, family) coping, ineffective breathing pattern, and knowledge deficit related to sleep hygiene practices.

Therapeutic interventions are aimed at promoting comfort, controlling physical disturbances, and maintaining a quiet, restful environment. Hypnotics (sleeping pills) may be administered as ordered, but only after all other methods of inducing sleep have failed. Special care must be taken when administering hypnotics or sedatives to older persons because they react strongly to these classes of medications.

Recent research has demonstrated that morning bright light therapy improves the sleeping patterns of older adults with dementia by helping reestablish natural biological rhythms (Mishima and others, 1994) and has revealed that the body has a naturally occurring sleep hormone, called *melatonin*, which helps to control our biological clocks. These findings may prove to be promising developments in the treatment of sleep disorders.

Box 23-4 Sleep Hygiene Strategies

Set a regular bedtime and wake-up time, 7 days a week.

Exercise daily; however, vigorous exercise too close to bedtime may make falling asleep difficult.

Schedule time to wind down and relax before bed.

Avoid worrying when trying to fall asleep.

Guard against nighttime interruptions. Earplugs may help with a noisy partner. Heavy window shades help to screen out light. Create a comfortable bed.

Maintain a cool temperature in the room. A warm bath or warm drink before bed often helps.

Excessive hunger or fullness may interfere with sleep. Avoid large meals before bed. If hungry, a light carbohydrate snack may be helpful.

Avoid caffeinated drinks, excessive fluid intake, stimulating drugs, and excessive alcohol in the evening and before bedtime.

Excessive daytime napping may make it difficult for some people to fall asleep at night.

Do not eat, read, work, or watch television in bed. The bed should be used only for sleep and sex.

Maintain a reasonable weight. Excessive weight may result in daytime fatigue and sleep apnea.

Get out of bed and engage in other activities if unable to fall asleep.

From Stuart GW, Laraia MT: *Stuart and Sundeen's pocket guide to psychiatric nursing,* ed 5, St. Louis, 1998, Mosby.

Become aware of the importance of keeping client environment dark during sleep and brightly lit during daylight hours. Read about the new developments in the treatment of sleeping disorders and apply them to yourself and your clients because we are learning more every day about the mysteries of sleep.

KEY CONCEPTS

◆ Body image is the collection of perceptions, thoughts, feelings, and behaviors that relate to body size and appearance.

◆ An eating disorder is an ongoing disturbance in behaviors associated with the ingestion of food.

◆ One of the most serious eating disorders is anorexia nervosa, a condition in which an individual refuses to maintain a normal body weight because of an intense fear of becoming fat.

◆ Bulimia is a disorder of binge eating and the use of inappropriate methods to prevent weight gain.

◆ Obesity is defined as an excess of body weight. Although not officially classified as an eating disorder, it presents problems for a great number of people.

◆ The main therapeutic goal for treating all eating disorders is to establish eating behaviors that promote health and to assist their clients in identifying and coping with the problems that lead to their inappropriate eating behaviors.

◆ A sleeping disorder is a condition or problem that repeatedly disrupts an individual's pattern of sleep.

◆ Dyssomnias are characterized by abnormalities in the amount, quality, or timing of sleep.

◆ Sleep disorders characterized by abnormal behavioral or physical events during sleep are called parasomnias.

◆ Sleep disorders can also result from medical, psychological, or drug-induced conditions.

◆ The first step in the treatment of sleep disorders is to teach good sleep hygiene habits.

◆ Therapeutic interventions to promote sleep are aimed at promoting comfort, controlling physical disturbances, and maintaining a quiet, restful environment.

Suggestions for Further Reading

Christine Gorman's article, "Get Some Sleep: Bothered by Insomnia," (*Time,* p. 225, March 29, 1999) offers effective habits for obtaining a good night's sleep without the use of drugs.

The American Anorexia Bulimia Association (www.aabainc.org) offers help lines, referral networks, support groups, and public information about anorexia and bulimia.

References

American Psychiatric Association: *Diagnostic and statistical manual of mental disorders,* ed 4, text revision, Washington, DC, 2000, The Association.

Biddle C, Oaster TRF: Adult sleep cycles, *Journal of the American Association of Nurse Anesthetists* 58(1): 36, 1990.

Carley J, Rooda L: Help for eating disorders, *Advances in Nursing Practice* 3(9):31, 1995.

Hobson JA, Silvestri L: Parasomnias, *Harvard Mental Health Letter* 15(8):1, 1999.

Irwin EG: A focused overview of anorexia nervosa and bulimia: part 1, etiological results, *Archives of Psychiatric Nursing* 7(6):342, 1993.

Insomnia: get a good night's sleep, *Harvard Health Letter* 24(12):1,1998.

Mishima K and others: Morning bright light therapy for sleep and behavior disorders in elderly patients with dementia, *Acta Psychiatrica Scandinavica* 89(1):1, 1994.

North American Nursing Diagnosis Association: *NANDA nursing diagnoses: definitions and classification 1999-2000,* Philadelphia, 1999, The Association.

Physicians of the Geisinger Health System: *Help for anorexia nervosa,* Philadelphia, 1997.

Potter PA, Perry AG: *Basic nursing: concepts, process, and practice,* ed 4, St. Louis, 1998, Mosby.

Seidel HM and others: *Mosby's guide to physical examination,* ed 4, St. Louis, 1999, Mosby.

Stuart GW, Laraia MT: *Principles and practice of psychiatric nursing,* ed 7, St. Louis, 2001, Mosby.

Stuart GW, Laraia MT: *Stuart and Sundeen's pocket guide to psychiatric nursing,* ed 5, St. Louis, 1998, Mosby.

Travis, J: The threat of a piece of pumpkin pie, *Science News* 154(23):367, 1998.

U.S. Bureau of the Census: Statistical abstract of the United States: 1998, ed 118, Washington, DC, 1998, U.S. Government Printing Office.

Walsh T: Eating disorders: progress and problems, *Science* 280(5368): 1387, 1998.

Williams SR: *Basic nutrition and diet therapy,* ed 10, St. Louis, 1995, Mosby.

Wong DL: *Whaley and Wong's nursing care of infants and children,* ed 6, St. Louis, 1998, Mosby.

Chapter 24

Dissociative Disorders

Learning Objectives

1. Examine the meaning of the term *self-concept*.
2. Describe the continuum of self-concept responses.
3. Compare the development of self-concept throughout the life cycle.
4. Classify the main characteristic of dissociative disorders.
5. Describe four types of dissociative disorders.
6. Explain the outstanding feature of a dissociative identity (multiple personality) disorder.
7. State the main goal of treatment for clients with dissociative disorders.
8. Plan three nursing diagnoses for clients with dissociative disorders.
9. Develop a care plan for a client who has been diagnosed with a dissociative disorder.

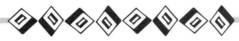

Key Terms

ageism

amnesia

body image

depersonalization

dissociation

dissociative disorder

dissociative identity disorder (DID)

fugue

identity diffusion

personal identity

role performances

self-concept

self-esteem

self-ideal

trance

Human beings differ from animals in a significant way: they have a concept of *self*. As children grow, they learn to identify and define themselves as individuals. They develop a picture (a point of view) of who they are, then they use that picture as a framework for perceiving, experiencing, and evaluating the world. This point of view becomes one's self-concept.

Self-concept is defined as all the attitudes, notions, beliefs, and convictions that make up a person's self-knowledge. "It includes the individual's perceptions of personal characteristics and abilities, interactions with other people and the environment, values, associated experiences and objects, and goals and ideals" (Stuart and Laraia, 2001).

The development of self-concept is influenced by many factors. The *culture* into which an individual is born and the *society* in which one lives have a strong impact on self-concept. The attitudes and beliefs of parents, siblings, and other *significant people* influence how an individual defines himself or herself. The *experiences* of life also shape and influence one's picture of the self.

Self-concept is the frame of reference through which people view the world. It is the sum of several components, including **body image** (the attitudes and feeling one has for his or her body), **self-esteem** (an individual's judgment of his or her own worth), **self-ideal** (personal standards of how one should behave), **personal identity** (an awareness of oneself as an individual), and **role performances** (socially expected behavioral patterns). All these parts of an individual fuse and blend over time into the unique characteristics called self-concept.

CONTINUUM OF SELF-CONCEPT RESPONSES

People behave in a manner based in large part on their self-concepts. The range of behavioral responses relating to self-concept can be seen as occurring on a continuum. At the adaptive end, a healthy self-concept leads one toward self-actualization. Low self-concept results in maladaptive behavioral responses as individuals struggle to define who they are (Figure 24-1).

The Healthy Personality

Persons with healthy personalities are able to effectively perceive and function within their worlds (Fortinash and Holoday-Worret, 1999). They have achieved a sense of peace and harmony within themselves that allows them to successfully cope with life's anxieties, traumas, and crises. A realistic self-ideal and a clear personal identity help to provide these individuals with a sense of purpose and direction in life. High self-esteem and confidence provide the strength to handle anxieties and learn from life's highs and lows. Socially they are satisfied with the roles they play in society. They have the ability to intimately relate to others and to share themselves without fear. In short, individuals with healthy personalities are able to struggle with life's problems while feeling good about living (see Think About box).

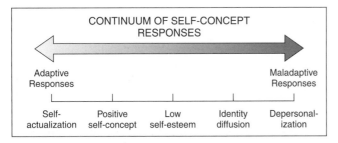

Figure 24-1 Continuum of self-concept responses. (Redrawn from Stuart GW, Laraia MT: *Principles and practice of psychiatric nursing,* ed 7, St. Louis, 2001, Mosby.)

Think About

Using the five components of a healthy personality described above, assess yourself.

◆ How do your results compare to the description of a person with a healthy personality?

SELF-CONCEPT THROUGHOUT THE LIFE CYCLE

Self-concept develops over time, shaped by the influences within one's environment. The theorist Erik Erikson, in describing his eight stages of human development, stated that a psychosocial crisis or core task must be resolved for further personality development. As each task is completed, one's self-concept is affected. Mastery of core tasks builds self-confidence, worth, and esteem (Wong, 1998). If, however, one is unable to cope with a core task, ineffective or maladaptive behaviors result. This process, according to Erikson, continues throughout life.

Self-Concept in Childhood

Infants do not view themselves as separate from the rest of the world. Only after a period of time do they begin to distinguish themselves as different from their mother or father. Infants learn to trust others when their needs are consistently met. After a series of social experiences, they develop stable relationships and learn to feel good about themselves. Rejection by parents or significant others at this time has a strong negative effect on an individual's self-concept.

Toddlers' tasks are to explore the limits of their abilities, and these tasks include the nature of their impact on others. Toddlers become independent by exploring their environments and testing their capabilities. They develop autonomy and sense of self through experimenting with a variety of behaviors. Actions that get results are effective, even if they are inappropriate, and they are added to the general knowledge of the child. Behaviors that are not rewarded or do not get results are discarded. In this way, children learn about "right and wrong," and then use this information as a framework for their self-ideal. When parental reactions are routine and consistent, children develop a stable sense of who they are and a stable self-concept. When the reactions of significant others change or differ, children become confused and have trouble establishing a positive identity and healthy self-concept.

School-age children become aware of different perspectives of life. They learn about social norms, peer pressures, and moral issues. Skill building and broadening social relationships keep them occupied with self-evaluations. Self-concept continues to develop as school-age children assess their skills and interactions with others and form mental pictures of themselves. If the picture is positive, the move into adolescence is graceful; but if self-concept is low or threatened, adolescence is filled with anxiety and turmoil.

Self-Concept in Adolescence

By the early teen years, the comfortable self-concept of childhood is challenged. As adolescents mature, they begin to develop a more complex picture of themselves. Self-concept becomes more individual and is based on one's special characteristics rather than on the similarities shared by others. Thinking becomes more abstract and much self-reflection is needed to digest all the physical, emotional, and social changes that are taking place.

During adolescence, self-concept is influenced by many things. Relationships with family and peers play an important role in helping to define teens' confidence levels. The development of a sexual identity and the adjustment to a new adult body image must be included in the new concept of self. The struggle is to define oneself by combining previous roles and new emotions into a reasonably consistent and pleasing sense of self. Without the love, nurturing, and guidance of concerned adults, many teens do not finish the task of developing a comfortable self-concept. They become ill-prepared to assume the many responsibilities of adult life because the struggle to find themselves continues.

Self-Concept in Adulthood

Adults with strong, positive self-concepts can freely explore their environments because they have a background of success and effectiveness. Positive experiences further enhance self-concept, and the cycle of learning, succeeding, and growth repeats itself.

If the concept of oneself is low or negative, individuals develop views of themselves as inadequate or unable. They become easily threatened, which in turn increases anxiety levels and forces them to become preoccupied with defending themselves. Soon this cycle becomes a way of life, and individuals find themselves caught in the trap of looking only at the negative or "down" side of life. The cycle of few successes and much negative reinforcement becomes established, and the adult suffers from a poor self-concept. Most adults, however, function somewhere between these two extremes.

Self-Concept in Older Adulthood

Self-concept is established in childhood, developed in adolescence, strengthened in adulthood, and refined in older adulthood. In later life many occurrences and situations can threaten a positive self-concept. **Ageism,** the stereotyping of older persons as feeble, dependent, and nonproductive, contributes to older adults' self-concepts. Threats to the stability of one's lifestyle, such as changes in occupation, social standing, or environment, often lead to changes in self-concept. Health care providers can enhance older clients' feelings of self-worth through active listening and demonstrations of concern.

DISSOCIATIVE DISORDERS

Dissociation is an attempt to cope with deep-seated emotional anxiety or distress. Low self-esteem is a problem for many persons. It is usually expressed through various levels of anxiety and involves feelings of being weak, inadequate, and helpless (Box 24-1). Low self-esteem is a common component of many mental health problems. Feelings of self-rejection and dislike are expressed through various behaviors.

Box 24-1 Behaviors Associated With Low Self-Esteem

Criticism of Self and Others

"Doomed to failure" outlook; negative thinking
Sees normal life stresses as impossible barriers

Decreased Productivity

Does not complete tasks; works below level of actual abilities
Postpones decisions

Denies Self Pleasure

Feels need to be punished, so refuses pleasure
Rejects personal strengths and assets

Destructive Toward Self and Others

May displace self-hate onto others
Becomes accident prone or engages in dangerous activities
Suicide is ultimate act of self-rejection

Disturbed Interpersonal Relationships

Exploits others
May be demeaning, cruel, withdrawn, or isolated

Exaggerated Sense of Self-Importance

Makes up for low self-esteem with grandiose thinking; may boast, brag, or describe special abilities
Sets unrealistic goals; has unrealistic dreams

Feelings of Guilt, Inadequacy, and Worry

Uses destructive activities to punish self
Rejects self through nightmares, obsessions, phobias, or reliving of distressing memories
Is irritable and easily angered

Negative Outlook About One's Body, Abilities, and Life

Has polarized view of life; everything is either right or wrong, good or bad
Rejects aspects of self that have potential for growth and refuses to consider real strengths and assets
Has physical complaints and problems

Withdrawal

Becomes socially isolated
May withdraw from reality when anxiety of self-rejection reaches severe levels
May have delusions, hallucinations, dissociation, jealousy, suspicion, paranoia

Modified from Stuart GW, Laraia, MT: *Principles and practice of psychiatric nursing,* ed 7, St. Louis, 2001, Mosby.

Identity diffusion is the failure to bring various childhood identifications into an effective adult personality. Individuals with identity diffusion are not sure of who they really are because they have been unable to build a "picture" of themselves. They drift through life, like a boat without a rudder, unable to set a course or steer themselves around obstacles.

Although these people have feelings of emptiness and anxiety, they often exploit others. Feelings of empathy are often lacking. This leads to problems with intimacy and a lack of caring. Because the self-ideal is confused, moral codes or standards of behavior are often missing (Keltner, Schwecke, and Bostrom, 1998). Frequently they are so desperate to define themselves that they attempt to bind their self-concepts to another. This type of identity diffusion is called personality fusing. When behaviors interfere with an individual's ability to function, a mental health problem exists. The mental health problems that relate to anxiety and self-concept are called the dissociative disorders.

Characteristics

Dissociation is an "interruption of a person's fundamental aspects of waking consciousness" (National Alliance for the Mentally Ill, 1996). It is a complicated neuropsychological process that ranges from normal, everyday experiences to those that disrupt everyday living. Dissociation is a common, natural experience. Examples of normal dissociations are daydreaming or becoming so absorbed in an activity that one loses a sense of time and surroundings. Dissociation is also used as a coping mechanism to protect us from trauma. The victim of a mugging or severe accident is often unable to remember events surrounding the incident, and individuals who were abused in childhood may have only a few small, unrelated memories.

Children dissociate more easily than adults. Faced with overwhelming abuse or trauma, children often psychologically flee their distresses by blocking emotionally damaging information from awareness. Dissociation, when used as a defense in childhood, can later grow into a dissociative disorder.

A **dissociative disorder** is a disturbance in the normally interacting functions of consciousness: identity, memory, and perception. With a dissociative disorder, the most anxiety-producing aspects of the self are walled off or split from the remainder of the personality in an attempt to cope with severe anxiety or emotional trauma.

Although they once were considered rare, new evidence reveals that dissociative disorders are becoming more common in the United States, especially in the many individuals who were neglected or abused in childhood. Dissociative disorders are diagnosed more frequently in women. In other countries, such as Japan, England, and France, the incidence of diagnosed dissociative disorders is low. In several cultures, dissociative trances and experiences are a part of religious or spiritual practices. Frequently the devout will enter into altered states in which they communicate or interact with spirits or beings. Nurses who work with clients from different cultural backgrounds must be alert to the customs and practices of the culture. Several interesting culturally defined mental health disorders involving dissociative states are described in Table 24-1.

When the disturbance of a dissociative disorder occurs primarily with memory or consciousness, amnesia or **fugue** (inability to remember important personal events or travels) results. If the disturbance is with one's identity, parts of the self assume separate personalities, and a dissociative identity (multiple personality) disorder is diagnosed. Posttraumatic stress disorder, although considered an anxiety disorder, is actually a recall of past traumatic events alternating with detachment or dissociation. All of the disorders are based in traumatic experiences. Behaviors are the result of repeated dissociations of traumatic memories. As the body walls off the infection of an abscess, the mind walls off the extreme distresses of trauma and anxiety. Four types of dissociative disorders are classified by the *Diagnostic and Statistical Manual of Mental Disorders* (DSM-IV–TR). They are depersonalization disorder, amnesia, fugue, and identity disorder.

Depersonalization Disorder

During an episode of depersonalization, one feels detached or unconnected to the self (Rollant, 1998). The individual may feel like a robot, working on automatic. There may be a sensation of being an outside observer and of not being involved. **Depersonalization** is a response to severe anxiety associated with a blocking of awareness and a fading of reality. One becomes unable to tell the difference between internal and external stimuli because the self-concept becomes disorganized. The body takes on an unreal quality, and the world becomes a dream.

Depersonalization serves as a defense mechanism but does nothing to relieve the cause of the distress, so it becomes a maladaptive behavior. In cases in which depersonalization becomes a mental health problem, individuals attempt to "escape" distress and anxiety by losing their identities. Table 24-2 lists the physical, emotional, intellectual, and behavioral characteristics of this behavioral pattern.

Depersonalization is commonly associated with other mental disorders, including acute stress disorder, panic disorder, obsessive-compulsive disorder, and schizophrenia. These mental health problems can suddenly follow a life-threatening event or develop slowly following years of distress.

Dissociative Amnesia

Amnesia is a loss of memory. Dissociative amnesia is characterized by an inability to remember personal information that cannot be explained by ordinary forgetfulness. It is an attempt to avoid extreme stress by blocking memories from consciousness. Individuals with dissociative amnesia usually have gaps in their ability to recall certain events during their childhood. Most of these memory lapses are related to extremely stressful events.

For example, a rape victim often has no memory of the attack but still experiences the emotional numbness and depression associated with the trauma. Sights, sounds, odors, and images can trigger emotional distresses long after the event has occurred. Actual memories are too

Table 24-1	Cultural Aspects: Culturally Defined Mental Health Disorders Involving Dissociative States	
Disorder	**Culture(s)**	**Description**
Amok	Malaysia, Laos, Philippines, Polynesia, Puerto Rico, Navajo	Period of brooding followed by outbursts of aggressive, violent behavior; found only in males
Ataque de nervios	Latinos	Uncontrollable shouting, crying, fainting, and suicidal gestures following stressful event
Falling out	Southern United States, Caribbean groups	Sudden collapse; eyes are open, but individual is unable to see; hears and understands but feels powerless to move
Latah	Japan (*imu*), Philippines (*mali-mali*), Thailand	Excessive reactions to sudden fright; trancelike behavior with command obedience, echolalia
Pibloktoq	Arctic and subarctic Eskimos	Extreme excitement and irrational behavior followed by seizures and coma lasting up to 12 hours
Qi-gong psychotic reaction	Chinese	Acute episode of psychotic behaviors following folk practice of *qi-gong*, the exercise of vital energy
Shin-byung	Korean	Anxiety and somatic complaints that progress to dissociation and possession by ancestral spirits
Spell	African-American, European, Americans from southern United States	Trance in which communication with deceased relatives or spirits takes place
Zar	Egypt, Ethiopia, Iran, Sudan	Spirit possession that interferes with daily activities; may develop long-term relationship with spirit and withdraw from reality

Modified from American Psychiatric Association: *Diagnostic and statistical manual of mental disorders*, ed 4, text revision, Washington, DC, 2000, The Association.

Table 24-2	Behaviors Associated With Depersonalization	
Areas of functioning	**Description**	
Affective (emotional)	Feels identity is lost	
	Lacks sense of inner togetherness	
	Unable to feel pleasure or pride	
	Feelings of detachment, fear, insecurity, shame, unreality	
Behavioral (social)	Affect blunted; emotionally unresponsive and passive; not lively or spontaneous	
	Communications odd or difficult to follow	
	Loss of drive, decision-making abilities, impulse control	
	Social isolation and withdrawal	
Cognitive (intellectual)	Confusion; distorted thinking and memory	
	Impaired judgment; disoriented to time	
Perceptual (physical)	Dreamlike experiences of world	
	Difficulty telling self from others	
	Disturbed body image and sexuality	
	May experience auditory and visual hallucinations	

Modified from Stuart GW, Laraia MT: *Principles and practice of psychiatric nursing*, ed 7, St. Louis, 2001, Mosby.

painful to consider, so they stay submerged—walled off but still capable of inflicting pain.

These clients require high levels of emotional support. Client safety becomes a primary therapeutic goal because suicide attempts are common. Although memory may be gone, the emotional distresses still remain. Clients' connections with other human beings are sometimes the only link on the road back to mental health.

Dissociative Fugue

One of the most interesting dissociative disorders is the rare, but dramatic, amnesiac fugue. The word **fugue** means to escape from reality. The main characteristic of dissociative fugue is sudden, unexpected travel with an inability to recall the past. A fugue occurs in response to an overwhelmingly stressful or traumatic event. It is an extreme expression of the fight-or-flight mechanism, engaged to protect the individual.

Persons with dissociative fugue may travel from a few miles away from home to another continent. Individuals behave quite normally during periods of travel but are confused about their personal identities, which is what frequently brings them to the attention of authorities. Some individuals assume entirely new identities, complete with a new occupation and significant others. The Case Study box describes an interesting case of fugue.

During an actual fugue, few personality changes are noticeable. Individuals may be more friendly and outgoing, but their behaviors remain appropriate. After the return to the prefugue state, individuals may experience aggressive impulses, conflict, depression, guilt, and suicidal wishes. There may be loss of memory of the events that occurred during the time of the fugue. Recovery is usually rapid, but some amnesia may remain. Psychosocial care and emotional support are important elements in recovery.

Dissociative Trance Disorder

A **trance** is defined as a state resembling sleep in which consciousness remains but voluntary movement is lost. In many cultures, trances are expressions of spiritual or religious beliefs. Cultural trances are entered into voluntarily and cause no distress or harm to the individuals. Channelers, psychics, spirit guides, shamans, and the like rarely suffer from mental impairments. Cultural influences also have an impact on the type of trance, the associated sensory disturbances, and the behaviors exhibited during the trance. Culturally normative trances involve signs, symptoms, and behaviors that are expected by other members of the culture. During these trances, individuals do not lose their identities.

Possession trances involve the appearance of one or more distinct identities, which direct the individual to perform sometimes complex behaviors and activities such as culturally appropriate conversations, gestures, or facial

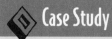

Amy was only 3 years of age when she was first abused by her father. By 4, she was hiding whenever she heard his footsteps coming down the hall; by 6, Amy slipped out the window to escape. On those occasions when he could not be avoided, Amy played a game in her mind in which she would fly away to a land where everyone was kind and carried no evil. She would wish and dream and hope during those times, ignoring the pain and distress of being repeatedly molested.

By the time Amy was 13, she had run away from home. Luckily she found a youth shelter early in her wanderings where staff members were understanding and had a genuine interest in seeing Amy survive her adolescence. She stayed at the shelter for about 7 months, learning the skills needed for adulthood. Soon Amy became very efficient in coordinating and supervising the daily household events.

Because of her newly learned organizational abilities, Amy was offered a position as a teacher's assistant at the local grade school where she remained for many years. By the time she was 30, Amy had buried the memories of her abuse and forgotten the pain of her childhood. She was married and looking forward to a bright future.

Amy's father became seriously ill the following year. He was alone and in need of care. After having no communication with Amy in 20 years, he wrote to ask if he could come and live with Amy and her family.

The letter arrived and Amy stared, horrified, at the return address. Six months later, she remembers nothing more: not the trip to San Francisco, not the bus ride to Colorado, not even her new fiancé. Today she can hardly remember who she really is.

◆ What happened after Amy read the return address on the letter?
◆ If Amy was admitted to your unit, what psychosocial interventions would you include in the care plan?

expressions. Amnesia following either type of trance state is not uncommon, but it occurs more frequently with possession trances.

A dissociative trance disorder exists when trances cause "clinically significant distress or functional impairment" (American Psychiatric Association, 2000). Dissociative trance disorders are listed in the DSM-IV–TR in the category of "diagnoses in need of further study." However, the fact remains that if trances cause a great deal of anxiety and distress in an individual, he or she can likely benefit from psychotherapeutic interventions.

Dissociative Identity Disorder

When stress or trauma is repeated and severe, the personality attempts to protect itself. Abused children use dissociation to escape, distance, and defend themselves from the anxiety, trauma, and helplessness of reality. Major studies have confirmed that dissociative identity disorders are the result of severe physical, sexual, and/or emotional abuse.

A **dissociative identity disorder (DID)** is defined as the presence of two or more identities or personalities that repeatedly take control of the individual's behavior. Dissociative identity disorder develops as a defense against prolonged and inescapable trauma. The diagnosis of DID, which was formerly called "multiple personality disorder," occurs more often in the United States than other countries. Some mental health professionals believe that this is a result of better diagnostic tools, whereas others think that DID is overdiagnosed or view it as a culturally related syndrome.

The essential features of DID are associated with the presence of other personalities in one individual. Individuals with DID often have a personal history full of time losses, unexplained possessions or changes in relationships, out-of-body experiences, and the awareness of other parts of the self. A history of abuse or trauma is not always identified because emotions are deeply buried.

When different personalities do emerge, each has its own way of thinking about and relating to the world. Each personality is unique and often represents the individual at different developmental stages. The identities may be helpful, controlling, seductive, or destructive, but each serves a specific protective purpose. They may differ in age, gender, knowledge, state of health, speech, and behaviors. The primary personality (called the *host*) may or may not be aware of the presence of the other personalities (called *alters*). Usually the transition from one personality to the other is sudden and related to stress. Sometimes the identities cooperate with each other, but more often they attempt to take control and refuse to share knowledge with the others. Hostility or open conflict can result among the more powerful personalities.

Individuals with dissociative problems, especially DID, often have symptoms of posttraumatic stress syndrome (nightmares, flashbacks, extreme startle responses). Other mental or physical health problems are frequently present, especially with some of the identities found in DID. The main goal of treatment is to help the client integrate or combine the personalities into one functional individual, capable of coping with life's stresses in a healthy manner.

THERAPEUTIC INTERVENTIONS

Treatment for dissociative disorders involves long-term therapy in an outpatient setting. Hospitalization is required only in three situations:

1. When anger, aggression, or violence is directed toward self or others and presents a danger

2. When individuals are unable to function because of memory loss, rapid switching between identities, flashbacks, or overwhelming emotions
3. When medications need to be evaluated or adjusted

The stages of treatment for dissociative disorders relate to assessment, stabilization, and reworking past traumas. The most effective results are seen when clients with dissociative disorders are able to work with stable, established multidisciplinary treatment teams.

Treatments and Therapies

Therapy for clients with dissociative disorders begins with assessment and stabilization. Because the work of coping with deeply seated trauma is difficult and emotionally demanding, an environment in which clients can safely examine their conflicts must first be established. A careful assessment includes the client's history, symptoms, support systems, medical status, relationships, and problems and the presence of substance abuse and sleeping or eating disorders. Family history should include both the family of origin and the current family situation. Videotaping the alters often results in more diagnostic information.

During the stabilization phase, the diagnosis is established as the client gradually reveals the complexities of his or her nature. After each treatment team member assesses the client, a plan for stabilization is jointly developed. Therapies are carefully chosen and may include individual psychotherapy, group therapy, family therapy, psychoeducation, and various expressive therapies, such as art, poetry, and dance. Contracts to ensure safety during therapy are established. During this time, clients and care providers develop trust in each other and build client support networks. Although this part of treatment may last for more than a year, it is an essential step for the work to come.

The next phase of treatment involves revisiting and reworking past traumas. Once the client develops an awareness of other personalities and their purposes, the painful material is slowly and gently analyzed. Each identity is treated equally with respect and is encouraged to communicate with the others. Feelings of shame, guilt, anger, and grief are encountered as each traumatic event is encountered. With time, patience, and hard work, the client eventually begins to integrate or combine the memories (or personalities) into a unique individual who is able to effectively cope with life's stressors, which is the main treatment goal for clients with dissociative disorders.

Pharmacological Therapy

No specific medication exists at this time to treat amnesia, fugues, or other dissociative behaviors. Treatment is often based on symptoms. If high anxiety is apparent, antianxiety agents may be prescribed. When depression is intense, an antidepressant may be ordered. If hallucinations or delusions are commonly present, an antipsychotic medication may be administered. All medications are prescribed for only short periods to encourage the use of inner coping skills.

Nursing Process

As with all other mental health clients, assessments are routinely performed on clients with dissociative disorders. Clients with dissociative disorders can present different pictures to various staff members to manipulate and divide their care providers. They may offer one side of themselves during one minute, then, in the next moment, a personality that wants to pick a fight emerges. Assessments should describe the client's behaviors, communications, anxiety, depression, social functioning, and the presence of amnesia (Shives, 1998). A much clearer picture is given with descriptions than with psychiatric "buzz words" or jargon.

Nursing diagnoses for clients with dissociative disorders are related to self-concept responses and depend on the identified problems of each client. The expected outcome for each diagnosis is a client who is able to obtain his or her maximum level of effective functioning and self-actualization. Primary or main nursing diagnoses include disturbances in personal identity, body image, self-esteem, and role performance. Refer to Box 24-2 for examples.

After clients have established trust with the staff, interventions are directed at helping them examine their situations and related feelings within an environment of safety and support. This process assists the growth of personal insight, the first step toward making behavioral changes. A problem-solving approach helps clients to gradually expand self-awareness, explore and evaluate the self, and eventually plan for actions that result in behavior changes. Clients are emotionally supported and encouraged to actively take part in therapy.

Some clients with dissociative disorders engage in self-destructive behaviors. They may cut, bite, or repeatedly hit themselves or pull out their hair. Self-destructive behavior is of great concern, and several interventions have been devised to assist clients in achieving control over these behaviors.

First, clients must be routinely assessed for self-destructive thoughts. The easiest way to find out if such thoughts are occurring is to ask the client. Contracts and agreements between client and staff help staff and client to develop trust in the therapeutic relationship and environment. During the admission process, ways of dealing with destructive behaviors should be discussed with the client. If necessary, one-to-one support is provided until the client can achieve self-control.

If the client is willing, a daily journal of thoughts and feelings is kept. This practice has been found to be a

> ### Box 24-2 NANDA Nursing Diagnoses Related to Dissociative Disorders
>
> Adjustment, impaired*
> Anxiety
> Body image disturbance
> Coping, ineffective individual
> Decisional conflict
> Denial, ineffective
> Environmental interpretation syndrome, impaired
> Family processes, altered
> Fear
> Hopelessness
> Memory, impaired*
> Personal identity disturbance*
> Powerlessness
> Role performance, altered
> Self-esteem disturbance
> Self-mutilation, risk for
> Social interaction, impaired
> Social isolation*
> Violence, risk for: self-directed

From North American Nursing Diagnosis Association: *NANDA nursing diagnoses: definitions and classification 1999-2000*, Philadelphia, 1999, The Association.
*Primary nursing diagnoses for dissociative disorders.

helpful self-control activity. Care providers should be limited to a few personnel to provide a stable therapeutic environment (see Sample Client Care Plan).

The care and treatment of individuals with dissociative problems is complex, time-consuming, and challenging. Individuals who have been diagnosed with dissociative disorders are suffering from one of the worst human fears—not knowing and being out of control over oneself. Although the behaviors may be odd, unusual, or dramatic, each serves a purpose and communicates something about the person. Health care providers are challenged with the twin tasks of accepting and understanding the messages sent by dissociated individuals. Treatment of clients with backgrounds of trauma is complex and at times frustrating. At the same time, it can be an extremely rewarding experience.

KEY CONCEPTS

◆ Self-concept is defined as all the attitudes, notions, beliefs, and convictions that make up an individual's self-knowledge. It develops over time, shaped by one's developmental level and influences within one's environment.

◆ Low self-esteem is a common component of many mental health problems and often represents feelings of self-rejection and self-dislike, which are expressed through various behaviors.

Sample Client Care Plan   Maladaptive Self-Concept

Assessment

History: Christine is a 35-year-old wife and mother of three children, ages 15, 10, and 7. Although she experienced severe sexual and physical abuse as a child, she has managed to complete college, marry, and raise her family. She is being admitted to the clinic's mental health services for "several episodes of losing myself" that she has experienced in the past 5 months.

Current Findings: A well-groomed woman who is distressed because she was unable to remember to pick up her daughter's dress at the cleaners yesterday. Because of this, her daughter refused to attend the school dance and threatened to run away. Lately Christine has felt like an "outside observer of my own life," "like a robot on automatic." During these episodes she is aware of reality but feels as though everything is mechanical. She feels that she may be "going insane" because the "spells" are becoming more and more frequent since her daughter has begun dating.

Multidisciplinary Diagnosis

Personal identity disorder related to increased anxiety and past history of abuse

Planning/Goals

Christine will decrease the number of depersonalization episodes to fewer than one a week by May 20.

Christine will be able to recognize her anxiety and take steps to decrease it before it progresses to a depersonalization episode.

Therapeutic Interventions

Intervention	Rationale	Team Member
1. Establish therapeutic relationship; confirm her identity; support adaptive behaviors, identify strengths	Provides a way of offering emotional support; builds trust; supports current adaptive behaviors.	All
2. Assist Christine to describe thoughts and feelings.	Identification is the first step toward focused change.	All
3. Identify stresses that bring about her "spells."	Known stressors can be handled more effectively.	Psy, Nsg
4. Help to clarify faulty beliefs about self.	Builds confidence; helps focus energies in positive direction.	All
5. Encourage Christine to make a plan for decreasing her anxiety during times her daughter is on a date, role play mother-daughter roles.	Recalling and using successful strategies helps to decrease anxiety levels, thus preventing depersonalization epidodes.	Psy, Nsg
6. Reinforce strengths, assets, and problem-solving abilities; encourage Christine to focus on her "positives."	Helps to improve coping abilities and ease the pain of feeling powerless.	All

Evaluation

Christine was able to decrease her episodes of depersonalization to less than one a week by May 29.

A complete client care plan includes several other diagnoses and interventions.

◆ Identity diffusion is the failure to bring various childhood identifications into an effective adult personality.

◆ Dissociation is an interruption of a person's fundamental aspects of waking consciousness.

◆ Dissociative amnesia is characterized by an inability to remember personal information that cannot be explained by ordinary forgetfulness.

◆ The main characteristic of a dissociative fugue is sudden, unexpected travel, with an inability to recall the past.

◆ A trance is a state resembling sleep in which consciousness remains but voluntary movement is lost.

◆ A dissociative identity disorder (DID) is defined as the presence of two or more identities or personalities that repeatedly take control of the individual's behavior.

◆ Treatment for dissociative disorders involves long-term psychodynamic/cognitive therapy.

◆ There are no specific psychotherapeutic drugs for the treatment of dissociative disorders.

◆ Therapeutic interventions for clients with dissociative disorders focus on safety, trust, communication, and problem solving.

Suggestions for Further Reading

This suggestion involves an old movie. The *Three Faces of Eve* is an old but very accurate portrayal of a woman who suffers from dissociative identity disorder with several interesting and conflicting personalities.

Disorders—Internet Mental Health (www.mentalhealth.com/fe20.html) offers information about dissociative disorders and American and European approaches to treatment.

References

American Psychiatric Association: *Diagnostic and statistical manual of mental disorders,* ed 4, text revision, Washington, DC, 2000, The Association.

Fortinash KM, Holoday-Worret PA: *Psychiatric-mental health nursing,* ed 2, St. Louis, 1999, Mosby.

Keltner NL, Schwecke LH, Bostrom CE: *Psychiatric nursing,* ed 3, St. Louis, 1998, Mosby.

National Alliance for the Mentally Ill: Dissociative disorders: what are they?, Arlington, Va, 1996, The Alliance.

North American Nursing Diagnosis Association: *NANDA nursing diagnoses: definitions and classification 1999-2000,* Philadelphia, 1999, The Association.

Rollant PD: *Mosby's review cards,* St. Louis, 1998, Mosby.

Shives LR: *Basic concepts in psychiatric-mental health nursing,* ed 4, Philadelphia, 1998, Lippincott.

Stuart GW, Laraia MT: *Principles and practice of psychiatric nursing,* ed 7, St. Louis, 2001, Mosby.

Wong DL: *Whaley and Wong's nursing care of infants and children,* ed 6, St. Louis, 1998, Mosby.

Chapter 25

Anger and Aggression

Learning Objectives

1. Explain the differences between anger, aggression, and assertiveness.
2. Describe how anger is expressed by children, adolescents, young adults, and older adults.
3. Examine the impact of anger and aggression on society.
4. Compare three theories that attempt to explain the causes of aggression.
5. Describe each of the five stages of the assault cycle.
6. Explain the main characteristics for three mental health disorders that relate to anger or aggression.
7. Outline the process for assessing clients who are angry or aggressive.
8. Develop four therapeutic interventions for clients who are experiencing anger or acting aggressively.
9. Consider seven techniques for recognizing and coping with your own anger.

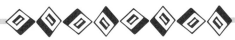

Key Terms

acting out

aggression

anger

assault

assertiveness

battery

impulse-control

passive aggression

violence

Anger is a normal emotional response to a perceived threat, frustration, or distressing event. It commonly occurs in reaction to feelings of being threatened or losing control. Anger is felt, experienced, suffered, and expressed in many ways. In a crisis situation, anger is often one of the first coping behaviors used.

Anger can be directed outward through aggressive or violent behaviors, or it may be expressed through passive-aggressive behaviors. Anger can also be focused on oneself. Some individuals turn their anger inward and become suicidal or depressed. Some live bouncing between aggression and helplessness, whereas others channel their anger into physical complaints and problems. Figure 25-1 illustrates the continuum of anger responses.

Anxiety and loss of control are associated with anger. Anger can include feelings of hopelessness, powerlessness, and regret. It can arise intentionally as one "stews" about an event or situation, or it can result from an unplanned situation. People tend to label anger as justified or unjustified according to their personal values. Anger can be rational and planned, or it can arrive in a blind fury of irrational rage.

Anger serves several purposes. It can be used as a coping mechanism by some people to meet their needs. According to Maslow's hierarchy (ladder) of human needs, when basic needs are threatened, a person may react with anger. The client who feels powerless at the news of his prolonged recovery may react by insulting others, or the child who flies into temper tantrums may be attempting to meet basic needs.

People can be motivated or encouraged to act by anger. Consider the college student who, as a child, felt the anxiety and helplessness of watching her mother being abused. Now she studies to become a lawyer and champion of abused people. In this case the use of anger motivated positive actions.

Table 25-1 lists many expressions of anger. Many of the listed emotions and actions are appropriate expressions of anger. However, when anger provides the motivation for inappropriate behaviors, it becomes defined as a problem.

Aggression is a forceful attitude or action that is expressed physically, symbolically, or verbally. Aggressive behaviors often are the result of angry feelings that are converted into action and expressed. Socially approved aggression is a basic element of many sports, such as

football, hockey, and soccer (Stuart and Laraia, 2001). Aggressive behavior is socially approved for certain groups, such as news people hot on the trail of some developing story. However, aggressive behaviors become inappropriate when they affect other people or their possessions. Several terms describe the characteristics of anger (Box 25-1).

The legal concepts of assault and battery were established to define inappropriate aggression and to protect people from those who act on their emotions in ways that are threatening to others. Finally, the term **assertiveness** defines the quality for which we strive. Assertiveness is the ability to directly express one's feelings or needs in a way that respects the rights of other people yet retains one's dignity.

ANGER AND AGGRESSION IN SOCIETY

Anger and its expressions have a strong impact on a society. The histories of many cultures are peppered with accounts of uprisings and wars. Children were often sacrificed to the gods of their parents to keep them from

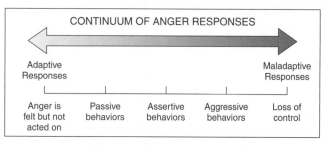

Figure 25-1 Continuum of anger responses.

Table 25-1	Expressions of Anger		
Turned Outward		**Turned Inward**	
Overt anger	**Passive aggression**	**Subjective**	**Objective**
Verbalization of anger	Impatience	Feeling upset	Crying
Irritation	Sulking	Tension	Self-destructive behavior
Pacing with agitation	Frustration	Unhappiness	Self-mutilation
Swearing	Tense facial expressions	Feeling hurt	Substance abuse
Hostility	Pessimism	Disappointment	Suicide
Contempt	Resentment	Guilt	
Clenched fists	Jealousy	Feelings of inferiority	
Insulting remarks	Bitterness	Low self-esteem	
Intimidation	Complaining	Sense of failure	
Bragging about violent acts	Deceptive sweetness	Humiliation	
Provoking behaviors	Unreasonableness	Somatic symptoms	
Sadistic acts	Intolerance	Feeling harassed	
Maliciousness	Resistance	Envy	
Verbal abuse	Stubbornness	Feeling violated	
Temper tantrums	Intentional forgetting	Feeling alienated	
Violation of others' rights	Noncompliance	Feeling demoralized	
Screaming	Procrastination	Feeling depressed	
Deviance	Antagonism	Resignation	
Rage	Belittling remarks	Powerlessness	
Argumentativeness	Sarcasm	Helplessness	
Overt defiance	Fault finding	Hopelessness	
Threats: words or weapons	Manipulation	Desperation	
Damage to property	Power struggles	Apathy	
Assault	Unfair teasing		
Rape	Sabotage of others		
Homicide	Domination		

From Keltner NL, Schwecke LH, Bostrom CE: *Psychiatric nursing*, ed 3, St Louis, 1998, Mosby.

becoming angry. Cultural expressions of anger differ, and care providers need the ability to recognize the signs of anger in the cultural groups with whom they work (see Cultural Aspects box).

Gender Aggression

"Violence against wives has been tolerated since the beginning of history" (Landers, Jacobs, and Siegel, 1995). Ancient and well-accepted beliefs that men were superior led to values that supported the abuse of women. Beatings and floggings of women were accepted practices throughout ancient Greek and Roman societies. By the fourteenth century, it was legal in France for a man to beat his wife as long as he did not maim or kill her. In 1427 a nobleman encouraged his fellow Italians to treat their wives with as much concern and consideration as they did their livestock and fowl.

In eighteenth-century America, the high incidence of violence against women and children became unacceptable. By 1871 states began to enact statutes that denied the husband's right to physically abuse his wife. Today in the United States, wives can legally sue their husbands for abusing them, but the problems of violence against women and children continue to occur far too often.

Gender aggression and abuse are still practiced all over the world. Many aggressive acts against women are centered around the concepts of virginity and fidelity. Young women in parts of Africa and the Middle East are forced to undergo circumcision and other mutilating genital surgeries. Women of all ages can suffer from the effects of gender violence (Table 25-2).

Aggression Throughout the Life Cycle

Expressions of anger begin in infancy and end with death. As infants, unmet needs are expressed through diffuse rage reactions with "loud, uncontrollable crying and screaming, profuse perspiration, difficulty in breathing

---

Box 25-1 Terms Relating to Anger

Expressions of anger depend on **impulse-control,** the ability to express one's emotions in appropriate or effective ways.

Acting out is the use of inappropriate or destructive behaviors to express emotions.
Passive aggression involves indirect expressions of anger through subtle, evasive, or manipulative behaviors.
Violence is behavior that threatens or harms other people or their property. A violent act is actions of force that result in abuse or harm.
Assault is a legal term that describes any behavior that presents an immediate threat to another person.
Battery is the unlawful use of force upon a person without his consent.

 Cultural Aspects

Koreans express anger and other distresses by becoming physically ill.
Oriental individuals may smile when angry.
Filipino people may react to anger by becoming passive-aggressive.

Table 25-2 Gender Violence Throughout the Life Cycle

Phase	Type of violence present
Prebirth	Sex-selective abortion (China, India, Republic of Korea); battering during pregnancy (emotional and physical effects on woman; effects on birth outcome); forced pregnancy (e.g., mass rape in war).
Infancy	Female infanticide; emotional and physical abuse; differential access to food and medical care for female infants.
Girlhood	Child marriage; genital mutilation; sexual abuse by family members and strangers; differential access to food and medical care; child prostitution.
Adolescence	Dating and courtship violence (acid throwing in Bangladesh, date rape in the United States); economically coerced sex (African secondary school girls with "sugar daddies" to afford school fees); sexual abuse in the workplace; rape; sexual harassment; forced prostitution; trafficking in women.
Reproductive age	Abuse of women by male partners; marital rape; dowry abuse and murders; partner homicide; psychological abuse; sexual abuse in the workplace; sexual harassment; rape; abuse of women with disabilities.
Elderly	Abuse of widows; elder abuse (in the United States, the only country where data are available, elder abuse affects mostly women).

(sometimes turning blue), and flailing of arms and legs" (Keltner, Schwecke, and Bostrom, 1998).

In toddlerhood, individuals engage in temper tantrums, during which they learn to focus their aggression on the person or thing they believe is responsible for their anger (Potter and Perry, 1998). Toddlers observe the behaviors of others in their environment and pattern their own actions after them. If shouting, fighting, or other forms of aggression are observed, toddlers understand that aggressive behaviors are acceptable. In some families, a show of aggression is encouraged in children as a way of teaching them to "stand up for their rights." Television is another source of aggression. Many studies have shown that violence on television has a direct effect on the children who watch the programs (Wong, 1998).

During preschool years, children often direct their anger toward others, especially peers or younger children. Children in the early school-age years assault or hit each other frequently. By preadolescence most children stop hitting and learn to channel their aggression into physical activities, such as competitive sports or physical conditioning. Slander, gossip, and practical jokes provide other outlets for aggressive feelings during the school years.

By adolescence, fighting is organized, controlled, and purposeful. The peer group becomes the greatest source of influence on the individual. If the activities of the peer group are illegal or disruptive to others, then the adolescent peer group is known as a gang.

As an individual's age increases, so does his or her control of emotional reactions and impulses. "Between the ages of 22 and 45 years, most expressions of aggression and fighting occur within the family" (Keltner, Schwecke, and Bostrom, 1998). After age 45, few people engage in physical aggression until into their 70s, when sensory and cognitive (intellectual) impairments may result in the expression of aggressive or hostile behaviors.

Scope of the Problem Today

Today aggression and violence are worldwide concerns. Wife beating is still common in many countries. In Papua, New Guinea, almost 67% of wives suffer from abuse. In the United States, 1,682,000 violent crimes were reported. Homicide (murder) is the tenth leading cause of death for all citizens. Injuries are the second leading cause of death for Native Americans. For black males and 5 to 15-year-old children, murder was the third leading cause of death (U.S. Bureau of the Census, 1998).

Statistics are impressive, but they cannot tell the stories of how aggression and violence have changed the lives of so many individuals. It is the task of each of us, as health care providers and human beings, to help people focus their acts of aggression into more effective (and less violent) ways of coping with today's complex world.

THEORIES OF ANGER AND AGGRESSION

Theories about human aggression and violence attempt to explain why certain persons behave the way they do. Many theories about the nature of aggression have been devised, but most fall into one of three basic models: biological, psychosocial, and sociocultural theories.

Biological Theories

Models that credit the causes of aggression and violence to physical or chemical differences are called biological or individual theories. Currently much research is being focused on the areas of the brain that influence emotional control and aggressive behaviors. The roles of certain neurotransmitters are being investigated as possible factors in the development of violent or aggressive behaviors. Biological theories explain aggressive behavior as a psychopathology—a disorder in the biological or physical makeup of a person. Charles Darwin favored his animal model, which stated that aggression strengthened human beings through natural selection. Sigmund Freud believed that the greater the death wish, the greater the need for aggressive behavior. Other biological theories explain aggression as an innate (instinctual) drive. One thing, however, is certain: physical problems that cause aggressive behaviors do exist.

Psychosocial Theories

The models based on psychosocial theories focus on individuals' interactions with their social environments. Violence arises from interpersonal frustrations. Psychosocial theories of aggression state that aggressive behaviors are learned responses.

Sociocultural Theories

With the sociocultural theories, aggression is explained from a social and cultural group viewpoint. *Cultural theories* state that aggressive or violent acts are a product of cultural values, beliefs, norms, and rituals. Many cultures have rules that endorse the use of violence.

The *functional model* states that aggression and violence fill certain functions in a society, serving as catalysts or motivators for action. Behaviors associated with aggression are often used to achieve fame, fortune, and power. For example, athletes must be aggressive if they are to excel.

Conflict theories assume that aggression is a natural part of all human interactions. They state that individuals, groups, and societies seek to further their own causes. This results in disagreements, conflicts, and aggressive actions. Because conflict is a natural part of human associations, conflict theories state that aggression will never be eliminated. It can only be controlled.

The *resource theory*'s premise is that aggression is a fundamental part of society. Therefore the person who has the most resources can muster the greatest force or power. With this model, aggression is the result of having many resources and the power that goes with them.

The last theory of aggression is the *general systems model*. Here the feedback loop is used to demonstrate how aggression and violence perpetuate (feed on) themselves. Violence is viewed as a product of a system that must be stabilized and managed.

Many factors contribute to the use of aggressive behaviors. Attitudes about work, education, the media, and religion all influence the development of anger, hostility, and aggression. Population problems, such as overcrowding, can influence aggressive behaviors. Available community resources or the lack of them also plays an important role in the occurrence of violent or criminal acts. Many attempts have been made to explain the nature of aggression and violence. No matter what the cause, though, society must learn to recognize and cope with the aggressive behaviors of some of its members.

THE CYCLE OF ASSAULT

Assaults are aggressive behaviors that violate others' person or properties. Behaviors that are considered assaultive in this society include hitting, biting, pinching, or causing physical pain; certain criminal acts, such as rape, murder, suicide, robbery, theft, assault and battery; subtle actions of passive-aggressive individuals; and many forms of emotional abuse.

Studies have demonstrated that assault and violence occur in a predictable pattern of emotional responses. Each pattern of responses is called a stage, and there are five stages in the assault cycle. These stages are called trigger, escalation, crisis, recovery, and depression. Figure 25-2 illustrates the cycle of assault. This section describes each stage.

Trigger Stage

During the trigger phase, a stress-producing event occurs. Stress responses, such as anger, fear, or anxiety then occur. Coping mechanisms—behaviors to deal with the situation—are chosen in an attempt to achieve control.

For most individuals these coping behaviors are appropriate reactions to stress. For persons who are assaultive, however, the choice of coping behaviors becomes automatic. Their abilities to problem solve or choose effective options decrease as aggressive responses increase. Crisis interventions are very successful if begun early in this stage.

Escalation Stage

The escalation phase is the building stage during which each behavioral response moves a step closer to total loss of control. Attempts to use aggressive behaviors to gain control are repeatedly ineffective, resulting in frustration and greater anger. These emotions further flame the fires of aggression. Intervention is crucial at this stage if violence is to be prevented.

Crisis Stage

During this phase the potential for danger is increased. This stage is a period of emotional or physical blowout during which the actual assaultive behaviors occur. Many individuals act out, physically harm other people and animals or destroy property. Others become verbally abusive or scream and shout. People in this stage of the assault cycle are unable to listen to reason, follow directions, or engage in mental exercises. They are so controlled by their emotional responses they cannot respond to most outside stimuli. The best interventions at this stage are to protect the individual and others in the environment from physical harm.

Recovery Stage

The recovery stage is the cooling-down period that follows an emotional explosion. The individual slowly calms and returns to normal behavioral responses and actions. Interventions during this stage include assessing for injuries or trauma and providing a safe, quiet environment in which the person can recover.

Depression Stage

The last phase of the assault cycle involves a period of guilt and attempts to reconcile (make up) with others. Aggressors are aware of the assault and genuinely feel bad about it. They may provide loving care for the person who was assaulted or spend large amounts of money on gifts or other offerings of forgiveness. With the passage of time, the assaultive event is slowly placed in the past. Life returns to normal; that is, until the next trigger is cocked, and the cycle repeats itself over and over again.

ANGER CONTROL DISORDERS

Anger and aggressive responses are elements of many mental health disorders. Aggressive behaviors are com-

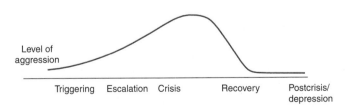

Figure 25-2 The assault cycle. (Redrawn from Keltner NL, Schwecke LH, Bostrom CE: *Psychiatric nursing*, ed 3, St. Louis, 1998, Mosby.)

monly encountered in clients with substance abuse, mood, anxiety, and depressive disorders. The potential for violence always exists in individuals with schizophrenia and other psychotic disorders. Clients with eating, sleeping, or somatoform disorders seldom behave aggressively toward others, but they are at a great risk for suicide because they focus their anger and aggression inward.

The *Diagnostic and Statistical Manual of Mental Disorders* (DSM-IV–TR) lists three categories of disorders relating to aggressive behaviors. Conduct disorders most often occur in childhood. Impulse-control disorders usually develop later in life, and adjustment disorders can occur at any time. The potential for aggressive actions is present in every client, regardless of diagnosis. Treating each person with respect and concern goes a long way toward removing that potential and helps to establish the groundwork for effective therapeutic interventions.

Aggressive Behavioral Disorders of Childhood

Being a child is like being a stranger in a foreign land, unable to speak the language and unaware of the proper behaviors for that world. To function as healthy adults, children need limits and rules that are lovingly, repeatedly, and consistently applied throughout their childhoods. They need to learn the customs, which behaviors are "right" or appropriate and which behaviors are "wrong," and they require the energies of adults in their environments to help guide them through the foreign lands of childhood and adolescence. Without this attention and guidance, children learn to cope in the best ways they can, even if these ways lead to ineffective or destructive behavioral disorders. Two diagnoses that relate to childhood and adolescent aggression are conduct disorder and oppositional defiant disorder.

Conduct disorder is characterized by a pattern of behavior "in which the basic rights of others or major age-appropriate societal norms or rules are violated" (American Psychiatric Association, 2000). The behaviors associated with this disorder fall into four main groups: aggressive conduct, nonaggressive conduct, deceitfulness, and serious rules violations. Individuals with conduct disorder naturally relate aggressively to others even when the situation is nonthreatening. They seldom have empathy for others, and they lack appropriate guilt feelings. The inability to tolerate frustration leads to temper outbursts and reckless behaviors. Inappropriate behavior patterns occur in homes, school, and communities.

Conduct disorders are usually diagnosed in late childhood or early adolescence. The majority of persons "outgrow" the problem by adulthood and are able to live effectively. However, a significant number of people go on to develop social and legal problems. Often they are diagnosed with antisocial personality disorders as adults.

Oppositional defiant disorder is a pattern of negative, aggressive behaviors that focuses on authority figures in the child's life. Children with this problem are constantly involved in power struggles, always fighting for control and attention. Their behaviors are stubborn, uncooperative, resistant, and hostile. The signs and symptoms of oppositional defiant disorder are often seen by 8 years of age and, without effective intervention, the behaviors often escalate or grow into conduct disorders. (See Chapter 14 for a discussion of conduct disorders in children.)

Impulse-Control Disorders

The essential feature of an impulse-control disorder is "the failure to resist an impulse, drive, or temptation to perform an act that is harmful to the person or to others" (American Psychiatric Association, 2000).

The typical individual with an impulse-control disorder begins to feel an increasing tension when presented with the "trigger" stimuli. Emotions continue to build and grow until the individual can no longer resist or control the impulse. He or she engages in the behavior (commits the act) and then experiences gratification, pleasure, and a release of tension. Guilt, remorse, or regret may or may not be felt after the impulse has been fulfilled.

Impulse-control disorders are named for the impulse that is related to the specific problem. Box 25-2 lists five types of impulse-control disorders. Although all types involve some form of aggression, the impulse-control problems encountered by health care workers most often relate to clients with intermittent explosive disorder.

Box 25-2 Impulse-Control Disorders

Intermittent Explosive Disorder

Repeated failures to resist acting on aggressive impulses, resulting in assaultive or destructive behaviors

Kleptomania

Repeated failure to resist the impulse to steal objects when they are not needed for personal use or survival

Pathological Gambling

Repeated episodes of maladaptive betting, wagering, playing games of chance, or gambling

Pyromania

Repeated behavioral pattern of starting fires for pleasure, relief of tension, or gratification

Trichotillomania

Repeated behavioral pattern of pulling out one's hair that results in noticeable loss of hair

Modified from American Psychiatric Association: *Diagnostic and statistical manual of mental disorders,* ed 4, text revision, Washington, DC, 2000, The Association.

The main feature of intermittent explosive disorder is a failure to resist aggressive impulses that result in the destruction of property or assault of another living being. Persons with intermittent explosive disorder have angry outbursts that are out of proportion to the stressor. For example, an individual may strike the teller at the bank for making him wait in line too long, whereas other people would sigh and continue to wait quietly for their turn.

Because these aggressive behaviors place others at risk for harm, people with these disorders often have difficulty with interpersonal, work, and social relationships. Intermittent explosive disorders more commonly occur in males and may appear during late adolescence through early adulthood.

Adjustment Disorders

The problems associated with coping with a new set of stressors can be overwhelming for any of us. The discomfort of adjusting from one situation to another can lead to certain mental health problems. Adjustment disorders are emotional or behavioral problems that develop in response to an identifiable source.

Persons with adjustment disorders have difficulty adapting to a new situation. These individuals become overwhelmed with the changes required of them during stressful times. Their distress is so great that it interferes with their activities of daily living. The stressor may be a single event (such as leaving a romantic relationship), continuous (such as living in a crime-filled neighborhood), or repeated (such as ongoing marital problems). Whatever the cause, the individual has difficulty coping effectively.

Adjustment disorders are also classified on the basis of their most frequent symptoms. The five subtypes are listed in Box 25-3.

By definition, an adjustment disorder lasts no longer than 6 months after the stressor(s) have stopped. Adjustment disorders are common, with most of us experiencing at least one episode during our lives. Fortunately human beings are adaptable, and most individuals learn to effectively cope with change. However, suicide attempts occur more frequently with persons who are having trouble adjusting to new situations. The

above diagnoses relate to mental health problems in which aggression plays an important part. Do not forget that anger, aggression, or hostility can be present in any individual.

GUIDELINES FOR INTERVENTION

It is important to keep in mind that diagnoses are only labels. You are working with individuals, real people with real problems. Therapeutic interventions should always be focused on the person, rather than on the diagnosis.

Assessing Anger and Aggression

The first step in controlling aggressive behaviors is to assess the client's potential for engaging in inappropriate behaviors. Obtain a mental status assessment as soon as possible after admission. Use therapeutic communication skills to help clients feel at ease. Try to establish trust and let clients know that they are respected even when angry.

Mental Status Assessment

Basic mental status examinations can be performed by any astute observer. Share your findings with other members of the health care team. During the mental status assessment, observe the client's *general appearance* and note the state of dress, cleanliness, and use of cosmetics or jewelry. Be sure to observe the client's *activity and behaviors*. Many times the clues to violence are being communicated nonverbally. Health care providers need to be alert enough to receive the messages. What about the client's *attitude*? Are interactions friendly and cooperative or resistive and hostile? Listen for the quality, rate, and amount of *verbal communications* in the client's speech. Pay particular attention to the individual's *mood, affect (emotional expressions), perceptions, and thoughts*. Have the client describe his or her mood at the time. Listen to the client's conversation for form and content. Does he or she speak logically, with a flow of ideas that are easily followed? What is the problem according to the client? Is the client's *judgment or insight* clear and easy to follow, or does it follow a twisted path of fuzzy explanations for past inappropriate behaviors? Is the client's *reliability* intact (does he or she give accurate information)?

Psychosocial Assessment

Next, perform a psychosocial assessment. Find out which internal or external *stressors* are present in the client's life. Which *coping skills* are being used to adapt to the stressors? Encourage the client to tell you about his or her important *relationships* and how they are affecting the situation. Do not forget to pay attention to the *cultural, spiritual,* and *occupational* areas of the client's life. Is he or she a member of a specific cultural group, organized religion, or occupation? Is there a *value and belief system*

Box 25-3 Types of Adjustment Disorders

1. Adjustment disorder with **depressed mood**
2. Adjustment disorder with **anxiety**
3. Adjustment disorder with **mixed anxiety and depressed mood**
4. Adjustment disorder with **disturbance of conduct**
5. Adjustment disorder with **disturbed emotions and conduct.**

that the individual feels is valuable, desirable, or worth following? Observe the client's *reactions and behaviors* during the interview. His or her reactions, behaviors, and attitudes during this time offer many clues concerning the potential for aggression or violent behaviors. Remember, the key to effective intervention begins with assessments. Assess clients often and report new behaviors. Troubleshooting is always an easier task than controlling a full-blown violent reaction. Possible nursing diagnoses are listed in Box 25-4.

Therapeutic Interventions

Therapeutic interventions for clients with anger and aggression focus on two basic areas: the client and the caregiver. Interventions for aggressive or potentially aggressive client behaviors can be viewed from three levels (Table 25-3).

Level one interventions focus on the *prevention* of violence. The goal of level one interventions (the best intervention for aggression) is to establish and maintain a trusting therapeutic relationship with clear and honest

communications. This is accomplished using a number of simple communication strategies.

Call the client and any family members by name. No one likes to be an anonymous face in the crowd. Explain what is happening, the reason for any delays, and why testing is needed. Most important, listen actively, with your whole body, not just the ears. Communicate your concern nonverbally while listening. Maintain good eye contact, while leaning forward slightly to communicate your interest. Give the client time to respond. Concentrate on the message he or she is trying to communicate to you. Paraphrase the problem to make sure that you have a good understanding of the client's point of view. Finally, help identify the emotions associated with the problem and explore appropriate options. Refer to Box 25-5 for an effective communication strategy.

Box 25-4 NANDA Nursing Diagnoses Related to Anger and Aggression

Adjustment, impaired*
Anxiety
Coping, ineffective individual
Denial, ineffective
Family processes, altered
Fear
Hopelessness
Noncompliance, specify
Powerlessness
Self-esteem disturbance
Self-mutilation, risk for
Social interaction, impaired
Violence, risk for: directed at others
Violence, risk for: self-directed

From North American Nursing Diagnosis Association: *NANDA nursing diagnoses: definitions and classification 1999-2000*, Philadelphia, 1999, The Association.
*Primary nursing diagnoses for anger and aggression.

Box 25-5 Communicating With Angry Clients

First, take a deep breath. Become calm and introduce yourself to the client. Speak slowly and do the following:

1. *Listen actively.* Use active listening skills to communicate interest in helping the client. Allow the client to define the problem that is causing the anger or aggression.
2. *Identify emotions.* Try to understand what is causing the problem and why the client is reacting with anger. Ask yourself what the client may be feeling and verbalize it. "You must be feeling pretty . . . " or "How do you feel about that?" allows the client to identify and discuss his or her emotions or problems.
3. *Explore options.* Help the client to regain some sense of control by brainstorming possible solutions to his or her problems. You may not be able to solve the problems, but you can assist the client in finding his or her own solutions.
4. *Offer positive comments.* Increase self-esteem by finding something the client does well and complimenting him or her. Many clients and their loved ones feel helpless, and the reassuring words of a concerned caregiver can provide great comfort.

Table 25-3 Levels of Intervention With Anger

Level	Goal
Level One—Prevent violence	Establish and maintain a trusting therapeutic relationship.
Level Two—Protect	Protect the client and others from potential harm.
Level Three—Control violence	Client is out of control. Protect client and others through seclusion, restraints, and intramuscular (IM) medication.

Level one interventions should be practiced routinely as preventive measures. They are also appropriate for clients who are in the "trigger stage" of the assault cycle. Very often just the caring concern of someone who is willing to really listen is enough to prevent anger from turning into aggression or violence.

Level two interventions focus on *protecting* the client and others from potential harm. These interventions are used when level one interventions are ineffective and signs of trouble are beginning to brew (see Case Study box). Learn to recognize the verbal and physical signs of impending violence.

>>> Sample Client Care Plan   Risk for Violence

Assessment

History: Bruce, a 15-year-old boy, has been sent to the mental health unit for psychiatric evaluation by the local police. Since age 13 he has been arrested several times for vandalism, drug possession, and menacing. His parents are cooperative but "feel helpless." His older sister is living away from home because she refuses "to be exposed to his violent behaviors."

Current Findings: An unkempt, sullen adolescent boy with tattoos on each knuckle of the right hand. Head is shaved in a pattern. Smoking cigarettes despite the "no smoking" sign posted on the wall.

Multidisciplinary Diagnosis	Planning/Goals
Risk for violence: directed at others	Bruce will demonstrate absence of aggressive or hostile threats or behaviors by October 10.

Therapeutic Interventions

Intervention	Rationale	Team Member
1. Approach Bruce with respect; avoid judging.	Adolescents need acceptance from adults as much as they need direction.	All
2. Orient to unit routine and policies; give clear, specific rules and the consequences for breaking them.	Assists Bruce until he is able to gain internal control over his aggressive behaviors.	Nsg
3. Assess for warning signs of increasing anger.	Behavioral changes often indicate an aggressive reaction; good assessment skills prevent injury to client and others.	All
4. Assess past acts of aggression and determine the potential seriousness of present actions.	Knowledge of previous patterns of violence helps assess Bruce's tolerance for current stresses.	All
5. Demonstrate acceptance of the painful feelings underlying Bruce's behaviors.	Helps to encourage Bruce's self-worth even though his behaviors are unacceptable.	All
6. Use open-ended questions; avoid asking "why."	"Why" questions call for an explanation or defensive reaction; open-ended questions help explore feelings, thoughts, and reactions.	All
7. Contract with Bruce for "no violence" while on unit.	Protects others from injury; encourages him to be responsible for his own actions.	
8. Teach stress management and problem-solving techniques.	Redirects energy created by anxiety and anger into healthier responses.	Psy, Nsg

---

Evaluation

By September 15, Bruce no longer required daily "time out" sessions. By October 2, Bruce was able to identify one source of his anger.

A complete client care plan includes several other diagnoses and interventions.

Case Study

Randy, a well-known, hot-tempered 24-year-old man, visits the clinic for weekly dressing changes for his right eye. Today he arrives seething with anger because his girlfriend just broke off their relationship.

"That _____ ! Just because we had a little fight she can't stand to be with me now. You women are all alike. I could punch you out right now and feel just fine," he snarls through clenched teeth as he glares into your eyes.

"You sound pretty upset. Tell me about it," you calmly reply. As Randy tells you about his relationship with his ex-girlfriend, you can see him becoming angrier by the moment. He begins to pound his fists on the table and stomp around the room. You signal for other staff members who have

been keeping an eye on the situation to be prepared to offer help, but so far Randy is acting out by ranting and raving. No damage is being done, and no person is in danger of harm.

After a few moments you reply, "Randy, I understand your anger, but stomping around is not appropriate. Let's take a couple of minutes to cool off, then maybe together we can think of some way to help solve the problem." Because you remained calm, quiet, and prepared, Randy responded to your request and took a few minutes to regain his composure.

◆ How do you think Randy would have reacted if he had encountered three staff members during his "ranting"?

Table 25-4	Client Education Plan: Modifying Impulsive Behavior		
Content	**Instructional activities**	**Evaluation**
Describe characteristics and consequences of impulsive behavior.	Select a situation in which impulsive behavior occurred. Ask the patient to describe what happened. Provide the patient with paper and a pen. Instruct the patient to keep a diary of impulsive actions, including a description of events before and after the incident.	Patient will identify and describe an impulsive incident. Patient will maintain a diary of impulsive behaviors. Patient will explore the causes and consequences of impulsive behavior.
Describe behaviors characteristic of interpersonal anxiety.	Discuss the diary with the patient.	Patient will connect feelings of interpersonal anxiety with impulsive behavior.
Relate anxiety to impulsive behavior.	Assist the patient to identify interpersonal anxiety related to impulsive behavior.	
Explain stress reduction techniques.	Describe the stress response. Demonstrate relaxation exercises. Assist the patient to return the demonstration.	Patient will perform relaxation exercises when signs of anxiety appear.
Identify alternative responses to anxiety-producing situations.	Using situations from the diary, and knowledge of relaxation exercises, assist the patient to list possible alternative responses.	Patient will identify at least two alternative responses to each anxiety-producing situation.
Practice using alternative responses to anxiety-producing situations.	Role-play each of the identified alternative behaviors. Discuss the feelings associated with impulsive behavior and the alternatives.	Patient will describe the relationship between behavior and feelings. Patient will select and perform anxiety-reducing behaviors.

From Keltner NL, Schwecke LH, Bostrom CE: *Psychiatric nursing,* ed 3, St. Louis, 1998, Mosby.

Interventions during level two include measures to maintain a safe environment. Take charge with a calm but firm attitude. Allow clients to act out as long as they limit their behaviors to verbal assaults and harmless physical movements. Assure clients that they have a right to express angry feelings but not to impose them on others. Gently, but firmly, set limits on the client's behaviors by suggesting that they take a "time out," a cooling-off period. If it appears that the "time out" is not effective,

offer prn medication. Only after all other measures have been tried are level three interventions implemented. "Nonviolent physical control and restraint should be used only as a last resort" (Stuart and Laraia, 2001).

The last level of therapeutic interventions (level three) is reserved for those clients who are out of control (escalation stage of the assault cycle). Clients who are out of control fight, bite, kick, scratch, spit, and throw things. They may be verbally abusive or physically aggressive.

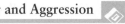
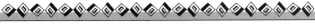

Think About

There are several techniques for managing your own anger.

1. **Vent your feelings.** Yell, scream, shout, but do it in a safe place.

2. **Change your focus.** Distract yourself for a moment or two—listen to the radio, take a walk. Move your energies from the anger to another topic. Playing with a pet is a great tranquilizer. Even counting to 10 can be very effective.

3. **Use your anger constructively.** Take the energy that is used to be angry and do something else with it. Clean the house. Organize the junk drawer. Exercise. Meditate.

4. **Discuss your anger** with those involved. Talking it out (after you are calm) lets people know what is on your mind and how you feel. Discussion also offers opportunities for personal learning and developing more therapeutic behaviors.

5. **Forgive** those with whom you are angry. If harsh words were exchanged, apologize. Apologies are free; they are not a sign of weakness, and they communicate a willingness to cooperate in the future. Forgiveness is an underused therapeutic tool.

6. **Relax.** Take slow, deep breaths and tell your body to relax and become calm. Remember the effects of our stress neurochemicals? Emotional responses have a strong impact on the physical body. Smile. It requires fewer muscles than a frown and promotes positive reactions in yourself and others.

Without intervention, both clients and their care providers are at an increased risk for injury. If level one and two interventions were effective, few clients reach this stage. However, for those who are engaging in violent behaviors, three interventions are available: seclusion, restraints, and intramuscular (IM) medication.

A point to remember here is that the use of restraints and seclusion as interventions for the control of assaultive behaviors must be planned ahead. Both strategies involve federal and state laws, institutional policies, and special procedures. Study the procedures for applying restraints and placing clients in seclusion (available in any nursing fundamentals text). Remember to monitor the condition of the restrained client at least every 15 minutes, and use other, less drastic measures as soon as the client has regained behavioral control. The Sample Client Care Plan on p. 293 offers suggestions for addressing aggressive behavior.

Once the assaultive event has subsided and the client is willing to discuss the problem, begin to enlist his or her help to modify the inappropriate behaviors. Table 25-4 offers an example of an educational plan for controlling impulsive, aggressive behaviors.

Interventions for caregivers focus on learning to effectively control your own feelings of anger. Even the most therapeutic care provider experiences anger. Learning to cope with your own feelings of anger or aggression allows you to be more successful in working with the angry emotions of others (see Think About box).

Practice your ability to cope with feelings and reactions at home and at work. As you improve, you will find yourself becoming more effective when working with the emotional responses of others.

KEY CONCEPTS

◆ Anger is a normal emotional response to a perceived threat, frustration, or distressing event.

◆ Anger serves as a coping mechanism, a motivator, or an opportunity for learning.

◆ Aggressive or hostile behaviors are angry feelings and impulses that are converted into action.

◆ Aggressive behaviors become inappropriate when they affect other people or their possessions.

◆ Assertiveness is the ability to directly express one's feelings or needs in a way that respects the rights of other people and retains the individual's dignity.

◆ Gender violence, which is the abuse of members of one sex by members of another, is seen in many cultural and social settings.

◆ The expression of anger occurs throughout the life cycle.

◆ Theories about the nature of aggression fall into one of three basic models: biological, psychosocial, and sociocultural theories.

◆ Assaults are aggressive behaviors that violate others' person or properties.

◆ Assault and violence occur in a predictable pattern of emotional responses called the assault cycle.

◆ The DSM-IV–TR lists three categories of disorders relating to aggressive behaviors: conduct disorders, impulse-control disorders, and adjustment disorders.

◆ The first step in controlling aggression is to assess the client's potential for engaging in inappropriate behaviors.

◆ Interventions for aggressive or potentially aggressive behaviors are divided into three levels: preventing violence, protecting the client and others, and secluding or restraining the out-of-control client.

◆ Learning to cope with your own feelings of anger or aggression allows you to be more successful in working with the emotions of others.

Suggestions for Further Reading

There are many good articles on this subject in various nursing, mental health, and social work journals, such as "Violence and Aggression in Psychiatric Patients" (*Harvard Mental Health Letter*, 15[10]:1, 1999).

Mental Health Net (www.cmhc.com) offers a wide range of information about many mental health problems.

References

American Psychiatric Association: *Diagnostic and statistical manual of mental disorders,* ed 4, text revision, Washington, DC, 2000, The Association.

Keltner NL, Schwecke LH, Bostrom CE: *Psychiatric nursing,* ed 3, St. Louis, 1998, Mosby.

Landers A, Jacobs NR, Siegel MA: *Violent relationships: battering and abuse among adults,* ed 7, Wylie, Tex, 1995, Information Plus.

Potter PA, Perry AG: *Basic nursing,* ed 4, St. Louis, 1998, Mosby.

Stuart GW, Laraia MT: *Principles and practices of psychiatric nursing,* ed 7, St. Louis, 2001, Mosby.

U.S. Bureau of the Census: *Statistical abstract of the United States: 1998,* ed 118, Washington, DC, 1998.

Wong DL: *Whaley and Wong's nursing care of infants and children,* ed 6, St. Louis, 1998, Mosby.

Chapter 26

Violence

Learning Objectives

1. Consider how violence influences the members of a society.
2. Explain three groups of theories that attempt to explain the cause of violence.
3. Describe six characteristics of a dysfunctional family.
4. Illustrate three consequences of abuse during pregnancy.
5. Identify two examples of abuse or neglect for each age group throughout the life cycle.
6. Outline the essential features of posttraumatic stress disorder and rape-trauma syndrome.
7. Discuss the special assessments for suspected victims of violence.
8. Describe three nursing interventions for helping clients recover from violence.
9. Explain how self-awareness can lead to a decrease in violent, abusive, or exploitive behaviors.

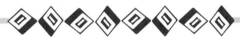

Key Terms

abuse

aggression

agitation

battering

domestic violence

exploitation

forensic evidence

homicide

incest

machismo

neglect

physical abuse

pornography

prostitution

rape

sexual abuse

shaken baby syndrome

violence

Aggressive, violent, and exploitive behaviors occur throughout the animal kingdom. Many animals battle violently for the right to mate and pass on their genes. Starlings exploit other birds by laying their single egg in another nest. These characteristics are also present in human beings, but they are expressed differently. There is a goal with animal aggression—to procure food, to mate, or to establish dominance in the group. Their use of violence is predictable and useful. Animals seldom risk injuring themselves just to be aggressive.

Human beings, however, engage in aggressive or violent behaviors for a variety of reasons, ranging from boredom to fear. In some instances, motives are clear and understandable. In others, however, all we are left with is uneasy questions. Human reactions exist on a continuum, ranging from calm to violent (Figure 26-1).

To discuss violence, one must be familiar with its related terms. **Agitation** describes behavior that is verbally or physically offensive. **Aggression** is defined as "a malicious act or threat directed toward others" (Littrell and Littrell, 1998). **Abuse** is the intentional misuse of someone or something that results in harm, injury, or trauma. Abuse can take place in the form of active harm or passive neglect. **Violence** is defined as "an ouburst of physical force that abuses, injures, or harms another" person or object (Littrell and Littrell, 1998). **Neglect** is harm to another's health or welfare through a failure to provide for basic needs or by placing the individual's

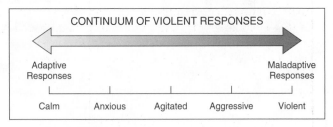

Figure 26-1 Continuum of violent responses.

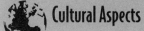

Cultural Aspects

Children as young as 4 years of age in poverty-stricken countries go to work in the rug mills and other manufacturing businesses. Many labor long hours in miserable working conditions for little pay. If a child does not work fast enough or has the courage to complain, he or she is physically punished. Children who are too outspoken about the poor working conditions have been known to "disappear."

health or welfare at unreasonable risk. Neglect often occurs to the more vulnerable members of society, such as children and elders. **Exploitation** refers to the use of an individual for selfish purposes, profit, or gain. Children who must labor with no time for study or play are examples of exploited individuals. Each of these terms describes some type of physical or psychological activity that is socially unacceptable.

The purpose of this chapter is twofold: (1) to help you understand the many ways in which violence is present in society and (2) to provide you with the tools to effectively assess, intervene, reduce, and prevent aggressive incidents.

SOCIAL FACTORS AND VIOLENCE

No one is certain exactly why violence occurs. We do know, however, that violent acts and their consequences are increasing with alarming frequency. Violence is a major cause of death and disability in most of the industrialized countries. For example, the murder rate in the United States has climbed from 17 murders per 100,000 people in 1970 to an alarming 27 murders per 100,000 by 1991. By 1996, the rate had dropped to 20 homicides per 100,000, but the United States still has the highest murder rate of all the "civilized countries" in the world. Finland and Hungary claim the sad distinction of having the highest number of suicides in the industrialized countries (U.S. Bureau of the Census, 1998).

These statistics mean that you will likely work with the victims of violence—as patients, parents of patients, friends, and relatives (Keltner, Schwecke, and Bostrom, 1998). Nurses and other health care providers accept and care for all people, but this philosophy also comes with the risk of violence. Therefore it is important to learn as much as possible about the problems and solutions related to the use of violence in society today.

Several cultural and social factors affect violence. Many societies promote the use of aggressive behaviors through beliefs, customs, and rituals. "The American culture of violence is reflected in the history, attitudes, belief systems, and coping styles of the population in dealing with conflicts, frustration, and the quest for wealth and power" (Schacter and Sienfield, 1994). In cultures in which the resources are scarce, violent acts become a way of life (see Cultural Aspects box).

Aggressive and violent acts are found in every group in society, and it appears that poverty plays a role in the development of aggressive behaviors. In many societies, productive and financially rewarding work is expected from most adults, especially men. A lack of fulfilling work often leads to poverty, frustration, and in many cases violence. To illustrate, the unemployment rate for young, minority men in the United States is "close to 50%. This group also has the highest rate of violence" (Stanhope and Lancaster, 1996).

THEORIES OF VIOLENCE

Several theories attempt to explain the nature of violence. The *psychiatric/mental illness model* views violence as a mental illness. Both victim and abuser are considered to be mentally disturbed. Recent evidence, however, has found that the incidence of mental illness is no greater in batterers or their victims than the rest of the population.

The *social learning theory* states that aggressive and violent behaviors are learned through role modeling others in the environment. Aggression is believed to be a learned behavior based on the values, attitudes, and actions of role models within the individual's environment.

Sociological theories credit environmental and social factors as causes for violence. Environmental factors, such as overcrowding, lack of adequate housing, and poor hygiene, can increase the incidence of aggression. The social factors of unemployment, poverty, crime, drug abuse, and isolation are believed to be related to violent acts.

Anthropological theories, which are based in the study of man's social history, explain violence and aggression as the result of cultural patterns, social organizations, or sexual differences. Because some cultures encourage the use of aggressive behaviors, their citizens learn to interact and cope aggressively. In other cultures, equality and harmony are stressed. Male and female roles are less

Box 26-1   Characteristics of Machismo

Has an attitude of male pride
Engages in thrill-seeking behaviors
Employs competition as his guiding principle
Is egocentric (self-centered)
Is unable to express emotions except anger and rage
Dislikes being gentle or vulnerable
Values sexual virility
Displays sexist attitudes
   Treats women as objects or commodities
   Sees women as objects of conquest
   Insists on being dominant to girls and women
   Holds to unwritten law that infidelity by a woman must
     be avenged
   Unable to cooperate with women
   Agrees to sexual use and abuse of women
Glorifies war and violence, supports the use of military
   force
Enjoys contact sports
Uses aggression to physically solve problems

defined in cooperative cultures than they are in cultures with hierarchies or degrees of power.

Finally, the *feminist theories* use the concept of "machismo" to explain the occurrence of violence against women. **Machismo** is defined as compulsive masculinity. Feminist theories state that males are socialized throughout childhood to behave more aggressively and violently. By the time boys have reached adolescence, they are preoccupied with physical strength and athletic prowess, attempts to demonstrate daring, violent, or aggressive behaviors. Men who have a high degree of machismo demonstrate certain social, behavioral, and sexual attitudes.

Machismo is found to be a strong influence on male behavior in many countries. These theories do not imply that every man with a high level of machismo abuses other people. They do, however, remind us that the potential for abuse lies within the machismo belief system (Box 26-1).

Dr. Sherry Turkle, a psychologist who studies cyberspace (the world of computers), believes that computer networks will change the way "people think about themselves and their role in society." Her particular fear is "that young people will succumb to the temptation to leave 'real life' behind for the ever-so-much more controllable realm of cyberspace" (Sessions, 1996). As more people become members of the computer network society, the number of "real," face-to-face relationships decreases. In these times of public isolation and anxiety over so many social forces, people are turning more and more to the Internet's "chat rooms" or other "information highways" in search of social interaction and supportive relationships.

Social connectedness is more than just an obligation or a desire—it fills the basic human need to belong. Social relationships are also important elements in preventing aggression and violence. The lack of supportive relationships has been linked to many negative consequences, including mental illness, crime, and suicide.

ABUSE, NEGLECT, AND EXPLOITATION WITHIN THE FAMILY

For far too long physical and emotional abuse within the family have remained unspoken issues. Traditionally victims suffer in silence, unable to seek help for fear of being revealed as less than a real person. Today communities are working to provide care and counseling for abused and exploited people. Family violence can take several forms.

Domestic Violence

In Western society the idea that a "man's home is his castle" has been inviolate. This principle has historically meant that the home is a private place. "What goes on inside one's home is nobody else's business" still remains a popular attitude today, even if the activities endanger family members.

Domestic violence is a term that describes abuse and battering within a family. **Battering** is a term that describes repeated physical abuse of someone, usually a woman, child, or elder. Victims of violent or abusive acts often suffer from posttraumatic stress disorder (discussed later in this chapter).

Accurate statistics on the incidence of domestic violence are unavailable because very few victims are willing to share their experiences. In 1994 only 40% of assaults were reported (U.S. Bureau of the Census, 1998). Today it is estimated that 1 American woman out of every 2 will be physically abused at some time in her life by the man with whom she lives. The Bureau of Justice National Crime Survey states that a woman is beaten in her home every 15 seconds (Statman, 1995). Studies conducted by the March of Dimes indicate that 1 of every 12 pregnant women suffer physical abuse (battering) during pregnancy.

A functional family unit is described by what it does (processes) to achieve its goals. These processes include clear and supportive communications among all family members, conflict resolution, the setting of goals, and the use of resources inside and outside of the family (Potter and Perry, 1998). A dysfunctional family is described by its inability or unwillingness to fulfill its basic functions. Box 26-2 lists several characteristics of a dysfunctional family.

Not all dysfunctional families have an element of abuse, but the inability of a family to meet the physical or psychological needs of its members greatly increases the opportunity for aggressive or violent behaviors.

Box 26-2 Characteristics of Dysfunctional Families

Family members are self-centered.

Authority is inconsistent or lacking; parents feel they cannot control children.

Roles are not clearly defined; it is unclear who is the parent, who is the child.

Members are unable to meet own or others' needs but each expects needs to be met.

Individualism is not encouraged; autonomy and trust are lacking.

No common goals can be identified; focus is on the present only.

Family appears chaotic, disorganized; no one is really aware of what is happening in the family.

Communications are cold and indifferent; family members feel pain and desperation; humor, caring, empathy, intimacy are absent; no clear communications exist.

Conflict is viewed as negative and is expressed through power struggles and sexual aggression.

Family may confuse violence with caring.

Family boundaries are rigid; threatened when outsiders try to enter group; family members are socially isolated; parents often married young and have few parenting skills.

Family violence is present.

Think About

Characteristics of Victims

Feels captive in the system (family, group, community)

Blames self for problems leading to abuse

Has low self-esteem; views self as unworthy

Feels helpless and powerless to change situation

Is financially, emotionally, or physically dependent on abuser

Is depressed, unable to see a future without abuse

◆ How many people do you know who demonstrate these characteristics?

◆ What interventions would you choose for a client who feels like a victim?

The family is considered a social unit that is entitled to privacy and freedom from intrusion. Unfortunately this doctrine has allowed untold numbers of women and children (and occasionally men) to suffer at the hands of their "loved ones." Violence within the family occurs in several ways. Common forms include physical, emotional, or sexual abuse and neglect of partners, children, and elderly.

Gender Abuse

No woman enters a relationship with the intent of becoming a battered partner, but wife beating is still considered an accepted part of marriage in many groups. Even in societies where domestic violence is condemned, individuals have their own attitudes, personal agendas, and faults that may cause conflict within the family. The notion that "all is fair in love and war" promotes the idea that marriage is a private relationship and the legal system should stay out of the picture—even when the picture includes assault, abuse, or injury.

There is no "typical" abused woman. The victims of violence do have some characteristics in common (see Think About box). Perhaps the most common trait is a trusting nature. Many women were raised to be nonaggressive and traditional; they were brought up to believe that the man is master and protector of the household.

These women, in turn, often feel that submission is the way to "please your man." The problem is that most abusive partners cannot be pleased.

When abuse occurs, guilt, anger, and terror shatter a woman's self-esteem. She suffers in silence, knowing that the consequences will be severe if she seeks help. Once a woman is battered, a vicious cycle of violence is soon established. Table 26-1 describes the cycle of domestic violence.

Abuser (batterer) behaviors have several characteristics. The profile of a typical abuser includes poor emotional control, a superior attitude toward women, a history of substance abuse, high levels of jealousy and insecurity, and the use of threats, punishment, and physical violence to control another's behavior. This profile may easily be the picture of a client, a client's partner, a parent, mate, neighbor, friend, or loved one. Early recognition of the characteristics of potential violence allows for more effective interventions. Box 26-3 lists several early signs of a potential abuser.

Abuse During Pregnancy

Pregnancy should be a time of great joy and anticipation, but for some women, pregnancy only increases their chances of being abused. It is difficult to believe that fathers would intentionally harm the mothers of their children, but trauma is the leading cause of maternal death during pregnancy. Statistics on prenatal violence are difficult to gather. Studies in public prenatal clinics reveal that more than 15% of clients are physically abused during the pregnancy and about 60% of the women questioned had suffered two or more assaults, indicating that episodes of abuse were recurrent. The frequency and severity of abuse, as well as the potential for homicide, are significantly increased for white women. In addition, abused women of all races were twice as likely to postpone beginning prenatal care until the third trimester of pregnancy, too late to prevent or treat many problems.

Table 26-1	Cycle of Domestic Violence
Man	**Woman**

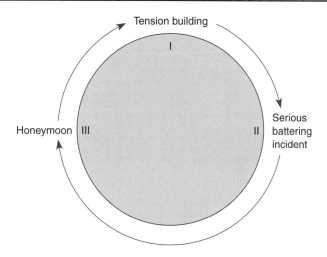

I. Tension Building

He has excessively high expectations of her.

He blames her for anything that goes wrong.

He does not try to control his behaviors.

He is aware of his inappropriate behaviors but does not admit it.

Verbal and minor physical abuse increase.

Afraid she will leave, he gets more possessive to keep her captive.

He gets frantic and more controlling.

He misinterprets her withdrawal as rejection.

She is nurturing, compliant, and tries to please him.

She denies the seriousness of their problems.

She feels she can control his behaviors.

She tries to alter his behavior to stay safe.

She tries to prevent his anger.

She blames external factors: alcohol, work.

She takes minor abuse, but does not feel she deserves it.

She gets scared and tries to hide (withdrawal).

She may call for help as the tension becomes unbearable.

II. Serious Battering Incident

The trigger event is an internal or external event or substance.

The battering usually occurs in private.

He will threaten more harm if she tries to get help (police, medical).

He tries to justify his behaviors but does not understand what happens.

He minimizes the severity of the abuse.

His stress is relieved.

In cases of long-term battering, she may provoke it just to get it over with.

She may call for help if she is afraid of being killed.

Her initial reaction is shock, disbelief, and denial.

Fearing more abuse if police come, she may plead for them not to arrest him.

She is anxious, ashamed, humiliated, sleepless, fatigued, depressed.

She may not seek help for injuries for a day or more and lies about the cause of injuries.

III. Honeymoon

He is loving, charming, begging for forgiveness, making promises.

He truly believes he will never abuse again.

He feels that he taught her a lesson and she will not "act up."

He preys on her guilt to keep her trapped.

She sees his loving behaviors as the real person and tries to make up.

She wants to believe it will never happen again.

She feels that if she stays, he will get help; the thought of leaving makes her feel guilty.

She believes in the permanency of the relationship and gets trapped.

Modified from Walker L: *The battered woman,* New York, 1979, Harper & Row.

Box 26-3 Early Signs of an Abusive Personality

1. A push for a quick involvement
2. Jealously controlling
3. Unrealistic expectations
4. Isolation
5. Blames others for own problems and mistakes
6. Makes others responsible for his feelings
7. Hypersensitive, easily insulted
8. Cruel to animals and children
9. "Playful" use of force during sex
10. Verbal abuse
11. Enforces rigid sex roles
12. Sudden mood swings
13. History of past batterings
14. Threatens violence

Modified from Carson VB: *Mental health nursing: the nurse-patient journey,* ed 2, Philadelphia, 2000, Saunders.

 Cultural Aspects

The following is popular saying in the red light district of Bangkok, where children are forced into prostitution:

At 10 you are a woman.
At 20 you are an old woman.
And at 30 you are dead.

The effects of abuse during pregnancy can be devastating. The frequency of low-birth-weight infants and preterm deliveries is almost doubled in women who have a history of abuse during pregnancy (Dickason, Schult, and Silverman, 1998). Because the mother is afraid to seek help, she often delays her entry into the health care system, thus denying both herself and her developing child the benefit of adequate prenatal care.

Child Abuse

Unfortunately the most vulnerable individuals in society, the children, are often the most abused. Child abuse occurs in many cultures and in many different manners (see Cultural Aspects box).

Child **pornography** (writings, pictures, or other messages pertaining to children that are intended to sexually arouse), child **prostitution** (selling of sexual favors by children), and child sexual abuse exist all over the world. In Brazil alone, it has been estimated that between 250,000 and 500,000 children are involved in the sex trade, but the numbers are even greater in Asia with more than a half million child prostitutes in Thailand. Most of them are girls under the age of 16, but in Sri Lanka, many child prostitutes are boys who cater to older men.

Many children are sold into prostitution with the belief that they will not be infected with acquired immunodeficiency syndrome (AIDS). Sadly, however, this is not the case. The Children's Rights Protection Center in Thailand claims that the AIDS rate among Thai child prostitutes approached 50%.

Children are also bought, sold, and exploited as objects of trade. They are purchased cheaply in one country and sold for a handsome profit in another. Young girls from the Philippines are imported to Japan for prostitution in a business that makes over a million dollars a day. Many gypsy children are forced into begging, often bringing in hundreds of dollars a day, and are under complete control of their abusers.

In some societies, female infants are undesirable. Girls commonly receive less food, attention, or education than their brothers. For example, according to the World Bank, the death rate for young girls in India outnumbers the death rate for young boys by more than 300,000 deaths per year. The majority of orphans in China are girls. After reviewing these facts, it is easy to understand why child abuse and neglect is an important issue of our time.

Spanking was, and still is in several countries, a main form of discipline for children. Unfortunately spanking and other forms of physical punishment teach children that power and violence are approved coping mechanisms. Today the countries of Sweden, Finland, Norway, Austria, and Switzerland, in an effort to curb the growing rates of child abuse, prohibit all forms of physical punishment in schools and homes. Most other industrialized countries, except the United States, South Africa, and parts of Australia and Canada, have banned physical punishment in schools.

Child abuse went almost unrecognized in the United States until the early 1960s. Since then, the number of reported incidents has swelled to almost 3 million children (U.S. Bureau of the Census, 1998). One can see why child abuse has been called a national emergency.

The mistreatment of children can take several forms. **Physical abuse** is defined as inflicted injury to a child, ranging from minor bruises and lacerations to severe trauma and death. **Sexual abuse** is the intentional engaging of children in sexual acts. Sexual abuse can take the form of rape, incest, fondling, intercourse, or other forms of sexual contact. Emotional abuse involves rejection, criticism, terrorizing, and isolation. Although the scars of this type of abuse are seldom seen objectively, they result in deep and penetrating wounds for many individuals.

Neglect is the failure to provide the necessities of life. Physical neglect is the failure to provide a child's basic needs, such as food, clothing, shelter, and a safe environment. Emotional neglect is characterized by a lack of parent-child attachment. Medical care neglect is the refusal to seek treatment when it is needed. Delays in treatment are common in abused children. A rare form of child abuse, called *Munchausen syndrome by proxy*, occurs when caretakers simulate or create the signs and symptoms of illness in the child in order to receive attention from health care providers.

Abuse or neglect occurs during every stage of childhood. In infancy, the **shaken baby syndrome** should be suspected in every infant with unexplained or vague injuries. Shaken baby syndrome is defined as vigorous shaking of an infant that leads to whiplash-induced bleeding within the brain with no external signs of head trauma. This syndrome is difficult to diagnose because of the lack of physical evidence and the parents' refusal to discuss the situation.

Every health care provider must be alert for the possibility of a "shaken baby" whenever there is a history of unexplained lethargy, fussiness, or irritability in an infant. Seizures or swelling in the head demand immediate investigation. Because the incidence of shaken baby syndrome is increasing, efforts must be made to educate parents and community members about the importance of handling our youngest members of society with gentleness and care.

Children are victimized more often than adults. The types of violent behaviors associated with abused children include pandemic aggression in which the majority of children are assaulted; acute aggression, in which children are abused, neglected, or exploited; and extraordinary aggression, which usually results in death.

Adolescent Abuse

The incidence of abuse in adolescence is greater than once thought. Recent studies have reported that the rate of abuse for adolescents surpasses that of younger children. Abuse of adolescents is often the most overlooked type of family violence. For this reason abused teens are less likely to receive needed services and counseling.

Adolescence is a time of emotional development, but not all teens have severe mood swings, periods of depression, or suicidal thoughts. Too often these signs of possible abuse go unnoticed by adults. At other times they are recognized as natural outcomes of adolescent misbehavior. "He or she had it coming" is still a widely held attitude when it comes to abusing adolescents.

Abused adolescents often have significant health risks. High on the list are emotional disorders, which often result from a history of insecurity and self-survival. The incidence of eating disorders, substance abuse problems, delinquent behaviors, posttraumatic stress disorders (PTSDs), and suicide attempts are increased in adolescents who suffer from abuse. Premature sexual activity is common and all too often leads to unwanted pregnancies, sexually transmitted diseases, and AIDS. Worse yet, adolescent abuse can result in fatal accidents, murder, and suicide, the three leading causes of death for all adoles-

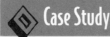

Case Study

Pete is a quiet, thoughtful, and charming young man whose intelligence shines through his sarcastic and tough demeanor. At 17 he is well developed and equipped to cope on the streets of Chicago. Pete is also the leader of a street gang and does not hesitate to use violence.

Pete comes from a family with two older brothers and a younger sister. In his early years it was common to see his mother and father arguing and hitting each other. By the time Pete was 6, his older brother had shot a neighbor and was "doing time." Throughout his childhood, Pete frequently vented his frustrations on his younger sister by hitting, pinching, and spitting on her.

At 8 Pete was initiated into his brother's gang. By 10 his intelligence and creativity had earned him the nickname of "the brain." By 14 he was destined for leadership. Today, at 17, Pete sits in a hospital bed with three bullet holes in his body. His bruised and pregnant girlfriend sits at his side. As soon as he can walk again, he plans to "make a little visit and even the score" with the guys he believes are responsible for his attack.

♦ Can you see any learned patterns of behavior in this family?

♦ What do you think could have been done to prevent this situation from occurring?

cents. One in four violent crimes are committed by adolescents (Wood, 1999).

Girls are more likely to be abused than boys, but boys are more likely to suffer abuse outside the home by peers and others. Sadly, studies have shown that many adults who were physically disciplined as children approve of the use of physical force for controlling another person's behavior. Individuals "who resort to acts of violence as adolescents are often the same people who end up in the nation's criminal system as adults" (Wood, 1999).

Adolescents are abused by parents, siblings, and persons outside the family. The most common form of violence within the home occurs between siblings. Violence between brothers and sisters is so common that it is often considered to be "normal behavior because parents take it for granted that "kids will be kids," and tend to ignore it. Yet this type of violence can have long-lasting effects.

Children learn to exploit and victimize each other during the early school years. By the teen years the use of violence can become interwoven with daily activities. Peer pressure can be great during adolescence, and those who are different suffer the consequences at the hands of their own peers.

Adolescents often receive the most severe abuse, the kind that results in serious disability or death (see Case Study box).

Often, though, the signs of family mistreatment are vague. A history of abuse is frequently found in teens who are runaways, homeless, or incarcerated (in jail or prison). The blossoming problems of teen violence and abuse can be prevented if health care providers are willing to invest their best therapeutic efforts into these "forgotten clients."

Elder Abuse

As the number of older people grows, the potential for their maltreatment or neglect increases. Each year more than 1 million elderly persons are victims of abuse or mistreatment, but only one in five cases is reported. Almost 5% of crimes involving victims occur in the elderly population (U.S. Bureau of the Census, 1998).

Vulnerable older adults include those with chronic or disabling illnesses, the aged, and those who are poor or have few resources. The "typical victim" of elder abuse is an older woman who is living with a relative and is physically or mentally impaired. She usually has a history of unexplained bruises or injuries, burns in unusual places, sexually transmitted disease, or poor personal hygiene. She may experience extreme mood swings, be depressed, fearful, and extremely concerned about the cost of health care. Many times the families of abused elders "health care shop," missing appointments and changing health care providers frequently.

Family members are the most frequent abusers of the elderly. The demands placed on caregivers often influence the development of abuse. Violence can erupt when caregivers feel stressed, pressured, or frustrated. In addition, many people who abuse their elders are coping with current substance-related or mental health problems themselves.

Neglect and exploitation are also common among the elderly. Neglect can take the form of not providing food, health care, or aids such as dentures, glasses, or hearing aids. Older adults who are unable to walk can suffer from long periods of isolation or abandonment. Neglect also includes deliberate efforts to cause emotional distress, such as threatening harm or withholding important information.

Exploitation of the elderly is often financial in nature. They are a favorite target for cons or extortionists. Many times, older adults are forced to sign over their properties, their pensions, or other assets. The elderly may be denied the right to vote or to make their own decisions. On some occasions they are placed in nursing homes without their consent.

Today many states have passed laws that require reporting of abusive incidents. Nurses can go a long way toward preventing elder abuse by recognizing the signs and symptoms of abuse, becoming familiar with the laws governing mandatory reporting of abuse, and working to prevent violence in all settings. It is every person's responsibility to protect the aging members of society.

Sexual Abuse

A particularly devastating form of abuse is sexual abuse, the unwanted sexual attentions of another. When sexual activities or intercourse occurs between members of the same family (other than the parents) it is called **incest.** Sexual violence has strong and lasting consequences for the victims. Children who are sexually abused suffer from a wide spectrum of mental health disorders, ranging from chronic headaches to depression, posttraumatic stress disorders, and severe personality disorders.

Sexually abused adults are most often women. Most sexual assaults are made by women's partners. Sexual assaults occur in 200 out of every 1000 people (Rose, 1998). The most violent form of sexual assault, rape, often occurs more frequently in relationships associated with other forms of physical aggression. Episodes of battering often include sexual and physical attacks—a deadly combination for many maltreated adult women.

Sexual abuse in the elderly, especially women, occurs with all-too-common frequency. Because sexual mistreatment of the elderly is still a "taboo" subject, it often goes unrecognized by health care providers. Clues to the presence of sexual abuse in the elderly include complaints of pain, itching, or soreness in the genital area; bruises or other evidence of injury around the genital area or elsewhere on the body; difficulty in walking, sitting, or moving; the presence of unexplained venereal disease or genital infections; and stained, torn, or bloody underclothing.

Health care providers, especially nurses, should routinely assess all clients for a history of abuse or victimization and report any suspicious signs, symptoms, or behaviors to supervisors and required authorities. An individual's well-being is worth the effort.

ABUSE, NEGLECT, AND EXPLOITATION WITHIN THE COMMUNITY

Aggressive and violent behaviors are fast becoming a common way of coping with problems. Violence against innocent bystanders continues to increase as more people approve of its use or turn a blind eye to its occurrence. No statistic can accurately record the number of violent acts that occur, but in 1996, an estimated 42 violent acts per 1000 people occurred in the United States (U.S. Bureau of the Census, 1998).

Violence, Trauma, and Crime

People use violence against each other in many ways, in both legal and illegal manners. Today society is confronted with a steady diet of violent behaviors. Although most **homicides** (taking the life of another person) are committed by family members or friends, a surprising number of them occur at the hands of complete strangers. Robbery has become commonplace in most communities, and an unsettling trend of murder in the workplace is rising. Car theft and drive-by crimes are increasing. Children are being kidnapped with greater frequency, and the incidence of violent crimes by and against children and adolescents continues to soar.

Acts of violence are becoming commonly accepted in society. Radio, television, and the "Net" (Internet) surround people with examples of violence. Our children are soaked in tales of aggressive actions from the time they are first exposed to cartoons. Studies by television's cable network group have revealed that over half the programs on television are violent or aggressive in nature. In most programs, the victims are not hurt, and the aggressor is seldom caught or punished. This steady diet has resulted in children who are more willing to solve their problems with the use of violence than with critical thinking or problem solving.

Acts of violence on television pale in comparison with those that occur daily in "real life." Daily newspapers and radio and television news programs announce a litany of the day's violent activities. People listen, shake their heads, and then continue with their own lives, unaware that they may be the next victims.

Violence breeds physical and emotional pain for its victims. The basic needs of trust and autonomy (control) are threatened when one is involved with violence. Victims react with anger, fear, denial, and shame. The well-meaning comments of friends and loved ones may even imply fault. Many victims of violence harbor feelings of unworthiness and contamination. Relationships with family and friends may become disturbed as victims attempt to put the pieces of their lives back together.

Crime is a natural vehicle for violence. Many crimes are committed on impulse, whereas others are well planned. Crime may or may not involve physical aggression and violence, but the impact of being victimized by crime leaves deep emotional scars on most individuals.

Group Abuse

Throughout history people have chosen certain groups of people to define as "being different" from themselves. Individuals within these groups may be kind and gentle, but association with the group stigmatizes them as "one of those people." This label somehow justifies the aggressive and violent reactions of persons who view the group members with hostility. Excellent examples of this twisted line of thinking can be found throughout history and in the "ethnic cleansing" occurring in many countries.

Aggression against certain groups also exists in more subtle ways. Admission to many schools or academic institutions often depends on belonging to the "right group." Job requirements may be structured to attract only a certain "kind" of applicant, and running for a political office can be done only if one "fits in." These forms of aggression against members of certain groups are all quiet, subtle, and usually unspoken, but they still exert influences over the lives of many good people.

MENTAL HEALTH DISORDERS RELATING TO VIOLENCE

Crisis is a part of every violent act. One's usual coping skills are ineffective when dealing with the effects of a violent act. To recover from an act of violence, new coping behaviors must be found and then applied. The victims of violence suffer through a number of emotional and behavioral experiences that may take months or even years to resolve. The process of putting one's life back together after a violent act involves many changes that take place over time (Table 26-2). The process of recovery from violence is influenced by the severity of the trauma, the resources of the victim, and the help and treatment received immediately following the traumatic event.

Aggressive and violent behaviors are a part of numerous mental health disorders; however, the *Diagnostic and Statistical Manual of Mental Disorders* (DSM-IV–TR) defines only one clinical syndrome as directly related to violence: posttraumatic stress disorder. Rape-trauma syndrome is a related nursing diagnosis that encompasses the essentials of care for the victims of this violent experience.

Posttraumatic Stress Disorder

"The essential feature of posttraumatic stress disorder (PTSD) is the development of characteristic symptoms following exposure to extreme traumatic stressors" (American Psychiatric Association, 2000). Posttraumatic stress disorder clearly relates to an actual traumatic event that was outside the realm of common human experience. Examples include war and military combat, violent assault, rape, torture, burglary, natural disasters, terrorist activities, fires, bombings, sudden destruction of one's home, and witnessing the assault, injury, or death of a loved one.

Typically people with PTSD persistently relive the traumatic event through intrusive thoughts or distressing dreams. Intense fear, horror, and hopelessness are experienced as individuals struggle to rid themselves of their memories. The sudden arrival of these intrusive thoughts (often called flashbacks) motivate individuals with PTSD to avoid any stimuli associated with the traumatic event. Emotional responses in general become blunted except for those related directly to the violent event. This "psychological numbing" effectively shuts

Table 26-2	Stages of Recovery From Violence	
Stage of recovery	**Time frame**	**Emotions, behaviors**
Impact: disorganization	Minutes to days	Initial reactions: crying, confusion, denial, disbelief, fear, hysteria, helplessness, shock; may have physical responses, eating or sleeping disturbances; may be calm with others and then react in private
Recoil: struggle to adapt	Weeks to months	Slowly becomes aware of impact of event on his or her life; immediate danger is past but emotional stress remains; may plan for revenge; tries to resume daily routines; needs to discuss details of violent event; may become dependent; needs much emotional support
Reorganization: reconstruction	Months to years	Emotions fade, but event is not forgotten; reviews event with "Why me?" questions; justifies own actions, then gains sense of control over life; grieves over losses; may experience lingering emotions, nightmares; realizes that life will always be different as result of violence; eventually integrates memories and learns to live with reasonable sense of safety and security; may develop mental health problems if reorganization is not successful

Modified from Keltner NL, Schwecke LH, Bostrom CE: *Psychiatric nursing,* ed 3, St. Louis, 1998, Mosby.

out the outside world until the person is exposed to an event, item, or situation that symbolizes some aspect of the traumatic event. For many survivors of war, just watching television can precipitate flashbacks and stress reactions.

People suffering from PTSD often feel removed and detached from other people, even those they love. The ability to feel emotions is reduced, especially those associated with love, intimacy, and sexuality. Often persons with PTSD believe that their lives will be short and wonder why they survived when others did not.

Rape-Trauma Syndrome

Rape is an act of sexual violence by one person against another. Although rape may involve sexual behaviors, it is an act of power that aims to cause pain at the most intimate level of one's being. Forced sexual attentions are a violation of one's person, whether they occur at the hands of a stranger or a loved one.

A woman may be raped at any age, but the ages of 15 to 24 are associated with the highest risk. Rape is an underreported crime, with estimates of one woman in three being raped at sometime during her life. Although not as common, the incidence of men being raped by other men is rising, but it is rarely reported (Keltner, Schwecke, and Bostrom, 1998).

Many of the victims of rape realize that they have lived through the experience but wish they had died. A threat on the life of the victim or the promise to return may have been made. Bodily injuries may be minor or severe. Some

individuals may have been tortured or injured during or shortly after the rape episode.

Survivors of sexual assaults feel severely violated. Feelings of anger, frustration, loss of control, fear, shame, and guilt haunt the victims of these violent acts. Following the rape, most individuals feel the need to retreat to a safe place, clean themselves thoroughly, and destroy all reminders of the event. To do this, however, destroys most of the evidence that may be useful in apprehending the offender.

Recovery from being the victim of a rape follows the same steps as the stages of recovery from other violent acts (see Table 26-2). Immediately following the incident, the individual becomes disorganized, then attempts to adjust are made, and finally the experience is integrated into his or her life. The greater the force or brutality, though, the greater psychological harm and recovery time. Many individuals do not report the assaults to the police. They carry the burden alone and suffer a silent rape-trauma syndrome.

Nurses may be the first health care providers with whom a rape victim interacts. Strong support, gentle understanding, and nonjudgmental acceptance have a powerful influence on how well the victim copes with and successfully recovers from this violent assault. Because rape is a reportable crime, evidence must be gathered, with the victim's permission. Nurses should make sure to follow the same protocol every time they care for a client who has been raped. Evidence that has been gathered carefully and good documentation are important tools if the case is taken to court.

THERAPEUTIC INTERVENTIONS

Health care providers are concerned with two major goals when working with the victims of violence. The first and longest-reaching goal is to prevent violence from occurring. The second goal revolves around early recognition and treatment for violated individuals.

Working with abused or victimized clients on a regular basis requires special education and training. Some nurses and other health care providers become rape counselors or advocates for the abused and exploited. However, every caregiver can apply special measures to care for the individuals who have the misfortune to become victims of violence.

Special Assessments

Whenever a suspected victim of violence is brought into the health care system, be it the emergency department or clinic, special attention is required. The first priority of care is to ensure the client's safety, but the preservation of evidence also is extremely important.

Forensic evidence is information that is gathered for legal purposes. It is the evidence that helps find and convict perpetrators of violent acts. When violence is suspected, the caregiver's most effective tools are accurate observations, precise documentation, and notification of the appropriate authorities. By law, health care providers are required to report these incidences. Although the victims of rape are not required by law to report it, all evidence is important and must be gathered carefully.

When assessing a client who has been a victim of violence, first obtain his or her consent (Rose, 1998). Then document the size, shape, color, and pattern of any wounds, bruises, scars, or other marks. The skin records evidence well. Human bite marks leave a history. Look for them on the ears, nose, nipples, armpits, back, and genitals. Rings, belt buckles, and other items leave telltale marks behind when they are used as weapons. Other physical signs or symptoms that may indicate violence or abuse include odd marks on the skin, hyperactive reflexes, and poor eye contact. Child abuse or neglect is not always easy to spot. Table 26-3 lists numerous signs and symptoms of child abuse and neglect.

Caregivers, especially nurses, must know how to assess suspicious injuries and describe their findings objectively. Box 26-4 offers an example of an abuse assessment documentation form. Document objective evidence as accurately as possible. Do not guess or draw conclusions about the cause of any injury. If the client is a rape victim, all specimens should be labeled and saved for analysis. It is wiser to err on the side of gathering too much information rather than not enough.

Treating Victims of Violence

Remember, the first priority of care for every victim of violence is to ensure his or her safety and security. Once a client feels safe, other therapeutic interventions can be more easily implemented.

Do not leave the client alone. Many victims believe that their abusers may attempt to hurt them again, even when they are seeking help. Explain all procedures simply, and ensure cooperation before proceeding. Allow the client to maintain as much control as possible.

The care plan is developed based on the individual client, the type of abuse, and the resources available. Nursing diagnoses are chosen according to identified problems. Refer to Box 26-5 for a list of possible nursing diagnoses.

It is important to remember that each diagnosis has many interventions, and the selection depends on each client and his or her particular circumstances. However, all clients who have been abused exploited, or neglected have certain care needs in common (see Sample Client Care Plan for a victim of violence).

Aggressive and violent actions are often seen in clients who are diagnosed with a mental illness. Treatment consists of assessing risk factors, developing interventions to reduce aggressive reactions, and helping clients learn more effective coping skills. Clients are often prescribed medications to help control aggressive and violent behaviors (see Table 26-4).

Preventing Violence in Your Life

Given the statistics, it is likely that each of us will be exposed to violence at some time during our lives. As members of the health care profession, the odds of being involved in violent acts are increasing. Health care providers are less immune to acts of violence than they were in the past. It is important to remain aware that violence can erupt in any client situation.

When interacting with clients, watch for signs of growing anxiety, frustration, or agitation and then intervene quickly to prevent problems from escalating. Refer back to Figure 26-1. Trust your own judgment or "gut-level feelings," and seek assistance from other care providers when needed.

Prevent yourself from becoming victimized by clients or their family members by enforcing your professional boundaries (see Chapter 12, discussion of helping boundaries) and working within your legal and ethical parameters. The goal of providing emotional/mental health care is to *assist* clients in successfully coping with *their* problems. Remembering "who owns the problem" allows care providers to remain therapeutic without becoming victimized.

Work to prevent violence in your life. Contact the sponsors of violent programs on television; write companies and protest. Support legislative actions that are designed to reduce violence. Volunteer at shelters, crisis hot lines, or support groups. Educate those who will listen about the effects of violence on children. Volunteer to teach a program on problem solving at local preschools.

Table 26-3	Signs/Symptoms of Child Abuse and Neglect
Category	**Child's appearance**
Physical abuse	**Bruises and welts:** on face, lips, or mouth; in various stages of healing; on large areas of torso, back, buttocks, or thighs; in unusual patterns, clustered, or reflective of instrument used to inflict them; on several different surface areas
	Burns: cigar or cigarette burns; glove or sock-like burns or doughnut-shaped burns on buttocks or genitalia indicating immersion in hot liquid; rope burns on arms, legs, neck, or torso; patterned burns that show shape of item (iron, grill, etc.) used
	Fractures: skull, jaw, or nasal fractures; spiral fractures of arms or legs; fractures in various states of healing; multiple fractures; any fracture in child under 2
	Lacerations and abrasions: to mouth, lip, gums, or eye; genitalia
	Human bite marks
Neglect	Consistently dirty, unwashed, hungry, or inappropriately dressed
	Without supervision for extended time or when engaged in dangerous activities
	Constantly tired or listless
	Has unattended physical problems or lacks routine medical care
	Is exploited, overworked, or kept from attending school
	Has been abandoned
Sexual abuse	Has torn, stained, or bloody underclothing
	Is experiencing pain or itching in genital area
	Has bruises or bleeding in external genitalia, vagina, or anal regions
	Has venereal disease
	Has swollen or red cervix, vulva, or perineum
	Has semen on mouth or genitalia or on clothing
	Is pregnant
Emotional maltreatment	Emotional maltreatment, often less overt than other forms of child abuse and neglect; indicated by behaviors of child and caretaker

Modified from *Interdisciplinary glossary on child abuse and neglect: legal, medical, social work terms,* DHHS Pub No 80-30137, Washington, DC, 1980, U.S. Department of Health and Human Services.

Child's behavior	Caretaker's behavior
Wary of physical contact with adults	Has history of abuse as child
Apprehensive when other children cry	Uses harsh discipline
Demonstrates extremes in behavior (e.g., aggressiveness or withdrawal)	Offers illogical, unconvincing, contradictory, or no explanation of child's injury
Seems frightened of parents	Seems unconcerned about child
Reports injury by parents	Significantly misperceives child (e.g., sees him or her as bad, evil, a monster)
	Psychotic or psychopathic
	Misuses alcohol or other drugs
	Attempts to conceal child's injury or to protect identity of person responsible
Engages in delinquent acts (e.g., vandalism, drinking, prostitution, drug use)	Misuses alcohol or other drugs
Begs or steals food	Maintains chaotic home life
Rarely attends school	Shows evidence of apathy or futility
	Mentally ill or of diminished intelligence
	Has long-term chronic illnesses
	Has history of neglect as child
Appears withdrawn or engages in fantasy or infantile behavior	Extremely protective or jealous of child
Has poor peer relationships	Encourages child to engage in prostitution or sexual acts in presence of caretaker
Unwilling to participate in physical activities	Has been sexually abused as child
Engages in delinquent acts or runs away	Experiencing marital difficulties
States he or she has been sexually assaulted	Misuses alcohol or other drugs
	Frequently absent from home
Appears overly compliant, passive, undemanding	Blames or belittles child
Extremely aggressive, demanding, or rageful	Cold and rejecting
Shows overly adaptive behaviors, either inappropriately adult (e.g., parents other children) or inappropriately infantile (e.g., rocks constantly, sucks thumb, is enuretic)	Withholds love
	Treats siblings unequally
	Seems unconcerned about child's problem
Lags in physical, emotional, and intellectual development	
Attempts suicide	

Box 26-4   Abuse Assessment Screen

1. Have you **ever** been emotionally or physically abused by your partner or someone important to you?

    Yes ☐   No ☐

2. **WITHIN THE LAST YEAR,**
    have you been hit, slapped, kicked, or otherwise physically hurt by someone?

    Yes ☐   No ☐

    If YES, by whom? _____ Total number of times _____

3. Since you've been pregnant, were you hit, slapped, kicked, or otherwise
    physically hurt by someone?

    Yes ☐   No ☐

    If YES, by whom? _____ Total number of times _____

MARK THE AREA OF INJURY ON THE BODY MAP, SCORE EACH INCIDENT ACCORDING TO THE FOLLOWING SCALE:

SCORE

1=Threats of abuse including use of a weapon   _____

2=Slapping, pushing; no injuries and/or
   lasting pain   _____

3=Punching, kicking, bruises, cuts and/or
   continuing pain   _____

4=Beating up, severe contusions, burns,
   broken bones   _____

5=Head injury, internal injury, permanent
   injury   _____

6=Use of weapon; wound from weapon   _____

If any of the descriptions for the higher number apply, use the higher number.

4. **WITHIN THE LAST YEAR,**
    has anyone forced you to have sexual activities?

    Yes ☐   No ☐

    If YES, by whom? _____ Total number of times _____

5. Are you afraid of your partner or anyone you listed above?

    Yes ☐   No ☐

Developed by the Nursing Research Consortium on Violence and Abuse. Readers are encouraged to reproduce and use this assessment tool. (Redrawn from McFarlane J, Parker B: Preventing abuse during pregnancy: an assessment and intervention protocol, *MCN: American Journal of Maternal Child Nursing* 19(6):321, 1994.)

Box 26-5 NANDA Nursing Diagnoses Related to Violence

Adjustment, impaired*
Anxiety
Coping, ineffective individual
Denial, ineffective
Family processes, altered
Fear
Hopelessness

Personal identity disturbance
Powerlessness
Rape-trauma syndrome
Self-esteem disturbance
Social interaction, impaired
Violence, risk for: directed at others
Violence, risk for: self-directed

From North American Nursing Diagnosis Association: *NANDA nursing diagnoses: definitions and classification 1999-2000,* Philadelphia, 1999, The Association.
*Primary nursing diagnosis for violence.

Table 26-4 Medications Used to Manage Aggression

Drug class	Example	Care implications
Atypical antipsychotics	Clozapine, risperidone	Can only be given by mouth
Beta-adrenergic blockers	Propranolol, nadolol, metoprolol, pindolol	Frequent side effects
Antianxiety agents	Buspirone, lorazepam, benzodiazepines	For short-term use only
Anticonvulsants	Valproic acid, divalproex sodium	Frequent side effects; interacts with other anticonvulsants, sedatives, and other medications

Learn to recognize aggression and violence in your personal thoughts, attitudes, and responses. Become aware of how you cope with feelings of anger, frustration, and aggression; practice developing more effective methods for working with your emotions. Howard Zinn, in his book *You Can't Be Neutral on a Moving Train* (1994), titled the epilogue "The Possibility of Hope." In it he states that "small acts, when multiplied by millions of people, can transform the world." The small acts of nurses and other health care providers help to nourish the human connections that weave us together. Perhaps, just perhaps, we can make a difference in relation to violence—if we are all willing to try.

KEY CONCEPTS

◆ Violence is a major cause of death and disability in most industrialized countries of the world.
◆ Theories that attempt to explain the nature of violence include the psychiatric/mental illness model, social learning theories, sociological theories, anthropological theories, and feminist theories.
◆ Battering is a term that describes ongoing physical abuse of someone, usually a woman, child, or elder.
◆ Trauma is the leading cause of maternal death during pregnancy.

◆ Since the early 1960s, the number of reported incidents of child abuse or neglect has increased dramatically.
◆ Adolescent abuse is often an overlooked type of violence.
◆ Each year over a million elderly persons are victims of abuse or mistreatment.
◆ Throughout history people have chosen certain groups of people to define as being different and therefore deserving of aggressive behaviors.
◆ The process of recovery from violence is influenced by the severity of the trauma, the resources of the victim, and the help and treatment received by the victim immediately following the traumatic event.
◆ The essential feature of posttraumatic stress disorder (PTSD) is the development of characteristic symptoms following exposure to an extreme traumatic stressor.
◆ Rape is an act of sexual violence by one person against another that involves the use of power.
◆ Two major health care goals for treating the victims of violence are to prevent violence from occurring and to provide early recognition and treatment for the violated individuals.
◆ The first priority of care for every victim of violence is to ensure safety and security.
◆ By law, health care providers are required to report incidences of suspected or actual abuse or neglect.

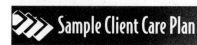

Sample Client Care Plan — Rape-Trauma Syndrome

Assessment

History: Sierra is a 19-year-old college student who lives at home. Three weeks ago she met Ben, a road maintenance worker who was visiting a mutual friend. After a short visit, Sierra said she was going to the club for her workout. Ben offered to drive her since he was going in the same direction. Sierra accepted, saying that she had to stop at her house first to change clothes.

On arrival Sierra left the car and walked into the house.

She was surprised to see Ben following her and asked him to wait in the car. Later that day Sierra's mother found her beaten and tied to her bed.

Current Findings: A stuporous young woman, lying in the fetal position. Numerous bruises and abrasions are noted on the face, both wrists, legs, and feet. Mother is at the bedside.

Multidisciplinary Diagnosis

Rape-trauma syndrome related to recent sexual attack and injury

Nursing diagnosis: as above

Planning/Goals

Sierra will be free of medical or physical complications of rape trauma.

Sierra will establish a therapeutic alliance with the primary nurse.

Therapeutic Interventions

Intervention	Rationale	Team Member
1. Allow Sierra's mother to remain with her at all times.	Mother has historically provided safety and security for Sierra.	Nsg
2. Assist with physical assessment and gathering of specimens after consent is obtained.	To assess the extent of her physical injuries, psychological trauma; to gather forensic evidence.	Nsg
3. Let Sierra know that she will not be blamed for the rape incident.	Violated persons often feel they will be held responsible for encouraging the assult.	Nsg, Psy
4. Convey an accepting, caring, non-judgmental attitude regardless of the circumstances.	Helps to establish therapeutic communications and builds trust.	All
5. Encourage Sierra to acknowledge the pain and anger of the rape experience.	Releasing painful emotions lessens their intensity and power.	Psy, Nsg
6. Explain the importance of seeking support and counseling for Sierra and her family.	Provides emotional support during the process of returning to "normal."	Psy, Nsg
7. Encourage Sierra to report the incident to the police.	May help to prevent other occurrences; may help to bring the perpetrator to justice.	Psy, Nsg
8. Make referrals to rape crisis center, family counselors (with permission).	Long-term emotional support will help Sierra and her family effectively adapt.	Soc Svc

Evaluation

Sierra tested negative for sexually transmitted diseases 3 weeks after the incident. Following 2 weeks of emotional support and encouragement, Sierra attended her first crisis support group.

A complete client care plan includes several other diagnoses and interventions.

Suggestions for Further Reading

The *Battered Woman's Survival Guide,* written by Jan Berliner Statman (Dallas, 1995, Taylor) is a must-read for every health care provider. The true stories contained within will give you a realistic and valuable look into the lives of battered women and their children.

A wealth of online trauma resources and support information can be found at David Baldwin's Trauma Info Pages (www.trauma-pages.com).

References

American Psychiatric Association: *Diagnostic and statistical manual of mental disorders,* ed 4, text revision, Washington, DC, 2000, The Association.

Carson VB: *Mental health nursing: the nurse-patient journey,* ed 2, Philadelphia, 2000, Saunders.

Dickason EJ, Schult MO, Sliverman BL: *Maternal-infant nursing care,* ed 3, St. Louis, 1998, Mosby.

Interdisciplinary glossary on child abuse and neglect: legal, medical, social work terms, DHHS Pub No. 80-30137, Washington, DC, 1980, U.S. Department of Health and Human Services.

Keltner NL, Schwecke LH, Bostrom CE: *Psychiatric nursing,* ed 3, St. Louis, 1998, Mosby.

Littrell KH, Littrell SH: Current understanding of violence and aggression: assessment and treatment, *Journal of Psychosocial Nursing* 36(12):18, 1998.

McFarlane J, Parker B: Preventing abuse during pregnancy: an assessment and intervention protocol, *MCN: American Journal of Maternal Child Nursing* 19(6):321, 1994.

North American Nursing Diagnosis Association: *NANDA nursing diagnoses: definitions and classification 1999-2000,* Philadelphia, 1999, The Association.

Potter PA, Perry AG: *Basic nursing: theory and practice,* ed 4, St. Louis, 1998, Mosby.

Rose VL: ACOG issues report on sexual assault, *American Family Physician* 57(5):1144, 1998.

Schacter B, Sienfield J: Personal violence and the culture of violence, *Social Worker* 39(4):347, 1994.

Sessions with a cybershrink: an interview with Sherry Turkle, *Technology Review* 99(2):41, 1996.

Stanhope M, Lancaster J: *Community health nursing,* ed 4, St. Louis, 1996, Mosby.

Statman JB: *The battered woman's survival guide: breaking the cycle,* ed 2, Dallas, 1995, Taylor Publishing.

U.S. Bureau of the Census: *Statistical abstract of the United States: 1998,* ed 118, Washington, DC, 1998, U.S. Government Printing Office.

Walker L: *The battered woman,* New York, 1979, Harper & Row.

Wood T: Defusing school violence, *UC Davis Magazine* 17(1):18, 1999.

Zinn H: *You can't be neutral on a moving train: a personal history of our times,* New York, 1994, Beacon Press.

Chapter 27

Suicide

Learning Objectives

1. Explain the range of self-protective behavioral responses.
2. Discuss three myths about suicidal behaviors.
3. Identify two cultural or social factors that relate to suicide.
4. Examine four categories of motivation for attempting suicide.
5. Explain how suicide affects family members and friends.
6. Describe three theories that attempt to explain the causes of suicide.
7. Discuss the occurrence of suicide throughout each life cycle.
8. Outline the process for assessing the suicidal potential of a client.
9. Choose three therapeutic goals and interventions for clients with suicidal behaviors.

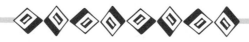

Key Terms

ambivalence

direct self-destructive behaviors

indirect self-destructive behaviors

parasuicidal behaviors

passive suicide

rational suicide

self-injuries

suicidal attempts

suicidal gestures

suicidal ideation

suicidal threats

suicide

suicide precautions

suicidology

Suicide is the action of intentionally taking one's own life. In England suicide historically was considered an offense against the king. During the 1930s many people in the United States took their own lives after the stock market crash in 1929 that began the Great Depression. During World War II Japanese kamikaze pilots intentionally sacrificed their lives for political and religious principles. In some societies suicide is acceptable, but Western societies generally consider suicide as an immoral act committed by desperate or mentally ill individuals.

Suicide has historically served as a solution to life's great obstacles. Today we struggle with the dilemmas of rational suicide, freedom of choice, and physician-assisted suicide. Discussions about the morality or legality of suicide will grow and fade, but the ending of life by one's own hands continues to occur as people struggle for control over their situations.

CONTINUUM OF BEHAVIORAL RESPONSES

According to Maslow's hierarchy of needs, safety and security are basic requirements for life. Individuals behave in many ways to secure these needs. Some people respond with behaviors that promote growth, whereas others begin a journey to self-destruction. Behaviors that are adaptive and help the individual cope result in a greater understanding and acceptance of oneself, but maladaptive self-protective responses, if not changed, can eventually lead to self-destruction. Figure 27-1 illustrates the continuum of self-protective responses.

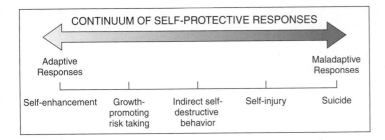

Figure 27-1 Continuum of self-protective responses. (Redrawn from Stuart GW, Laraia MT: *Principles and practice of psychiatric nursing*, ed 7, St. Louis, 2001, Mosby.)

Self-destructive behaviors commonly take two forms: direct and indirect. **Direct self-destructive behaviors** are defined as any form of *active* suicidal behavior, such as threats, gestures, or attempts to end one's life. In this case the individual intends to commit suicide. Although he or she may waver between wanting to live and longing to die, the behaviors communicate an active wish to end the suffering.

Many more people, however, engage in **indirect self-destructive behaviors**, which are the more subtle responses to self-protection. Indirect self-destructive behaviors are described as any behaviors or actions that may result in harm or death to the individual's well-being. In this case, people have no actual intention of ending their lives. They may be unaware of the potential for self-harm when engaging in harmful activities and deny the possibility of danger when confronted. Examples of indirect self-destructive behaviors include substance abuse, engaging in inappropriate or dangerous activities, and an unwillingness to change negative thoughts and actions. Because many of these behaviors are legal or socially accepted, people do not realize their potential for harm.

As the continuum of self-protective responses (see Figure 27-1) moves more toward maladaptive behaviors, indirect self-destructive behaviors progress to active attempts to injure oneself. **Self-injuries** reaffirm to individuals that they are still alive. Pain serves as a reminder of their connection with the body and its physical world. The last and ultimate maladaptive self-protective response is **suicide**, the ending of one's own life. Suicide is a complex and emotional issue, but it is one with which most health care providers must cope. Although overt suicidal attempts receive the most attention, indirect self-destructive behaviors carry risks as great as those of individuals who actually attempt to end their lives.

Myths About Suicide

Many half-truths and misconceptions about suicide still continue to exist despite educational efforts to promote accurate understanding. Although suicide has always been present in society, little effort was made to understand its nature until the beginning of this century. Today many false ideas about suicide still exist. Table 27-1 explains several of these myths and offers facts to more accurately reflect the nature of suicide.

IMPACT OF SUICIDE ON SOCIETY

Over 1000 suicides occur throughout the world every day. To illustrate, the number of suicides in the United States is growing. In 1980 approximately 29,000 suicides per 100,000 people were documented. By 1997 the number had grown to over 31,000 suicides per 100,000 citizens (U.S. Bureau of the Census, 1998). Suicide is the eighth leading cause of death in the United States, "the third leading cause of death among people ages 15 to 24, and the suicide rate of children ages 10 to 14 has doubled since 1980" (Phan, 1999). Twenty percent of all suicides occur in white men over 65. The true number of persons who end their own lives is unknown because many motor vehicle accidents, murders, and other mishaps are actually intentions to commit suicide. For this reason it is important for nurses and other health care providers to be well versed in recognizing and intervening with clients who are suicidal.

Cultural Factors

No one knows exactly why a person chooses suicide, but many cultural, social, and individual factors have an influence. The laws, customs, beliefs, values, and norms of a culture usually include a view of suicide. In some cultures, such as ancient Japan, suicide was considered an honorable atonement for transgressions committed during one's life. When a pharaoh king of Egypt died, it was an expected custom for the widow(s) to commit suicide and join him on his journey across the heavens.

Religious beliefs and customs have an impact on the incidence of suicide. Some Christian faiths, for example, forbid suicide under any circumstances, whereas the taking of one's life may be justified in the beliefs of another religious group.

Customs and rituals may play a role in suicide. The "evil eye" or voodoo practiced by Caribbean islanders is very real for the victim of the curse. Suicide is not a surprising outcome for an individual who has been hexed or cursed in these societies.

Hungary routinely comes in first in the World Health Organization's statistics on suicide (see Cultural Aspects box). Since 1993 with their cultural upheaval, Russia and the Baltic republics have surpassed Hungary in the number of suicides. Providers of health care must

Table 27-1 Myths and Facts About Suicide

Myth	Fact
People who talk about it will not commit suicide.	Most people communicate their intent.
One does not need to take a suicide threat seriously.	Every threat of suicide is serious.
A failed suicide attempt is manipulative behavior.	Manipulation is usually not a factor.
People who are really serious about suicide give no clues.	Many people communicate warnings of their intent by tidying up their affairs, giving away possessions, or being preoccupied with death.
It is harmful to discuss the subject of suicide with clients.	Most suicidal persons need acceptance and emotional support; discussing the topic demonstrates interest and concern.
Only psychotic or depressed people commit suicide.	Depression is a high risk factor for suicide, but not all suicidal persons are depressed. Mental illness is a risk factor for suicide.
Suicide occurs only in the lower socioeconomic classes, the poor.	Although poverty is a risk factor, suicide occurs in all socioeconomic classes.
Young children never commit suicide.	Suicidal behavior is the leading cause of psychiatric hospitalization for young children. Suicide can occur in children as young as 4 years of age.
When people show signs of an improved mood, the threat of suicide is over.	Depressed people often show improved moods, attitude, and behaviors before their deaths because the decision to commit suicide has been made

Modified from Fortinash KM, Holoday-Worret PA: *Psychiatric mental health nursing*, ed 2, St. Louis, 1999, Mosby.

Cultural Aspects

In some societies, suicide is an accepted, centuries-old tradition. In Hungary, for example, villages dwindle as their residents choose suicide over the uncertainty of living an isolated, lonely life. When people in Hungary "get fed up, they hang themselves, cut their wrists, or swallow pesticides, just like their fathers and grandfathers did," states Dr. Jorge Ulloa, a psychiatrist who runs a suicide clinic near Budapest.

From Beck E: In gloomy Hungary, suicide takes on a life of its own, *Wall Street Journal* 48(132):A1, May 10, 1995.

remember that people hold strongly to their cultural beliefs and practices. An awareness of a cultural group's attitude relating to suicide may someday help prevent suicide from happening to one of your clients.

Social Factors

There are many influences in society that have an effect on the incidence of suicide. Chief among them is a sense of social isolation felt by members of fast-paced, goal-oriented societies. Family and community support systems have dwindled as mobility, politics, and finances move people away from the safety and security of family and friends. The support of kind neighbors and friends has been replaced by the generic, ready-made support of massive and complicated governmental systems. Crime and other aggressive actions force people to mistrust the intentions of others and barricade themselves behind locked doors and secured communities, but the price for security is paid with isolation and its ensuing sense of hopelessness.

The inability to meet basic needs has a strong influence on the occurrence of suicide. Since the emptying of state psychiatric hospitals, the number of homeless has swelled. It is now estimated that persons with mental illnesses make up over one third of the homeless population. The risk of suicide, for both healthy and mentally troubled individuals, skyrockets when one is unable to meet food, shelter, and clothing needs. Poverty and homelessness lead to depression and hopelessness in the long run. Suicide becomes an acceptable alternative when one is continually hungry, cold, ill, or living in fear.

The availability of weapons, especially firearms, has proven to be a significant factor in relation to the occurrence of suicide. In countries where the ownership of guns is prohibited, suicide rates are lower. To illustrate, in the United Kingdom, owning a handgun is illegal. According to the U.S. Bureau of the Census (1998) the suicide rate for England and Wales was 6.7 people per 100,000. In the United States, where gun ownership is hotly debated and defended, the rate is 31.3 suicides per 100,000 persons. The availability of firearms is reflected in a country's statistics on violence and suicide (see Think About box).

One's state of health or illness influences suicidal considerations. Losses associated with old age can lead to depression and feelings of futility. Why struggle when tomorrow is a sad repeat of today? Suicide rates climb as age, infirmity, and illness take their toll.

The appearance of human immunodeficiency virus (HIV) and acquired immunodeficiency syndrome (AIDS) has had a profound influence on the suicide rates of many countries. In the United States the "death-with-dignity" philosophy has influenced many AIDS sufferers to choose the time and place of their passing. This form of suicide is called "**rational suicide**" because the choice to end one's life was made freely and rationally with a sound mind.

Other social factors play a role in a society's suicides. The number, availability, and kind of community-based resources for health promotion and treatment have an influence on a society's mental as well as physical health. Without these resources and the support they offer, the stresses of life can overwhelm a society's citizens. Be aware of the social changes in this world because hidden among them are clues to caring for clients who are thinking of ending their lives.

DYNAMICS OF SUICIDE

The act of attempting suicide has a profound impact on the lives of individuals, families, friends, and communities. When many suicides occur, the society becomes affected. Because human beings dynamically function in several realms or dimensions at any given time, it is important to consider suicide from a holistic point of view.

Characteristics of Suicide

Suicide is an act of individual meaning. The actual reasons for choosing such a final course of action will probably never be known to anyone but the individual. However, it is likely that more than one motive drives a person to suicide.

In the physical dimension, thoughts of suicide produce many of the same biochemical changes in the body as depression. Chronic fatigue and vague complaints are common in both depressed and suicidal individuals. Often suicidal persons will not eat, drink, or rest enough to maintain required energy levels. Recent studies have suggested a link between low serum cholesterol levels and suicide attempts in men. At this time there appears to be no such correlation for women and cholesterol.

One's method of choice for committing suicide differs by gender. Men prefer to rely on firearms, hanging, or drowning, whereas women prefer to overdose with pills or to inhale carbon monoxide.

The emotional dimension of functioning for the suicidal person is filled with feelings of ambivalence, anger, aggression, guilt, helplessness, and hopelessness. **Ambivalence** is a state in which an individual experiences conflicting feelings, attitudes, or drives. For the suicidal person, the struggle is between self-preservation (life) and self-destruction (death). Often, suicidal individuals threaten or attempt suicide and then behaviorally act out their feelings of ambivalence by seeking treatment.

Anger and aggression are turned inward in suicidal persons. Fears of being abandoned or rejected add to the dynamics. Many persons who feel trapped in frustrating relationships commonly react with rage that becomes self-directed and harmful.

Guilt can also lead to suicide. Suicidal individuals often shoulder the guilt of the world. They feel sinful and carry around the belief that they must have done something very wrong to deserve their misfortunes. Often personal guilt is exaggerated until the only way to make up for one's transgressions is to offer the final sacrifice—the self.

For the suicidal individual, the emotional dimension is marked by overwhelming feelings of helplessness and hopelessness. Nothing the person tries to do works out the way it was expected. The individual becomes unable to emotionally function. Life is bleak and hopeless as its meaning and purpose slip from the suicidal person's control. Self-esteem sinks to an all-time low.

In the intellectual dimension, intense emotional suffering leads to distorted thinking and self-defeating thoughts. The self becomes devalued and worth little. Everything is glum and depressing, which leads individuals to a negative and pessimistic view of the future. One's self-talk becomes self-defeating, which soon leads to negative behaviors. Thinking is self-centered rather than oriented toward solving problems. Why continue when the future looks so bleak?

The social dimension of functioning includes one's views of others. Many suicidal individuals depend on the feedback of others to frequently reaffirm their self-worth. Self-esteem is very low in suicidal people. Their feelings of inferiority, of being less than others, interfere with social relationships and lead to the isolation and loneliness that accompanies suicide.

In the last area of functioning, the spiritual dimension, suicidal individuals grapple with the cultural, religious, and ethical dilemmas associated with bringing about one's own demise. Many respond by blaming other people, their society, or their religious practices. Others "make their peace" with the spiritual sides of themselves and experience a spiritual calm and serenity before committing suicide. Some people believe they will be reunited with loved ones in a new life after leaving this reality.

Categories of Motivation

People are motivated to take their own lives for many reasons. All suicide victims, however, seem to share two major viewpoints. The first is a deep, inner, disturbance of hopelessness, despair, poor self-esteem, and feelings of being trapped. The other is described as a logic whereby suicidal individuals consider the act as a way of relieving themselves from the miseries of this life and connecting with a sense of immortality or a life beyond the one they are leaving behind.

There are several categories of motivation for suicide. The first motive is called *a cry for help.* Most commonly, suicidal persons bounce between the wish to live and the need to die. They feel trapped in a situation from which they believe there is no other escape. Killing oneself is seen as an effort to break out and take control and to do something about one's life. These individuals are communicating their need for the kind of help that will radically change their lives and alter their present existence. The Case Study box illustrates this type of motivation.

The second motive for considering suicide is the *refusal to accept a diminished quality,* style, or pace of life. This motive causes persons to commit rational suicide. They assess their situation in a clear and unemotional manner, consider all the options, and then decide to take steps that will end their lives. Decisions and plans are made logically, with little or no emotion. The decision to commit suicide is seen as a logical one. An example would be the 80-year-old man who kills his 78-year-old blind and bedridden wife and then ends his own life after making arrangements for their funerals and property settlements.

The third motivation centers around the *need to affirm one's soul.* These persons believe that there are values more important than life and that suicide is a way of fulfilling one's existence. The 18-year-old who takes his life one summer evening when everything is going well and the future is bright may be searching for that fulfillment.

The fourth motive for suicidal behavior is to *relieve distress* related to situations that threaten the intactness of a person. The 70-year-old businessman with prostate cancer who chooses suicide over potentially life-prolonging surgery is an example of this type of motivation.

Last are those individuals who are *preoccupied with suicide.* They derive comfort knowing that they will control the time and circumstances of their death. These

Case Study

Sandy was young, alone, pregnant, and scared. She knew that she was not welcome at home because her father told her when she left for college, "If you get into trouble, don't come crying to me. You'll have to take care of it by yourself."

Her boyfriend, who swore love and devotion, denied that he was the father of her baby and then left town. Even her new friends deserted her when they heard she was pregnant. Now the school officials were asking about her plans.

In desperation Sandy sought to terminate the pregnancy but found that she was "too far along." She decided that there was only one course of action that could end her troubles. She really did not want to die, but there seemed to be no other way out. The thought of facing life alone with a new baby was more than she could tolerate.

As she made her final plans, a feeling of calm came over Sandy. She would handle the situation in her own way. At least this way, she rationalized, "I am in control. I am the one who will do something about this."

Later that night Sandy connected a rubber hose from the exhaust system to the interior of her car, rolled up all the windows, and sat quietly with the motor running. The next morning, when her body was discovered, she held a small note in her hand. It read: "Daddy, I took care of it myself. Love, Sandy."

◆ What do you think motivated Sandy to commit suicide?

◆ Do you think this was her only or best course of action?

◆ If Sandy had come to you for help, what could you have done?

people are usually unwilling to accept life on any terms but their own. They set conditions for living and refuse to continue with life unless it is on their terms. Often suicide is the only form of real control they feel they have.

When working with suicidal clients, remember that no matter what the motivation, each individual is experiencing deep discomfort and very low self-esteem. Compassion and understanding become valuable therapeutic tools when working with suicidal clients.

Theories About Suicide

Because suicide is an end result, it is difficult to understand all the factors that led up to one's decision to end his or her life. The study of the nature of suicide is called **suicidology.** Several theories attempt to explain the causes of suicidal behavior.

The *psychoanalytical theory* states that all humans have the instinct for life and death within them. Suicidal persons experience much ambivalence between wanting to live and wanting to die. Anger turns inward, and when stressful life events activate their death wish, suicide becomes an option.

Sociological theory looks at the relationship between the number of suicides and the social conditions of an area. These theorists believe that suicide rates are affected by group support (or the lack of it), social changes, regulations, religion, legal sanctions or limitations, and philosophical beliefs. In short, the sociological theories consider the impact of social factors on the occurrence of suicide.

Last is the *interpersonal theory,* developed by H.S. Sullivan. Suicide is viewed as the outcome of a failure to work with or resolve interpersonal conflicts. These three theories formed much of the foundation for further studies into the nature of suicide. However, recent research into the psychobiological nature of the human being is revealing many new facts about suicide and its motivation.

New Biological Evidence

Depression, anxiety, and impulsive behaviors are common in suicidal individuals. As scientists are now able to study the structure and functions of the living human brain, new connections between physical and behavioral activities are being rapidly discovered.

Anxiety and depression are often the forerunners of suicidal thoughts. Researchers have demonstrated that when certain chemicals in the brain (neurotransmitters) are not in balance, people have difficulty regulating their moods. For example, irregularities in a certain neurotransmitter pattern, called the *serotonin system,* have been found in depressed and suicidal persons. These findings have implications for health care providers. As our understanding of the dynamics of suicide grows, so does our ability to recognize the potential for suicide and effectively intervene.

Effects of Suicide on Others

Suicide, like natural death, has a strong effect on those left behind. Following the suicide, the lives of the survivors can be filled with questions, anger, sadness, shame, guilt, and health problems. The grieving process is further complicated by social attitudes about taking one's own life.

Survivor Guilt

Because of the emotions attached to a suicidal act, the loss of a loved one through suicide is considered to be a much more stressful event than the grief reaction to a natural death. Guilt is a main response because survivors often think they could have done something to prevent the suicide. Guilt may also stem from the unexpressed anger toward the deceased for abandoning family and friends. Depression, posttraumatic stress disorder (PTSD) with flashbacks, and somatic complaints are the common prob-

lems of most suicide survivors. Impaired immune system functioning may accompany the emotional disturbances.

Anger may be expressed as "agonized questioning," which helps the survivors cope with their emotional turmoil and disorganization. Some may hide their resentment, anger, and rage, turning it into depression. Children often feel responsible for the suicide. Unless they receive much love, support, guidance, and permission to be angry, depression or other behavioral problems may develop.

Socially the stigma of suicide is soon felt. Forced interactions with health care providers, the police, or the media soon after death can bring home the feelings of rejection that are often experienced by the family members of suicide victims. Friends and relatives, unsure of how to help, withdraw or do nothing. This reaction limits the social contact and support that is so needed after the suicide of a loved one. The survivors of a suicide victim may also withdraw from social interactions to protect themselves from the gossip and intrusion of inconsiderate others. Thus begins a cycle of guilt, withdrawal, and blame between the survivors of a suicide and others in their world. With support and understanding, survivors eventually recover and accept the fact that the responsibility for the suicide rests with the individual who committed it and not with those left behind.

Health care providers are not immune to the effects of suicide. When a client, especially an inpatient, commits suicide, staff members and other clients may experience guilt, anger, or helplessness. Both clients and staff members need to grieve and express the emotions that follow a suicide. Often other clients on the unit will express anger at the staff, act out, or become self-destructive. Sharing emotions about the suicide allows both staff and clients the opportunity to express themselves and cope with the experience. The survivors of suicide, no matter who they are, must grieve and learn to heal.

SUICIDE THROUGHOUT THE LIFE CYCLE

Attempts to end one's life occur in every age group. Although the motivations for suicide may vary with the developmental level, the act remains the same: an effort to die. Understanding how suicide is used at different developmental levels is important. Recognition and treatment of the problems underlying suicidal behaviors are much more effective when begun early.

Suicide and Children

Although depression is usually a component of suicide, with children it may be different. Some experts believe that suicide in children is most often the result of family conflict or disruption. The children of depressed mothers think about and attempt suicide more often than those of emotionally healthy mothers (Klimes-Dougan and others, 1998). Children commit suicide as a cry for help, to change their situations, or to act out a sincere wish to die. Children with existing mental health problems, such as conduct disorders, attention-deficit hyperactivity disorders, or psychoses, are at a greater risk for committing suicide than other children. Because they are impulsive, many suicides in children are not planned. Often the loss of a parent triggers suicidal behaviors in children who were not encouraged to grieve. Because very young children cannot understand the concept of death as a permanent state, their wishes to join their lost parent may lead to suicidal behaviors.

The key to recognizing the signs of suicidal intent lies in a *change in the child's behavior.* Any child whose attitudes or behaviors change dramatically in a short period of time, especially following a stressful event or situation, is a candidate for suicide.

Suicide and Adolescents

The rate of adolescent suicide has risen dramatically in the past 30 years. The suicide rate for 10- to 19-year-olds has almost doubled, from 6.5 per 100,000 people in 1970 to an astounding 14.2 suicides per 100,000 people in 1995 (U.S. Bureau of the Census, 1998). Young men are the most affected by violence and suicide in adolescence. These figures may not accurately reflect the actual number of adolescent suicides because many suicidal deaths are listed as accidental.

During adolescence any long-standing family or social problems may continue to worsen as they experience the difficulties of growing up. If coping skills or resources are insufficient, adolescents, especially those with low self-esteem, may consider suicide as an option for solving their problems. Adolescents commit suicide when they feel there is no other way out of their problems. They see their problems as genuinely unsolvable, now or in the future.

Many factors come into play in adolescent suicide. Depression, poor impulse-control, and emotional isolation are related to suicide in adolescents. Dysfunctional or disrupted family interactions, such as divorce or separation of parents, can devastate many teens. Adolescents with anorexia nervosa have higher rates of suicide. In fact, many theorists believe that anorexia is a slow attempt at suicide.

Social problems with peers, the use of drugs or alcohol, and a lack of consistent relationships also add to the risk of suicide. When the environment lacks security or presents dangers, many teens feel that their lives will be short and they will not live until adulthood. The outlook for the future holds little promise with this attitude.

The incidence of suicidal behaviors is also increased in children and adolescents who suffer from chronic disease. Children and adolescents with immune-mediated (or type 1) diabetes, for example, have a higher risk of suicide than healthy individuals. Those diabetics who actually try to commit suicide often do so by some method relating to their diabetes, such as overdosing on insulin. Health care

providers should routinely assess every client (including those with medical diagnoses or problems) for the presence of suicidal thoughts. Become aware of the risk factors that can play an important role in an individual's choice to commit suicide (Box 27-1).

Suicide and Adults

Suicide is a significant problem in adulthood, especially for white men. Women attempt suicide three times more frequently than men, but men are more successful at completing the act. In 15- to 24-year-old men, suicide ranks as the third leading cause of death (U.S. Bureau of the Census, 1998)

In young adults suicide occurs when individuals are unable to cope with the pressures of adulthood. Some experience problems associated with interpersonal relationships, whereas others lack personal resources and are poor, hungry, or unemployed. All, however, are dissatisfied with their lives.

Loneliness is a factor in adult suicides. The loss of a family or significant relationship, whether through divorce or death, increases the risk of suicide. In addition, certain professions and occupations are associated with higher rates of suicide.

Most adult suicides can be prevented if the clues are uncovered early enough. Do not hesitate to ask clients if they ever think about suicide. The answer to that question may offer an opportunity to help save an individual's life.

Suicide and Older Adults

As age increases, so does the rate of suicide. Many studies show that the incidence of suicide increase with age. The

Box 27-1 Risk Factors for Suicide

Abuse, neglect, exploitation
Accident prone
Academic pressures, school problems
Chronic or terminal illness, disability, HIV/AIDS
Dysfunctional family relationships
Family or self history of anxiety, depression
History of alcoholism and/or substance abuse
Other mental health problems*
Profession/occupation: policeman, fireman, air traffic controller, physician, psychiatrist, college student, dentist
Inadequate childrearing practices
Loss of parent or significant other
Low socioeconomic status, poverty, or homelessness
Male gender, unmarried, unemployed
Member of certain religious cults
Negative outlook for future
Previous suicide attempts*
Social isolation, lack of social support
Stressful or unhappy personal

*Highest risk for suicide.

actual number is difficult to determine because only active suicides are counted. Many older adults choose to commit a **passive suicide** by refusing to eat, drink, or cooperate with care.

The causes and risk factors of suicide in the elderly are poorly understood. Although many of the elderly who commit suicide have had contact with a health care professional within a month before their deaths, their risk was not identified or treated. Older adults tend not to communicate their intentions unless directly asked, and suicidal attempts in older adults are more successful. One out of every two suicide attempts in the elderly results in death. These sobering statements must alert every care provider to perform a suicidal risk assessment for all older adults.

Most older adults view the timing of death in one of three ways—God controlled, physician and individual controlled, or controlled by the individual alone. Older males have the highest suicide rates in the elderly (Stanhope and Lancaster, 1996). Risk factors for suicide in the elderly are advanced age, male gender, low socioeconomic status, chronic pain or illness, and fear of becoming dependent or helpless. A lack of relationships appears to be a driving force behind many suicides in older persons. Other researchers believe that intolerable life circumstances is the main motive for suicides in the elderly.

Social attitudes about suicide in the elderly differ. Some people think that all suicides in the elderly are irrational decisions, based in depression or physical illness. They believe aggressive interventions are always required. Others view elder suicide as the last rational decision, the last act of control over one's life.

The concept of rational suicide in the United States is "at odds with the legal system," but in other countries, such as the Netherlands, suicide is an acceptable way to achieve "death with dignity." It may seem that the important questions and issues surrounding the control of one's own death are issues for philosophers and discussions of medical ethics; however, health care providers will be addressing many of these questions in daily practice.

THERAPEUTIC INTERVENTIONS

Thoughts about suicide can be described on several levels. **Suicidal ideation** is described as thoughts or fantasies that are expressed but have no definite intent. Ideas may be expressed directly or symbolically. **Suicidal threats** are verbal or written expressions of the intent to take one's life, but they are without actions. As the seriousness increases, **suicidal gestures** may be observed. These are suicidal actions that result in little or no injury but communicate a message of suicidal purpose. **Parasuicidal behaviors** are unsuccessful attempts and gestures associated with a low likelihood of success. **Suicide attempts** are serious self-directed actions that are intended to do harm

or end life. The last level is *completed suicide,* the successful attempt to end one's life. Motivation for the successful suicide may be conscious or unconscious (Fortinash and Holoday-Worret, 1999).

The surgeon general of the United States has declared suicide to be a serious public health threat (Meckler, 1999). Prevention is thus the most important health care action for clients who may be suicidal. Preventing a suicide from occurring means saving a life. Prevention requires a knowledge of the dynamics of suicide and the ability to recognize the potential for suicidal actions in every client. Applying the nursing (therapeutic) process is an excellent method for working with clients who may be considering suicide.

Assessment of Suicidal Potential

Because suicide is becoming so prevalent, it is important to evaluate every client for its potential. To accomplish this, assess the risk factors for the age of the client. Then ask the client directly if he or she has any thoughts relating to suicide. Asking clients will not encourage them to take any suicidal actions. On the contrary, it gives them permission to discuss their feelings and attitudes. Box 27-2 offers a list of questions for assessing suicidal intentions.

Hospitalization may be required for the client's safety and protection if he or she feels unable to control suicidal behaviors. Not every question may be appropriate for every client, but a series of questions like these will usually bring out expressions of suicidal thoughts if they are present.

Suicidal intentions can exist with any medical or psychiatric diagnosis. Clients who are depressed must be

---

Box 27-2 Questions That Assess the Potential for Suicide

What has been the most difficult moment for you in the recent past?

Have things been so bad that you have thought about escaping? If so, how?

Are there times when death seems like an attractive option to you?

Have you thought of harming or killing yourself?

If you were to harm yourself, how would you do it?

Do you have access to the items you would need to carry out your plan? (This includes a gun, medications, a rope, an enclosed garage.)

Have you thought about or attempted to harm yourself in the past?

What has kept you from harming yourself thus far?

What might keep you from harming yourself in the future?

"Do you think you can control your behavior and refrain from acting on your thoughts or impulses?" *is the most important question to ask.*

Drug Alert

Many medications can cause changes in mood. Much publicity has been given to the drug fluoxetine hydrochloride (Prozac), an antidepressant that has been reported to cause violent and suicidal reactions in some individuals.

The side effects of certain steroids (prednisolone) have been known to cause elation and feelings of well-being in some individuals. The same drug, administered to others, can result in severe depression and suicidal thoughts.

Elderly persons who are taking potent analgesics (pain medications) are at a high risk for feelings of depression.

Obtain a drug and medication history for each and every client. Sometimes something as simple as discontinuing or changing a medication can lift spirits and decrease suicidal thoughts.

Box 27-3 NANDA Nursing Diagnoses Related to Suicide

Adjustment, impaired*
Anxiety
Body image disturbance
Coping, ineffective individual
Denial, ineffective
Grieving, dysfunctional
Hopelessness
Pain, chronic
Powerlessness
Self- esteem, chronic low
Self-mutilation, risk for
Social interaction, impaired
Spiritual distress
Violence, risk for: self-directed

From North American Nursing Diagnosis Association: *NANDA nursing diagnoses: definitions and classification 1999-2000*, Philadelphia, 1999, The Association.
*Primary nursing diagnosis for suicide.

Table 27-2 Suicide Assessment

Assessment	Description
Suicide ideation (thoughts)	Client talks about wanting to be dead, imagines AIDS or other serious illness, seems gloomy, brooding.
History of suicide attempts	Client has tried to end own life before; there may be family history of suicide.
Present suicide plan	The more detailed a suicide plan, the more likely it will be carried out.
Availability of items to carry out plan	What guns, rifles, knives or other weapons are available? How difficult is it to obtain such items?
Substance use or abuse	Suicide rates are higher in people who abuse alcohol or other chemical substances.
Level of despair	Ask about the future; when despair is high, hope is low.
Ability to control own behavior	Inpatient hospitalization is indicated for individuals who are unable to control their suicidal impulses.

Box 27-4 Suicide Precautions

Protect client from harming him or herself.
Determine if client has specific suicide plan.
Determine history of suicide attempts.
Make a no-suicide contract.
Remove dangerous items from the environment.
Place client in least restrictive environment that allows for necessary level of observation.
Place client in room with protective window coverings, as appropriate.
Observe closely during suicidal crisis.
Escort client during off-ward activities, as appropriate.
Demonstrate concern about client's welfare.

Refrain from criticizing.
Facilitate discussion of factors or events that precipitated the suicidal thoughts.
Facilitate support of client by family and friends.
Instruct client and significant others in signs, symptoms, and basic physiology of depression.
Instruct family that suicidal risk increases for severely depressed clients as they begin to feel better.
Instruct family on possible warning signs or pleas for help client may use.
Refer client to psychiatrist, as needed.

Modified from: McCloskey JC, Bulechek GM, editor: *Nursing interventions classification (NIC)*, ed 3, St. Louis, 1997, Mosby.

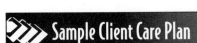

Sample Client Care Plan   Self-Directed Violence

Assessment

History: Joe, a 19-year-old man, recently lost his best friend in an auto accident. For several weeks he has been saying that he should have been killed instead of his friend. In the past 2 weeks Joe has refused to work, eat, or engage in any social activities. Yesterday he bought a gun.

Current Findings: A depressed-looking young man sitting between two worried parents. Grooming is unkempt; shirt and denims are ragged and dirty. He volunteers no information but states "It's not worth it" to the nurse. After obtaining the past history from parents, Joe was admitted to the unit for assessment and observation.

Multidisciplinary Diagnosis

Risk for violence, self-directed, related to loss of significant other

Planning/Goals

Joe will refrain from making any suicidal gestures or attempts during his inpatient stay.
Joe will discuss his feelings of loss by August 28.

Therapeutic Interventions

Intervention	Rationale	Team Member
1. Establish contact and rapport.	Open communication and trust must be established before work can begin.	All
2. Establish a no-harm contract as soon as possible.	Helps prevent Joe from acting impulsively.	Psy, Nsg
3. Implement necessary suicide precautions; watch closely.	Protects Joe from self-injury or death.	All
4. Evaluate and document Joe's suicide potential at least twice daily.	Helps assess for changes in seriousness of client's intent.	Psy, Nsg
5. Help Joe identify and discuss sources of distress.	Increases awareness of feelings; helps to plan effective interventions.	All
6. Offer emotional support and acceptance.	Encourages Joe to think more highly of himself; helps develop self-worth.	All
7. Involve Joe and his family in the treatment plan.	Promotes active decision making; provides emotional support and resources.	All
8. Explore coping strategies that worked in the past.	Helps Joe to apply successful coping mechanisms to prevent problems.	All

Evaluation

During the course of hospitalization Joe made no attempts at suicide. By August 18 Joe was able to share his sorrow and anger with the unit chaplain.

An actual client care plan includes several other diagnoses and interventions.

carefully monitored for expressions of hopelessness. Table 27-2 lists the basic components of a suicide assessment. Do not hesitate to use this data-gathering tool whenever problems with the client's emotional state are suspected.

When used as part of a health history, the suicide assessment will yield valuable information about the client's suicidal intentions (if any) along with numerous clues about the individual. The Drug Alert box offers an important reminder.

Nursing diagnoses for suicidal persons are based on each client's identified problems and needs (Box 27-3).

Therapeutic Interventions for Suicidal Clients

The first priority for the care of suicidal clients is *protection from harm*. If the client is actively attempting suicide, he or she must be physically prevented from doing so. If the risks are so high that a serious attempt may be made, **suicide precautions** are implemented. These precautions are standard interventions to prevent a suicide attempt from occurring. They are listed in Box 27-4.

Clients with strong suicidal intents may require *constant observation*. "Constant, one-to-one observation is practiced in a psychiatric inpatient setting and requires a nursing staff member to watch the patient's actions and listen to his statements—24 hours a day" (Robie and others, 1999).

One of the most important therapeutic interventions (after ensuring safety) with suicidal persons is to establish rapport with the client. Many suicidal people are alone, and most have little self-esteem. These individuals are distressed and experiencing enormous emotional reactions, but they will usually agree to make a *no-self-harm agreement* (a promise not to engage in self-destructive behaviors) with their caregivers (Stuart and Laraia, 2001). Establishing a therapeutic relationship with a health care provider is important for clients. The focused communications and concerned actions of caregivers help suicidal individuals to feel self-worth. With the encouragement and advocacy of their caregivers, many suicidal clients are able to develop more effective strategies for living satisfying lives. The Sample Client Care Plan box illustrates a client care plan, for an individual who may be suicidal.

Suicide and its associated effects are problems in today's society. Many of us will be or have been touched by the suicide of a loved one or friend. As health care providers, it is our duty and responsibility to protect our clients, even from themselves, when we must. Hopefully, through all our efforts, the tide of senseless loss of life can be turned, and choices will be made looking toward life instead of away from it.

KEY CONCEPTS

- Suicide is the action of intentionally taking one's own life.
- Many misconceptions about suicide continue to exist despite efforts to promote an accurate understanding of the problem.
- Many cultural, social, and individual factors influence the occurrence of suicide.
- The act of suicide has a profound impact on the lives of individuals, families, friends, and communities.
- Thoughts and actions directed at self-destruction affect every dimension of human functioning.
- There are several categories of motivation for suicide, including a cry for help, a refusal to accept a diminished quality of life, a need to affirm one's soul, an attempt to relieve the distress related to situations that threaten the intactness of a person, and an act of those who are preoccupied with suicide.
- Theories that attempt to explain the causes of suicidal behavior include the psychoanalytical theory, sociological theory, and interpersonal theory.
- New connections between physical and behavioral activities are being rapidly discovered.

- After the suicide of a loved one, the lives of the survivors can be plagued with anger, sadness, shame, guilt, health problems, and agonizing questions.
- Some experts believe that suicide in children is most often the result of family conflict or disruption.
- Adolescents commit suicide when they feel there is no other way out of their problems.
- Adult women attempt suicide three times more frequently than men, but men are more successful at completing the act.
- The incidence of suicide in older adults continues to increase with age.
- Prevention is the most important therapeutic action for clients who may be suicidal.
- Because suicide is becoming so prevalent, it is important for nurses to assess every client for its potential.
- The first priority for the care of clients who may be suicidal is protection from harm.
- With encouragement and the advocacy of their care providers, many suicidal clients are able to develop effective strategies for living more satisfying lives.

Suggestions for Further Reading

Survivor Guilt: A Self-Help Guide (1999, New Harbinger Publications) is written by a PTSD psychotherapist who shows survivors how to overcome the chronic guilt and other emotional problems associated with the suicide of a friend or loved one. It is highly recommended reading.

Suicide Awareness/Voices of Education (www.save.org) is an excellent source for information relating to suicide.

References

Beck E: In gloomy Hungary, suicide takes on a life of its own, *Wall Street Journal* 48(132):A1, May 10, 1995.

Fortinash KM, Holoday-Worret PA: *Psychiatric mental health nursing*, ed 2, St. Louis, 1999, Mosby.

Klimes-Dougan B and others: Suicidal ideation and attempts: a longitudinal investigation of children of depressed and well mothers, *Journal of the American Academy of Child and Adolescent Psychiatry* 38(6):651, 1998.

McCloskey JC, Bulechek GM, editors: *Nursing interventions classification (NIC)*, ed 2, St. Louis, 1996, Mosby.

Meckler L: Suicide in U.S.: a "national tragedy," Associated Press, July 28, 1999.

North American Nursing Diagnosis Association: *NANDA nursing diagnoses: definitions and classification 1999-2000*, Philadelphia, 1999, The Association.

Phan A: Harsh reactions to mental illness shatter the innocence of youth, *USA Today* 18(14):10D, 1999.

Robie D and others: Suicide prevention protocol, *American Journal of Nursing* 99(12):53, 1999.

Stanhope M, Lancaster J: *Community health nursing: promoting health of aggregates, families, and individuals*, ed 4, St. Louis, 1996, Mosby.

Stuart GW, Laraia MT: *Principles and practice of psychiatric nursing*, ed 7, St. Louis, 2001, Mosby.

U.S. Bureau of the Census: *Statistical abstract of the United States*, ed 118, Washington, DC, 1998, U.S. Government Printing Office.

Chapter 28

Substance-Related Disorders

Learning Objectives

1. Define five terms relating to substance use and treatment.
2. Explain how chemical dependency affects persons from different age groups.
3. Describe four serious consequences of substance abuse.
4. Classify four categories of abused substances, and give an example from each group.
5. Identify three reasons why inhalants are abused by adolescents and young adults.
6. Describe the three stages or phases of becoming addicted.
7. Compare the three criteria for the diagnosis of a substance-related disorder.
8. Explain what is meant by the term *relapse*.
9. Plan at least four interventions for clients who are diagnosed with substance-related disorders.

Key Terms

abstinence

abused substances

addiction

alcohol

amphetamines

caffeine

cannabis

cocaine

crack

detoxification

disulfiram (Antabuse)

dual diagnosis

habituation

hallucinogens

heroin

inhalants

intoxication

methadone

narcotics

nicotine

phencyclidine (PCP)

relapse

substance

substance (drug) abuse

substance (chemical) dependency

substance use

The practice of using substances to make one feel better is as old as human beings themselves. Even animals have been noted to eat certain plants that change their behaviors. Alcohol has played a role in many cultures throughout recorded time, and various drugs, potions, solutions, and formulas have been developed as humans have attempted to cope with the problems of disease and illness. Drugs have also played a role in political history. For example, the Opium Wars of the nineteenth century between China and Britain and the drug movement of the 1970s in the United States changed the course of history. Even today we are struggling with political and social events that relate to drugs and other illicit substances (see Cultural Aspects box).

The world of substance use and abuse is always changing. As health care providers become familiar with current chemical fads, new and more potent drugs are being introduced. The focus of this chapter is to provide an understanding of substance use, abuse, and addiction; its effects on society; and the current interventions used to

Cultural Aspects

Today, in the drug-producing countries of Central and South America, the growing of cocaine plants is the only means of making a living for many poor farmers. Prices for coca leaves far outstrip the money paid for corn, wheat, or other agricultural products. When officials spray or otherwise destroy their illicit crops, many men, women, and children suffer from hunger and malnutrition as a consequence. What do you think could be done to outlaw drugs and prevent the starvation of farmers at the same time?

treat and educate clients suffering from substance-related problems.

VOCABULARY OF TERMS

To communicate about substance-related disorders, an understanding of terms is necessary. Several terms are used to describe addictive disorders. A **substance** is defined as a "drug of abuse, a medication, or a toxin" (American Psychiatric Association, 2000). Substances are also called chemicals, drugs, or toxins. **Substance use** is the ingesting (eating, drinking, injecting, or inhaling) of any chemical that affects the body. This includes legal, illegal, and medicinal substances. **Abused substances** are those chemicals that alter the individual's perception by affecting the central nervous system (CNS). They are often referred to as *mind-altering substances* because of their ability to enhance or depress moods or emotions.

Substance (drug) abuse is culturally and socially defined. In some cultures, the use of certain drugs is expected to fulfill religious obligations or some other culturally defined duty, whereas in other societies the use of the same substance is considered illegal or immoral. In the United States, Canada, Great Britain, and other industrialized societies, for example, laws define which substances are socially approved and legal and those that are illegal. In other cultures the use of substances that are deemed illegal in the industrialized countries is acceptable and even provides economic opportunities. A broad but workable definition of **substance (drug) abuse** is the "excessive use of a substance that differs from societal norms" (Keltner, Schwecke, and Bostrom, 1998). No matter which culture, however, when the use of a substance falls outside society's definition of approved use, a drug problem exists.

Drug or chemical **habituation** occurs when an individual depends on a substance to provide pleasure or relief from discomfort. **Substance (chemical) dependency** occurs when a user must take his or her usual or an increasing dose of the drug to prevent the onset of withdrawal signs and symptoms. When the dependence on the substance is physical, the term **addiction** is used. Today, the term *substance (chemical) dependency* is preferred for describing addictions. **Abstinence** occurs when an addicted individual is not using an addictive substance.

ROLE OF CHEMICALS IN SOCIETY

Chemical substances are important in modern societies. Without them, we would be unable to produce food, fight disease, or develop the products that allow us to live comfortably. The use of different chemical substances has increasingly become a part of everyday life.

Children are unconsciously taught to solve problems by using substances. The doctor prescribes a medicine to help a family member recover from an illness, and the child learns that drugs can be beneficial. Children observe their parents taking pills or drinking beverages that change their actions and unconsciously register approval of those behaviors.

We are constantly bombarded with encouragement to ingest chemicals in advertisements on televisions, radios, and the Internet. Commercials are routinely encouraging us to cope with constipation, heartburn, or hemorrhoids by taking drugs, and many of society's athletes and role models freely admit to using body-enhancing chemicals. No wonder so many people, young and old, are having to cope with the problems of chemical use today.

Substance Use and Age

The use of chemical substances occurs throughout the life cycle, from the fetus to the elderly. Even the growing life protected within the mother's uterus is not safe from the effects of chemicals. A national study of pregnant women (National Pregnancy and Health History, 1996) found that 18.8% drank alcohol and 5.5% used drugs at least once during pregnancy.

There are no safe drugs for pregnant women. Every chemical ingested by a pregnant woman poses a potential danger to her unborn child, especially during the first trimester of pregnancy, when the developing fetus is highly sensitive. Chemicals that are taken during pregnancy can seriously interfere with normal fetal growth and development. They may also alter the placenta itself or interfere with its ability to perform its life-promoting functions.

A sad but common example of the effects of maternal drug use can be seen in infants and children with fetal alcohol syndrome (FAS)—the result of excessive alcohol use during pregnancy. Fetal alcohol syndrome affects an estimated 1 child per 1000 live births (Fetal alcohol

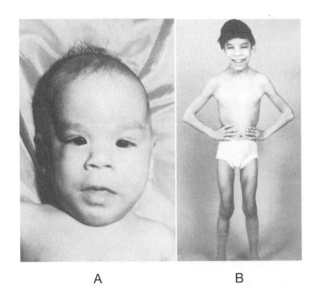

A   B

Figure 28-1 Fetal alcohol syndrome (FAS). **A** and **B,** Child of chronically alcoholic mother, diagnosed at birth with FAS. Although he was raised his entire life in one excellent foster home and participated in various remediation programs, he continues to have an IQ around 45 (more severe retardation than most FAS children), with accompanying hyperactivity and distractibility. (From Streissguth AP: *Ciba Foundation Symposium No. 105: mechanisms of alcohol damage in utero.* By permission of AP Streissguth and the Ciba Foundation, Pitman, London.)

syndrome, 1997). In countries in which the intake of alcohol is high, the incidence of FAS is greater. Children with FAS are smaller at birth, have small heads (microcephaly), and fail to develop normally (Dickason, Silverman, and Schult, 1998). Figure 28-1 illustrates the physical effects on the child of a chronically alcoholic mother. The less obvious effects include CNS deficits, various degrees of mental retardation and hyperactivity, irritability, and poor feeding habits. These children also have slow rates of growth, developmental delays, behavioral problems, intellectual impairment, poor judgment, and certain facial characteristics common to the children of alcoholic mothers.

Infants who have been exposed to cocaine in utero have sleeping and eating problems, unusual levels of irritability, and high-pitched cries. Other syndromes and developmental problems result from the use of different drugs, but all drugs have one thing in common: pregnancy and substance use do not mix.

Children who live with substance-abusing parents are at increased risk for injuries and developing drug problems themselves. Research has demonstrated that many children of parents who use both legal and illegal chemicals do poorly in school, have difficulty controlling their emotions, and exhibit low self-esteem. Many of these individuals repeat the cycle of substance use and child abuse when they reach adulthood. Some choose alcoholic or drug-abusing spouses.

Children abuse substances too, but often the substances are legal and easily available. The 9-year-old who demands cola drinks every day demonstrates the same signs of a caffeine addiction as an adult. The 8-year-old boy who has grown up with beer in the house can become an alcoholic just as quickly as his adult counterpart. Admissions to substance treatment units by children younger than the age of 12 is increasing. This reminds us that drug abuse problems really do exist among children.

Adolescent substance use, abuse, and dependence is becoming an ever-increasing problem. Eighty-two percent of high school seniors have used alcohol, 65% have smoked cigarettes, 50% have smoked marijuana, and 9% have used cocaine (National Institute on Drug Abuse, 1996). For people in the 15- to 24-year-old age group, alcohol-related accidents are the leading cause of death.

Because of their developmental levels, teens are encouraged to explore the adult world, but their ability to exercise sound judgment is still limited. Adolescents experiment with a variety of attitudes, behaviors, and lifestyles, and often substance use becomes a part of that experimentation. The younger an individual begins to use substances, the more likely that abuse problems will occur later in life.

Adolescents have various patterns of substance abuse. They may experiment by using drugs on a few occasions. They may use substances (usually alcohol, tobacco, or marijuana) in recreational ways, in social settings for the purpose of relaxation or intoxication. If actual addiction occurs, teens are likely to also become involved in illegal activities, such as drug trafficking, prostitution, or criminal behaviors.

In adults substance abuse is common, with about 10% of the adult population regularly abusing alcohol. This statistic is low because episodes of frequent binge drinking are not documented. Substance use and abuse occur most commonly between 18 and 35 years of age, but significant numbers of older adults abuse alcohol and prescription medications.

Older adults are not immune to substance-related problems, but they are often misdiagnosed or treated inappropriately. Older drinkers and elderly persons who misuse drugs are often isolated within their social groups or families. Although the incidence of substance abuse in older adults is unknown, more than 40% of all drug reactions occur in persons older than 65 (National Institute on Drug Abuse, 1996). This fact should alert nurses and health care providers who work with the elderly to the possibility of substance abuse in every older client.

Substances for abuse vary according to minority group. For example, the use of cocaine is higher among blacks, whereas whites and Hispanics prefer alcohol.

Drug use also varies with the location. For example, drug use in the United States is highest in the West and lowest in the North Central region.

Scope of the Problem Today

The abuse of chemical substances presents many problems for people in today's society. Alcohol and drug abuse have an impact on every citizen, in both financial terms and human costs. There are more women using street drugs during pregnancy than available drug treatment programs can accommodate. Infants exposed to cocaine and other drugs are filling health and foster care systems as the children of addicted parents are born. There are millions of children of alcoholics living in the United States today. Children of problem drinkers also have three times the risk of serious injury as children of nondrinking parents.

Substance use and dependence cost society dearly. The suicide rate for 15- to 24-year-olds has more than doubled since 1960 (Meckler, 1999). The use of alcohol and drugs often results in trauma, violence, and mental health problems. Alcohol-related motor vehicle accidents are one of the leading causes of death among people younger than age 45. Many deaths attributed to falls, drowning, and burns may be related to substance use.

Society's homeless and mentally ill people often use and abuse chemicals. Homeless persons with alcohol, drug, or mental disorders are one of the most disadvantaged and underserved groups in the United States. People with serious mental illness who also are addicted to or use chemicals are defined as having a **dual diagnosis**. The number of people with dual diagnosis is estimated to be as high as 75% of the mentally ill population.

CATEGORIES OF ABUSED SUBSTANCES

Every chemical has the potential for abuse. For example, the current concern over the effectiveness of antibiotic drugs stems from a form of abuse. As people routinely insisted on being treated with antibiotics for illnesses that did not actually require them, the microorganisms the antibiotics were designed to kill grew stronger and increasingly resistant. The repeated abuse of antibiotics has resulted in serious consequences for us all. Not all abused substances are illegal. In this text, however, the discussion of abused substances is limited to those that are currently considered illicit or harmful.

Chemicals of Abuse

The most popular substance of abuse in the United States and most developed countries is alcohol. Other substances increase and decrease in popularity, but the fact that more than 10% of the adult population in the United States abuses alcohol has remained constant for over 20 years.

Alcohol has been used since the beginning of recorded time. The effects of different alcoholic beverages are caused by the presence of ethanol (ETOH), a chemical that results from the fermentation of yeast and grains, malts, or fruits. "Hard liquor," such as whiskey, brandy, gin, and vodka, is derived from distilled spirits, whereas beer and wine are not. The process of distillation increases

Table 28-1	Effects of Alcohol on the Nervous System	
Blood alcohol content	**Approximate number of drinks**	**Central nervous system (behavioral) responses**
0.05%	1 or 2 (½-1 oz of alcohol)	Thought, restraint, judgment slowed; more socially at ease; reaction time slowed; unable to do complicated tasks
0.10%	3 or 4 (1½ oz of alcohol)	Voluntary motor actions clumsy; depth perception altered; reaction time to stimuli slowed; eye movement and focus affected; judgment and control continue to decrease; legal limit for driving
0.20%	5 or more (≥2½ oz of alcohol)	Entire motor area of brain depressed; may want to lie down; staggers; loses conscious control of reason; easily angered; may weep, shout, fight
0.30%	6 or more (≥3 oz of alcohol)	Acts confused; may be in a stupor; unresponsive to most external stimuli; losing ability to control involuntary responses; decreased heart rate, blood pressure, respiratory rate
0.40%-0.50%	7 or more (≥3½ oz of alcohol)	Comatose; medulla severely depressed; death from respiratory failure; death can occur with 0.40% if blood alcohol rises too rapidly; blood alcohol level of 0.50% is fatal without immediate medical attention

*Consumed within a 4-hour period.

the alcohol content of the beverage. To illustrate, ½ ounce of alcohol is found in one shot of distilled alcohol, 5 ounces of wine, and 12 ounces of beer.

Many people think of alcohol as a stimulant because they feel relaxation, alertness, and pleasure when they drink. Actually these feelings are caused by the depressant effects of alcohol on the central nervous system. Once swallowed, alcohol is rapidly diffused to all the body's organ systems. Because of its high solubility in water, alcohol collects in organs that have a high content of water (brain, heart, liver, and gastrointestinal tract). Alcohol is metabolized in the liver and excreted by the kidneys and lungs.

Low doses of alcohol cause a rise in blood pressure and pulse, but large doses can affect the pumping action of the heart, resulting in cardiac dysrhythmias. Surface blood vessels dilate, producing flushing of the skin and rapid loss of body heat. Alcohol also causes numbness of the hands and feet, which creates a false sense of warmth. In large doses, alcohol can actually reduce body temperature. The effects of alcohol on the CNS are directly related to the amount (dose) consumed (Table 28-1).

With repeated and continued use, tolerance develops and individuals become dependent on (addicted to) alcohol. If drinking is not stopped, death from multiple organ failure (especially the liver) results, usually after a series of assorted chronic health problems.

Narcotics are central nervous system depressants. They occur naturally, semisynthetically, and synthetically. Some natural narcotics have been altered to produce new artificially produced (synthetic) drugs. Natural narcotics are opium and its principal ingredient, morphine, which is used for medicinal purposes. These substances are often called *opioids* or *opiates* and are obtained by milking a flower called *Papaver somniferum,* the opium poppy.

The use of opium was documented 4000 years before Hippocrates, and it continues to be a commonly used substance in many countries today. Before the 1900s opium was readily available in the United States and a common ingredient in many patent medicines. Today there is little opium use in the United States as a result of the restrictive laws governing the drug.

Opium can be found in several forms. The fluid scraped from the base of the poppy flower and rolled into dark brown chunks is called raw opium (Figure 28-2). Processed opium can appear as a fine white powder.

The semisynthetic narcotics include heroin, hydromorphone, and thebaine derivatives. The Bayer Company of Germany first marketed heroin in 1898 as a new pain reliever. In the United States heroin was legally available to the public until the passage of the Harrison Narcotic Act of 1914.

Pure **heroin** is a white, bitter-tasting powder, which is usually put into solution and injected. Today potent forms of heroin are available. Some are so strong that they need only to be smoked or inhaled to produce the same effect as injecting. Street heroin is found in colors ranging from white to dark brown depending on the additives. A new form, called "black tar heroin," has become available throughout the western United States. This crudely processed form of heroin is manufactured in Mexico and may contain as much as 80% impurities. It is most commonly diluted and injected. The signs and symptoms of heroin use, overdose, and withdrawal are listed in Table 28-2.

Stimulants are another group of commonly abused substances. They include caffeine, cocaine, and certain prescription drugs, such as amphetamines, appetite suppressants, and methylphenidate (Ritalin).

Caffeine is found in every supermarket. It is the main active ingredient in coffee, black teas, most cola drinks,

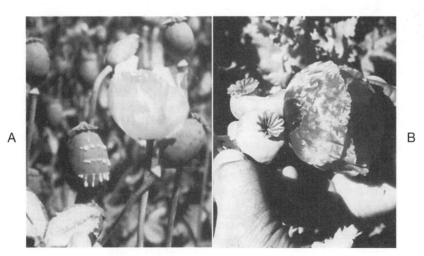

Figure 28-2 Opium. **A,** The fluid oozes form the seedpod of the poppy. **B,** An incision is made in the Mexican poppy to release opium. (Courtesy Drug Enforcement Agency.)

Table 28-2	Signs/Symptoms of Heroin Use, Overdose, and Withdrawal	
Heroin use	**Heroin overdose**	**Heroin withdrawal**
Constricted pupils	Shallow respirations	Watery eyes
Depression	Clammy skin	Runny nose
Drowsiness	Convulsions	Sweating
Euphoria (feelings of great well-being)	Coma	Muscle cramps
Nausea		Loss of appetite, nausea
Respiratory depression		Chills
		Tremors
		Panic

and other bottled beverages. Caffeine stimulates the nervous system, relieving fatigue and increasing alertness and the body's metabolic rate. In large amounts, it can produce tremors, tachycardia, nervousness, and insomnia. The most prominent withdrawal symptom from caffeine is headache.

Cocaine is a potent natural stimulant. For centuries the natives of the South American Andes Mountains chewed the weakly psychoactive leaves of the coca plant to relieve fatigue and hunger. Today coca is grown, processed into cocaine, and shipped to many countries throughout the world.

Cocaine is available "on the street" as a white, crystalline powder that is commonly contaminated with local anesthetics or sugar. It is either injected or "snorted" by inhaling. Cocaine produces an immediate rush of energy, vigor, and feelings of well-being that last less than an hour. The intense pleasurable feelings can lead to a mental dependency that can ultimately destroy one's life as more and more doses are sought and used. Repeated use of cocaine overstimulates the nervous system and can dissolve the nasal septum, resulting in a collapsed nose.

Crack is a type of processed cocaine. Combining cocaine with ammonia or baking soda and heating it removes the hydrochloride molecule and produces chips or chunks of highly addicting cocaine, called rocks. These are usually vaporized in a pipe or smoked with tobacco or marijuana. Because of its concentrated form, crack reaches the brain immediately and produces a more intense but shorter lasting high. Tolerance and addiction to the drug develops quickly as users chase the feeling of that first, intense experience.

Amphetamines were originally pharmaceutically manufactured medicines developed to treat depression, narcolepsy, hyperactivity in children, and obesity. Amphetamines were initially sold without a prescription in inhalers and diet pills. Today they are available only by prescription, but many are illegally manufactured. They are strong stimulants with addictive properties.

The last category of abused chemicals, the **hallucinogens,** are natural and synthetic substances that alter one's perception of reality. The active ingredient of the

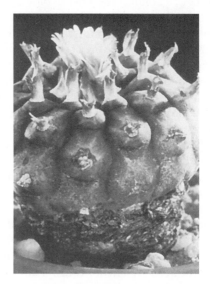

Figure 28-3 Peyote cactus. (Courtesy Drug Enforcement Agency.)

peyote cactus, mescaline, has been used in the religious ceremonies of certain Native Americans for many years (Figure 28-3).

Lysergic acid diethylamide (LSD), an ergot fungus, was discovered by accident in the 1940s, but the introduction of laboratory-designed hallucinogens in the United States did not occur until the early 1970s. Today, "designer drugs," such as synthetic hallucinogens LSD (acid), methylenedioxyamphetamine (MDA), 2,5-dimethoxy-4-methamphetamine (STP), and "ice" are easily available in all areas of the country. Most are taken orally or inhaled, and they are frequently contaminated. These hallucinogens vary in onset, duration of action, and potency, but all produce a sense of altered reality.

Phencyclidine (PCP) was originally developed for use as an animal tranquilizer. When taken by humans, it produces mild depression with low doses and a schizophrenic-like reaction with higher amounts. Phencyclidine is a dangerous drug because it causes people to behave in unpredictable, often violent, ways (Table 28-3).

Table 28-3	Signs/Symptoms of PCP Use	
	Physical signs/Symptoms	**Psychological signs/Symptoms**
	Increased blood pressure	Belligerence (wants to fight)
	Increased temperature	Bizarre behaviors
	Muscle rigidity, ataxia (uncoordinated, staggering)	Hallucinations
	Repeated jerking	Impaired (poor) judgment
	Agitated movements	Impulsive behaviors
	Vertical and horizontal nystagmus (eye tremors)	Paranoia
		Unpredictable behaviors

Modified from Taylor CM: *Essentials of psychiatric nursing*, ed 14, St. Louis, 1994, Mosby.

Users of hallucinogens experience everything from profound mind-expanding experiences to "bad trips" in which dangerous behavioral reactions occur. The mind-altering effects of hallucinogens include a heightened awareness of reality; distortions in time, space, and body image; feelings of depersonalization; and the loss of a sense of reality. *Flashbacks,* which are a return to the psychedelic experience after the drug has worn off, can occur with the use of hallucinogens. The repeated use of hallucinogens can lead to various mental health problems.

Cannabis (marijuana) is a term applied to the hemp plant, *Cannabis sativa,* which grows wild in many tropical and temperate climates all over the world. The hemp plant has been used for centuries by many cultures in folk remedies and other medicines. Historically it has been used to treat pain, decreased appetite, muscle and gastrointestinal tract spasms, asthma, and depression. It has also been used as an antibiotic and a topical anesthetic. Commercially, rope, clothing and paper are made from hemp (marijuana) (see Think About box).

Cannabis is available in several forms. The dried tops and leaves are called *marijuana.* Hashish (hash) is the dried resin that seeps from the top and leaves, and hash oil is the distilled oil of hashish. All are usually smoked, but they may also be eaten.

Marijuana and other cannabis products produce a sense of well-being and relaxation. They alter time perception and affect short-term memory and concentration. Motivation, especially for distasteful tasks, may be decreased. Frequently an increase in hunger occurs. Large doses can result in feelings of anxiety and paranoia. There are no proven withdrawal signs or symptoms, but anxious moods, irritability, and sleep disturbances have been reported.

Medications

Many chemicals that were developed to save lives and ease suffering have the potential for being abused. For example, almost all the opium arriving in the United States today is broken down into its most useful alkaloids, morphine and codeine. These substances are then refined into powerful pain-relieving medications (narcotic anal-

gesics). They are available in the United States only with the prescription of a licensed physician, dentist, or nurse practitioner, but they remain a source of abuse.

Morphine is one of the most effective painkillers available. It is marketed as a white powder or in solution for injection. It is administered by injection under the direction of a licensed health care practitioner.

Hydromorphone and the thebaine derivatives are semisynthetic narcotics made from opium. Hydromorphone is commonly called Dilaudid. It is used as an analgesic and is produced in liquid or more potent tablet form. It is shorter acting, more sedating, and up to eight times more powerful than morphine. Although available only by prescription, it is highly sought by addicts. Thebaine derivatives, another opium product, are up to a thousand times more potent than morphine. Because of the danger of overdose, these drugs are used by veterinarians for the care of large animals only.

Commonly abused stimulants include the amphetamines, diet pills, and the appetite suppressants. Methylphenidate (Ritalin), a medication used to treat attention-deficit hyperactivity disorders, is another often abused stimulant. The signs and symptoms of stimulant use include changes in personality, anxiety, tension, anger, restlessness, and rapid speech and movement.

Laxatives and diuretics are commonly abused by people trying to lose weight and the elderly. Individuals with eating disorders or altered body images often use these drugs to keep themselves excessively thin or to atone for an eating binge. Elderly people can develop a dependence on laxatives when they are used too frequently.

The sedative, hypnotic, and antianxiety drug classes are commonly used in ways other than therapeutic. During the 1950s, many people were unknowingly addicted to the drug diazepam (Valium) and other sedatives. The individual who is unable to sleep without hypnotic medications may be abusing sleeping pills, and many people reach for their "nerve pills" when they feel anxious or upset. The importance of obtaining a thorough history of every client's medication use cannot be overemphasized.

Inhalants

The breathing in of volatile substances or chemical gasses (**inhalants**) has become popular with adolescents and young adults for several reasons: they are legal, inexpensive, and easily available, and they have a rapid onset of effects. Unfortunately the practice is also associated with significant complications, such as sudden death caused by cardiac dysrhythmia or respiratory depression. The use of inhalants can also result in hyperactive motor responses, loss of coordination, and seizures.

The most commonly inhaled substances are alcohol solvents, gasoline, glue, paint thinner, hairspray, and spray paints. Less frequently used chemicals used as inhalants include cleaning fluids, typewriter correction liquids, and spray can propellants.

Inhalants are most often used by adolescents in group settings. Several methods are used to inhale the vapors, such as soaking a rag and then holding it to the nose and mouth. The substance may be inhaled directly from the container or placed in a bag or other closed container and then inhaled. Soon after inhaling, the individual feels a "high" that is associated with feelings of great well-being (euphoria), excitement, sexual aggressiveness, a lessened sense of right and wrong, and loss of judgment. Signs and symptoms of inhalant intoxication include delusions, hallucinations, anxiety, and confusion. Although no withdrawal syndrome has been recognized, the repeated use of inhalants can result in profound physical and psychosocial harm.

Nicotine is currently a legal inhalant. It is present in all forms of tobacco (cigarettes, chewing tobacco, pipe tobacco, cigars, and snuff) and certain medications (nicotine patch and gum). It produces relaxation, increases alertness, and helps to relieve feelings of hunger. Nicotine is frequently used as a method to control body weight.

Although its popularity is declining, tobacco is still a commonly used substance. Tobacco is either smoked or held between the gum and lip and absorbed through the mucous membranes of the mouth. It is never swallowed because of its toxic effects. Tobacco is addictive, and its continued use is associated with many health complications. Recently in the United States, Canada, and other industrialized countries, a movement to restrict the sales and use of tobacco products (especially to children and teens) has arisen.

There are many substances that have the potential for abuse. Some clients may be addicted to more than one substance. Many practice binge drinking, in which short periods of ingestion are followed by periods of abstinence. For these reasons, it is important to obtain an accurate history of every client's substance use patterns.

CHARACTERISTICS OF SUBSTANCE USE AND ABUSE

It is important to remember the differences between substance use and abuse. Some people can use various chemicals to change the way they feel, but the use does not affect their abilities to perform the activities of daily life. This is substance *use*. Substance *abuse*, however, occurs when use of the chemical becomes more important than the activities of daily living.

The causes of substance abuse are unknown, but several theories have attempted to explain why people use mind-altering chemicals. Biological theories state that there are variations between ethnic groups that offer genetic and biochemical explanations for substance abuse. Theories relating to psychological factors explore the roles of personality and emotional problems as causes, and environmental theories concentrate on the individual, the family, and sociocultural surroundings in which substance abuse takes place.

Stages of Addiction

Many individuals use alcohol, tobacco, or other chemicals and function very well. Those who move from use to dependency (addiction) follow a fairly predictable course. During the early stage, individuals are able to use and enjoy their chosen substance. A desire to repeat the first pleasurable experience leads to a frequent pattern of use where one prefers being "high" to other activities.

Soon a habit of excessive use develops as the individual begins to ignore responsibilities and obligations. The person may deny that a problem exists, ignore others' comments, lie to cover up the activity, or conceal the problem by sneaking drinks or doses. During these periods the individual may also become intoxicated.

Intoxication is defined as a state of maladaptive behavioral or psychological changes resulting from exposure to certain chemicals. Intoxicated people are frequently belligerent (looking for a fight or an argument) and have wide emotional swings. They often lack sound judgment, and their ability to think critically is reduced. Commonly they will stagger or show other signs of impaired motor abilities. The actual picture of an intoxicated individual varies greatly. Psychological effects are based on the person's expectations of what the chemical will do and the setting or environment in which the substance is taken.

During the middle (crucial) stage of addiction, the intoxicating episodes increase as the body attempts to compensate by adapting to the substance. Tolerance develops as increased amounts of the chemical are needed to produce the same effects that one dose once produced. Physical tolerance occurs when the body has adjusted to living and functioning with the substance in its system. Psychological tolerance develops when individuals feel that they cannot function without the use of their chosen chemical.

By the time one has progressed to the chronic late stage, tolerance for the chemical is usually quite high. Now the need for the substance leads to a loss of control over one's behavior. Without the chemical, life is miserable. Daily living becomes a nightmare, and every waking effort and energy is focused on obtaining and using the now required substance. The Case Study box offers a vivid example.

Criteria for Diagnosis

For a substance-related disorder to be diagnosed, individuals must meet certain criteria. The pattern of substance use must be disabling and lead to significant impaired functioning and distress. The individual must demonstrate signs of tolerance, withdrawal, and dependence (American Psychiatric Association, 2000).

Clinical Presentation

Unlike physical illness, there is no classic presentation of a substance abuser. Each person has a unique variety of signs and symptoms, depending on chemical use and individual characteristics. However, because substance abuse affects every body system, there are some common indicators, such as alterations in neurological functioning or appearance, that can help with the assessment and monitoring of clients. Refer to Tables 28-1 through 28-3 for specific signs and symptoms.

GUIDELINES FOR INTERVENTION

The three most commonly abused types of drugs are alcohol and sedative-alcohol combinations; opiate narcotics, chiefly heroin; and stimulants, chiefly cocaine and amphetamines.

The costs and consequences of substance abuse are high. As individuals progress with their drug abuse, their world narrows as the individual becomes isolated from occupational and community relationships (see Drug Alert box).

Absenteeism from work, unpaid bills, and job loss frequently result when chemical use is out of control. Involvement with the legal system can occur with drunken driving or domestic violence charges. Some people completely deplete their financial resources to obtain their substances. Accidents, trauma, crime, domestic violence, child abuse, prostitution, suicide, disease, and the loss of safe communities are associated with substance abuse. Therefore it is important for all health care providers to be alert to the possibility of substance-related problems in every client.

◆ Case Study

Ernie's father was 15 years old when Ernie was born. His mother, who was 14 years old, gave custody to the father after the first 6 months of Ernie's life. To keep Ernie quiet during his infant and toddler years, his father would blow marijuana smoke into Ernie's face. It worked. Ernie would sleep for hours while his father "partied."

By the time Ernie was 5 years old, he was drinking beer. At 8, he graduated to vodka, gin, and tequila. By 10, Ernie was mixing alcohol with cocaine. School became impossible, so he dropped out at 12. By the time he was 14 years old, Ernie was hustling drugs and trying to sell the sexual favors of three neighborhood girls.

Where is Ernie today? Fortunately he overdosed one evening when he was about 17 years old. The nurse in the emergency department, recognizing the potential in this young man, took the time to tell him that he had choices. Ernie listened. His detoxification was painful, and his recovery slow and difficult, but he persisted, knowing there was something more in life than a fog of consciousness.

Today, despite several setbacks, Ernie has been clean for more than 10 years. He is a college graduate, happily married, and the father of two boys. The strongest thing he drinks now is orange juice.

◆ How do you think the nurse made an impact on Ernie's life?

Drug Alert

Remember, elderly persons are at risk for becoming drug dependent. When an older adult becomes less social and begins to isolate himself or herself, suspect a problem with drugs. The usual drugs of abuse in the elderly are pain medications and drug combinations.

Have your elderly clients bring all their medications to you in a paper bag. These medications should include all over-the-counter and herbal preparations. In this way, an accurate assessment of their medication use can be obtained. Do not forget to ask about alcohol use, especially in combination with their medications.

Assessment

The physical examination, patient history, and emotional assessment should focus on the following aspects:

Central nervous system: Assess for orientation, level of consciousness, balance, gait, and ability to follow instructions.

Head and neck: Examine eyes and check pupils and sclera (whites) of the eyes. Note ruddy or pale complexion, distended neck veins, or petechiae (small red dots) on the face. Observe for evidence of injections under the tongue, and inspect the area between the gums and lips.

Chest: Do not forget to take vital signs. Count pulse and respirations for a full minute. Palpate pedal and radial pulses. Observe for any difficulty in breathing. Auscultate the heart for irregular rates or rhythms. Listen to the breath sounds, and note any abnormal sounds.

Abdomen: Inspect the size, shape, and contours of the abdomen. Auscultate all four quadrants and count the bowel sounds. Check for ascites (water in the abdomen), distention, or enlarged organs. Look for bruising, petechiae, and other signs of bleeding. Have the client describe the color and consistency of stool.

Skin: Observe and document the size, location, and characteristics of any skin lesions or marks. Check for needle marks on the client's arms, fingers, legs, and toes. Note the skin turgor and muscle mass of the arms and legs.

Nutritional status: Many chemically dependent persons do not eat regularly and run a risk of becoming malnourished. Observe the client's body build and appearance. Ask the client to list everything he or she ate yesterday and tell you how the meals were prepared. Ask if there have been any recent appetite or weight changes. Inspect the client's skin color, hair, and fingernails. If the client lives alone or is homeless, find out how food is obtained on a daily basis.

The psychosocial assessment includes the following:

General appearance: Is the client tidy or unkempt? Note the client's manner and style of dress, jewelry, makeup, hairstyle, and body marks (e.g., tattoos or symbolic scars).

Behaviors: Note rate of speech, motor activity, and interactions during the interview. Observe for signs of memory loss, difficulty following directions, and problems with communication.

Emotional state: Watch for signs of depression, emotional instability (mood swings), suspiciousness, anger, agitation, self-pity, or jealousy. Ask clients if they have ever had a hallucination, a blackout (period of time during which the user cannot remember events), any violent impulses, or suicidal ideas.

Social support: Have clients identify the most important people in their lives. Are these people willing to become involved in treatment with the client? If possible, observe how clients interact with their family and friends. Remember that family members may also need support and treatment.

Motivation: Obtain a description of the chemicals currently being used: how often, how much, when was last dose? When did use begin? What (if anything) has been tried to decrease or stop using the chemical? Describe clients' history of treatment for substance-related or emotional problems. Ask what motivated them to seek treatment now. Is the court, the job, or the family insisting on treatment, or are they seeking relief from the problems associated with the chemical use? The motivation level of clients plays an important part in recovery.

Diagnostic tests: Diagnostic testing usually includes standard blood and urine examinations. A complete blood count (CBC), urinalysis, and chemistry panel is done to assess for organ damage. Frequently tests for hepatitis, human immunodeficiency virus (HIV), tuberculosis (TB), and other infectious diseases are performed. Clients are also assessed for nutritional or bleeding problems. Other diagnostic tests, such as a computed tomography (CT) scan, magnetic resonance imaging (MRI), x-ray films, or an electroencephalogram (EEG) may also be ordered.

Treatments and Therapies

The treatment of substance-related disorders continues to change and grow. Consequently a broad range of approaches are available today. Most treatment programs are based on a certain philosophy, although they may offer many different types of therapy.

The *disease model* of treatment states that substance abuse is a disease and should be treated as such. Substance abuse has acute and chronic signs and symptoms, a certain pattern of progression, and physical pathological conditions associated with continued use. Two types of treatment programs based on the disease model are the 12-step programs and residential treatment programs.

The first *12-step program* was a self-help, group-centered program developed by two alcoholics in 1935. The 12-step process involves admitting one's powerlessness to control drug use and then seeking help from a higher power through prayer or meditation, moral inventories, confessing wrongs, asking for forgiveness, and carrying the message to others. The first 12-step program was Alcoholics Anonymous (AA). Many other 12-step programs are based on this model and revised to fit the beliefs of the population they serve. Box 28-1 offers a general listing of self-help groups available in many countries throughout the world. Self-help groups can be very effective when the individual wants them to be.

The *medical model* considers addictions from a public health, chronic and acute infectious disease perspective.

Box 28-1 Self-Help Groups for Recovering Abusers

Alcoholics Anonymous—for individuals recovering from alcoholism; founded in 1935

Al-Anon—for families of alcoholics

Alateen—for 12- to 20-year-olds who are affected by someone else's drinking problem

Association of Recovering Motorcyclists—support group for motorcyclists recovering from alcohol or drug addiction

Calix Society—Catholic alcoholics who maintain sobriety through participation in AA

Christian Addiction Rehabilitation Association—provides support and ministry to individuals with addictions

Cocaine Anonymous—for those recovering from cocaine addiction; a 12-step program

Drug-Anon Focus—for families and friends of persons addicted to mind-altering drugs; a 12-step program

Drugs Anonymous—for individuals addicted to drugs; a 12-step program

Dual Disorders Anonymous—for people with both alcohol or drug addiction and mental or emotional disorders; a 12-step program

Families Anonymous—for parents, relatives, and friends of drug addicts

Gay AA—provides support for gay and lesbian alcoholics

Impaired Physician Program—provides assistance to physicians and their spouses who have problems with alcohol, drugs, or codependence

International Nurses Anonymous—for nurses, nursing students, and former nurses who are involved in a 12-step recovery program

Naranon—provides assistance to drug-dependent individuals and their families

Narcotics Anonymous—for individuals recovering from drug abuse; a 12-step program

Rational Recovery Systems—uses rational emotive therapy (versus a spiritual approach) to assist people in their recovery from substance abuse

From Keltner NL, Schwecke LH, Bostrom CE: *Psychiatric nursing*, ed 3, St. Louis, 1998, Mosby.

The *biopsychosocial framework* for treating clients is a medical model that attempts to explain substance abuse. New understanding of neurotransmitters and other biochemical activities of the brain is leading toward the development of medications that may someday help people cope with their chemical dependencies.

Psychiatric models view substance abuse as an expression of an underlying emotional conflict or mental disorder. Several therapies are based on this framework.

Sociocultural models state that substance abuse can be treated by changing an individual's environment and teaching people how to develop new responses to their current environments. This view has led to the establishment of long-term residential treatment programs and therapeutic communities.

Regardless of the type of substance used, the goals of care remain the same. The first step in treatment is for the individual to recognize the need for help. Denial is a strong part of most substance-related disorders. For any treatment to be effective, the client must be truly willing to work toward living without his or her addiction.

Before treatment of the addiction can actually begin, many persons must first go through **detoxification,** the process of withdrawing a substance under medical supervision. Clients who are addicted to opium, narcotics, alcohol, or sedatives are often hospitalized because of potentially fatal complications, such as seizures and respiratory and cardiac problems. Sometimes medications, such as phenobarbital, Dilantin, and Valium, are given to ease physical discomforts and prevent complications. **Methadone** (drug used to treat heroin addiction) has been administered to ease the effects of withdrawing from heroin, but methadone itself is addicting, and it is difficult to "detox" from methadone.

Once clients are physically free from their addictions (practicing abstinence), the focus turns to uncovering and treating existing emotional or mental health problems. The incidence of psychiatric disorders is very high in substance users. Anxiety and depression are often found in clients with substance-abuse problems (Scott, Gilvarry, and Farrell, 1998). These disorders must also be treated if the individual is to remain drug-free.

The last, and perhaps the most difficult, goal of treatment is to assist individuals in changing their behaviors. Individual psychotherapy is very effective for clients with certain dependencies (cocaine addictions), but it is expensive and unavailable to many people. Group therapy can offer peer support from individuals "who have been there." It also offers people the opportunity to experiment with and explore their new, drug-free behaviors.

Medications are prescribed with extreme care. Two specific medications used in the care of substance-addicted clients are methadone and disulfiram (Antabuse). Methadone is a chemical relative of heroin. Taken orally once a day, it prevents the symptoms of withdrawal and helps to stabilize the lives of these substance abusers. Recently a new form of methadone, called LLAM, has been developed. It requires that a dose be taken only once every 72 hours.

Disulfiram (Antabuse) is a medication taken daily by nonpracticing (dry) alcoholics. It causes very unpleasant physical reactions when combined with alcohol, including intense headache, flushing, nausea, vomiting, low blood pressure, and blurred vision. It is prescribed as a preventive measure to help reduce the desire for alcohol. It is very important to thoroughly research each of these medications and routinely monitor your clients for therapeutic and adverse reactions of these chemicals.

Relapse

Long-term recovery is often marked by periods of relapse. **Relapse** is the recurrence of the substance-abusing behaviors after a significant period of abstinence. In other words, the client returns to "using" after he or she has been "dry" for a period of time. Not only do people return to the chemical-abusing behaviors, but they also readopt the psychological and emotional mind-set that brought about the abuse in the first place. Many treatment therapies and programs concentrate on preventing and treating relapses. Remember that clients who have relapsed feel many distressing emotions. True therapeutic care is given when these clients are accepted and respected, even when they are the least accepting and respecting of themselves. Remember, you are a therapeutic agent.

Nursing Process

An important intervention for clients with substance-related problems is to act as a therapeutic agent. Practice effective listening skills to gain an understanding of who the client really is. Use your knowledge of the therapeutic relationship to establish trust and cooperation. Learn to act as a role model and teacher, quietly demonstrating problem solving and other effective coping skills; be willing to look beyond the addiction to see the person.

Nursing diagnoses that relate to clients with substance abuse problems are based on identified problems and goals. Box 28-2 lists several possible diagnoses.

A Sample Client Care Plan summary for the diagnosis of ineffective individual coping is presented.

Although the actual care for each client is individually planned, certain key nursing actions are common to all substance-dependent clients (Box 28-3).

Caring for clients with substance-related problems is challenging and frustrating. Nurses and other caregivers are in valuable positions to influence their clients' well-being. Demonstrations of respect, acceptance, and concern can offer many clients the connection that encourages them to work toward freedom from their chemicals. The personalized approaches of nurses allow for discussions about diet, health, problem solving, and other health concerns. Drug therapists work with clients to develop long-term strategies for coping with their dependency. Clients are offered opportunities for learning, changing, and developing new and more effective skills for living. Work to become familiar with the subject of substance abuse. Learn as much as you can because you will be caring for clients whose problems are related to the use of chemical substances.

KEY CONCEPTS

◆ Substance use is the ingesting (eating, drinking, injecting, or inhaling) of any chemical that affects the body.

◆ Abused substances alter the individual's perception by affecting the CNS; they are often referred to as

>>> Sample Client Care Plan

Ineffective Coping

Assessment

History: Mary is a 34-year-old housewife with three children and a husband who works long hours. Two years ago, she complained of feeling jittery and tense to her physician. He prescribed a mild sedative, which Mary took religiously every evening before bed. Lately she has begun to take her "nerve pill" during the day and uses alcohol to help "stabilize" her. She is being admitted for evaluation and treatment after her husband found her unconscious on the sofa yesterday.

Current Findings: A well-groomed woman with flattened speech. Mary answers questions when asked but volunteers no information. She stated she does not belong here because she is not really addicted to anything and resents "being treated like a drugger."

Multidisciplinary Diagnosis

Ineffective individual coping related to increasing use of sedatives and alcohol.

Planning/Goals

Mary will abstain from using all mood-altering chemicals. Mary will identify and seek help for her problem.

Therapeutic Interventions

Intervention	Rationale	Team Member
1. Confront Mary with her substance-abusing actions and their consequences and assist her in identifying the problem.	Denial is very common with persons who have a substance-related problem, identifying problems is the first step toward change.	Psy, Nsg
2. Encourage Mary to agree to participate in the treatment program.	Therapeutic interventions are not effective unless the client wants to cooperate.	All
3. Work with Mary to develop a written contract for behavioral changes.	A personal commitment enhances the likelihood of success.	Psy, Nsg
4. Assist Mary in identifying and adopting more effective coping behaviors.	Encourages problem solving and the use of more effective behaviors.	Nsg, Psy
5. Assess the social support systems available for Mary.	Supportive significant others are often unavailable for substance abusers.	Nsg, Soc Svc
6. Educate Mary and her family about chemical abuse and resources for help.	Knowledge helps Mary and her family cope more successfully with problems.	Nsg, Soc Svc
7. Refer Mary to a treatment center and provide support until Mary is involved in the program.	Specialized drug treatment programs are likely to be more effective if clients are willing to participate.	Soc Svc

Evaluation

During her entire stay Mary remained chemical free but expressed many discomforts. Mary was able to identify her drug-using behaviors during her stay but refused to participate in an outpatient treatment program.

A complete client care plan includes several other diagnoses and interventions.

mind-altering drugs because of their ability to enhance or depress mood and emotions.

◆ Every chemical ingested by a pregnant woman poses a potential danger to her unborn child.

◆ The younger an individual begins to use substances, the more likely that abuse problems will occur later in life.

◆ The most popular substance for abuse in most developed countries today is alcohol.

◆ Narcotics are CNS depressants that occur naturally, semisynthetically, and synthetically.

◆ Stimulants include caffeine, cocaine, and certain prescription medications, such as the amphetamines, appetite suppressants, and methylphenidate (Ritalin).

◆ Hallucinogens are natural and synthetic substances that alter one's perception of reality.

◆ Cannabis is a term applied to the hemp plant. Marijuana is usually dried and smoked.

◆ Many medications have the potential for being abused.

◆ Abused medications include morphine and its derivatives, amphetamines, sedatives, hypnotics, antianxiety agents, laxatives, and diuretics.

- The use of inhalants is associated with significant complications, such as cardiac dysrhythmia or respiratory depression.
- Nicotine is currently a legal inhalant present in all forms of tobacco and certain medications.
- Substance abuse occurs when the use of the chemical becomes more important in the individual's life than the activities of daily living.
- The movement from use to dependency (addiction) follows a fairly predictable course.
- For a substance-related disorder to be diagnosed, the pattern of substance use must be disabling and lead to significant impaired functioning and distress, and the individual must demonstrate the signs of tolerance, withdrawal, and dependence.
- The assessment of clients with substance-related problems should include a thorough history and physical examination.
- Most treatment programs for clients with substance-related disorders are based on a certain philosophy, although many different types of therapy may be offered.
- Detoxification is the process of withdrawing a substance under medical supervision.
- Relapse is the recurrence of the substance-abusing behaviors after a significant period of abstinence.
- The most important intervention for clients with substance-related problems is to act as a therapeutic agent.

Suggestions for Further Reading

The following websites are filled with current information about alcohol and drug abuse:

Council on Alcohol and Other Drug Abuse (CAODA) (www.caoda.org/)

National Clearinghouse for Alcohol and Drug Information at (www.health.org/index.htm)

Alcohol Problems and Solutions at (www2.potsdam.edu/alcohol-info/)

References

American Psychiatric Association: *Diagnostic and statistical manual of mental disorders,* ed 4, text revision, Washington, DC, 2000, The Association.

"Fetal alcohol syndrome," fact sheet, Atlanta, 1997, Centers for Disease Control and Prevention.

Dickason EJ, Silverman BL, Schult MO: *Maternal-infant nursing care,* ed 3, St. Louis, 1998, Mosby.

Keltner NL, Schwecke LH, Bostrom CE: *Psychiatric nursing,* ed 3, St. Louis, 1998, Mosby.

Meckler L: Suicide in U.S.: a "national tragedy," Associated Press, July 28, 1999.

National Institute on Drug Abuse (NIDH): *National household survey on drug use,* Bethesda, Md, 1996, The Institute.

National pregnancy and health history, NIH Publication No. 96-3819, 1996, National Institute on Drug Abuse.

North American Nursing Diagnosis Association: *NANDA nursing diagnoses: definitions and classification 1999-2000,* Philadelphia, 1999, The Association.

Scott J, Gilvarry E, Farrell M: Managing anxiety and depression in alcohol and drug dependence, *Addictive Behaviors* 23(6):919, 1998.

Siegel MA, Landes A, Jacobs NR, editors: *Information plus: illegal drugs and alcohol,* 1995 edition, Wylie, Tex, 1995, Information Plus.

Streissguth AP: *Ciba Foundation Symposium No. 105: Mechanisms of alcohol damage in utero,* London, 1984, Pitman.

Taylor CM: *Essentials of psychiatric nursing,* ed 14, St. Louis, Mosby.

U.S. Public Health Service: *State resources and services related to alcohol and other drug problems,* Washington, DC, 1994.

Chapter 29

Sexual Disorders

Learning Objectives

1. Describe the continuum (range) of sexual responses.
2. Explain how self-awareness affects the care of clients with psychosexual problems.
3. Illustrate how sexuality is expressed through each life stage.
4. Describe four modes of sexual expression.
5. Examine three possible causes of sexual problems.
6. Compare the difference between a sexual dysfunction and a sexual disorder.
7. Define paraphilia and list three examples of paraphiliac behaviors.
8. Apply the nursing process to the care of a client with a psychosexual problem.
9. Explain the importance of human immunodeficiency virus (HIV)/acquired immunodeficiency syndrome (AIDS) counseling for every client with a psychosexual problem.

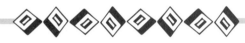

Key Terms

bisexuals

dyspareunia

erotic

exhibitionism

gay

gender identity

gender perceptions

gender role

heterosexual

homosexuality

lesbian

masochism

paraphilias

prostitution

sadism

sexual disorders

sexual dysfunction

sexuality

sexual orientation

transsexualism

transvestism

vaginismus

voyeurism

According to Maslow's hierarchy of needs, sex ranks as a basic physiological need. Humans, like most other creatures, have strong sexual drives; but unlike other creatures, human sexual expression is defined by the social customs, norms, and laws of society. A number of terms are used when discussing sex, and several are listed in Box 29-1.

People express their sexuality through a variety of thoughts, attitudes, and behaviors. Sexuality is important in every dimension of functioning. The physical dimension of sexuality includes anatomy and physiology—the characteristics that physically define us as men or women.

Sexuality in the emotional and intellectual dimensions encompasses our thoughts, beliefs, and values about sexuality. The social dimension of functioning is associated with sexuality. Interactions with others may range from the intimacy of sexual intercourse, to discussions of sexual attitudes with trusted friends, to passing feelings generated by attractive strangers. Sexuality and its expressions are social in nature.

Cultures have an impact on sexuality. All societies have laws, rules, or customs that regulate sexual behavior. Attitudes, beliefs, and rituals help define what is appropriate sexually. Religious institutions have a strong impact

Box 29-1 Terms Relating to Sexuality

Human **sexuality** is the combination of physical, chemical, psychological, and functional characteristics that are expressed by one's gender identity and sexual behaviors.

Sexuality is comprised of one's:

gender identity: the physical makeup of an individual
gender perception: a view of one's maleness or femaleness
gender role: cultural and social obligations relating to one's sex
sexual orientation: gender to which one is romantically attracted

From Stuart GW, Laraia MT: *Principles and practice of psychiatric nursing,* ed 7, St. Louis, 2001, Mosby.

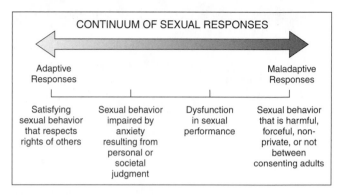

Figure 29-1 Continuum of sexual responses. (Redrawn from Stuart GW, Laraia MT: *Principles and practice of psychiatric nursing,* ed 7, St. Louis, 2001, Mosby.)

 ## Cultural Aspects

In her book titled *Growing up in Samoa,* Margaret Mead describes children with few sexual restraints. Although sexual play and experimentation are accepted methods of expression, the pregnancy rate of the islanders is no greater than other populations.

In Malaysia, children born out of marriage are common. It is the custom for the father to quietly provide for the child's welfare.

Think About

What is your definition of "normal" sexuality?

◆ How does your view compare with the views of a relative, a friend, and a classmate?
◆ What is your opinion of those who practice different means of sexual expression?
◆ How do you think your personal beliefs and opinions affect your interactions with clients?

on views of what is right or wrong sexual behavior. In some cultures, the sexual act is considered a religious ritual, with taboos and regulations governing the experience. Evidence of the practice of religious **prostitution** (the selling of sexual services in exchange for [spiritual] gain) has been found dating as far back as 5000 years ago. Cultural attitudes, beliefs, and behaviors toward sexuality and its expressions have changed throughout the years, and they will continue to change in the future (see Cultural Aspects box).

CONTINUUM OF SEXUAL RESPONSES

Even experts have difficulty agreeing on what is normal sexual behavior. For years the norm was defined as a married man and woman who engaged in sexual relations for the purpose of procreating (for having children). Today a wider range of sexual behaviors is considered socially acceptable.

Sexual behaviors can be viewed as occurring along a continuum (Figure 29-1). At the adaptive end of the spectrum lie satisfying sexual behaviors that respect the rights and wishes of others. As the continuum moves toward maladaptive, sexual behaviors become impaired or dysfunctional. The opposite end of the continuum is

marked by sexual actions that are harmful to self or others in some manner.

Perhaps a useful definition of adaptive or healthy sexual responses is sexuality that is (1) between two consenting adults, (2) satisfying to both, (3) not forced or coerced, and (4) conducted in privacy (Stuart and Laraia, 2001). Maladaptive or unhealthy sexual responses are those behaviors that do not meet these criteria. They are, in some way or degree, physically or psychologically harmful for the individual or others. Labeling sexual behaviors must be done with caution because judgments are easy to pass on those who behave differently (see Think About box).

Self-Awareness and Sexuality

Because nurses and other health caregivers work with the human condition, each of us must strive to develop an awareness of our thoughts, attitudes, values, and beliefs toward sexuality and its various modes of expression. One's level of self-awareness has a strong influence on discussing sexual issues with clients. Values that may be unconscious to the caregiver can be transmitted loudly and clearly to clients. Nonverbal messages of disapproval dampen the effectiveness of the therapeutic relationship and all other interventions.

Individuals who feel judged are not likely to cooperate with the plan of care.

Developing an awareness of your views about sexuality involves the process of defining and clarifying attitudes and values. Each of us carries a sexual point of view, a way of looking at sexuality. Much of the foundation for this view was unconsciously established during childhood and adolescence as a part of growing up and interacting with others.

Refer to Chapter 3 for the values clarification process. Apply each of the steps to the topic of sexuality, and then think about how your values may affect the care of clients with sexual disorders. Choose your positions and prize your choices. Know that values are not static; they change as one learns and develops. Remember, when it comes to working with sexually disordered clients, the caregiver's effectiveness is directly related to personal self-awareness and comfort. No client should ever have to endure the ignorance of his or her health care provider.

SEXUALITY THROUGHOUT THE LIFE CYCLE

The expression of one's sexuality begins at birth and ends with death. Sexual differences define roles in society, attitudes about the dynamics of living, relationships with others, and views of who we are. Sex roles develop as new knowledge, attitudes, and behaviors are added to life experiences. A basic knowledge of sexuality throughout the life cycle is important for care providers.

Sexuality in Childhood

"From the moment of birth, children are treated differently by their families based on their biological sex" (Wong, 1998). Female infants are dressed in pink, males in blue. Each is assigned a name, which usually indicates a gender. For example, girls are seldom named Bruce or Joseph, and few boys are addressed as Sarah or Sally.

Families treat boys differently from girls, even in infancy. Female infants are seen as delicate. They are handled and spoken to more tenderly, whereas male infants are stimulated by boisterous voices and play involving motor activity.

Young children are unaware that sex is a permanent attribute. Around the age of 2, children learn to label themselves according to their sex. Most respond to being called "good girls" or "brave boys" by the adults in their environment and soon internalize the label of male or female, boy or girl.

By age 3, the majority of children can accurately label the sex of other persons, but they still believe that their sex can be changed with time if they want it. By about age 7, children understand that one's sex is permanently assigned and will not naturally change. Between 7 and 9, they learn that one's sex is identified by genital appearance.

Children learn about sex roles in relation to themselves first and then apply their learning to members of the same sex. Finally, their knowledge is applied to persons of the opposite sex. By about 3 years of age, children can identify the simpler aspects of sex roles. They know, for example, that boys and girls differ in appearance, toy preference, and choice of activities.

By the time they enter school, it is thought that most children identify with the same-sex parent. School is the time to learn about the expected behaviors associated with each sex role. In the past this identification involved much stereotyping. Girls could not play certain sports, for example, whereas boys were discouraged from taking home economics or engaging in other "sissy" activities. Fortunately this attitude is fading as individual qualities become more important than playing appropriate sex roles.

By the middle elementary school years, children are aware of most aspects of their sex-role stereotypes. Future goals, occupational choices, personality traits, and sexual behaviors are influenced by sex roles that were established early in childhood.

Sexuality in Adolescence

During the early teen years, close relationships with same-sex peers intensify. "Through these relationships, children learn about the possibility of intimacy between equals and are exposed to peer standards for appropriate sex-role behavior" (Wong, 1998). As relationships progress, adolescents begin to encounter expectations for mature sex-role behavior from both peers and adults.

Although 12-year-olds are intensely involved with same-sex friends, opportunities for mixed-group activities and dating increase. Dating activities in the United States usually begin in the seventh or eighth grade with group social activities, such as dances, picnics, or organized school functions. Group dating moves to double-dating, and by the twelfth grade, most adolescents have been on single-pair dates.

Teens have difficulty believing that sex can exist without love, so each boy-girl attachment is seen as "true love." Because adolescence is an emotionally stressful time for most individuals, steady dating can offer some relief from insecurity and loneliness and provide a sense of belonging.

In the United States, sexual activity among adolescents has become the norm rather than the exception. Most teens begin experimenting with sexual activity through kissing and petting. As adolescents get older, most become sexually active. Many teens have experienced multiple sexual relationships by the time they are 19. Unfortunately most adolescent girls use ineffective or no contraception at all, and most adolescent boys do not use condoms. Because of this practice, the sexually transmitted disease rate (including HIV/AIDS) and the rate of pregnancy are higher for adolescents than the general population of sexually active adults. Adolescence is a time of intense searching and learning. Much information related to sexuality is gained from peers and other inexperienced or unknowledgeable persons. Nurses should always be alert for the opportunity to assess and correct, if necessary, adolescents' misconceptions about sexuality and its expressions.

Sexuality in Adulthood

The age of first intercourse has decreased and the age at marriage has increased over the years. As a result, there are more unmarried, sexually active young adults than ever before. Most young adults are sexually active, but many are now willing to assume responsibility for preventing pregnancy and disease. Between ages 18 and 24, most adults engage in sexual activity with multiple partners and serial relationships. Women tend to be less sexually aggressive than men, who are more likely to seek out and experience sexual relationships with a number of persons.

Among adults 25 to 59 years of age, relative monogamy (the practice of having only one partner) appears to be the norm. Sexuality becomes shared with one special person as many adults commit to marriage and family relationships. However, as divorce rates continue to climb, more adults are involved with multiple sexual partners.

Sexual behaviors during adulthood change to accommodate the situation. After the birth of children, for example, parents are usually less likely to act on spontaneous sexual expression. The fear of another unplanned pregnancy on a limited income has a strong effect on the sexual behaviors of many adults who are already coping with all they can financially handle.

The sexuality patterns of middle-age adults have recently changed. More women in their 30s and 40s are bearing children and beginning families. Single parenthood is not uncommon. Satisfying patterns of sexual functioning are continued throughout the middle years. As children leave home and menopause occurs, many women experience a feeling of sexual freedom. The fear of pregnancy is over. The couple is once again alone and able to spontaneously interact.

Sexuality in Older Adulthood

The typical picture of the older adult is one of an asexual and uninterested individual. Nothing could be further from the truth. Older adulthood, for many people, is a time of pursuing one's own interests and desires, including sexuality.

Sexual expression in older adults shifts "from procreation to an emphasis on companionship, sharing, touching, and intimate communication, not just the physical act of coitus" (Edelman and Mandle, 1998). The closeness, intimacy, and sharing of sexuality becomes more impor-

tant than the physical act for most older adults. Sexuality can also be communicated through touching, stroking, or other means of expression when intercourse is not desirable or possible.

Sexuality persists throughout one's life and, although sexual activity may decrease in frequency as one ages, established sexual patterns continue. Unfortunately the sexual expression of older adults meets many cultural and social barriers, attitudes, and expectations. Poor health, medications, disabilities, and the normal aging process may influence one's sexual behaviors, but sexuality is a basic need that will be with us until the day we die.

Sexuality and Disability

Many permanently disabled persons are able to enjoy rich and satisfying sexual lives with some adaptation. People with spinal cord injuries, for example, can still be lovers, partners, and parents. Any condition that affects well-being, mobility, or self-esteem has an impact on sexuality and its expressions. Health problems such as diabetes, arthritis, cancer, and cardiovascular disease can affect one's sexuality. However, these conditions only affect the expression of sexuality, not one's sexuality itself.

Men and women who are disabled learn to adapt to their conditions. Most must also cope with society's negative attitudes and stigmas toward the disabled. People with disabilities have the exact same needs as the rest of the population. Remember, everyone is an individual first; some of us just happen to be different. Improving the quality of life for people with disabilities involves changing social attitudes that limit the disabled.

MODES OF SEXUAL EXPRESSION

An individual's sexual attraction to others is referred to as one's *sexual orientation* or *sexual preference*. In 1948 one of the first researchers into human sexual responses (A.C. Kinsey) developed a scale of human sexual preference, ranging from exclusively heterosexual to exclusively homosexual. He stated that most people were not exclusively one or the other because many had experienced both heterosexual and homosexual expressions of sexuality (Kinsey, Pomeroy, and Martin, 1953). Today, several modes of sexual expression are seen (Table 29-1).

Heterosexuality

Persons who express their sexuality with members of the opposite sex are known as **heterosexual**. Heterosexual relationships are the foundation for procreation (bearing children) and family. Today it is not uncommon to encounter families with homosexual or bisexual parents.

Historically, heterosexual relationships have been the norm—the culturally and socially acceptable form of coupling. However, variations of the man-woman relationship have existed throughout history. For example, in ancient Greece it was customary for men to regard the women they married as useful for having children and taking care of household affairs. The social, emotional, and **erotic** (sexually desiring) needs of husbands often were filled by other men, especially adolescent boys. In this culture, both heterosexuality and homosexuality were considered socially appropriate expressions of sexuality. History is filled with examples of sexual restrictions and permissions, but it appears that heterosexual relationships are here to stay because biology still requires a male and a female to produce the next generation of human beings.

Homosexuality

The sexual desire or preference for members of one's own sex is known as **homosexuality.** People who prefer homosexuality are often referred to as **gay** (applies to both sexes) or **lesbian** (applies to female homosexuals). Historically, same-sex relationships have been around as long as opposite-sex relationships, but cultural and social attitudes toward them have changed as history has evolved.

One's sexual orientation is established in late childhood and continues to develop through adulthood. For adolescents who are homosexual, adolescence is a particularly difficult time because, in addition to the average development tasks, these individuals are faced with "their own unique issues of identity formation" (Wong, 1998). The process of establishing an integrated or complete identity as a homosexual is known as "coming out," and it occurs in fairly predictable stages (Table 29-2).

Homosexuality has historically been considered a maladaptive mode of sexual expression, but many studies of both sexes have revealed that homosexuals commonly function as well with their love relationships as heterosexual persons. Studies of homosexual couples (Bell and Weinberg, 1978) have found that homosexual relationships or behaviors tend to fall into one of five categories: close-coupled, open-coupled, functional, dysfunctional, and asexual.

Close-coupled relationships are akin to a married couple. Each individual looks to the other for emotional and sexual satisfaction. These couples spend the majority of their evenings at home and do not seek sexual experiences outside the relationship. They are less likely to visit gay bars, and they report few sexual problems. Couples in this type of homosexual relationship are usually well adjusted and more accepting than average individuals.

Open-coupled relationships consist of two persons living together while continuing to have sexual experiences or relationships with others. These couples are less committed to their primary relationship and seek the company of a larger circle of homosexual friends. They

Table 29-1 Modes of Sexual Expression

Term	Definition
Heterosexuality	Sexual desire or preference for members of opposite sex
Homosexuality	Sexual desire or preference for members of same sex
Bisexuality	Sexual desire or preference for members of both sexes
Transvestism	Practice of receiving sexual satisfaction from dressing in clothes of opposite sex; also called cross-dressing
Paraphilia	Sexual preference for or obsession with objects or situations that are not normally arousing; considered socially undesirable behaviors or disorders

Table 29-2 Identity Formation Process of Gay Adolescents

Approximate age/stage	Steps in process	Description
Childhood to early adolescence	Identity awareness	Becomes aware of feeling differently about stereotyped gender activities; feels discomfort with gender stereotypes and the expected behaviors that accompany them
Middle to late adolescence (about age 17 in boys, 18 in girls)	Identity recognition	Discomfort with sex-role behaviors increases as attraction to same-sex persons begins to emerge; begins to feel that he or she is probably homosexual; period of identity confusion, isolation, depression, and great discomfort
Early to middle twenties	Identity assumption	Acknowledges homosexual identity; begins to experiment with sexuality; socializes within homosexual community and subculture
Midtwenties and beyond	Commitment	Individuals assume homosexual lifestyle; state to themselves and world that they are homosexual; give themselves permission to be who they are

Modified from Wong DL: *Whaley and Wong's nursing care of infants and children,* ed 6, St. Louis, 1998, Mosby.

visit gay baths and bars and report higher levels of sexual activity than close-coupled homosexuals.

The third type of homosexual relationship is called *functional*. These persons have no special sexual partner, and they are usually not interested in finding one. Their lives appear to be organized around sexual activity, and they report a greater number of sexual partners than any other group. Many are unconcerned with homosexuality and are openly involved in the gay community. Both open-coupled and functional homosexuals are at high risk for contracting sexually transmitted diseases.

Dysfunctional homosexuals have a number of worries and problems. They regret their sexual orientation and are often more unhappy, depressed, or paranoid than most people. Although they try, dysfunctional homosexuals have great difficulty in establishing a permanent relationship. Problems can extend to other areas of their lives, as evidenced by the high number of mental health problems and crime rates in this group. Many are involved in long-term counseling or receiving mental health care.

Last is the category called *asexual*. Individuals in this group feel sexually unattractive, lonely, and unhappy with themselves. They report few sexual partners, little sexual experience, and low levels of sexual activity. They are not likely to visit gay bars or other gathering places, so much of their time is spent alone and withdrawn. Mental health problems are often present.

It appears that both homosexual and heterosexual behavior styles have much in common. Homosexuality is now receiving acceptance as a mode of sexual expression, but many health care providers still carry attitudes and stereotypes that can interfere with the care provided to gay and lesbian patients. We must all work to develop the self-awareness that enhances our therapeutic effectiveness, especially with persons of different sexual orientations. The Case Study box illustrates this point.

Bisexuality

Persons who are attracted to and engage in sexual activities with members of both sexes are known as **bisexuals.** These individuals identify themselves as bisexual as compared with homosexuals or heterosexuals. Little research has been done on bisexuals because they do not receive the research attention that is focused on homosexuals or heterosexuals. Most bisexual individuals appear to be as well adjusted as those who prefer other modes of sexual expression, but they are at high risk for contracting HIV/AIDS and other sexually transmitted diseases.

Transvestism

Transvestism is commonly referred to as cross-dressing. It is defined as sexual excitement from wearing the clothing of the opposite sex. Two types of transvestism are usually practiced. In the first, a man is aroused by a certain article of clothing, such as shoes or undergarments. With the second type, the individual dresses completely in women's clothing (Figure 29-2). The typical transvestite is a married man with children who is rather secretive about

Case Study

It is evening in a busy medical-surgical unit. You have just received notice that a 42-year-old man, Jim S., is being admitted for injuries suffered in a motor vehicle accident. Because of the severity of his injuries, the physician has ordered that he be visited by immediate family only.

Jim is admitted to the unit and made comfortable. As you glance around for family members who accompanied him from the emergency department, you see only one youngish-looking gentleman, peering anxiously at your client. "I'm sorry, but immediate family only is allowed in here," you say politely, as you usher him out the door.

Later that evening, Jim begins to respond. He keeps calling out for "my love, J.J." and asking you where J.J. is, so loudly that you are sure everyone on the floor can hear. Finally Jim quiets down only after he extracts a promise from you to find J.J. Exhausted, you agree, hoping she would somehow arrive and help to keep this man quiet.

As you open the door to leave the room, the youngish-looking man from earlier in the evening almost falls through to the floor. With tears in his eyes, he glares intently at you but says nothing. Quietly you ask if his name could possibly be J.J.

◆ What is the lesson to be learned from this case study?

◆ How could this experience help you to be more sensitive and therapeutic?

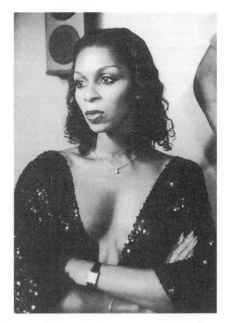

Figure 29-2 Male transvestite. (From Denney NW, Quadagno D: *Human sexuality,* ed 2, St. Louis, 1992, Mosby.)

his cross-dressing. He is heterosexual, and his behaviors are usually accepted by his wife. Although few reliable statistics are available, transvestism may be more common than once thought.

Factors Relating to Psychosexual Variations

Although no one understands exactly why an individual prefers a certain mode of sexual expression, many theories and explanations have been offered.

Biological theories explain sexual variations as differences in chromosomes, the genetic material that determines hereditary traits. Some studies have "suggested that homosexuality may be inherited from the maternal side of the family through the X chromosome" (Stuart and Laraia, 2001). Other researchers suggest a correlation between brain structure and sexual orientation, whereas others are pursuing the notion that hormones wire the brain for sexual orientation during the prenatal period. Researchers (Dessens and others, 1999) have found that certain anticonvulsant medications alter the hormone levels of developing fetuses and lead to disturbances in sexual orientation.

Psychoanalytical theories as proposed by Freud and his followers consider sexual variations (other than heterosexuality) as behaviors with neurotic or psychopathic motivations (Fortinash and Holoday-Worret, 1999). Problems arise early in life as a result of the child's Oedipus/Electra complex, in which children experience sexual feelings for the opposite-sex parent and resent the same-sex parent. According to this theory, persons with different sexual behaviors also exhibit problems in other areas of their lives. Aspects of the psychoanalytical point of view have been criticized for being male oriented and viewing women as inferior. Little scientific evidence has been found to justify Freud's psychoanalytical view of sexual orientation.

Finally, the *behavioral theories* consider the various modes of sexual expression as learned, measurable responses. The *learning theory* states that individuals are introduced to a certain sexual variation by an accidental experience that is sexually stimulating. When other sexual experiences lead to feelings of inadequacy, the "pleasurable accident" experience encourages continued use of the sexual variation. Behavioral theorists also believe that the sexual behaviors of adults in the child's environment have a strong influence on the sexual preferences and behaviors of an individual. Significant emotional, adjustment, and mental health problems are common in adults who were sexually abused as children.

PSYCHOSEXUAL DISORDERS

Because knowledge of human sexuality is still evolving, a broad definition of psychosexual problems is needed. **Sexual disorders** are those problems that cause distress and impaired functioning in an individual or others who are exposed to the sexual behavior. These disorders include problems with sexual functions, gender identity disorders, and socially inappropriate or illegal methods of sexual expression.

Sexual Dysfunctions

The average person experiences four stages of sexual excitement and pleasure: appetite, excitement, orgasm, and resolution. A **sexual dysfunction** is a disturbance anywhere during these four stages of the sexual response cycle (American Psychiatric Association, 2000). Its definition also includes any discomfort or pain associated with sexual intercourse. Sexual dysfunctions may be lifelong or acquired after a period of normal functioning. They may be limited by certain situations, partners, or types of stimulation, or they may be generalized to every sexual experience. The causes are often related psychological distresses, medication or illicit drug use, and many physical conditions. Arthritis, diabetes, and chronic illness can result in various sexual dysfunctions or alterations in sexual desire. Impaired hormonal functioning and neurological problems can also lead to difficulties with sexual functioning. Problems with relationships or unrealistic attitudes about sex may also contribute (Gregoire, 1999). Table 29-3 describes the most common sexual dysfunctions in men and women.

Paraphilias

The **paraphilias** are a group of sexual variations that depart from society's traditional and acceptable modes of seeking sexual gratification. When the word *paraphilia* is taken apart, the suffix *philia* means "an attraction to." When used to describe a specific behavior, the descriptive term replaces the prefix *para*. For example, pedophilia refers to a person who is sexually attracted to children (*pedo*, meaning "child"). Several of these behaviors, such as exhibitionism, pedophilia, and voyeurism, are considered illegal in some countries, including the United States. Others are harmless when practiced in private with other consenting adults. Box 29-2 names and briefly describes the more common paraphilias.

Gender Identity Disorder

One of the first things an individual develops is a **gender identity**, the knowledge that one is a boy or a girl. When there is an inconsistency between the child's biological sex and his or her gender identity, a gender identity disorder is usually diagnosed.

Children with gender identity disorder are unhappy with their own sex. They want to eliminate their sexual characteristics and trade them for those of the opposite sex. Many truly believe they have been born into the wrong body and reject any expectations or behaviors associated with their biological sex. Older children often

Table 29-3 DSM-IV–TR Classification of Sexual Dysfunctions

Classification	Disorder	Description
Sexual desire disorders	Hypoactive sexual desire disorder	Absence of sexual fantasies and desire for sexual activity
	Sexual aversion disorder	Active avoidance of sexual contact with partner; reacts to sexual opportunity with anxiety, fear, or disgust
Sexual arousal disorders	Female sexual arousal disorder	Inability to attain or maintain sexual excitement during sexual activity; has little sexual arousal
	Male erectile disorder	Inability to attain or maintain adequate erection during sexual activity
Orgasmic disorders	Female/male orgasmic disorder	Delay in or absence of orgasm following normal excitement
	Premature ejaculation	Ejaculation that occurs with minimal stimulation before person wishes it to occur
Sexual pain disorders	**Dyspareunia**	Pain associated with sexual intercourse; may occur in both females and males
	Vaginismus	Persistent involuntary contractions of muscles around vagina when penetration is attempted
Sexual dysfunction caused by medical condition	Dependent on medical diagnoses	Significant sexual problems caused by direct effects of medical condition
Substance-induced sexual dysfunction	Dependent on substance used	Significant sexual problems caused by direct physical effects of substance

Modified from American Psychiatric Association: *Diagnostic and statistical manual of mental disorders*, ed 4, text revision, Washington, DC, 2000, The Association.

Box 29-2 DSM-IV–TR Description of Paraphilias

Exhibitionism

Exposure of one's genitals to unsuspecting person(s) followed by sexual arousal.

Fetishism

Utilization of objects (e.g., panties, rubber sheeting) for purposes of sexual arousal.

Frotteurism

Rubbing up against nonconsenting persons to heighten sexual arousal.

Pedophilia

Fondling and/or other types of sexual activities with prepubescent child (usually under age 13 having not yet developed secondary sex characteristics).

Sexual Masochism

Sexual arousal is achieved by being receiver of pain (either physical or emotional), humiliation, or being made to suffer.

Sexual Sadism

Sexual arousal is achieved by infliction of pain (either physical or emotional) or humiliation onto another person.

Transvestic Fetishism

The act of cross-dressing (heterosexual men wearing female clothing) to achieve sexual arousal.

Voyeurism

Sexual arousal is achieved by observing unsuspecting persons who are naked, in act of disrobing, or engaging in sexual activity ("peeping Tom").

Paraphilia NOS (Not Otherwise Specified)

These disorders do not meet criteria for aforementioned categories:

Telephone scatologia: obscene phone calling; "900" sex lines
Necrophilia: sexual activity with corpses
Partialism: exclusive focus on particular body part for sexual arousal
Zoophilia: sexual activity involving participation with animals (bestiality)
Coprophilia: sexual arousal by contact with feces
Klismaphilia: sexual arousal generated by use of enemas
Urophilia: sexual arousal by contact with urine
Ephebophilia: fondling and/or other types of sexual activities with pubescent children who are developing secondary sex characteristics (e.g., pubic hair, breasts); these children are usually between ages 13 and 18
Paraphilic coercive disorder: rape; aggressive sexual assault involving act of sexual intercourse against one's will and without consent

Modified from American Psychiatric Association: *Diagnostic and statistical manual of mental disorders*, ed 4, text revision, Washington, DC, 2000, The Association.

fail to develop same-sex relationships in school, leading to isolation and loneliness. Adolescents and adults with gender identity disorder commonly find that their desire to be another sex interferes with work and social relationships. Separation anxiety disorders are common in children with gender identity disorder, and mental health problems are often seen in both parents and children (Bradley and Zucker, 1997).

Transsexualism is the persistent desire to become a member of the opposite sex. Transsexuals are discontented with their biological sex and desire to actually become an opposite-sex person to fit their gender identity. This is accomplished by a series of psychological counseling, hormonal treatments, and major surgeries. Because decisions made by the individual are irreversible, the process of changing one's sexual identity is deliberately prolonged and can take as long as 2 years.

THERAPEUTIC INTERVENTIONS

Treatment of sexual problems depends on the cause, the distressing signs and symptoms, and the type of disorder. Group or individual therapy may help clients explore their emotions, behaviors, and coping mechanisms. Behavioral therapies, such as positive reinforcement or aversive therapy, focus on changing or managing sexual behaviors in a more acceptable way. Hormonal drug therapy is sometimes employed to reduce sexual drives (see Drug Alert box).

Environmental controls for sexually undesirable behaviors include incarceration (prison or jail). The individual is removed from society and may or may not be accepted into a special program for sexual offenders while in prison.

Most clients with sexual problems are treated on an outpatient basis. However, many medical-surgical nurses work with problems of sexuality in relation to clients and their surgical procedures or medical conditions.

An important point to remember: if you are uncomfortable with any aspect of a client's sexuality, your professional judgment and behaviors could be affected. Some psychosexual problems are complex and require the skills of specially educated nurses or sexual therapists. Discuss the situation with your supervisor because the goal is still to provide the client with the best possible care. As with other clients, therapeutic interventions remain the same: accept, assess, intervene, and educate.

Psychosexual Assessment

Sexuality is a sensitive topic for most persons. For this reason, nurses must be aware of the client's level of comfort when assessing sexual functioning. Barriers to obtaining a sexual history also lie with the nurse or other care provider. They include inadequate training, embarrassment, and a fear of offending the client (Warner, Rowe, and Whipple, 1999). Hopefully, both client and caregiver will establish enough trust in the therapeutic relationship to honestly share information.

Nursing Process

Nursing diagnoses for psychosexual disorders are based on each client's identified problems. The primary nursing diagnoses for problems with sexuality are sexual dysfunction and altered sexuality patterns. Other nursing diagnoses are selected to help to enhance the client's physical, emotional, social, and spiritual functioning, and several are listed in Box 29-3.

The quality of care for clients with psychosexual problems is dependent on each caregiver's abilities to remain nonjudgmental and accepting of his or her clients. The team treatment approach is usually more effective in treating individuals with sexual problems because it helps

---

 Drug Alert

Hormones that reduce the sexual drive have many side effects. Be familiar with each medication and remember to monitor clients routinely for any unusual symptoms.

Many medications prescribed for various medical problems can cause sexual problems.

Examples include the following:

Antihypertensives

Antidepressants, anticonvulsants, and other psychotropic medications

Medications used for problems of the stomach and small intestine, pain-relieving medications

A complete and accurate history should include an assessment of each client's medication (including over-the-counter and street drugs) history, and current use.

Box 29-3 NANDA Nursing Diagnoses Related to Sexual Disorders

Anxiety
Community coping, ineffective
Coping, ineffective individual
Denial, ineffective
Injury, risk for
Noncompliance, (specify)
Self-esteem disturbance
Sexual dysfunction*
Sexual patterns, altered
Violence, risk for: directed at others
Violence, risk for: self-directed

From North American Nursing Diagnosis Association: *NANDA nursing diagnoses and classification 1999-2000*, Philadelphia, 1999, The Association.
*Primary nursing diagnosis for sexual disorders.

to maintain objectivity and prevents any one member from becoming too involved in a client's treatment. The box describes a Sample Client Care Plan for a client with a sexual dysfunction.

Assessment and treatment are only two important functions of client care. Advocacy and education are also important in relation to providing effective care for clients with sexual difficulties. Advocacy allows care providers to provide an atmosphere of acceptance where clients feel safe in discussing sexuality. It also encourages us to discover our prejudices and refine our own professional and personal values about sexuality.

Perhaps most important is the nurse's ability to educate, to share information that could spell the difference between life and death for people. Education about the prevention of HIV/AIDS and other sexually transmitted diseases, appropriate methods of preventing unwanted pregnancies, and various means of

---

⏩ Sample Client Care Plan   Sexual Dysfunction

Assessment

History: Brian, a 31-year-old man, has been treated for chronic depression for the past 2 years. Since his medications were changed 3 months ago, Brian has been complaining of a lack of sexual interest. He has been married for approximately 10 months, and his wife is "worried."

Current Findings: An anxious-appearing man. General appearance, speech, motor activity, and interactions are appropriate. Brian describes his problem as a "growing lack of interest" and fears that it will interfere with his marriage.

Multidisciplinary Diagnosis

Altered role performance related to treatment for depression

Planning/Goals

Brian and therapist will identify the medications he is taking and list their side effects.

Brian's anxiety will decrease as he works to solve his problems.

Therapeutic Interventions

Intervention	Rationale	Team Member
1. Assess degree of sexual frustration and dysfunction; begin with less personal statements.	Builds trust and rapport; helps determine extent of problems and plan effective therapeutic interventions.	Psy, Nsg
2. Reassure that symptoms are troubling but not unique.	Provides reassurance that no physical problems exist.	Nsg
3. Develop a list of every medication (including over-the-counter drugs) that Brian is currently taking.	Certain medications, or combinations of medications can lead to changes in sexual functioning.	Nsg, Psy
4. Consult with physician for possible dosage regulation of Brian's medications.	Adjustment of dosages may decrease or correct the problem.	Nsg, Psy
5. Educate Brian about each medication's effects on sexual functioning.	Learning to recognize side effects early lessens their intensity and offers opportunities for early interventions.	Nsg
6. Refer Brian and his wife for sexual counseling.	Increases knowledge regarding sexuality and its expressions.	Psy

Evaluation

Brian listed each medication and demonstrated great interest in learning about side effects.

Brian reported a decrease in his level of anxiety as his knowledge of his medications and their effects grew.

A complete client care plan includes several other diagnoses and interventions.

sexual expression are within the realm of nursing. If we are to save a population from the ravages of HIV/AIDS, sexual abuse, and mental illness, all health care providers should teach about sexuality at every opportunity. It is up to us in the helping professions to care for us all.

KEY CONCEPTS

◆ Human sexuality is the combination of physical, chemical, psychological, and functional characteristics that are expressed by one's gender identity and sexual behaviors.

◆ Healthy sexual responses are those that occur between two consenting adults, are satisfying to both, are not forced or coerced, and are conducted in privacy.

◆ The expression of one's sexuality begins at birth and ends with death.

◆ Many permanently disabled persons are able to enjoy rich and satisfying sexual lives with a little adaptation.

◆ Persons who express their sexuality with members of the opposite sex are known as heterosexual.

◆ The sexual desire or preference for members of one's own sex is known as homosexuality.

◆ Persons who engage in sexual activities with members of both sexes are known as bisexuals.

◆ Transvestism, referred to as cross-dressing, is defined as the practice of wearing the clothing of the opposite sex for sexual excitement.

◆ Theories that attempt to explain why an individual prefers a certain mode of sexual expression include biological, psychoanalytical, and behavioral viewpoints.

◆ Sexual disorders are those problems that cause distress and impaired functioning in an individual or others who are exposed to the sexual behavior.

◆ A sexual dysfunction is a disturbance anywhere in the sexual response cycle and includes any discomfort or pain associated with sexual intercourse.

◆ Problems with sexual expression can be caused by medication or illicit drug use and many physical conditions.

◆ The paraphilias are a group of sexual behaviors considered to be socially undesirable.

◆ A gender identity disorder is an inconsistency between a child's biological sex and his or her gender identity.

◆ Transsexualism is the persistent desire to become a member of the opposite sex.

◆ Treatment of sexual problems depends on the cause, distressing signs or symptoms, and type of disorder.

◆ An important point to remember: if a care provider is uncomfortable with any aspect of a client's sexuality, his or her professional judgment and behaviors may be affected.

◆ Nurses must be sensitive to the client's level of comfort when assessing sexual functioning.

◆ The quality of care for clients with psychosexual problems depends on care providers' abilities to remain nonjudgmental and accepting of the client.

◆ Assessment, treatment, advocacy, and education are important nursing activities in relation to caring for clients with sexual difficulties.

◆ Education about the prevention of HIV/AIDS and other sexually transmitted diseases, appropriate methods of preventing unwanted pregnancies, and various means of sexual expression is an important health care responsibility.

Suggestions for Further Reading

An article by Rochelle Scheela, titled "Working with Sex Offenders" (*Journal of Psychosocial Nursing* 37(9):25, 1999), offers insight into the world of sex offenders and their rehabilitative processes.

The Sexual Assault Information Page (www.cs.utk.edu-bartley/ sainfoPage.html) is a nonprofit information and referral service that covers a number of topics.

References

American Psychiatric Association: *Diagnostic and statistical manual of mental disorders*, ed 4, text revision, Washington, DC, 2000, The Association.

Bell AP, Weinberg MS: *Homosexuality: a study of diversity among men and women*, New York, 1978, Simon & Schuster.

Bradley SJ and Zucker KJ: Gender identity disorder: a review of the past ten years, *Journal of the American Academy of Child and Adolescent Psychiatry* 36(7):872, 1997.

Dessens AB and others: Prenatal exposure to anticonvulsants and psychosexual development, *Archives of Sexual Behavior* 28(1):31, 1999.

Edelman CL, Mandle CL: *Health promotion throughout the lifespan*, ed 4, St. Louis, 1998, Mosby.

Fortinash KM, Holoday-Worret PA: *Psychiatric-mental health nursing*, ed 2, St. Louis, 1999, Mosby.

Gregoire A: Assessing and managing male sexual problems, *British Medical Journal* 318(7179):315, 1999.

Kinsey AC, Pomeroy WB, Martin EC: *Sexual behavior in the human female*, Philadelphia, 1953, WB Saunders.

Stuart GW, Laraia MT: *Principles and practice of psychiatric nursing*, ed 7, St. Louis, 2001, Mosby.

Warner PH, Rowe MS, Whipple B: Shedding light on the sexual history, *American Journal of Nursing* 99(6):34, 1999.

Wong DL: *Whaley and Wong's nursing care of infants and children*, ed 6, St. Louis, 1998, Mosby.

Chapter 30

Personality Disorders

Learning Objectives

1. Explain the continuum of social responses.
2. Describe how personality develops throughout the life cycle.
3. Compare four theories relating to the development of personality disorders.
4. Discuss four characteristics of a personality disorder.
5. Explain the meaning of the term *dual diagnosis*.
6. Classify ten types of personality disorders and their most significant associated behaviors.
7. Describe the main goal of therapy for clients with personality disorders.
8. Compare four classes of drugs used to treat clients with personality disorders.
9. Plan nursing diagnoses and therapeutic interventions for a client with a personality disorder.

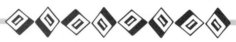

Key Terms

antisocial personality

avoidant personality

borderline personality

deceit

dependent personality

dual diagnosis

gregarious

histrionic personality

ideas of reference

impulsivity

manipulation

narcissistic personality

object constancy

obsessive-compulsive personality

paranoia

personality

personality disorder

psychopath

schizoid personality

schizotypal personality

splitting

temperament

The social realm of human functioning is a vital part of being human. People are **gregarious** (sociable and in need of the company of others). Although some individuals are able to live in isolation as hermits, the vast majority of us need interactions with other people throughout our lives.

During childhood, individuals establish their personalities. **Personality** is defined as the composite of behavioral traits and attitudes that identify one as an individual. Personality is the unique pattern of thoughts, attitudes, values, and behaviors each individual develops to adapt to a particular environment and its standards. In short, our personalities define who we are.

To find satisfaction in life, people establish relationships with other people. Some relationships assume a special degree of closeness and sharing that becomes important. These relationships develop intimacy, as another person becomes significant in one's life.

Developing intimate relationships requires a willingness to reveal the private side of oneself: the emotions, beliefs, attitudes, dreams, and anxieties that describe one's personal nature. Most people are able to develop and sustain their social relationships. Families are established, maintained, and transformed. Relationships outside the family grow and fade as individuals interact and life progresses. For many individuals, however, the intimacy of important relationships is not achieved because of lifelong patterns of maladaptive thoughts, social responses, and behaviors.

CONTINUUM OF SOCIAL RESPONSES

Interactions with others (social responses) range from autonomy and interdependence to the disordered behaviors of manipulation, intimidation, aggression, and hysteria. People who are highly functional move freely along the continuum, recognizing and balancing their needs for intimacy with their needs for solitude. Those with ineffective behaviors cope with feelings of dependence, loneliness, and the need to withdraw from others. Individuals with personality problems struggle to define and meet their social needs (Figure 30-1).

PERSONALITY THROUGHOUT THE LIFE CYCLE

The human personality is shaped and influenced throughout life. Personalities are unique patterns of being. They are established early in childhood and molded through experience. Personality expresses the emotional, intellectual, social, and spiritual realms of an individual. A basic understanding of personality and the factors that influence its development helps health care providers assess and plan for more effective and therapeutic care.

Personality in Childhood

Infants do not see themselves as separate beings until about 18 months (Wong, 1998). The majority of infants experience their environments as warm, nurturing, and unconditionally accepting. When needs for water, food, comfort, warmth, safety, and socialization are consistently met, infants develop a sense of trust and self-worth. Refer back to Table 5-4 in Chapter 5. Infants who are denied unconditional love and nurturing have difficulties in forming and maintaining significant relationships in adulthood because they have not learned to trust in others.

During the early years of toddlerhood, much of the personality is still fluid, changeable, and undefined. As children age, the personality gradually takes shape. Between 18 months and 3 years of age, toddlers begin to learn to separate from their caregivers and explore the world about them. During this time, they develop a sense of **object constancy,** which is the knowledge that a loved person or object continues to exist, even though it is out of sight or cannot be perceived. For example, a child learns that his toys are still there in the toy chest, even though he cannot see them at this time.

Toddlers often seek out their parents for support, encouragement, and approval. If responses to their independent exploratory behaviors are positive, children build a solid sense of self and develop the capacity for interacting successfully with others. Most researchers believe that, once established, personality traits and temperament are consistent, stable, and generally predictable.

Feelings of morality begin to develop between 6 and 10 years. These years are marked by a preoccupation with self, a strong sense of right and wrong, and interactions with peers. Trust grows into the capacity for empathy (understanding the feelings and behaviors of others), which is an important ingredient for later relationships. Thinking (intellectual development) moves from here and now to thoughts of the future, from concrete to abstract. The focus of fantasies changes from imagined objects to real ones, and the use of fantasy becomes a primary way of coping with anxiety.

During the early school years, children learn about cooperation, competition, and compromise. Peer relationships begin to assume more importance, and approval from persons outside the family is sought. Conflicts with parents begin to occur in later childhood as the child's search for independence is tempered by the parents' limits on behavior. "During this period a supportive environment that encourages the budding sense of self fosters development of a positive, adaptive self-concept" (Stuart and Laraia, 2001). Without support and encouragement, children's needs for guidance and approval go unmet, and this helps set the stage for numerous problems later in life.

Personality in Adolescence

By the time an individual reaches the teen years, the personality is well established. Relationships with others (especially their peers) help adolescents assert their independence from their parents. Best friend relationships offer chances for sharing, clarifying values, and learning about the differences in people. These relationships become very interdependent and often include efforts to exclude others. Within their peer group, adolescents sup-

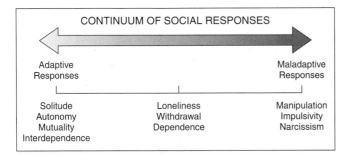

Figure 30-1 Continuum of social responses. (Redrawn from Stuart GW, Laraia MI: *Principles and practice of psychiatric nursing,* ed 7, St. Louis, 2001, Mosby.)

port each other in their struggles to assert themselves and cope with the distresses of becoming adults.

As adolescents grow, their relationships expand to include members of the opposite sex. Sexual issues produce anxiety as teens struggle to assume a sexual identity. Sexual activity is experimental and spontaneous. Struggles continue over autonomy within the family. By the early 20s, most have weathered the emotional ups and downs of adolescence and emerge with identities that can carry them into adulthood.

Personality in Adulthood

By young adulthood, most persons are making decisions, are self-sufficient, and are involved in give-and-take relationships. Occupational choices are made, and families may be started. Self-awareness grows as individuals learn the balance between personal independence and meeting the needs of others. Sensitivity to and an acceptance of the feelings of other persons is a critical characteristic of mature relationships in adulthood.

By middle adulthood, most persons are comfortable enough with themselves and their personalities to encourage independence in others. Relationships with friends and significant others grow and evolve. Demands on time and resources change as children mature, and many middle-age adults enjoy new freedoms to pursue their own wishes.

Many experts believe that, once established, the personality remains stable and constant. However, adulthood offers many opportunities for individuals to look within and decide which aspects of their personality they wish to keep and develop, and which aspects they would like to change. People are dynamic, always in physical or psychological motion, and change does occur—even within one's "well-established" personality.

Personality in Older Adulthood

Older adults must cope with loss and change. Old friends are lost. Family members move away. Occupational careers end, and friendships from the workplace fade as time passes.

The personality, however, remains intact as individuals age. Life takes on a deeper meaning as personal accomplishments and contributions to society are reviewed. Older adults with strong, integrated personalities are able to cope with their losses by maintaining what independence they can and accepting their limitations. Their strength of personality carries them through life's rougher times.

An important reminder about older adults: *a sudden change in personality is not a normal sign of aging.* By older adulthood, the personality is deeply entrenched. Patterns of thinking and behaving remain intact until death. Do not assume that a personality change in an older adult is normal. Changes in emotional control, responses, and levels of interest must be investigated. Many physical and biochemical problems first appear as subtle changes in personality. Alert investigations by nurses and all health care providers can often spell the difference between functional living and dementia.

THEORIES RELATING TO PERSONALITY DISORDERS

Interest in disordered personalities dates back to the time of the ancient Greeks. During the Middle Ages, individuals who behaved in unusual ways were thought to be possessed by evil spirits. The term **psychopath** was introduced in 1891 to describe a gross disturbance in social behavior with no impairment in mental state. Today the differences between normal personality and a personality disorder are being hotly debated, but clear definitions are rarely found in nature, and mental disorders are no exception.

It is difficult to tell the exact point at which a blood pressure reading becomes abnormal. It is just as difficult to establish the point at which a normal personality becomes a disordered one. Theories of personality development and disorder have been developed to help understand the complex nature of human beings. Currently there are four general theories of personality disorders: biological, psychoanalytical, behavioral, and sociocultural.

Biological

As research continues to investigate a possible connection between behavior and body, evidence mounts. Studies of families, twins, and relatives of individuals with personality disorders have demonstrated that behavior and personality are under a strong genetic influence. Researchers have found that one's **temperament** (the biological bases that underlie moods, energy levels, and attitudes) is genetically linked. Several studies of twins raised in separate environments have shown remarkable consistency in temperament when tested.

Cardiovascular responses, brain wave tracings, and brain dysfunctions have been studied as possible causes (Marshall and Cooke, 1999). Other biological evidence is beginning to establish a neurophysical basis for the behaviors seen in individuals with personality disorders. For example, abnormalities in certain neurotransmitters, such as dopamine and serotonin, are linked to maladaptive behaviors. Brain imaging studies suggest a possible physical basis for a failure to appreciate the emotional significance of words and images. In other words, the brain mechanism that connects emotions and intellect may be missing or inefficient in persons with personality disorders. Further studies into the biobehavioral connection are currently being conducted, and new developments will influence the treatment of persons with problem personalities (see Think About box).

Psychoanalytical

According to psychoanalytical theories, infants begin to discover the nature of "good/bad" and "love/hate" as the superego grows. If the mother responds to the child in ways that cause frustration, distress, or pain, the child will have difficulty finding the proper fit between aggression and love. Certain patterns of parental responses, ranging from overinvolvement to neglect, prevent the child from developing a strong sense of self and balance among the three forces of the personality (ego, id, and superego).

Behavioral

Theorists from the behavioral school of thought see personality disorders as the result of conditioned responses caused by previous events. The separation-individuation theory states that the average 1- to 3-year old is able to achieve object constancy. Personality disorders occur in persons who are not able to hold a consistent, stable image of the mother when she is absent. This results in fears that range from abandonment and separation to a complete loss of connection with others. Other behaviorists view personality disorders as the result of unmet needs during critical developmental periods.

Sociocultural

Sociocultural theories find the causes of personality disorders embedded in one's culture and society. One researcher (Paris, 1998) has demonstrated that "a lack of social structure, normlessness, and a lack of available social roles, are risks for the development of personality disorders." Numerous cultural expectations are seen to influence the use of adaptive or maladaptive behaviors.

The Cultural Aspects box offers an interesting historical enigma.

Many social stressors can lead to difficulties with relationships. Family instability, divorce, and mobility often isolate people from those they love. Traditions that once bound people together are no longer practiced, adding to the sense of isolation. Rates of violent crime and aggression force persons to seclude themselves from other people for protection. Unemployment, homelessness, and AIDS add to the powerlessness felt by many persons. Sociocultural theorists believe that the foundation for personality disorders is built on society's social and cultural stresses.

PERSONALITY DISORDERS

Personality disorders are defined as long-standing, maladaptive patterns of behaving and relating. All personality disorders "are characterized by persistent difficulties in interpersonal relations" (Brennan and Shaver, 1998). Many individuals have maladaptive behaviors but are not diagnosed as mentally ill because their actions do not deviate from or go beyond the limits of society's expectations.

The most important criterion for a personality disorder is that behaviors are "inflexible and maladaptive and cause significant functional impairment or subjective distress" (American Psychiatric Association, 2000). The inflexible, ineffective behavior patterns must occur throughout a broad range of occupational, social, and personal situations. The onset of the maladaptive patterns can be traced back to childhood or adolescence, and no medical or other mental health problem can account for them. Box 30-1 describes of the common characteristics

---

Think About

The defense "not guilty due to mental incompetence" has been used in many cases of murder and other crimes. Arguments in favor of this defense state that many individuals with diagnosed personality disorders did not know what they were doing at the time of the crime and therefore should not be held responsible for their actions.

Arguments in favor of abolishing the mental illness defense state that an individual is always responsible for his or her actions, no matter what the mental state.

◆ What do you think about the "mental illness" defense?

◆ How should people be held accountable for their behaviors?

 Cultural Aspects

In some cultures individuals with personality disorders are considered gifted or connected to spirits. The wife of Russia's last czar, Alexandra, was highly criticized for associating with a monk called Rasputin, a man with a supposed "connection to God." Because of concern for her hemophiliac son's health, she sought his guidance. Rasputin would spend his days in the company of priests, royalty, and generals, but nights were spent in drunken sexual parties with prostitutes and other street people.

While the czar was at the front with the troops, Rasputin met his demise. For his unusual behaviors and profound influences on Alexandra, he was poisoned, then shot, beaten, and thrown into a river by a group of noblemen. Rasputin is a compelling historic example of a man with a personality disorder.

Box 30-1 Characteristics of Personality Disorders

Cognition (Intellect, Perception, View)

Impaired self-perceptions: Distorted picture of self; tends to hate or idealize self

Impaired thought processes: Thinking concrete, difficulty abstracting; impaired concentration, memory; poor attention span

Impaired reality testing: Distorts and confuses inner and outer reality; projects own feelings onto others

Impaired judgment: Ability to problem solve is impaired; does not understand consequences of behaviors; does not learn from past behaviors

Affect (Emotional Responses, Mood)

Impaired stimulus barrier: Unable to filter out or regulate incoming sensory stimuli; easily excited; responds excessively to noise or light; easily agitated; anger escalates rapidly

Characteristic Moods

Dysphoric feelings, depression; abandonment when significant others are absent; emptiness; fear; guilt; rage

Interpersonal Functioning (Social Responses)

Impaired object relations: Has rigid and inflexible patterns of relating to others; has difficulty with intimate relationships

Poor impulse-control: Has uncontrollable pressures to act on internal urges; copes with internal pain by a acting out

Examples of acting-out behaviors: verbal and physical aggression, attacks on things or others, physical abuse; psychological abuse; manipulation; inappropriate sexual behaviors, casual sex; suicide attempts.

Modified from Rollant PD: *Mosby's review series: mental health nursing*, St. Louis, 1996, Mosby.

of personality disorders. Study it well because clients with these problems are often encountered in health care situations.

The DSM-IV–TR has classified 10 separate personality disorders. For the sake of discussion, personality disorders are grouped into three clusters based on similar behaviors: eccentric, erratic, and fearful. Table 30-1 lists the main feature of each disorder. Remember that individuals can exhibit behaviors from different clusters because human beings seldom fit neatly into any category.

Eccentric Cluster

The group of personality disorders called the eccentric cluster is characterized by odd or strange behaviors. Persons with problems in this cluster (group A) find it difficult to relate to others or socialize comfortably. Often they live in isolation and interact only when necessary.

Diagnoses in this cluster include paranoid, schizoid, and schizotypal disorders.

Paranoia is a suspicious system of thinking with delusions of persecution and grandeur. Individuals with a paranoid personality disorder have developed a pattern of behaviors marked by suspiciousness and mistrust. They automatically assume that everyone is out to harm, deceive, or exploit them. The loyalty and trustworthiness of friends are often questioned for hostile intentions. The search for hidden meanings can turn a casual remark into a conflict. Sharing information or becoming close to someone is avoided because it may provide information (ammunition) that may be used against them. Individuals with paranoid personality disorders become constantly alert for harmful intentions from other persons and are quick to counterattack if they feel wronged or slighted. Often a minor event arouses intense hostility and aggression.

These persons are very short-tempered and unwilling to forgive even the slightest error. Feelings of tenderness or respect are nonexistent. Many suffer from pathological (extreme) jealousy and often accuse their significant others of secretly having sexual relationships. Problem solving is difficult, and high anxiety levels keep these individuals resistant to change.

Paranoid personality disorders are diagnosed in up to 2.5% of the population. Men are diagnosed more often than women, and substance abuse is common. Ten percent to 30% of all psychiatric inpatients are diagnosed with paranoid personality disorders (Fortinash and Holoday-Worret, 1999).

Schizoid and schizotypal personality disorders are marked by an inability to develop and maintain relationships with other people. Persons with **schizoid personality** disorder lack the desire or willingness to become involved in close relationships. They are society's "loners" who prefer solitary activities and their own company. These people are emotionally restricted and unable to take pleasure in activities, friendships, or social relationships. Often individuals communicate emotional detachment, coldness, and a lack of concern for others. Sexual experiences hold little interest. Schizoid personality disorders are slightly more common in men and families with an already diagnosed member.

Persons with **schizotypal personality** disorder have the same interaction pattern of avoiding people as schizoid personalities, but the behaviors here are characterized by distortions and eccentricities (odd, strange, or peculiar actions). These individuals often have **ideas of reference** (incorrect perceptions of causal events as having great or significant meaning) and they commonly find special, personal messages in everyday events.

Schizotypal people are often superstitious or believe in the paranormal (events outside human understanding). Many think they have special powers to foretell events or

Table 30-1	Clusters of Personality Disorders	
Cluster/Disorder	**Main characteristic**	
A: Eccentric		
Paranoid	Distrust and suspiciousness; sees others' motives as malevolent (intend to do harm)	
Schizoid	Detachment from social relationships; emotional expression is restricted	
Schizotypal	Acute discomfort with close relationships; sensory distortions; odd behaviors, thinking, and speech	
B: Erratic		
Antisocial	Disregards/violates rights of others	
Borderline	Unstable self-image, affect, and interpersonal relationships	
Histrionic	Excessive emotional expression and attention-seeking behaviors	
Narcissistic	Grandiose, no empathy, needs to be admired	
C: Fearful		
Avoidant	Social distress, feelings of inadequacy, oversensitivity	
Dependent	Excessive need to be cared for, resulting in clinging, submissive behaviors	
Obsessive-compulsive	Preoccupation with control, orderliness, and perfectionism	

Modified from American Psychiatric Association: *Diagnostic and statistical manual of mental disorders,* ed 4, text revision, Washington, DC, 2000, The Association; and Rollant PD, Deppoliti DB: *Mosby's review series: mental health nursing,* St. Louis, 1996, Mosby.

read people's minds. Some claim to have magical control over others and are able to make people do their bidding just by wishing or thinking about it. These persons commonly experience perceptual alterations such as sensing that there is another person present (when there is not). Speech is often loose and vague, but it can be understood. Often they will use words in odd combinations or unusual ways.

As with the other disorders in the eccentric cluster, schizotypal personalities are marked by suspiciousness and paranoid ideation, the idea that people are "out to get them," to undermine their efforts or do them harm. Emotional expressions (affect) are usually inappropriate or restricted. Because of unusual mannerisms, style of dress or grooming, and inattention to appropriate social behaviors, these individuals are considered odd or eccentric. They have problems relating to other people and are very anxious in social situations. They have few if any friends because they feel different and just do not "fit in" with others. As many as 50% have signs of major depression. Schizotypal personality disorders are diagnosed more frequently in men.

Erratic Cluster

The main characteristic for the group of disorders called the erratic cluster is dramatic behavior. Each disorder in this cluster (group B) is associated with a dramatic quality in the way in which these individuals live and conduct their lives. The erratic cluster consists of four separate disorders: antisocial, borderline, histrionic, and narcissistic.

One of our most pressing mental health problems today is with people who have antisocial personality disorders. "The central feature of **antisocial personality** disorder is a pervasive pattern of disregard for, and violation of, the rights of others" (American Psychiatric Association, 2000).

These persons are often referred to as **psychopaths** or **sociopaths** because they rely on deceit and manipulation to get their way. **Deceit** is lying. It is the act of representing as true something that is known to be false. **Manipulation** is defined as controlling others for one's own purposes by influencing them in unfair or false ways.

The hallmark of psychopaths is a stunning lack of conscience. "Psychopaths use charm, manipulation, intimidation, and violence to control others and satisfy their own selfish needs" (Hare, 1995). They have a stunning lack of conscience and no feelings for others. Because of these traits, it is important for nurses to remain alert for these behaviors and investigate sources other than the client when performing assessments. The Case Study box describes an antisocial personality.

Antisocial personality disorders are rooted in childhood. Some children have trouble controlling their impulses so they become disruptive and antisocial as a way of coping. Many of these maladaptive behaviors can be seen as early as 4 years of age.

Children with conduct disorders usually express their distress by being aggressive to animals and people; deceiving, lying, stealing; destroying property; and/or breaking important rules. Many become bullies in school. They are impulsive, quick to anger, and have no regard for

◆ Case Study

Rusty was the youngest of two boys born to an older, loving couple. As a child, he was always in some type of trouble. When he was about 7, he broke his femur and was required to wear a body (spica) cast for 6 weeks. Although his mother checked on him frequently, he managed mobility. One day Rusty walked out of the house and was seen propelling his casted hips and legs down the street, disinterested in the fact that he could have harmed himself.

By 12 years old Rusty was self-centered, demanding, and intolerant of his parent's wishes. He often threatened to burn the house down or kill the dog when he did not get his way. Soon his father was bailing him out of jail for various minor offenses like skipping school and stealing. His parents, unable to control him and afraid for their safety, allowed him free run of the house.

At 18 Rusty joined the Army. By 19 he had received a general discharge for not following orders. Much to his parents' dismay, Rusty returned home and announced that he would attend the local college. By this time, however, he was deeply involved with cocaine, alcohol, and a crowd of thrill seekers. His arrest record continued to grow.

One night at a party, Rusty strangled the homeowner's pedigreed cat. The owner became angry and threatened to have him arrested. Rusty coldly looked into the homeowner's eyes, pulled a gun, and fired.

Later, when asked why he did it, he calmly replied, "What else could I do? That guy was in my face, and his stupid cat was in my way. I didn't hurt him bad."

◆ What are your reactions to Rusty's behaviors?
◆ How would your feelings affect the care of the client?
◆ Do you think anything could have prevented this event? If so, what?

the feelings of others. If the child is seen by mental health care providers at this time, a conduct disorder is usually diagnosed.

During adolescence, maladaptive behaviors become well established. Truancies from school, open disregard for rules, and thrill-seeking behaviors often get these teens into trouble with authorities and the law. Fighting and physical and verbal abuses are common in adolescents with antisocial personalities.

By adulthood, psychopaths are usually adept at manipulating and deceiving others. They gain money, power, or influence at the expense of others and feel no guilt. They lie, cheat, con others, and malinger (pretend to be ill) to achieve their goals, but they are unable to plan ahead and act because they are too impulsive. Decisions are made with no thought to the consequences. Often they are able to inflict great pain and suffering in others and feel no remorse or guilt.

Individuals with antisocial personality disorders (psychopaths) are often charming. They are glib and clever conversationalists, complete with compliments and entertaining statements. An inflated view of their own importance makes them the center of attention and justifies living by different rules.

Psychopaths have a remarkable ability to rationalize their own actions. That, coupled with a lack of guilt and empathy, allows them to shrug off any responsibility for their behaviors. Their emotions are shallow and their behaviors are impulsive, and the need for excitement often involves breaking rules.

Individuals who are psychopathic have a "hair trigger" on their emotions; they can fire off with very little cause. However, when they are violent, it is "cold," without the intense emotional arousal that other perpetrators of violence experience. There is little remorse, and victims are often blamed for being weak, stupid, or in the wrong place.

Men are more affected by antisocial personality disorders than women. They may abuse chemicals. Commonly they fail to become self-supporting and spend years being impoverished, homeless, or institutionalized. Psychopaths constitute a large portion of the populations in prisons and psychiatric institutions.

A **borderline personality** disorder can be summarized as a pattern of instability in mood, thinking, self-image, behavior, and personal relationships. Intense fears of being abandoned motivate these persons to avoid being alone. Relationships with others are marked by rapid shifts from adoring and idealizing to devaluing and cruel punishment. These extreme shifts are also seen in the area of self-image. Sudden, dramatic changes in career plans, values, types of friends, and even sexual identities are characteristic of these individuals.

Impulsivity, acting without forethought or regard to the consequences, is a feature of personality disorders. Persons with borderline personality disorders may gamble, abuse food or drugs, engage in unsafe sex with multiple partners, spend money irresponsibly, and engage in self-mutilating or suicidal behaviors. Cutting, burning, pulling out hair, or scratching oneself is very common, and 8% to 10% of these individuals actually commit suicide.

Moods (affect) are unstable. Although people with borderline personality disorders experience chronic feelings of emptiness, they commonly express intense anger and frequent displays of aggression or temper. Emotions range from great joy to deep depression and frequently change within minutes or hours. They express inappropriate anger and have difficulty controlling their aggression. These individuals become easily bored, so they are always busy. During stressful times, individuals with borderline personality disorder may develop paranoid delusions and feelings of depersonalization (loss of contact with the self).

The most important feature of histrionic and narcissistic personality disorders is attention-seeking behaviors. Individuals with these disorders are often highly emotional and self-centered. They feel inadequate and unappreciated when not the center of attention.

Histrionic personality disorder is defined as a pattern of excessive emotional expression accompanied by attention-seeking behaviors. Histrionic persons may be flashy or dramatic in style of dress, mannerisms, and speech. A **narcissistic personality** disorder is characterized by a pattern of grandiosity and the need to be admired. These individuals believe they are special, unique, or extra important. Often, they fantasize about unlimited money, power, or love and take advantage of others without guilt or remorse. It is interesting to note that more women are diagnosed with histrionic personality disorder, whereas 50% to 75% of persons diagnosed with narcissistic personality disorder are men (Fortinash and Holoday-Worret, 1999).

Individuals with personality disorders are often the perpetrators of violence in our culture. Children who were bullies commonly grow up to be abusive to their partners. Individuals who had problems with anger control and impulsive urges as children find themselves unable to express themselves appropriately as adults. Teens with histories of being "difficult" or "temperamental" often engage in illegal activities. Even within the criminal population, psychopaths stand out because their antisocial and illegal activities are more varied and frequent than those of other criminals. Psychopaths tend to try every type of crime and then wonder what all the fuss is about when they are caught.

Fearful Cluster

The common characteristic of the fearful cluster (group C) is anxiety. The three personality disorders in the fearful or anxious cluster are avoidant, dependent, and obsessive-compulsive. Each disorder is related to certain expressions of anxiety.

In **avoidant personality** disorder, anxiety is related to a fear of rejection and humiliation. To prevent possible rejection, individuals narrow their interests to a small range of activities. They have a minimal support system because they are so afraid of the reactions of others. Often their tension does not allow for new friends who may be critical, so they withdraw into a world of isolation and self-pity. "When all else fails, they retreat into daydreaming and fantasy" (Personality Disorders, 1996a). Often individuals with avoidant personality disorders also suffer from general anxiety, depression, or hypochondria.

The anxiety of a **dependent personality** disorder is associated with separation and abandonment. People with this problem carry a deep fear of rejection, which expresses itself as the need to be cared for. To avoid turning people away, they become overcooperative and docile and do not make demands or disagree with others. When alone, they feel helpless and will go to great lengths to find someone to care for them.

Individuals with dependent personality disorder refuse to take responsibility for their own actions. They are unwilling to begin a task alone, take any independent actions, or assume responsibility for their activities of daily living. Feelings of worthlessness often motivate them to seek out overprotective, dominating, or abusive relationships.

Dependent personality disorder is one of the most commonly diagnosed personality disorders. Men and women are equally diagnosed, although some studies show a higher incidence in women. Cultural factors must be considered before a diagnosis is made because many societies consider certain dependent roles as appropriate.

Persons with **obsessive-compulsive personality** disorder relate their anxiety to uncertainty about the future. They are extremely orderly and so preoccupied with details that little is actually accomplished. Delegating tasks to others is impossible because no one "can do it as well." Commonly these individuals are devoted to work, have few leisure activities, and are consumed by the need for perfection. "About two-thirds of compulsive personalities are men" (Personality Disorders, 1996b).

Dual Diagnosis

Many individuals with personality disorders are also suffering from substance abuse problems. They are categorized as having a **dual diagnosis.** Substance abuse problems occur as individuals attempt to cope with their problems with alcohol or street drugs. Many dual-diagnosed persons are also homeless, unemployed, or involved in legal troubles. Many mental health care facilities have units dedicated to clients with dual diagnoses. Those who care for such clients must be aware of the multiple problems involved with dual diagnosis clients. Thorough assessments and careful planning are necessary to address the numerous problems present in this population. Issues of housing, employment, and socialization, as well as treatment for substance abuse and mental illness, must be considered. The multidisciplinary treatment team uses many resources in the care of these individuals.

THERAPEUTIC INTERVENTIONS

The treatment for individuals with personality disorders is complex because these individuals have extremely diverse treatment needs, and no single treatment is appropriate for every client. Unfortunately, many do not seek treatment or refuse to accept it when it is recommended due to their basic mistrust of others intentions.

Treatment and Therapy

Treatment decisions are guided by the client's presenting symptoms, complaints, and problems. Persons with personality disorders may have significant impairments in functioning, but they seldom present for treatment because they are usually unable to recognize their problems. When they do cooperate with treatment, a combination of various psychotherapies and medications are used only after any physical causes are ruled out.

A number of different psychotherapies are selected to treat clients with personality disorders. Types of psychotherapy that have been used with success include psychodynamic, cognitive, behavioral, and group therapy. Cure is not the goal of therapy. Care providers "can hope only to make patients more aware of how their habits affect their lives, modifying their behavior enough so that a personality disorder becomes a more adaptive personality type or style" (Personality Disorders, 1996b).

Medications are used with great caution in the treatment of people with personality disorders. They are prescribed to help relieve some of the distressing symptoms associated with these disorders. Most psychotherapeutic medications are prescribed in limited amounts for short periods of time because their effectiveness in treating personality disorders is still under investigation (Kapfhammer and Hippius, 1998) (Table 30-2).

Nurses must exercise great care when administering medications to individuals with personality disorders. Compliance must be monitored frequently, and safeguards to prevent or reduce the risk of suicide must be in place. If the client is being seen on an outpatient basis, the amount of any prescribed medication must never be large enough to allow a successful suicide.

Also, be alert to the fact that suicidal clients will "hoard" their medications until they have a lethal dose on hand. Do not hesitate to assess every medicated client for suicidal thoughts or plans. Finally, be familiar with each class of drugs and their side effects. The prudent nurse does not wait to research a medication until a client must take one.

Box 30-2 NANDA Nursing Diagnoses Related to Personality Disorder

Anxiety
Adjustment, impaired
Coping, ineffective family
Coping, ineffective individual
Loneliness
Noncompliance, (specify)
Personal identity disturbance
Role performance, altered
Self-esteem disturbance
Self-mutilation, risk for
Social interactions, impaired
Violence, risk for: directed at others

From North American Nursing Diagnosis Association: *NANDA nursing diagnoses: definitions and classification 1999-2000*, Philadelphia, 1999, The Association.

Table 30-2 Drugs Used to Treat Personality Disorders

Class	Example	Common side effects
Antianxiety agents	Ativan, Valium BuSpar	Monitor kidney function; side effects are usually minimal; fatigue, sedation, dizziness, and orthostatic hypotension (a drop in blood pressure upon standing); long-term use can result in dependence.
Antidepressants	Elavil, Prozac	Side effects vary according to class but include dry mouth, nausea, vomiting, constipation, diarrhea, anorexia, differences in taste; headache, changes in alertness, tremor, dizziness, weakness, fatigue, increased sweating, sexual dysfunction; visual disturbances, urinary disturbances. Refer to Chapter 7.
Anticonvulsants	Dilantin, phenobarbital	Bone marrow depression is most serious; gastrointestinal (GI) symptoms; gingival hyperplasia (gum tissue growth); slurred speech, confusion.
Antipsychotics	Haldol, Thorazine	Extrapyramidal side effects (EPSEs) characterized by abnormal movements; dry mouth, blurred vision, and photophobia (sensitivity to bright light), tachycardia, and hypotension (see Chapter 7).
Lithium	Eskalith, Lithane	*Mild side effects* are fine hand tremor, increased thirst and urination, nausea, anorexia, and diarrhea or constipation. *Serious side effects* of lithium include vomiting, extreme hand tremor, sedation, muscle weakness, and dizziness.

Monitor and assess clients frequently for therapeutic responses and the many side effects of these medications.

Nursing Process

The goals of care for clients with personality disorders are twofold: (1) to help clients identify and then become responsible for their own behaviors and (2) to assist clients in developing satisfactory interpersonal relationships.

Possible nursing diagnoses are listed in Box 30-2.

Short-term goals are based on each individual's assessed problems. They usually focus on the discomforts or ineffective behaviors associated with daily living activities.

The assessment of every client should include a mental status examination, but for the client with a personality disorder, this examination is extremely important. A nursing history and observation of client behaviors will reveal how individuals cope with the many aspects of daily life, including interpersonal relationships.

The therapeutic relationship is begun at this time, so it is important for nurses to remain nonjudgmental. Remember, however, many clients use manipulation, charm, or other subtle behaviors to achieve their purposes. They often use a technique called **splitting,** emotionally dividing the staff by complimenting one group and degrading another. Consistent limit setting and reinforcement help clients to define their

---

⟫⟫⟫ Sample Client Care Plan — Personality Disorders

Assessment

History: Sophie was 6 years of age when her parents divorced after years of fighting and abuse. She, her mother, and her older brother, Sam, were forced to find shelter in a small hotel room. Shortly after moving in, her mother began to leave Sophie alone for long periods. Once Sophie set the room on fire. Another time she strangled the neighbor's canary. On one occasion, she was molested by a drunken visitor.

At 13 she dropped out of school and began living in the streets. Occasionally she would return home.

Current Findings: Today 19-year-old Sophie has been admitted to the medical unit for recovery from repeated attempts to "cut herself apart." She is suicidal, angry, and has difficulty in identifying her actions and their consequences.

Multidisciplinary Diagnosis

Risk for self-directed violence related to feelings of abandonment, depression and worthlessness.

Planning/Goals

Sophie will verbally identify the emotions associated with her self-destructive activities.

Sophie will not engage in self-destructive behaviors during her inpatient stay.

Therapeutic Interventions

Intervention	Rationale	Team Member
1. Inform Sophie that self-harm is not acceptable behavior while she is here.	Setting limits lets her know which behaviors will not be tolerated.	All
2. Have Sophie sign a no-harm contract.	Offers objective data of agreed-on behaviors.	Nsg
3. Establish trust and rapport with Sophie.	Allows Sophie to identify current behaviors and explore new ones within an atmosphere of safety and trust.	All
4. Institute suicide precautions; monitor continuously if acting out.	Provides safety, prevents self-harm, encourages therapeutic relationships.	All
5. Assess skin on arms and legs daily for new wounds or signs of trauma.	To monitor for further evidence of self-harm behaviors.	Nsg

Evaluation

Sophie expressed relief at knowing limits are set on her behaviors 2 days after admission.
During the first week, Sophie was able to identify her emotions following a dispute with another client.

A complete client care plan includes several other diagnoses and interventions

limits, but care providers must keep in mind their own therapeutic boundaries and communicate with each other frequently.

Clients with personality disorders often have several problems at once. The most important ones are identified and linked to the appropriate multidisciplinary and nursing diagnoses. Interventions and evaluations are developed for each diagnosis based on the individual client. The Sample Client Care Plan box presents a plan for an individual with a personality disorder. Caring for these clients can be a challenge, but the process can promote growth in both client and caregiver when they are willing to work together.

KEY CONCEPTS

◆ Personality is the composite of behavioral traits and attitudes that identifies one as an individual.

◆ The social responses of humans can range from autonomy and interdependence to the ineffective, disordered behaviors of manipulation, intimidation, aggression, and hysteria.

◆ The human personality is shaped and influenced throughout life.

◆ Currently there are four general theories of personality: biological, psychoanalytical, behavioral, and sociocultural.

◆ Personality disorders are defined as long-standing, maladaptive patterns of behaving and relating to others.

◆ The eccentric cluster (group A) of personality disorders is characterized by odd or strange behaviors and includes the paranoid, schizoid, and schizotypal personality disorders.

◆ The erratic cluster (group B) of personality disorders is characterized by dramatic behaviors and consists of four personality disorders: antisocial, borderline, histrionic, and narcissistic.

◆ The fearful cluster (group C) of personality disorders is characterized by anxiety and includes the avoidant, dependent, and obsessive-compulsive personality disorders.

◆ Individuals with personality disorders who are also suffering from drug abuse or some other form of mental illness are categorized as having a dual diagnosis.

◆ People with personality disorders may have significant impairments in functioning, but they seldom present for treatment because they are unable to recognize their problems.

◆ Types of psychotherapy that have been used with success for different personality disorders include psychodynamic, cognitive, behavioral, and group therapy.

◆ Medications are used with great caution in the treatment of people with personality disorders and only to help relieve some of the distressing symptoms associated with these disorders.

◆ The goals of care for clients with personality disorders are (1) to help clients identify and then become responsible for their own behaviors and (2) to assist clients in developing satisfactory interpersonal relationships.

Suggestions for Further Reading

Internet Mental Health (www.mentalhealth.com) offers interesting information about the diagnosis and treatment of personality disorders. Other resources include Psychiatry On-line (www.priory.co.uk/psych) and KEN—Knowledge Exchange Network (www.mentalhealth.org).

References

American Psychiatric Association: *Diagnostic and statistical manual of mental disorders,* ed 4, text revision, Washington, DC, 2000, The Association.

Brennan KA, Shaver PR: Attachment styles and personality disorders: their connections to each other and to parental divorce, parental death, and perceptions of parental caregiving, *Journal of Personality* 66(5):835, 1998.

Fortinash KM, Holoday-Worret PA: *Psychiatric mental health nursing,* ed 2, St. Louis, 1999, Mosby.

Hare RD: Psychopaths: new trends in research, *Harvard Mental Health Letter* 11(9):1, 1995.

Kapfhammer H-P, Hippius H: Pharmacology in personality disorders, *Journal of Personality Disorders* 12(3):288, 1998.

Marshall LA, Cooke DJ: The childhood experience of psychopaths: a retrospective study of familial and societal factors, *Journal of Personality Disorders* 13(3):211, 1999.

Paris J: Personality disorders in sociocultural perspective, *Journal of Personality Disorders* 12(4):289, 1998.

Personality disorders: the anxious cluster, part I, *Harvard Ment Health Letter* 12(8):1, 1996a.

Personality disorders: the anxious cluster, part II, *Harvard Ment Health Letter* 12(9):1, 1996b.

Rollant PD, Deppoliti DB: *Mosby's review series: mental health nursing,* St. Louis, 1996, Mosby.

Stuart GW, Laraia MT: *Principles and practice of psychiatric nursing,* ed 7, St. Louis, 2001, Mosby.

Wong DL: *Whaley and Wong's nursing care of infants and children,* ed 6, St. Louis, 1998, Mosby.

Chapter 31

Schizophrenia and Other Psychoses

Learning Objectives

1. Compare the differences between a psychosis and other mental health disorders.

2. Describe the continuum of neurobiological responses.

3. Outline the signs and symptoms of psychosis in childhood, adolescence, and adulthood.

4. Discuss three theories relating to the causes of schizophrenia and other psychoses.

5. Compare and contrast four subtypes of schizophrenia.

6. Describe the signs, symptoms, and behaviors exhibited by a person with schizophrenia.

7. Outline the main pharmacological treatments and mental health therapies for persons with schizophrenia.

8. Apply the therapeutic process to clients suffering from schizophrenia or another psychosis.

9. Plan three nursing responsibilities related to antipsychotic medications.

Key Terms

agnosia
akathisia
akinesia
alexithymia
anhedonia
apathy
bradykinesia
delusions
derealization
dyskinesia

dystonia
extrapyramidal side effects (EPSEs)
hallucinations
ideas of reference
illusions
laryngeal-pharyngeal dystonia
negative symptoms
neuroleptic malignant syndrome (NMS)

oculogyric crisis
perseveration
positive symptoms
poverty of thought
psychosis
schizophrenia
tardive dyskinesia
torticollis

To function effectively in society, individuals must be able to process information and to adapt to countless internal and external stimuli. Information is tested or validated through interactions with people and the environment. The result is a logical flow of thoughts and actions that allow human beings to function effectively.

Most people who experience mental health problems are able to think and act logically, even when their behaviors are maladaptive. However, for a certain group of people, reality is distorted and disturbed. These individuals suffer from a **psychosis:** the inability to recognize reality, relate to others, or cope with life's demands.

The most common psychosis is **schizophrenia,** a group of related disorders characterized by disordered thinking, perceptions, and behaviors. Other psychotic disorders include brief psychotic disorder, delusional disorder, and psychoses related to medical conditions or drug use. All these disorders involve a change in the individual's perception of reality. Since individuals with psychotic behaviors are often encountered in general health care settings, care providers who can recognize and intervene appropriately with these clients are more effective than those who work in ignorance.

CONTINUUM OF NEUROBIOLOGICAL RESPONSES

Highly adaptable persons are able to integrate all aspects of human functioning into a workable framework for coping with the world. In other words, the physical, emotional, intellectual, social, and spiritual realms work in combination and allow individuals to function effectively.

The ability to function, change, and adapt depends, in part, on certain physical brain functions, their connections, and their chemical messengers. In psychiatry these interactions are called *neurobiological functions.* They can be viewed as existing along a continuum of behavioral responses ranging from highly adaptive, effective responses to maladaptive, even destructive behaviors (Figure 31-1).

When everything is functioning in harmony, people are able to successfully adapt to their environments. They use logical thought, have clear perceptions, and are able to socially relate in appropriate ways. This state of functioning represents the adaptive end of the neurobiological continuum.

People who do not adapt as well are placed at the middle of the spectrum. These persons function within reality, but they may have emotional overreactions,

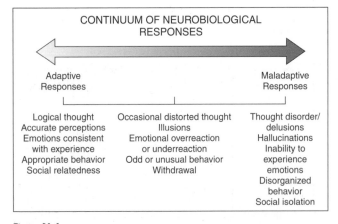

Figure 31-1 Continuum of neurobiological responses. (Redrawn from Stuart GW, Laraia MT: *Principles and practice of psychiatric nursing,* ed 7, St. Louis, 2001, Mosby.)

distorted thoughts, or odd behaviors. Many will never seek mental health services because their behaviors are not recognized as problems. Individuals at the maladaptive end of the spectrum are disorganized in their thought, emotions, and social behaviors.

PSYCHOSES THROUGHOUT THE LIFE CYCLE

As human beings grow and develop they learn to integrate new information into their knowledge stores. Infants begin to unify information at birth, and the process continues throughout life. Because of certain physical, social, or environmental factors, some individuals have difficulty in relating to new information. Although most cases of psychoses are encountered primarily in late adolescence or adulthood, some do begin in childhood. An awareness of the early signs of possible psychosis assists both client and care provider in providing early interventions.

Psychoses in Childhood

Children learn about their worlds through observation and experience. Senses develop, and infants become interested in the world around them. By 10 months, children have developed a wide range of complex behaviors and interactions with their caregivers. At 2 years of age, they begin to integrate emotional and behavioral patterns, and by 4, there is a rich and complex fantasy life.

Also at this time children are beginning to discover their intellectual side. Basic personalities emerge, and social experiences become important. During the school years, relationships and experiences are combined into the personality as children engage in more complex activities and behaviors.

For some children, however, processing or combining information is a near-impossible task. Infants with failure to thrive syndromes have slowed physical growth because of an inability to integrate the physical, emotional, and sensorimotor realms of functioning (Wong, 1998). Most often, this problem is related to neglect, environmental problems, or severe family stress. Whatever the cause, children with failure to thrive do not have a consistent opportunity to experience the activities and conditions for normal growth and development.

Psychotic disorders can occur in children as young as 5. The actual cause of childhood schizophrenia is unknown, but three risk factors have been identified:
1. Genetic influences. Studies have found that schizophrenia and other psychoses occur more often in families who have parents, siblings, or other relatives with schizophrenia.
2. Complications during pregnancy or birth. Exposure to the influenza virus during the second trimester of pregnancy has been linked to some cases of schizophrenia (Schultz and Andreasen, 1999).
3. Biochemical imbalances. Problems with a neurotransmitter, dopamine, upset the normal neurochemical

system (Stuart and Laraia, 2001), so the child perceives and acts differently.

Signs, symptoms, and behaviors of schizophrenic children vary considerably depending on each child's age, developmental stage, quality of previous experiences, and coping mechanisms. A core of behaviors generally indicate an increasing lack of contact with reality and withdrawal into a world of their own. There is an impaired ability to process visual information, regulate attention, and sort out incoming information. The child's affect (behavioral display of emotions) changes. Impaired interpersonal relationships and language or communication disturbances arise. Because schizophrenia involves every area of functioning, the child has problems with motor control, emotional control and expression, perception and understanding, thinking logically, and communicating effectively.

Psychoses in Adolescence

The unpredictable, up-and-down behaviors of adolescence are intensified in teens with schizophrenia or other psychotic problems. Where the average teen is in contact with his or her reality, the adolescent with schizophrenia is not. Even before the onset of a full-blown psychosis, family members may notice certain changes in behavior. Poor hygiene and grooming habits are most noticeable. Strange, vague speech and a lack of interest soon lead to social withdrawal. Odd behaviors such as hoarding food or talking to oneself occur. Thoughts and beliefs may be bizarre. Unusual superstitions, the belief that one is able to read others' minds (telepathy), and ideas that one is remotely controlled by others are common. Self-injury and destructive behaviors often begin in adolescence with these teens. The Case Study box describes an adolescent with a psychotic disorder.

Most psychotic adolescents are first treated in the inpatient setting, where their behaviors can be assessed, monitored, and controlled. Therapeutic interventions focus on decreasing acute symptoms and behaviors, improving relationships with significant others through family therapy, and educating client and family about the illness and its management.

Psychoses in Adulthood

The onset of acute symptoms most often occurs in men during the middle 20s, whereas women usually do not present with symptoms until the late 20s. Both want to seek treatment, but men endure their symptoms longer before seeking help. With continued treatment, one third of schizophrenic persons improve; without treatment, one third improve; with or without treatment, one third progress into a chronic downhill course.

The prognosis (long-term outlook) for schizophrenic individuals is improved if adaptive interpersonal relationships, school performance, and work histories were present before the onset of symptoms. The outlook is also better for women. On the average, men with schizophrenia respond less well to treatment, have higher relapse rates, and spend more time in inpatient settings.

Families with schizophrenic members face enormous demands. Because the length of institutional stays has sharply decreased, many individuals with schizophrenia return to the home while still psychotic, thus requiring constant observation and support. This places great strain on family resources. Social and occupational activities of caretakers are limited by the demands of the illness. The ability to communicate with the schizophrenic family member is limited. Family members, especially parents, struggle with guilt and frustration as they attempt to explain "why." Parents suffer the grief of losing a normal child and then must cope with the stigma of having a child who is "mentally ill." Brothers and sisters are strongly affected by their sibling's behaviors. Then there are the repeated role changes that occur with each hospitalization and each return home. Most families have difficulties because of the enormous amount of energy required to cope with a psychotic family member.

Psychoses in Older Adulthood

Schizophrenia is seldom diagnosed in the elderly. "Most older people with schizophrenia will have developed the illness before the age of 45" (Rodriquez-Ferrera and Vassilas, 1998). Most have long-standing problems, and many suffer from the irreversible side effects of

---

 Case Study

Rob was a model child, cooperative, pleasant, and enjoyable—until he turned 17. It all seemed to start when he began a campaign to see every science fiction movie ever made. Soon he was speaking an "interplanetary space language" that no one but himself could understand.

About 6 months into his outer space–oriented lifestyle, Rob quit school and began to spend his days "attending intergalactic conferences of great minds." His family became worried when Rob refused to bathe or change his clothes for weeks at a time. Often they would enter the

room to find Rob arguing animatedly with the lamp or listening with interest to the wall. When an outburst of unprovoked anger resulted in injuries to his younger sister, the family sought counseling.

- What do you think is the family's first priority with Rob?
- What do you think the mental health care team's first priority would be?
- What signs do you think would indicate a need for an inpatient psychiatric setting?

long-term antipsychotic drug use and other chronic medical problems.

Often the hallucinations and delusions of younger years decrease or disappear. Many older schizophrenics become more withdrawn or paranoid. They are frequently homeless. The fortunate elderly with schizophrenia spend the remainder of their days in long-term care facilities.

An important reminder: *The acute onset of psychotic behavior in elderly clients must be investigated.* Older clients who lose contact with reality, experience impaired interpersonal relationships, suddenly have difficulty communicating, or experience great emotional changes may be suffering from some physical or biochemical change. Changes in electrolyte balances, reactions to medications, drug interactions, and nutritional deficiencies can cause signs, symptoms, and behaviors that appear psychotic. The causes of most acute-onset psychoses in older adults are physical problems.

THEORIES RELATING TO PSYCHOSES

"Schizophrenia is a condition that exists in all cultures and socioeconomic groups" (Fortinash and Holoday-Worret, 1999). The first theory of psychosis was that individuals who were not in contact with reality were possessed by demons, spirits, or devils. Evidence of this belief is found in early Chinese, Egyptian, Greek, and Hebrew writings. The Cultural Aspects box offers an interesting insight.

The possession theory existed until the nineteenth century, when the work of two psychiatrists began to define schizophrenic behaviors. Emile Kraeplin (1856-1926) described the syndrome of hallucinations and delusions seen in schizophrenics. In 1911 a Swiss psychiatrist (Hans Bleuler, 1857-1939) coined the word *schizophrenia* (meaning "to split the mind") to describe the disconnection between the intellectual and emotional

aspects of a personality. Today confusion about the term exists because the general public often uses the word to describe someone with multiple personalities.

Once psychoses were thought to be the result of faulty parent-child interactions or failure of the ego to combine the drives of the id with reality. Today scientific evidence points to possible physical causes for psychotic behaviors. Other theories that attempt to explain schizophrenia relate to psychosocial and sociocultural factors. A brief explanation of each theory group helps in the understanding of clients suffering from psychotic disorders.

Biological Theories

Evidence for viewing schizophrenia as a brain disorder is building. Studies of fetal development have demonstrated that cell connections in the area of the brain that coordinates thinking and motivation has trouble communicating with other areas of the brain in schizophrenics (Bower, 1996). Neurochemical production and transmission problems are being investigated as having a possible role in the development of schizophrenia. Research with identical twins found that schizophrenic twins develop differently by the age of 5. Such data have led to the development of the *genetic/heredity model* as an explanation of schizophrenia.

The *stress/disease/trauma model* looks at the effects of stress on the individual, especially during the prenatal period. Immune reactions to viral infections during pregnancy and severe malnutrition during pregnancy have been shown to contribute to the development of schizophrenia in the children, especially the females, of these mothers (Bower, 1996). Complications occurring during birth, such as prolonged labor, difficult birth, or umbilical cord prolapse, have been related to the development of schizophrenia. Cocaine and other drug use during pregnancy has been linked to schizotypal behaviors in the children of users.

Because of the many refinements in brain-imaging technology, scientists have been able to pinpoint certain parts of the brain that are different in schizophrenic people. Other studies have found that certain chemical messengers (neurotransmitters) are altered in persons with schizophrenia The neurotransmitters serotonin, norepinephrine, and dopamine have been implicated as possible causes of schizophrenia. Theories developed from this type of research are called *neurochemical models*.

Other Theories

Until recently schizophrenia was thought to result from certain environmental or social factors. *Psychological models* view schizophrenia as being caused by a basic character flaw combined with poor family relationships. Overprotective, anxious mothers; cold, uncaring fathers; and couples who "stayed together for the sake of the

---

Cultural Aspects

In India a man with schizophrenia is often considered a "wise man" because of his ability to speak with spirits. He is usually honored and sought out for his advice.

In Haiti many people believe that humans can communicate with spirits and deities (gods) and have religious ceremonies to induce spirit possession. The group considers being possessed not as a shameful experience, but a privilege. Psychotic persons are believed to be victims of the "evil eye," called *maldyok,* or to be possessed by supernatural beings. Their behavior is tolerated by members of the community, but they are expected to consult native healers "who treat with amulets, packets of herbs and spices, liquids, baths, powders, rubbing, and massage" (Giger and Davidhizer, 1999).

children" were implicated. The child's failure to accomplish a developmental task, such as trust or intimacy, was also thought to be related to schizophrenia.

Sociocultural theories consider the effects of environment on the development of psychoses. Poverty, homelessness, unstable families, and cultural differences have been suggested as factors relating to schizophrenia. Some researchers believe that individuals become psychotic as a way of coping with problems. Although environmental and social factors may influence the development of psychoses, evidence for a neurobiological cause of psychosis is becoming more and more convincing.

PSYCHOTIC DISORDERS

Schizophrenia

Schizophrenia affects about 1% of the world's population. It is found equally in men and women. Although it occurs in every socioeconomic class, it is found more commonly in lower socioeconomic levels. "An estimated 10 to 15 percent of homeless people are schizophrenic" (Herbert, 1998). Because of the intense discomfort associated with the disorder, 10% of all schizophrenic individuals commit suicide.

The costs of treating schizophrenia are enormous—in terms of lost productivity, continued medical care, and social maintenance. In this day of scarce mental health resources, treatment for the disorder account for 2.5% of all health expenditures (Amadio, Cross, and Amadio, 1997). The costs in terms of distress and suffering cannot even be estimated.

Subtypes of Schizophrenia

Because schizophrenia is a cluster of related behaviors, it can be classified into different groups based on the clinical picture. Although many persons have symptoms of more than one cluster, diagnosis is made based on the most prominent symptoms or behaviors. The five subtypes of schizophrenia are catatonic, disorganized, paranoid, undifferentiated, and residual. Table 31-1 explains each subtype and its characteristics.

Signs, Symptoms, and Behaviors

The main characteristic of psychotic disorders is loss of contact with reality to the point where it grossly impairs functioning. Although each individual behaves uniquely, many appear to share certain basic symptoms. Table 31-2 describes the signs and symptoms of schizophrenia in each area of function.

The physical appearance of individuals with schizophrenia is one of an unkempt person. Focus on inner matters prevents them from routinely seeking out food or shelter. Personal hygiene is often poor, and body images are distorted. Motor activity ranges from agitated to immobile.

The signs and symptoms of schizophrenia affect perception, the way that one views the world. Individuals suffer from **hallucinations** (false sensory input with no external stimulus), **illusions** (false perceptions of real stimuli), and **agnosia** (an inability to recognize familiar environmental objects or people). Hallucinations may take the form of smells, sounds, tastes, sight, touch, or feelings of altered internal workings of the body.

Table 31-1 Subtypes of Schizophrenia	
Subtype	**Description**
Catatonic	Characterized by marked psychomotor problems: immobility or excessive activity with no purpose; odd movements, rigid posture, stereotyped movements, echopraxia (mimics movements of others); may be extremely negative or mute, echolalia (echoes others' speech) automatic obedience; may suffer from malnutrition, dehydration, exhaustion; prognosis is fair.
Disorganized	Disordered thinking, speech, and behavior; affect is flat or inappropriate; primitive, uninhibited behaviors, unusual mannerisms, distorted facial expressions, giggles or cries out; loosely organized hallucinations, delusions; withdrawn, socially inept; unable to perform activities of daily living; onset is early, prognosis is poor.
Paranoid	Organized delusions of grandeur or persecution, auditory hallucinations; high anxiety levels, guarded, suspicious, aloof, hostile, angry, can be violent or suicidal; onset is late, prognosis is good with treatment.
Undifferentiated	Does not meet criteria for other subtypes; disorganized speech, behavior; hallucinations, delusions, negative symptoms; prognosis is fair.
Residual	Has had at least one acute episode of schizophrenia, is free of acute psychosis but still has negative symptoms of withdrawal, emotional changes, disorganized thinking, and odd behaviors; schizophrenia present for many years; time is limited between acute episodes; prognosis is poor.

Table 31-2 Clinical Symptoms of Schizophrenia

Perceptual	Intellectual	Emotional	Behavioral	Social
Hallucinations: 1. Auditory: May be commanding; content matches delusions 2. Visual 3. Tactile: For example, may feel surrounded by spider webs 4. Olfactory and gustatory: May refuse to eat because food smells or tastes bad *Illusions:* False perceptions due to misinterpretations of real objects *Altered internal sensations:* 1. Formication: Sensation of worms crawling around inside 2. Chill: Feeling of chills in the marrow of one's bones *Agnosia:* Failure to recognize familiar environmental stimuli such as sounds or objects seen or felt; sometimes called "negative hallucinations" *Distortion of body image:* Relating to size, facial expression, activity, detail, exaggeration or diminution of body parts *Negative self-perception:* Relating to ability and competence	*Delusions:* Unusual ideas, not reality based: 1. Omnipotence 2. Persecution 3. Control *Derealization:* Loss of ego boundaries; cannot tell where own body ends and environment begins; feeling that the world around one is not real *Ideas of reference:* Notion that other people or the media are talking to or about one *Errors in recall of memory:* Due to incorrect categorization *Difficulty sustaining attention:* 1. Unable to complete tasks 2. Errors of omission *Incorrect use of language:* 1. Neologisms (invented words) 2. Incoherence, verbigeration 3. Echolalia, word salad 4. Concrete, restricted vocabulary 5. Poor comprehension 6. Loose associations *Flight of ideas:* Abrupt change of topic in a rapid flow of speech	*Labile affect: range of emotions:* 1. Apathy, dulled response 2. Flattened affect 3. Reduced responsiveness 4. Exaggerated euphoria 5. Rage *Inappropriate affect:* Laughing at sad events, crying over joyous ones *Disruption in limbic functioning:* Inability to screen out disruptive stimuli and loss of voluntary control of response	*Little impulse-control:* 1. Sudden scream as a protest of frustration 2. Self-mutilation, to substitute physical for emotional pain 3. Injury to a body part believed to be offensive 4. Responds to command hallucinations *Inability to cope with depression:* 1. Depressed client has a 50% risk for suicide 2. Frequent ups and downs in one who has insight 3. Lack of social support to help *Inability to manage anger:* Anger and lack of impulse-control lead to violence: verbal aggression, destruction of property, injury, homicide *Substance abuse:* Dulls painful psychological symptoms *Noncompliance with medication:* May feel it is not needed or has too many side effects	*Poor peer relationships:* 1. Few friends, as a child or teen 2. Preference for solitude *Low interest in hobbies and activities:* 1. Daydreamer 2. Not functioning well in social or occupational areas 3. Preoccupied and detached 4. Behavioral autism *Loss of interest in appearance:* 1. Careless grooming 2. Introversion *Not competitive in sports or academics:* 1. Poor adjustment to school 2. Withdrawal from activities *May suffer from:* 1. Attention deficit disorder 2. Somatic symptoms

Modified from Fortinash KM, Holoday-Worret PA: *Psychiatric mental health nursing*, ed 2, St. Louis, 1999, Mosby.

In the cognitive (intellectual) area of functioning, schizophrenics usually have problems with attention, memory, and use of language. Thinking may involve **delusions,** fixed false ideas that are not based in reality; **ideas of reference,** the idea that people or the media are talking about oneself; and **derealization,** a loss of ego boundaries with an inability to tell where one's body ends and the environment begins.

Language difficulties involve incorrect usage. The speech of persons with schizophrenia include a number of unusual characteristics: clang associations, concrete thinking, echolalia, flight of ideas, loose associations, ideas of reference, mutism, neologisms, verbigeration, and word salad. Table 31-3 explains each term and offers an example of each communication difficulty.

Thought processes in schizophrenics vary widely, from contact with reality to fantasy thinking. Negative experiences are remembered more than positive ones. Individuals may demonstrate **perseveration,** the repeating of the same idea in response to different questions, or **poverty of thought,** a lack of ability to produce new thoughts or follow a train of thought. People with chronic schizophrenia have little insight into their problems. Often their judgment is impaired. Usually there is a general decline in intellectual abilities as the disorder progresses.

In the emotional realm, persons with schizophrenia experience a range of inappropriate emotions. Affect, the outward expressions of one's emotions, is described as blunted, flat, inappropriate, or labile. Other emotional responses include **alexithymia,** a difficulty in identifying and describing emotions; **apathy,** a lack of concern, interest, or feelings; and **anhedonia,** the inability (or decreased ability) to experience pleasure in life.

Behaviorally, schizophrenics display little impulse-control and an inability to manage anger. They may injure themselves and others or act in response to hallucinations commanding them to do something. A lack of energy or motivation *(avolition)* often leads to poor performance at work or school, unemployment, and homelessness. The inability to cope with depression, plus a lack of social supports, lead to a high risk for suicide. Many refuse to comply with treatment by not taking their medications. Others abuse alcohol and street drugs. These dual-diagnosis individuals present many challenging health care situations.

Socially, schizophrenics are unable to establish or maintain relationships with others. Self-esteem is low, and gender identity confusion may exist. They have few friends and little interest in hobbies or other activities. Social behaviors are often inappropriate. Many prefer to be alone because of hallucinations or feelings of paranoia. The few family and social relationships that do exist usually follow a rocky course. Refer to Table 31-2 and review the description of symptoms in schizophrenia.

Table 31-3 Speech Disturbances in Schizophrenia

Speech problem	Description
Clang associations	Repeating words or phrases that sound alike or substituting a word that sounds like the appropriate word *Example:* "Honey, money, sunny" or "I need some honey to buy the paper"
Concrete thinking	Inability to consider the abstract meaning of a phrase; frequently tested by having clients interpret proverbs *Example:* "A stitch in time saves nine" may mean "sew the holes in your clothes" to a schizophrenic
Echolalia	Repeating words of another after one has stopped talking *Example:* Nurse: "How is your day going?" Client: "Day going, day going, day going."
Flight of ideas	Rapid change in topics with a rapid flow of speech *Example:* "The sky is blue. The dog is dead, and I have two eyes."
Ideas of reference	The belief that some events have special personal meaning *Example:* "The United States is sending satellites into space so that they can spy on me."
Loose associations	Thinking characterized by speech that moves from one unrelated idea to another *Example:* "I'm hungry, but the desert has no rain so it's cold outside."
Mutism	Refusal to speak
Neologisms	Words or expressions invented by the individual *Example:* "The ispy is not happy when the fulgari is green."
Verbigeration	Purposeless repetition of phrases *Example:* Client repeats for days: "Prepare to launch the orbiter."
Pressured speech	Rapid, forced speech *Example:* "I must prepare. There's no time to waste. Can't talk now."
Word salad	A random, jumbled set of words that have no connection or relationship to each other *Example:* "Hot happies are spying on me but no men love short feet."

The characteristic symptoms of schizophrenia can also be described as falling into two broad categories: positive and negative symptoms. **Positive symptoms** are related to maladaptive thoughts and behaviors. They include hallucinations, speech problems, and bizarre behaviors. **Negative symptoms** are related to the lack of adaptive mechanisms. They include flat affect, poor grooming, withdrawal, and poverty of speech. Mental health care team members commonly refer to the symptoms of schizophrenia using the terms positive and negative symptoms.

Most of the terms used to describe schizophrenic behaviors are not a part of everyday vocabulary. For this reason it is important to focus more on accurately describing clients' behaviors, communications, and interactions than finding the best label. If you are not sure of the meaning of the term, do not use it. One good behavioral description is worth many psychiatric terms.

Phases of Becoming Disorganized

The course of schizophrenia is marked by episodes of acute psychosis alternating with periods of relatively normal functioning. The symptoms of schizophrenia must occur for at least 1 year before a diagnostic label is assigned.

The slide into schizophrenia commonly occurs through four stages. The *prodromal phase* begins with withdrawal, a lack of energy, and little motivation. Individuals may appear confused and in a world of their own. They may complain about multiple physical problems or show a new, excessive interest in religion or philosophy. Affect becomes blunted. Ideas and beliefs become odd or unusual, and personal hygiene is ignored. Some individuals become agitated or angry. Speech may be difficult to follow. These symptoms can occur during both the prodromal and the residual stages of the disorder (see Think About box).

In the *prepsychotic phase,* individuals are usually quiet, passive, obedient, and prefer to be alone. They have few if any friends because of their odd, suspicious, or eccentric behaviors. Hallucinations and delusions may be present, but behaviors are not completely disorganized. Family members may report that they can sense the individual "slipping away" in front of their eyes.

Signs, symptoms, and behaviors during the *acute phase* vary widely but include disturbances in thought, perception, behavior, and emotion. Frequently individuals lose contact with reality and become unable to function even in the most basic ways.

The *residual phase* follows an acute episode. It is marked by a lack of energy, no interest in goal-directed activities, and a negative outlook. Many of the behaviors seen in the prodromal phase are also present during the residual phase.

Following the residual phase is a period of relative remission. The ability to manage some basic activities of daily living returns, and the individual experiences some relief from the distresses of psychosis. The course of schizophrenia alternates between acute episodes and periods of decreased symptoms. The outlook for recovery is fair to poor because of the many complex aspects of this disorder.

Other Psychoses

Besides schizophrenia, the *Diagnostic and Statistical Manual of Mental Disorders* (DSM-IV–TR) lists other psychoses. A *brief psychotic disorder* is a psychotic disturbance that lasts for more than a day but less than a month. A *delusional disorder* is characterized by more than a month of nonbizarre (reality-based) fixed ideas, and a *shared psychotic disorder* is defined as "a disturbance that develops in an individual who is influenced by someone else who has an established delusion with similar content" (American Psychiatric Association, 2000). *Schizoaffective disorder* is diagnosed when depression or mania are also present. Psychotic behaviors are also related to the abuse of street drugs and several medical conditions.

The alert care provider is always observant for changes in client's behavior or affect. Early detection of behavioral changes frequently prevents later complications from occurring.

THERAPEUTIC INTERVENTIONS

Because of impaired judgment and other problems, many individuals with schizophrenia do not receive treatment. Those who do cooperate with treatment are most often cared for by a multidisciplinary mental health team consisting of psychiatrists, nurses, psychologists, and psychiatric social workers. Individuals are admitted to an inpatient unit during episodes of acute psychoses, when they are a danger to themselves or others, or for stabilization of disorganized or inappropriate behaviors. The goals of inpatient, short-term care are to stabilize the client, prevent further decline in functioning, and assist the client in coping with his or her disorder. Long-term

---

Think About

The prodromal signs and symptoms of schizophrenia often begin in adolescence. As the teen's behavior becomes more bizarre, friends and family become uncomfortable with and afraid of the individual, so they respond by limiting their interactions with him or her.

◆ What are your feelings and reactions about people who are unable to share reality?

◆ How would you cope with being afraid of someone whose behaviors are out of contact with reality?

goals include psychosocial and vocational rehabilitation. When available, family members are included in the care and education of the client.

Treatments and Therapies

Clients with acute psychoses are treated with a combination of therapies and medications. The multidisciplinary treatment team may recommend "personal therapy, social skills training, vocational rehabilitation, and behavioral therapy. In addition, stress reduction, family education, and early intervention are important in the treatment of schizophrenia" (Kane and McGlashan, 1995). Although psychotherapies may focus on different areas of treatment, each relies on the therapeutic interactions of care providers.

Pharmacological Therapy

Medications used to treat psychoses are called *antipsychotic* or *neuroleptic drugs*. They are listed in Table 31-4.

The desired effects of antipsychotic drugs are to slow the central nervous system (CNS). These effects include an emotional quieting, slowed motor responses, and sedation. Antipsychotics exert their influence on the body by interrupting the dopamine (neurotransmitter) pathways in the brain, thus producing a calming effect throughout the entire nervous system. After an antipsychotic drug is taken, hallucinations and delusions are decreased, thought processes are changed, and hyperactivity subsides. Mental clouding clears, and previously withdrawn people begin to socialize.

Antipsychotic drugs interact with many other chemicals. They also have additive effects, that is, the combination of different drugs produces an enhanced effect, thus increasing CNS depression. The side effects

and adverse reactions of this group of medications are numerous and troublesome for the client. In fact, as many as half the clients who are prescribed antipsychotics do not actually take them or do not take them according to directions because of the side effects. Individuals who abuse alcohol and drugs are more likely to neglect taking their antipsychotic medications. Refer to Antipsychotic (Neuroleptic) Medications in Chapter 7 for a discussion of side effects and adverse reactions.

Nursing Process

Caring for clients with psychoses requires a team effort. First, a thorough physical and mental assessment is obtained. Histories include a description of the client's most distressing problems and a complete review of systems if the client is able to communicate appropriately. Interpersonal relationships and support systems are also explored.

The mental status examination is performed (see Chapter 13). Safety risks for violence and suicide are assessed, and a past medication history is taken. After the data are obtained and organized, both care team and nursing diagnoses are established. Primary nursing diagnoses include altered thought processes, social isolation, impaired communications, and ineffective management of therapeutic regimen. Box 31-1 offers several important general principles for working with schizophrenic and other psychotic clients.

Table 31-4	Drugs Used to Treat Psychosis (Antipsychotics)
Class	**Examples**
High-potency antipsychotics	fluphenazine (Prolixin), haloperidol (Haldol), thiothixene (Navane), trifluoperazine (Stelazine).
Moderate-potency antipsychotics	loxapine (Loxitane), molindone (Moban), and perphenazine (Trilafon).
Low-potency antipsychotics	chlorpromazine (Thorazine), mesoridazine (Serentil), and thioridazine (Mellaril).
Atypicals	clozapine (Clozaril), olanzapine (Zyprexa), quetiapine (Seroquel), and risperidone (Risperdal).

Box 31-1 Interventions for Clients With Psychotic Disorders

Maintain health and safety.
Establish a trusting interpersonal relationship.
Confirm the client's identity.
Orient the client to reality.
Assist the client in communication to help the client understand and be understood.
Decrease psychosocial stressors and demanding situations.
Help the client manage anxiety.
Encourage responsibility for self.
Promote compliance with prescribed therapeutic regimen.
Assist with activities of daily living.
Promote social interaction.
Regulate activity levels.
Encourage and praise socially acceptable behaviors.
Encourage family involvement and understanding.
Teach the client to identify stressors and how to recognize, manage, and prevent symptoms.
Educate client and family about side effects and toxic effects of antipsychotic medications.

Modified from Fortinash KM, Holoday-Worret PA: *Psychiatric nursing care plans*, ed 3, St. Louis, 1998, Mosby.

The basic goals of care are to assist clients in controlling their symptoms and achieving the highest possible level of functioning. For this to happen, clients and their families must be actively involved in the treatment. The expected outcome is for the client to live, learn, and work at the maximum possible level of success as defined by the individual. Short-term goals relate to keeping the client safe, restoring adequate nutritional and rest habits, establishing and maintaining contact with reality, and fostering open communications. A Sample Client Care Plan for schizophrenia is described.

Special Considerations

Because antipsychotic medications affect the body's nervous system, they are potentially harmful chemicals. Several special nursing assessments, interventions, and evaluations are required for clients who are receiving these powerful chemicals. Some side effects are harmless, some are uncomfortable, and others are life-threatening. The most common side effects of antipsychotic medications are alterations in the CNS and peripheral nervous system functions. Central nervous system alterations include **extrapyramidal side effects (EPSEs),** best described as "abnormal involuntary movement disorders [that] develop because of a drug-induced imbalance between two major neurotransmitters, dopamine and acetylcholine, in portions of the brain" (Keltner and Folks, 1997). As many as 75% of clients will experience EPSEs while taking these medications. The low-potency antipsychotics, such as chlorpromazine (Thorazine), are more likely to cause sedation and anticholinergic side effects (dry mouth, blurred vision or urinary retention). The high-potency antipsychotics, such as haloperidol (Haldol), are less sedating and anticholinergic, but they have an increased risk of extrapyramidal side effects.

Extrapyramidal side effects include akathisia, akinesia, dyskinesia, dystonia, and drug-induced parkinsonism. The most serious side effects are neuroleptic malignant syndrome and tardive dyskinesia. All these symptoms arise from a lack of dopamine in the brain and the subsequent blocking of nerve transmissions.

Akathisia is an inability to sit still. Clients experiencing akathisia report that they feel nervous and jittery or have lots of nervous energy. Assaultive behaviors can result if they are forced to remain in one position for even a short period of time. Many clients stop taking their medications because of these side effects. The best treatment for akathisia is to reduce the dose of antipsychotic medication. Nurses must be careful not to evaluate the signs and symptoms of akathisia as a worsening of the client's psychosis. If a prn antipsychotic drug is administered at this time, it will cause an *increase* in the client's symptoms.

Akinesia means the absence of movement, both physically and mentally. Actually, clients who are experiencing this unwanted effect demonstrate **bradykinesia** (slowing of body movements and a diminished mental state). Clients lack spontaneity and do not try to move or speak. They may assume bizarre postures and maintain them for long periods. Here is another case for careful assessment because many of the behaviors associated with EPSEs are very similar to the behaviors for which the clients sought treatment. Astute nurses who routinely observe their clients' behaviors stand a better chance of distinguishing between drug-induced or psychosis-induced behaviors.

Dyskinesia is characterized by involuntary abnormal skeletal muscle movements. They are usually seen as jerking motions and sometimes seriously interfere with the client's ability to walk and perform other voluntary movements.

Dystonia is impaired muscle tone. Dystonic reactions produce rigidity in the muscles that control gait, posture, and eye movements. When dystonia involves the muscles that control eye movements, the eyes involuntarily roll to the back of the head. This side effect is called **oculogyric crisis,** and it is a frightening experience for the client.

Another unsettling dystonic reaction is **torticollis,** in which contracted cervical muscles force the neck into a twisted position. But the most serious and potentially life-threatening side effect is **laryngeal-pharyngeal dystonia.** When the muscles of the throat become rigid, the client begins to gag, choke, and become cyanotic. Respiratory distress and asphyxia result if immediate intervention does not occur. Anticholinergic drugs are used to treat all of these reactions.

Drug-induced parkinsonism is a term used to describe a group of symptoms that mimics Parkinson's disease. Tremors, muscle rigidity, and difficulty with voluntary movements are seen in clients with Parkinson's disease and some individuals undergoing antipsychotic drug therapy. Other unwanted CNS effects of neuroleptic drugs include seizures, which can occur at any time during therapy. The drug clozapine (Clozaril) appears to be associated with a higher incidence of seizures, so clients taking this medication must be carefully monitored for signs of seizure activity.

Neuroleptic malignant syndrome (NMS) is a potentially fatal extrapyramidal side effect of antipsychotic medications. The condition is poorly understood and frequently underdiagnosed. Death can occur from respiratory failure, kidney failure, aspiration pneumonia, or pulmonary emboli. Although NMS is usually associated with the high-potency antipsychotics, it can occur with many other dopamine-altering drugs.

Neuroleptic malignant syndrome occurs more often when two or more psychotherapeutic drugs are combined. When lithium is used with a psychotherapeutic drug or depot (oil-based, long-acting) injections are given,

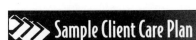

Sample Client Care Plan   Schizophrenia

Assessment

History: Terry, a 22-year-old man, was found wandering naked in the streets talking to himself. He seems preoccupied and appears to be listening to voices. Further history is unobtainable because Terry is unable to communicate understandably at this time.

Current Findings: A wild-eyed, unkempt young man who is preoccupied. Clothes are ragged and dirty. Speech is unintelligible; he carries on animated conversations with himself. Since admission, 24 hours ago, Terry has refused to eat, drink, or bathe because "someone is trying to poison" him. He is polite but responds only when addressed. No family or friends can be located.

Multidisciplinary Diagnosis

Sensory/perceptual alteration related to social isolation and lack of adequate support systems.

Planning/Goals

Terry will communicate in a logical manner within 15 days after admission.

Terry will carry out his activities of daily living independently within 25 days after admission.

Therapeutic Interventions

Intervention	Rationale	Team Member
1. Establish therapeutic relationship; be available, listen actively; do not pass judgment.	Trust must be established if therapy is to be effective.	All
2. Establish and reinforce a daily routine.	Increases security by knowing what to expect; helps refocus on the activities of daily living.	Nsg, All
3. Use clear, direct statements when talking; make sure body language is in keeping with the message being sent.	Unclear or confusing communications can increase Terry's distorted perceptions.	All
4. Intervene with active hallucinations; move Terry to quiet area, focus on reality, assure client that he will be safe, identify needs filled by the hallucination.	Decreases sensory input; helps divert attention to reality, provides reassurance; helps decrease anxiety.	Nsg, All
5. Accept and support Terry's feelings and appropriate expressions of emotion.	Communicating empathy and understanding decreases anxiety.	All
6. Encourage Terry to take his medications routinely.	Medications must be taken regularly to control psychotic symptoms.	Nsg, MD
7. Carefully monitor Terry's response to his medications.	Early recognition prevents serious side effects and complications.	Nsg
8. For discharge planning, explore the possibility of placement in an assisted living home.	A stable and predictable environment decreases acute psychotic episodes.	Soc Svc

Evaluation

Fifteen days after admission, Terry stated he was in control of his hallucinations. Twenty-five days after admission, Terry was independently eating, drinking, and performing his own activities of daily living, but he still required routine encouragement to bathe.

A complete client care plan includes several other diagnoses and interventions

clients are assessed frequently for signs of NMS. The development of NMS may occur suddenly after a single dose or after years of drug treatment. It is often associated with other extrapyramidal reactions such as dystonia and akathisia.

Symptoms of neuroleptic malignant syndrome begin with a sudden change in the client's level of consciousness and a rapid onset of rigid muscles. Often there is an associated respiratory difficulty, tremors, and an inability to speak; however, the cardinal sign of NMS is a high body temperature. Temperatures can reach as high as 108° F but usually range between 101° and 103° F. The temperatures of all clients receiving psychotherapeutic drugs must be frequently and routinely monitored. Without intervention, the client's physical condition declines rapidly.

Signs of autonomic nervous system dysfunctions are evident in NMS: tachycardia, rapid changes in blood pressure, increased perspiration (diaphoresis), incontinence, and rapid, labored respirations. Central nervous system alterations include sudden agitation, confusion, delirium, combativeness, and rigid posturing. The severe muscle rigidity leads to tissue breakdown, an increased white blood cell count, and possible kidney failure. No specific treatment exists for neuroleptic malignant syndrome. Supportive measures, including intensive respiratory care, are instituted, and administration of all medications that may be implicated in the development of NMS are stopped.

Subclinical (mild) cases of NMS have been reported. Nurses should suspect NMS in any client with signs or symptoms of pneumonia or urinary tract infection. Clients who have diaphoresis, tachycardia, an elevated white blood cell count, or any muscle rigidity may be experiencing NMS. Sudden changes in consciousness should always be investigated and reported.

Those who care for clients who are taking psychotherapeutic medication must be aware of the potential for the development of NMS. An action as simple and routine as obtaining vital signs may save the life of a client. Do not hesitate to notify your supervisor or physician if the client develops a sudden fever, changes in blood pressure, sudden changes in alertness, confusion, or altered levels of consciousness.

Tardive dyskinesia is a serious, irreversible side effect of long-term treatment. The word *tardive* means "appearing later." Dys means "difficult," and kinesis means "movement" in Greek. So the literal translation, "late difficult movement," explains the condition. Tardive dyskinesia is a drug-induced condition that produces involuntary, repeated movements of the muscles of the face, trunk, arms, and legs. Many clients exhibit the signs of tardive dyskinesia after several months or years of drug treatment. Others develop signs and symptoms after discontinuing their medications.

After a period of antipsychotic drug use, the body attempts to compensate for the lack of dopamine by developing hypersensitive receptors in the brain. When the brain is stimulated by dopamine, it overreacts and produces abnormal muscle movements. The elderly, especially women, and those who have had a stroke are at the greatest risk for developing tardive dyskinesia, but the symptoms are most severe in young men.

The signs and symptoms of tardive dyskinesia usually involve the facial muscles first. Box 31-2 lists the major signs and symptoms. Appendix C lists the AIMS assess-

> ### Box 31-2 Signs and Symptoms of Tardive Dyskinesia
>
> Protrusion of the tongue (fly-catcher sign)
> Puffing of cheeks or tongue in cheek (bonbon sign)
> Grinding of teeth, chewing, lateral jaw movements
> Lip smacking, puckering
> Grimacing, making faces, tics
> Blinking, squinting
> Impaired gag reflex (choking, aspiration)*
> Shrugging of shoulders
> Thrusting of pelvis
> Twitching of trunk, legs, and arms
> Toe movements, foot tapping
> Impaired diaphragmatic movements (breathing difficulties)*

*Potentially life threatening

ment tool. People who experience the effects of tardive dyskinesia are frightened at their lack of control. In addition, the sight of a person engaged in these unusual movements and behaviors can be unnerving for care providers. Sensitive, caring staff can help to ease the client's distress.

This condition is difficult to treat, and the effects are persistent. At this time tardive dyskinesia is considered irreversible except in the very early stages. Nursing measures for tardive dyskinesia include routine assessments and measures to prevent injuries. Clients with impaired gag reflexes may require soft foods. Be sure oropharyngeal suction devices are readily available. Teach every client and family member how to recognize the signs and symptoms of tardive dyskinesia.

Most medications are not effective for the treatment of tardive dyskinesia, but some success has been reported with the drugs bromocriptine (Parlodel), reserpine, and clonazepam (Klonopin). Vitamin E was recently found to be effective.

Undesired effects of antipsychotic drugs also influence the peripheral nervous system. The anticholinergic effects of dry mouth, blurred vision, urinary retention, and photophobia (sensitivity to bright light) are common, especially during the first few days of therapy. Tachycardia is a more serious side effect and can cause sudden death.

Hypotension is another potentially serious anticholinergic side effect. Nurses must protect clients from falls during the first few weeks of therapy because the hypotensive response is greatest when clients stand or change positions suddenly. These hypotensive episodes cause tachycardia as the body attempts to adapt to a lower blood pressure. Antipsychotic drugs are contraindicated in clients who have a history of low blood pressure, cardiac dysrhythmias, or heart failure. Table 31-5 lists the major side effects of antipsychotic medications.

Table 31-5 Side Effects of Antipsychotic Drugs and Nursing Care

Side effects	Interventions
Peripheral Nervous System Effects	
Constipation	Encourage high-fiber diet; increase water intake; give laxatives as ordered.
Dry mouth	Sip of water frequently; provide sugarless hard candies, sugarless gum, and mouth rinses.
Nasal congestion	Give over-the-counter nasal decongestant if approved by physician.
Blurred vision	Advise client to avoid potentially dangerous tasks. Reassure client that normal vision typically returns in a few weeks when tolerance develops. Pilocarpine eyedrops can be used on a short-term basis.
Mydriasis	Advise client to report eye pain immediately.
Photophobia	Advise client to wear sunglasses outdoors.
Hypotension or orthostatic hypotension	Ask client to get out of bed or chair slowly. Client should sit on the side of the bed for 1 full minute while dangling feet, then slowly rise. If hypotension is a problem, measure blood pressure before each dose is given.
Tachycardia	Tachycardia is usually a reflex response to hypotension. When intervention for hypotension (previously described) is effective, reflex tachycardia usually decreases. With clozapine, hold the dose if pulse rate is greater than 140 pulsations per minute.
Urinary retention	Encourage voiding whenever the urge is present. Catheterize for residual fluids. Ask client to monitor urine output and report output to nurse. Older men with benign prostatic hypertrophy are particularly susceptible to urinary retention.
Urinary hesitation	Provide privacy, run water in the sink, or run warm water over the perineum.
Sedation	Help patient get up early and get the day started.
Weight gain	Help patient order an appropriate diet; diet pills should not be taken.
Agranulocytosis	A high incidence of agranulocytosis (1% to 2%) is associated with clozapine. White blood cell count (WBC) should be performed weekly.
Central Nervous System Effects	
Akathisia	Be patient and reassure client who is "jittery" that you understand the need to move. Since akathisia is the chief cause of noncompliance with antipsychotic regimens, switching to a different class of antipsychotic drug may be necessary to achieve compliance.
Dystonias	If a severe reaction such as oculogyric crisis or torticollis occurs, give antiparkinson drug (e.g., benztropine mesylate [Cogentin]) or antihistamine (e.g., diphenhydramine [Benadryl]) immediately, as needed, and offer reassurance. Call the physician at once to obtain an order for intramuscular administration. For less severe dystonias, notify the physician when an order for an antiparkinson drug is warranted.
Drug-induced parkinsonism	Assess for the three major parkinsonism symptoms—tremors, rigidity, and bradykinesia—and report to physician. Antiparkinson drugs may be indicated.
Tardive dyskinesia	Assess for signs by using the abnormal inventory movement scale. Drug holidays may help prevent tardive dyskinesia. Anticholinergic agents will *worsen* tardive dyskinesia. Young men taking large doses of high-potency antipsychotic drugs (e.g., haloperidol) may be prescribed prophylactic antiparkinson drugs.
Neuroleptic malignant syndrome	Be alert for this *potentially fatal* side effect. Routinely take temperatures and encourage adequate water intake among all clients on a regimen of antipsychotic drugs, and routinely assess for rigidity, tremor, and similar symptoms.
Seizures	Seizures occur in approximately 1% of clients receiving antipsychotic drug treatment. Clozapine causes an even higher rate, up to 5% of patients taking 600 to 900 mg/day. Use seizure precautions. Document and report any seizure activity.

Special Considerations

Nurses have three major responsibilities when caring for clients who are receiving antipsychotic drug therapy. The first relates to drug administration. Nurses should review the desired actions, side effects, and incompatibilities for each medication prescribed. If the drugs are administered intramuscularly, choose a large muscle mass, warn the client of a burning sensation on injection, and rotate injection sites. If liquid preparations are ordered, be sure to follow the instructions for dilution. Some neuroleptic drugs cannot be mixed with water, so read the manufacturer's instructions before diluting any liquid medication.

Box 31-3 Client and Family Education: Antipsychotic Drugs

Review the expected benefits and possible side effects of drug therapy with the patient and family. Review extrapyramidal side effects. Because there is no effective treatment for tardive dyskinesia, signs or symptoms should be reported immediately. Fine vermicular (wormlike) movements of the tongue may be the first sign of this side effect.

Instruct client and family to *report any new signs or symptoms*.

Help clients understand that several weeks of drug use may be necessary before a benefit is received.

Instruct clients to swallow extended-release forms whole; do not crush or chew.

Warn clients to avoid driving or operating hazardous equipment and notify the physician if vision changes or sedation occurs.

Instruct client to report signs of agranulocytosis, including sore throat, fever, and malaise. Tell clients to report signs of liver dysfunction, including jaundice, malaise, fever, and right upper quadrant abdominal pain.

These drugs may interfere with the body's ability to regulate temperature. Warn clients to avoid prolonged exposure to extreme temperatures, allow for frequent cooling-off periods when exercising or in hot environments, and dress warmly for exposure to the cold.

Review possible endocrine side effects with client and family. Assess carefully and tactfully for these side effects. Provide emotional support as appropriate. If side effects are intolerable, consult the physician for possible drug or dosage change.

Instruct clients to monitor weight (if possible). If weight gain is a problem, counsel about low-calorie diets. Refer to a dietitian as needed.

Stress the importance of informing all health care providers of all drugs being taken.

Warn clients to avoid over-the-counter drugs unless first approved by the physician.

Caution clients to avoid alcoholic beverages while taking antipsychotics.

Warn diabetic clients that antipsychotics may alter blood glucose levels. Monitor blood glucose levels carefully. Consult the physician about changes in dietary or drug treatment for diabetes.

Tell clients not to discontinue therapy abruptly or without discussion with the physician.

Instruct clients to keep these and all drugs out of the reach of children.

The drugs may produce false-positive pregnancy results. Women who suspect they are pregnant should consult the physician. Women may desire to use contraceptive measures while taking these drugs; counsel as appropriate. As always, pregnant or lactating women should avoid all drugs, if possible.

If additional drugs are prescribed to treat side effects of antipsychotic agents, review their use and side effects with the client and family.

Modified from Clark JF, Queener SF, Karb VB: *Pharmacological basis of nursing practice*, ed 5, St. Louis, 1997, Mosby.

Read all labels carefully. Some parenteral drugs are water based, and others are oil based. Oil-based medications are never given intravenously. They are intended for intramuscular use only. The drug class called the phenothiazines has been known to cause contact dermatitis, so avoid getting it on the skin. Wash your hands after every contact, and wear gloves if you frequently handle phenothiazines.

The second major nursing responsibility relates to monitoring client responses to each medication. During the first week or two of therapy, assess the client's vital signs every 4 hours, record fluid intake and output, and routinely assess skin condition. Assess frequently for signs or symptoms of side effects.

Nurses must constantly remain vigilant to the occurrence of side effects with each medication prescribed. Thoroughly assess clients before administering any prn drug because a medication will actually worsen symptoms if the nurse is not able to tell a side effect from a behavior. Clients who are receiving antipsychotic drugs are at risk for developing neuroleptic malignant syndrome and tardive dyskinesia. Accurate identification of their signs and symptoms early helps prevent permanent problems.

The third nursing responsibility, client and family education, has a direct impact on the client's level of functioning. One of the primary tasks of nurses is to assist clients in coping with their daily living activities. When the client and family learn about the client's medications, treatment can be more successful. Box 31-3 lists the most important points of client and family education.

Keep these general guidelines in mind. Get to know the clients for whom you are caring. The more you know about the person, the better you will be able to tell the difference between behaviors that are related to the effects of medication and those that belong to the client. Antipsychotic drugs are powerful medications. They demand to be treated with respect and require knowledge from those who receive them and those who work with them.

Caring for persons with psychoses is one of the most challenging areas of mental health. Hospitalization and education are only the beginning steps in a long road toward optimal functioning. Relapse is common. Continued treatment and support are needed for family members and clients alike if we are to cope with the devastating effects of schizophrenia and other serious psychotic mental illnesses.

KEY CONCEPTS

- A psychosis is a disorder in which there is an inability to recognize reality, relate to others, or cope with life's demands.
- Neurobiological responses can range from adaptive contact with reality to disorganized thoughts, emotions, and behaviors.
- Although the majority of psychoses are encountered primarily in late adolescence or adulthood, some do present in childhood.
- Today scientific evidence points to possible biological (physical) causes for psychotic behaviors.
- Schizophrenia is a group of related mental health disorders characterized by disordered perceptions, thinking, and behavior.
- The five subtypes of schizophrenia are catatonic, disorganized, paranoid, residual, and undifferentiated.
- Other psychotic disorders include brief psychotic disorder, delusional disorder, and psychoses related to medical conditions or drug use.
- The treatment goals for inpatient, short-term care are to stabilize the client, prevent further decline in functioning, and assist the client in coping with his or her disorder.
- Long-term goals include psychosocial and vocational rehabilitation when possible.
- Clients with acute psychoses are treated with a combination of therapies and medications.
- Antipsychotic drugs, which may take weeks to become effective, help to stabilize behaviors.
- Psychosocial therapies include personal therapy, social skills training, vocational rehabilitation, and behavioral therapy, stress reduction, and family education.
- Several special nursing assessments, interventions, and evaluations are required for clients who are receiving powerful antipsychotic medications.

Suggestions for Further Reading

If you are interested in how people live with schizophrenia, read E. Fuller Torrey's *Surviving Schizophrenia: A Family Manual* (New York, 1983, Harper & Row).

The Schizophrenia Home Page (www.schizophrenia.com) offers much information relating to psychotic conditions and treatments.

References

Amadio PB, Cross LB, Amadio P: New drugs for schizophrenia: an update for family physicians, *American Family Physician* 56(4): 1149, 1997.

American Psychiatric Association: *Diagnostic and statistical manual of mental disorders,* ed 4, text revision, Washington, DC, 2000, The Association.

Bower B: New culprits for schizophrenia, *Science News* 149(5):68, 1996.

Clark JF, Queener SF, Karb VB: *Pharmacological basis of nursing practice,* ed 5, St. Louis, 1997, Mosby.

Fortinash KM, Holoday-Worret PA: *Psychiatric mental health nursing,* ed 2, St. Louis, 1999, Mosby.

Fortinash KM, Holoday-Worret PA: *Psychiatric nursing care plans,* ed 3, St. Louis, 1998, Mosby.

Giger JN, Davidhizer RE: *Transcultural nursing: assessment and intervention,* ed 3, St. Louis, 1999, Mosby.

Herbert W: Fearsome madness: schizophrenia remains frustratingly hard to control, *U.S. News & World Report* 125(6):53, 1998.

Kane JM, McGlashan TH: Treatment of schizophrenia, *Lancet* 346(8978):820, 1995.

Keltner NL, Folks DG: *Psychotropic drugs,* ed 2, St. Louis, 1997, Mosby.

Rodriquez-Ferrera S, Vassilas CA: Older people with schizophrenia: providing services for a neglected group—it's the quality of their environment that matters, not where it is, *British Medical Journal* 317(7154):292, 1998.

Schultz SK, Andreasen NC: Schizophrenia, *Lancet* 353(9):1425, 1999.

Stuart GW, Laraia MT: *Principles and practice of psychiatric nursing,* ed 7, St. Louis, 2001, Mosby.

Wong DL: *Whaley and Wong's nursing care of infants and children,* ed 6, St. Louis, 1998, Mosby.

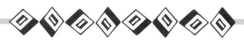

Chapter 32

Chronic Mental Health Disorders

Learning Objectives

1. Describe the experience of mental illness from a client's viewpoint.
2. Explain how deinstitutionalization has affected the delivery of mental health care in the United States.
3. Outline three psychological and three biological characteristics of chronic mental illness.
4. Explain how children and adolescents can be affected by chronic mental health problems.
5. Examine the connection between human immunodeficiency virus (HIV)/acquired immunodeficiency syndrome (AIDS) and mental illness.
6. Summarize the care for clients with multiple mental health problems.
7. Discuss three principles of psychiatric rehabilitation.
8. Apply the nursing (therapeutic) process to clients with chronic mental health disorders.
9. Plan seven basic interventions for clients who are chronically mentally disordered.

Key Terms

chemical restraint
chronic mental illness

comorbidity
exacerbations

psychiatric rehabilitation
remissions

The word *chronic* means long-lasting, persistent, or continual. Most chronic mental health problems are characterized by periods of exacerbations and remissions. **Exacerbations** are periods of dysfunction marked by an increase in the signs, symptoms, and seriousness of a problem. **Remissions** are times of partial or complete disappearance of symptoms. The course for chronic mental health problems follows this type of up-and-down pattern.

Many mental health problems are acute. They begin abruptly, increase in intensity, then subside after a short period of time. Persons with phobias, anxiety disorders, or depression often respond well to therapeutic interventions and have no further problems. However, for a certain group of individuals, being mentally ill becomes a way of life.

Chronic mental illness is the presence of one or more recurring psychiatric disorders that results in significantly impaired functional abilities. Individuals with chronic mental health problems are often referred to as CMI (chronic mentally ill) persons. Many people with chronic mental illness are contributing members of society, struggling to hold onto some degree of mental health. They are also the homeless, the criminals, and the odd neighbors down the street. They are our relatives, friends, and members of our community.

SCOPE OF MENTAL ILLNESS

Chronic mental disorders are disabling for people in every society and culture. Each year millions of individuals seek help for mental health problems. In the United States

Think About

Did you know that in any given year:

52 million adults experience a mental health disorder
28% seek mental health treatment
9 million people develop a mental disorder for the first time
8 million individuals suffer a relapse
35 million persons have continuing symptoms
The number of chronically mentally ill persons is relatively stable at about 28% of the total population

♦ What possible trends does an analysis of these statistics reveal?

2.8% of adults (more than 5 million) experience a mental disorder, but only a quarter of those affected seek help. "One in every five families is affected in their lifetime by a severe mental illness" (NAMI, 1999). See Think About box.

The estimated costs of treating persons with mental disorders is about 4% of total U.S. direct health care costs. Inpatient stays cost about 12 billion dollars a year (U.S. Bureau of the Census, 1998). When the social costs of lost productivity, shortened lives, and implementation of criminal justice are factored in, total costs are enormous.

The costs in terms of suffering cannot be estimated. Society encourages people to recover from acute mental disorders and resume normal daily activities, but it tends to ignore the needs of those persons who are (and will be) unable to cope independently with life. Chronic mental illness has social stigmas attached and being labeled as "crazy" keeps many people from seeking help.

Individuals with chronic mental health problems have much higher rates of suicide. Because mental health problems affect every area of functioning, each chronically mentally troubled person has a unique life experience. Many individuals handle their distressing symptoms by using alcohol, street drugs, or other chemicals. They must cope with an addiction in addition to their illness. Remember, though, that underneath every chronically mentally ill person lies a real person who is coping with personal problems and suffering from the stigmas of being labeled mentally ill.

PUBLIC POLICY AND MENTAL HEALTH

Today, chronically mentally ill individuals are cared for in the community. They are expected to provide for their basic needs, protect themselves, and seek help for their problems—all rather complex behaviors. The reality is that most of the chronically mentally ill are unable to meet these expectations.

Effects of Deinstitutionalization

When the first antipsychotic medications became available in the 1960s, chemical restraints replaced physical ones. A **chemical restraint** is a medication that reduces or eliminates psychotic symptoms and quiets behavior. People no longer had to be physically controlled, and the state psychiatric hospitals began to discharge long-term patients into the community through a practice called *deinstitutionalization*. The thought was that most people released from the state hospitals could live in the community with the proper support and aftercare. Unfortunately the aftercare, which was a critical part of the overall plan for providing community psychiatric services, failed to be implemented. Changing political parties and government policies chose to ignore the chronically mentally ill, thinking that everything would eventually work itself out. Today the consequences of our federal mental health policy can be seen in the ever-increasing numbers of homeless persons, prisoners, and county jail inmates.

EXPERIENCE OF CHRONIC MENTAL ILLNESS

What is it like to be chronically mentally ill? To face each day knowing the struggle ahead? To wonder if this day will bring acceptance and hope or the slide into "madness"?

Persons who face mental illness must cope with problems that are unknown to the rest of us. Individuals are often lumped into a group labeled CMIs and stripped of their identity, dignity, convictions, and feelings. They lack choice, respect, and control, and they are expected to cooperate with therapies that make them feel sick. The Case Study box allows a glimpse into the world of one chronically mentally ill individual. Hopefully, this true account will serve as a reminder that each client is truly a unique individual and should be viewed as such.

Meeting Basic Needs

The issues facing mentally troubled individuals are the same as those with which the rest of us must cope: adequate food, shelter and clothing; gainful employment; and access to health care. People with chronic mental illness must strive to meet their needs on a daily basis. The majority live with their families. Because their disorders prevent them from planning or logically carrying out an activity, many of the chronically mentally ill are homeless, hungry, and unable to care for themselves. The seriously mentally ill, who make up one third of the total homeless population (Torry and Zdanowicz, 1999), can be seen on street corners chatting amiably with or responding to voices in their heads.

Many of our society's mentally ill are now housed in county jails and prisons, awaiting available beds in the few state institutions that remain. Other mentally ill

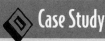

Case Study

The following was modified from the words of Betty Blaska (1991):

You spend the whole first night crying because you don't want to be here. There must be some awful mistake. You are very naive, only 18. You're not yet a CMI (chronic mentally ill). Next day the "staffing" (as they call it) is very intimidating. The hospital's brass are all there, and they just chuckle when you tell them you do not want to stay. They patronize you: "Oh, we think we will just keep you here for a while." You don't know it yet, but you are on the way to becoming a CMI.

◆ ◆ ◆

The first time you experience dystonia from the drugs they've given you, you are extremely frightened. Your tongue is rigid and you can't control its movements. You rush to the nurse's station where they are huddled inside their little cage. No one comes out for fear of contamination. They are puzzled by your presence, but you can't speak because of your tongue's movements. They wait impatiently for you to tell them what is wrong. You wonder what is wrong with them. Can't they see your problem? But, no—it's not that they don't see. They don't feel, because you don't count. You are on the way to becoming a CMI.

◆ ◆ ◆

After your first discharge, you are loaded up on medications, and your follow-up therapist announces that he will not continue with you unless you come in with your family for therapy. But there are eight of you scattered all over the state. And they don't want to come, anyway,

because they have been belittled and browbeaten too much already. So the therapist refuses to see you. And he refuses to refill your prescriptions. So you go through withdrawal. And you end up back on the same psych ward. And then they say to you accusingly: "Why did you go off your medicines?" It's then you realize: You're a CMI.

◆ ◆ ◆

You've been in and out of hospitals, seen numerous mental health professionals (some stranger than you), and been off and on loads of psychoactive drugs, given in doses you complain are too high, and in combinations that you complain are too much. And there are the side effects—nausea, diarrhea, dizziness. Vision so bad that you are afraid to cross the street. Drug-induced psychoses so bad you can't leave your bed or look out the window because of the terror you feel. Blood pressure so low that you can't stand for very long, and a voice so weak that you can't be heard across a telephone.

Oh great! Now you're without a job. So they send you to a place called Vocational Rehabilitation where they "help" you get a clerical job. Never mind that you have a degree—or two. You get the clerical job because you are a woman. A woman CMI. But the men CMIs are just as lucky. They get to become janitors! Now you are truly a full-fledged CMI.

◆ What "labels"(stigmas and stereotypes) is this person coping with?
◆ How has reading this case study changed your impressions of the mentally ill experience?

persons are jailed on "dine-and-dash" charges (eating a restaurant meal they cannot pay for) or as "mercy bookings" just to get them off the streets and provide some basic needs. State prisons are also feeling the increase in mentally ill inmates. It is estimated that 10% to 15% of inmates in state prisons suffer from mental illness.

The chronically mentally ill persons who do manage to provide for their own basic needs must struggle with the labels and expectations of others. Often it is difficult for them to remain employed for long periods because of the occasional relapse. As one chronic mental health client put it, "I am an effective, loyal worker for over 90% of the time, but the 10% of the time I have troubles are all that's remembered."

Poverty and mental illness go hand in hand. Although many mentally troubled persons receive some financial assistance, most are unable to plan or use the money wisely. Because about half the severely mentally ill population abuse alcohol or drugs, few dollars are spent on life's necessities. Today it is estimated that more than a quarter million severely mentally ill individuals are

living on the streets, in public shelters, in jails, and in prisons (Figure 32-1).

Access to Health Care

Until the time of community psychiatric care, people with severe or chronic mental health problems were treated (or at least provided with custodial care) through state programs. With ongoing therapy and medications, many people with chronic mental disorders could be returned to their communities and function effectively. However, community support was often not available after hospitalization, and many individuals once again fell victim to their psychoses.

Only this time the tightened admission policies of most institutions did not allow most of the chronically mentally ill back, and they were forced to cope with their disorders the best they could. Other mentally ill persons became involved in the revolving door syndrome, a cycle of repeated short hospital admissions and discharges. This in-and-out-of-the-institution behavior is also called *recidivism*.

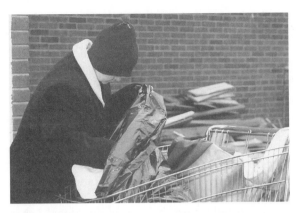

Figure 32-1 A "bag lady" with her personal belongings. (Copyright © Cathy Lander-Goldberg, Lander Photographics.)

Today a new generation of chronically mentally ill persons is emerging, known as the young chronically mentally ill. These individuals are young (18 to 35) and severely ill. Most have never sought treatment. Those who do receive treatment commonly refuse to follow therapeutic advice. "They lack internal controls, rarely take psychotropic medications, and exhibit excessive drug and alcohol abuse" (Fortinash and Holoday-Worret, 1999). Many self-medicate to relieve distressing symptoms. Cocaine is often used by persons with mood disorders, whereas alcohol is likely to be used by schizophrenics. Heroin is usually preferred by individuals with conduct disorders. Many of the young mentally ill are polysubstance abusers, that is, they use a variety of different chemical substances, sometimes in combination.

Access to health care is limited in the United States today. Currently as many as 25% of the population have no health insurance at all (U.S. Bureau of the Census, 1998). For many of those who do, mental health services are capped or limited to a certain amount of money per person. Individuals who are suffering from chronic mental problems are often unable to plan for or manage their health care because of their illness, even if they are fortunate to have some sort of insured coverage. Many refuse shelter or treatment because of their paranoia, believing people will harm them.

People with mental health problems also have physical problems. It is estimated that 50% of the mentally ill suffer from a medical disorder. People with mental illness live an average of 10 to 15 years less than the general population (Farnam and others, 1999).

On the other hand, people who want to receive treatment often find that services are inadequate or unavailable. Even when they are admitted to an institution, their stay may not be long enough to improve their condition. Supportive outpatient services that are the basis for supporting the mentally ill person in the community either may not be available or may be refused by the individual. Access to comprehensive mental health care remains a problem today. That is why every health

care provider must be prepared to recognize and assist those individuals whose only crimes are being too mentally disordered to effectively care for themselves.

CHARACTERISTICS OF CHRONIC MENTAL ILLNESS

Each person's experiences with mental illness is unique. Diagnoses serve only to group together and label certain behaviors. The real meaning of being "depressed" or "schizophrenic" can be found only within the individual who suffers from the distresses associated with the particular label.

Many mentally troubled persons can be labeled with more than one psychiatric diagnosis. Schizophrenics frequently suffer from severe depression after an acute psychotic episode. Suicidal gestures increase as depressed persons begin to stabilize from their medications and see the hopelessness of their situations. Persons with personality disorders may have disturbing phobias or anxiety. However, the experience and suffering of living with these labels is unique with each individual. Certain features are common to all persons who must live with mental illness. For the sake of discussion, these characteristics are divided into two categories: psychological characteristics and behavioral characteristics.

Psychological Characteristics

Chronically mentally ill individuals have several intellectual, emotional, social, and spiritual features in common. Intellectually, altered thought processes disrupt their abilities to think clearly, solve problems, or make plans. Hallucinations, delusions, and obsessive thoughts are unwelcome intrusions that routinely disrupt the flow of logical, reality-based thinking. Fear, mistrust, and paranoia can complicate the picture by presenting problems with daily living activities.

Chronic low self-esteem follows the label of mental illness everywhere. The ability to make logical sense out of life is hampered by the many distresses of being mentally ill. Even when one is adapting effectively, the stigma of being odd, crazy, or eccentric is dragged behind each action. Other people feel uncomfortable and avoid interacting, thus reinforcing the differences between "sick" and "well."

Mentally troubled people often see themselves as helpless, ineffective, and incapable of change. The experience of a small success will often prevent them from making any further attempts because they "just know" that they will eventually fail. When the self-concept is that low, it is difficult to convince someone that a brighter future can exist.

Depression is a partner of many mental health disorders, which makes a difficult life even more distressing. Depressive episodes can occur when an individual is coping with stress or in association with a psychotic episode. Even when they are functioning effectively, depression can be a companion for many mentally troubled persons. Prudent nurses assess each client for the presence of depressive symptoms.

Loneliness is the suffering that results when one is isolated from other people. People need associations, and they suffer when removed from the company of others. Individuals with chronic mental health problems are usually very lonely. Their basic needs for love and belonging go unmet, and they respond by becoming more emotionally paralyzed.

Starved for social interactions, some chronically mentally ill persons go to great lengths, such as criminal or violent activity, to gain attention. Others withdraw from society, fearing further rejection, and live a life of mistrust and solitude. Those who do have social interactions often are unable to express themselves, make decisions, or adapt to certain social roles. As the distress of attempting to cope socially increases, many find that retreating into their illness is an easier course to follow than struggling with the complexities of interacting with other people.

Another characteristic of chronic mental illness is hopelessness, the catalyst for suicide. The struggle for mental health consumes much energy. Feelings of worthlessness plague self-esteem and lead to depression. Hopelessness brings with it the feeling that there are no solutions to one's problems, that life is destined to remain distressful, and that the only way to relieve the pain is to destroy the sufferer.

Behavioral Characteristics

The nature of one's mental disorder determines the level of disability. Persons who suffer from chronic mental illness often have difficulty assuming the behaviors and activities that are required for successful living. Impaired judgment, lack of motivation, or altered realities often lead to an inability to perform even the most basic activities. Individuals may lack a knowledge of personal grooming habits, table manners, or expected social behaviors. They may have difficulty relating to others. Often they are unable to function socially or occupationally, and assaultive behaviors or criminal activities may be present. The majority of chronically mentally ill individuals are dependent on others for their care. Many times, this involves living with family members or in group homes. For those who try to live independently, it all too often means a life of homeless shelters and nameless streets.

Sexuality and the sexual behaviors of chronically mentally disordered persons pose a concern for health care providers because the sexual practices of this group place them at an increased risk for contracting and sharing sexually transmitted diseases, such as human immunodeficiency virus (HIV)/acquired immunodeficiency syndrome (AIDS). Research into the sexual behaviors of the chronically mentally ill revealed that

more than half of the clients screened were at a high risk for contracting HIV infection because of drug use and sexual practices. Studies regarding the knowledge of HIV/AIDS and its risk behaviors demonstrated that the chronically mentally ill participants "knew significantly less about AIDS than a comparison sample of public high school students" (Katz, Watts, and Santman, 1994). Clearly these individuals need education to prevent the increase of HIV infection, and this is one of the greatest challenges for nurses today.

Violence is an unfortunate aspect of many chronically mentally troubled people. The inability to solve problems, make sound judgments, or control emotional behaviors makes some individuals a threat to the safety and well-being of others. Family members, especially children, frequently become the targets for anger and aggression. Life within the community becomes difficult for persons who behave violently because violent behavior almost always leads to extensive contact with the criminal justice system. Stays in county jails or prisons do little to address the issues underlying violence. Many potentially dangerous individuals are released back into the community under the banner of self-determination and individual rights (Howd, 1998). Society's response to the problems posed by these individuals reflects the attitude toward people with severe chronic mental illness in general.

SPECIAL POPULATIONS

Chronic mental health problems can begin at any stage in life, but they are often not noticed until early or middle adulthood. Children, adolescents, adults, and the elderly all suffer from the difficulties of chronic mental illness, but each group poses some unique and special problems that affect their abilities to respond to mental health interventions.

Children and Adolescents With Chronic Mental Illness

The seeds of many adult mental health problems are planted in childhood. However, some children must learn to cope with psychological impairments early in life. Children with mental retardation (an IQ below 70 with impairments in functioning) have problems with the intellectual and emotional aspects of life. Also, people who are mildly or moderately retarded "are believed to be more susceptible to mental illness" (Fortinash and Holoday-Worret, 1999). Emotional problems, such as anxiety or depression, often accompany the challenges faced by these individuals. Also, conflicts between expectations and actual abilities may result in the development of a personality disorder or psychosis.

Children with autism are in a world of their own. Because they do not develop the ability to respond to and communicate their needs, they remain dependent on others, sometimes throughout their lives. Without the help and care of others, these children could not survive reality.

Health care providers play important roles in the care of autistic individuals and their families. Occupational therapy teams and nurses focus on the skills needed for daily activities. Psychologists and special education teachers measure functional abilities and encourage skill development, and psychiatrists monitor clients' overall progress. All provide emotional support and information.

Childhood schizophrenia, although uncommon, does occur and almost always develops into a chronic mental health problem. Other children at risk for developing chronic mental health problems include those who have been neglected, repeatedly abused or mistreated, and those who have witnessed or experienced violence. Children with conduct disorders, attention-deficit hyperactivity disorders, and depression also have a greater risk of developing a chronic mental health disorder.

During adolescence many maladaptive behaviors become ingrained and new ones are developed. Because all parts of an individual are related, adolescents with chronic physical health problems, such as arthritis, diabetes, and cystic fibrosis, commonly experience psychological problems as well. Teens with diabetes have high rates of depression and suicidal behaviors.

Several chronic mental health problems develop during adolescence. Eating disorders, personality disorders, and schizophrenia can begin during the teenage years. Depression can become a long-standing problem with adolescents who have not learned to cope successfully. The road to chemical dependency most frequently begins in adolescence. The effects of posttraumatic stress can lead teens to stress-reducing but maladaptive behaviors that, over time become daily patterns of ineffective functioning.

Older Adults With Chronic Mental Illness

The elderly with chronic mental illness fall into two groups: those who have had mental health problems for decades and those who were diagnosed with a mental disorder after age 50. The most common acquired mental health problems in older adulthood are Alzheimer's disease and other dementias. "As many as 20% of elderly persons over the age of 80 suffer from some form of dementia" (Fortinash and Holoday-Worret, 1999). Depression is another frequent chronic mental health problem of older adults, especially if it is accompanied by sensory losses and communication impairments.

The social epidemic of crack cocaine and other drug use has resulted in a whole new group of primary care providers in this country: grandparents who must raise a second family, their grandchildren. Because of the increase in drug abuse, violence, and chronic behavioral problems that leave adult children incapable of raising their children, many older adults have assumed the primary responsibility and care for their grandchildren.

At a time when individuals should be looking forward to personal freedom and decreased responsibilities, the prospect of spending another 15 to 20 years raising more children can be overwhelming. Health care providers work to address the issues of grandparents suffering from the strain of caring for the children of addicts. The mental health of at least two generations depends on timely and supportive health care interventions.

Persons With Multiple Disorders

The word **comorbidity** refers to the presence of two or more mental health disorders. Individuals with a dual diagnosis are suffering from two mental health disorders, one of which is usually substance related. The depressed person who uses cocaine is an example. Substance abuse and mental illness result in an interactive process that can be seen in physical, psychological, and behavioral patterns that are different from those of persons with just an addiction or serious mental illness.

As many as 75% of individuals with chronic mental illness use or abuse drugs. These people present a significant challenge for treatment because of the complexity of their disorders. The multidisciplinary treatment team seems to be the most promising approach for helping clients with comorbid disorders cope with their problems in each area of functioning.

PROVIDING CARE FOR THE CHRONICALLY MENTALLY ILL

People with chronic mental health problems are found everywhere in society. Today the majority of mental health care is provided within the community, outside the world of the institution. For this reason, each interaction between health care providers and clients usually addresses some issues or problems relating to mental health.

Inpatient Settings

Persons with chronic mental health problems are hospitalized only when their behaviors pose a threat to themselves or others. Even then it is often for only a short time. The average length of stay for mental illness is about 10 days (U.S. Bureau of the Census, 1998). Inpatient treatment settings for the chronically mentally ill include the acute care hospital, psychiatric unit of an acute care facility, state psychiatric institution, and private mental health facility.

State psychiatric institutions still provide care for more than 50% of all psychiatric inpatients; however, stays in all inpatient treatment settings are shorter, and readmissions more frequent. The pattern of admission, short stay in the institution, discharge, short stay in the community, and readmission (recidivism) remains a problem for many health care professionals and their chronically mentally ill clients. Frequently, high levels of stress precipitate acute psychotic behaviors. Table 32-1 lists several of the most common stressors that can trigger acute reactions and thus readmissions to inpatient care settings.

Outpatient Settings

Once an acute psychiatric episode has subsided, many chronically mentally disordered clients are discharged from the inpatient setting to halfway houses or other group-living environments. Aftercare programs range from partial hospitalization to sheltered living arrangements or home care, depending on the size, economics, and support of the community (see Cultural Aspects box).

The majority of people with chronic mental illness live with their families, who require much support to cope effectively. In some communities chronically mentally ill individuals live with therapeutic families in foster care programs. Unfortunately, more mental health care is need in settings such as homeless shelters, health clinics for the poor, jails, and prisons.

Psychiatric Rehabilitation

The concept of **psychiatric rehabilitation** focuses on assisting individuals with serious mental illness to effectively cope with their life situations. A multidisciplinary approach uses the special talents of physicians, psychologists, nurses, occupational and physical therapists, dietitians, and other specialists.

Each realm of human functioning is addressed during treatment. Physically, clients are assessed for and taught the skills needed to effectively perform the activities of daily living, including proper nutrition, activity, and rest habits. Emotional problems are explored, and clients are taught how to identify their feelings, control their anger, and reach their goals. Intellectually, clients are encouraged to problem solve and set goals. Occupational or vocational training allows individuals the opportunity for employment.

Involvement with psychiatric rehabilitation programs offers many opportunities for people with severe mental illness to meet their often neglected social needs. Many programs offer group therapies and opportunities to learn more socially appropriate behaviors. Some psychiatric rehabilitation programs lend spiritual help in the form of staff members, clergy, or referrals to the religious

---

 Cultural Aspects

When chronic mental health clients are cared for in community group housing situations, make sure to perform a complete cultural assessment. People from different cultures have different points of view about mental illness. Living with people from other cultures requires open communication and a willingness to accept other points of view. These qualities are often difficult to achieve, especially when one is mentally troubled.

Table 32-1	Common Triggers of Acute Psychotic Episodes	
Health	**Environment**	**Attitudes/Behaviors**
Poor nutrition	Hostile/critical enviornment	"Poor me" (low self-concept)
Lack of sleep	Housing difficulties (unsatisfactory housing)	"Hopeless" (lack of self-confidence)
Out of balance circadian rhythms		"I'm a failure" (loss of motivation to use skills)
Fatigue	Pressure to perform (loss of independent living)	"Lack of control" (demoralization)
Infection	Changes in life events, daily patterns of activity	Feeling overpowered by symptoms
Central nervous system drugs		"No one likes me" (unable to meet spiritual needs)
Impaired reasoning	Stress (lack of survival skills)	
Impaired information processing	Interpersonal difficulties	Looks/acts different from others same age, culture
Lack of exercise	Disruptions in interpersonal relationships	
Behavioral disorder		Poor social skills
Mood abnormalities	Loneliness (social isolation, lack of social support)	Aggressive behavior
Moderate to high levels of anxiety	Missed environmental cues	Violent behavior
	Job pressures (poor occupation skills)	Poor medication management
	Poor social skills	Poor symptom management
	Poverty	
	Lack of transportation (resources)	

From Stuart GW, Laraia MT: *Stuart and Sundeen's pocket guide to psychiatric nursing,* ed 4, St. Louis, 1998, Mosby.

organizations of the client's choice. Unfortunately there are too few psychiatric rehabilitation programs for the many individuals who truly need them.

THERAPEUTIC INTERVENTIONS

In 1978 the President's Commission on Mental Health recommended that persons with chronic mental disorders be treated in the least restrictive environment, which was defined as a setting that encouraged the "greatest degree of freedom, self-determination, autonomy, dignity, and integrity." However, the concept is not so easily implemented when clients are unable or unwilling to seek out or consent to treatment, and the funding for mental health care remains unstable.

Treatments and Therapies

Basic goals for chronically disordered mental health clients are to achieve stabilization and maintain the highest possible level of daily functioning. Therapies are designed for the individual based on identified problems, available resources, and the client's willingness to cooperate with the therapeutic regimen. Various individual and group therapies along with certain medications are usually recommended by the treatment team after a complete health assessment and consultation with the client.

With support and assistance many chronically mentally ill individuals are able to function outside the institution. However, a number of problems or situations can disrupt their stability and trigger an acute psychiatric episode. When hospital stays are shorter and acute episodes occur frequently, individuals bounce between living in the community and the institution. In 1991 the average length of hospitalization for psychiatric problems was 23 days. Today it is 9. Many hospital stays allow even less time for clients to stabilize and begin treatment.

Pharmacological Therapy

Persons with chronic mental disorders are treated with a variety of medications depending on symptoms and distress levels. Antianxiety agents and antidepressants are often prescribed to improve emotional comfort. Antipsychotic (neuroleptic) drugs are prescribed to help control hallucinations and other symptoms of psychosis. Drug therapy is an important part of treatment; however,

---

Table 32-2 Basic Interventions: Chronic Mental Illness

Nursing interventions	Rationale
Relating to Risk of Danger	
Assess risk for harm to self or others.	Ensure safety and prevent violence.
Encourage client to notify staff when feeling angry/when destructive thoughts begin.	Helps prevent violence before it actually occurs.
Frequently orient client to reality in nonthreatening way.	Reduces risk of violence, decreases client anxiety.
Sensory/Perceptual Alterations	
Assess for delusions and hallucinations.	Helps to determine the level of psychosis.
Ask client to share the meaning of his or her hallucinations, delusions.	To determine client's point of view and intent.
Teach client distraction techniques, such as whistling, clapping hands, telling hallucination to go away when hallucinating.	Offers client strategies for controlling hallucinations.
Activities of Daily Living	
Establish a schedule for grooming, eating, sleeping.	Increases self-esteem, encourages responsibility, and helps client appear more socially acceptable.
Monitor intake, output, personal hygiene activities.	
Communication	
Use active listening; establish trust; encourage conversation; praise attempts to speak clearly and effectively.	Helps to assess client's communication style and patterns; increases understanding of and respect for client.
Social Skills	
Encourage good social skills, such as table manners, personal grooming, appropriate communications, behaviors.	Promotes client's acceptability by other persons; increases self-esteem; helps to teach effective social behaviors.

Modified from Fortinash KM, Holoday-Worret PA: *Psychiatric mental health nursing*, ed 2, St. Louis, 1999, Mosby.

 **Sample Client Care Plan**   # Chronic Mental Illness

Assessment

History: Tom is a 34-year-old man with a history of at least 11 admissions to psychiatric units of various general hospitals. Today he is being readmitted after he was found wandering the streets arguing with himself and threatening to kill someone else if they "don't stop calling me names." He was medicated with 1 mg of haloperidol (Haldol) intramuscularly in the emergency department.

Current Findings: An unkempt man with a strong body odor and soiled clothing; speech is slow and disjointed; responds verbally without external stimuli. Emotional state (affect) is flat except for verbal responses to hallucinations. Tom states that he is and has been hallucinating for the past 3 days. The hallucinations are auditory; the voices want Tom to kill himself. He thinks they may be right because during the time he is in the community, he feels forced to spy on other people for the FBI and the voices tell him that he is better off dead than being a spy. When asked what made him take to the streets, Tom replied that he thought he could "outwalk the out talk." He has not taken his prescribed medications since he last saw his therapist about 4 weeks ago.

Multidisciplinary Diagnosis

Sensory/perceptual alterations, related to impaired perceptions.

Planning/Goals

Tom will seek out a staff member when he begins to hallucinate. Tom will not harm himself or others. Tom will report the absence of auditory hallucinations within four days after admission.

Therapeutic Interventions

Intervention	Rationale	Team Member
1. Orient Tom frequently to place, time, current activity.	Presents reality; reminds Tom of this reality.	All
2. Speak slowly; use clear, simple messages.	Helps to increase Tom's understanding, thus decreasing his anxiety.	All
3. Reassure often that he will not be harmed by the voices or other people.	Helps Tom to trust the safety of his environment, presents reality as safe.	All
4. Listen to and accept descriptions of his feelings, hallucinations.	Conveys respect and acceptance of the person and encourages communication.	All
5. Set limits on aggressive behaviors; contract with Tom for a no-harm contract.	Promotes a safe environment for all clients and staff, helps Tom to be responsible for his own behaviors.	Nsg, All
6. Encourage Tom to take his medications; make copy of the daily medication schedule and encourage Tom to follow it.	Medications help to control psychotic symptoms, reduce anxiety, improve functioning; developing a daily medication routine in the hospital helps increase compliance after discharge.	Nsg, MD
7. Discharge planning for Tom to return to his foster home.	A stable and predictable environment helps decrease acute psychotic episodes.	Soc Svc

Evaluation

After the fourth day of hospitalization, Tom sought out staff members when he was beginning to hallucinate. With the exception of one acting-out episode, Tom abided by his no-harm contract. Reports of hallucinations have decreased from "continually" on admission to once or twice a week the second week of his stay.

A complete client care plan includes several other diagnoses and interventions.

the side effects of many of these medications are uncomfortable, and clients often stop taking them as soon as the acute symptoms subside. Several antipsychotic medications are available in long-acting injectable forms called decanoate. One of the most powerful predictors of medication refusal is one's insight into the illness (Torry, 1996), and most chronically or severely mentally ill individuals have little insight. Nurses must carefully monitor clients routinely for compliance with medications.

Nursing Process

The first step in working with severely mentally disordered clients is to obtain the most complete database possible. Because mental health problems affect every area of functioning, nurses must perform thorough histories and assess clients' physical status, perceptions, and behaviors.

After each member of the treatment team completes his or her assessment, client problems are identified, and therapeutic interventions are designed. Nurses focus on helping clients cope with each activity of daily living. Multidisciplinary and nursing diagnoses are chosen, and basic interventions are agreed on by the treatment team and (when possible) the client. Nursing diagnoses for chronically mentally ill clients are selected according to the client's identified problems.

Therapeutic interventions are then designed to help the client solve the identified problems. Although each client requires a unique combination of interventions, several fundamental therapeutic actions apply to all clients. Table 32-2 lists each intervention and its rationale.

A care plan for a chronically mentally ill client is presented in the Sample Client Care Plan box.

Care plans for long-term psychiatric clients are adapted to the particular care setting—be it the home, community day center, clinic, or institution. If the mental health care services are well coordinated, care plans are moved with the client. That is, the care plans established in the institution move to a different care setting when the client does. This method encourages the continuity of care that is so important for coping with severe mental problems.

Once returned into the community, mental health centers provide clients with the ongoing care needed to help them function effectively, but many services are unavailable due to unstable sources of funding. Community mental health centers with strong financial bases are able to provide their clients with such services as medical care, medication supervision, individual and family therapy, crisis intervention services, family support services, skills training, and vocational counseling or training in addition to continued emotional support and encouragement. With the long-term support, many individuals with severe mental illness and their families are able to effectively cope with the numerous problems associated with their disorders.

KEY CONCEPTS

◆ Most chronic mental health problems are characterized by periods of exacerbations and remissions.
◆ Chronic mental disorders are disabling for people in every society and culture.
◆ Many chronically mentally ill individuals are homeless, hungry, and unable to care for themselves.
◆ Access to comprehensive mental health care remains a problem in the United States today.
◆ Each person's experiences with mental illness are unique.
◆ Chronic mental health problems can begin at any stage in life, but they are often not noticed until early or middle adulthood.
◆ The social epidemic of violence, crack cocaine, and other drug use has resulted in a new group of primary care providers: grandparents who must raise a second family, their grandchildren.
◆ Substance abuse and mental illness result in an interactive process that is seen in physical, psychological, and behavioral patterns uniquely different from those of persons with only an addiction or serious mental illness.
◆ Psychiatric rehabilitation is a multidisciplinary treatment approach that focuses on assisting individuals with serious mental illness to effectively cope with their life situations.
◆ The basic goals for chronically disordered mental health clients are to achieve stabilization and maintain individuals at their highest level of daily functioning.
◆ Persons with chronic mental disorders are treated with a variety of medications depending on symptoms and distress levels.
◆ Nurses focus on helping the chronically mentally ill client cope with each activity of daily living.
◆ Once returned into the community, the chronically mentally ill require aftercare or rehabilitation services.
◆ Because all areas of human functioning are deeply interwoven, mental health nursing is a critical component of every nursing situation.
◆ The mental health of a society depends on the mental health of each of its individual citizens.

Suggestions for Further Reading

Ruth Schofield's "Empowering Education for Individuals With Serious Mental Illness" (*Journal of Psychosocial Nursing* 36(11), 35, 1998) offers an excellent argument for interventions that enable people to increase control over their own lives.
Websites with information about chronic mental illness include the Alliance for the Mentally Ill (www.schizophrenia.com), Dual Diagnosis (www.erols.com), and Mental Health Education (www.metrolink.net).

References

Blaska B: What it's like to be a CMI, *Schizophrenia Bulletin* 17(1):173, 1991.

Farnam CR and others: Health status and risk factors of people with severe and persistent mental illness, *Journal of Psychosocial Nursing* 37(6):16, 1999.

Fortinash KM, Holoday-Worret PA: *Psychiatric-mental health nursing,* ed 2, St. Louis, 1999, Mosby.

Howd A: Trapped between the law and madness, *Insight in the News* 14(34):18, 1998.

Katz RC, Watts C, Santman J: AIDS knowledge and high-risk behaviors in the chronic mentally ill, *Community Mental Health* 30:395, 1994.

NAMI: The facts on severe mental illness, *National Alliance for the Mentally Ill* (10):1, 1999.

Stuart GW, Laraia MT: *Stuart and Sundeen's pocket guide to psychiatric nursing,* ed 4, St. Louis, 1998, Mosby.

Torrey EF: *Out of the shadows: confronting America's mental illness crisis,* ed 2, London, 1996, J Wiley.

Torrey EF, Zdanowicz MT: How freedom punishes the severely mentally ill, *USA Today,* July 7, 1999.

U.S. Bureau of the Census: *Statistical abstract of the United States: 1998,* ed 118, Washington, DC, 1998, U.S. Government Printing Office.

Chapter 33

Challenges for the Future

Learning Objectives

1. List three challenges that health care providers face in delivering mental health care in the United States.
2. Explain the purpose of the Americans with Disabilities Act of 1990.
3. Discuss the characteristics of a typical "old" and "new" homeless person.
4. Explain what is meant by "the right to self-determination."
5. Examine three obligations of the therapeutic partnership for the client and the care provider.
6. Describe three expanded roles for nurses who care for mentally ill people.

7. Examine two challenges involved with the change process.
8. Outline two techniques for coping with information overload.
9. Describe the roles, functions, and interactions of the mental health care team.
10. Examine the role of the mental health team in providing care for clients with human immunodeficiency virus (HIV)/acquired immunodeficiency syndrome (AIDS).

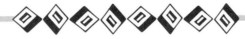

Key Terms

change
competent
entrepreneur

homelessness
information overload
mental health care team

nurse case managers
psychosocial rehabilitation

The need for mental health applies to us all. Every person experiences periods of emotional turmoil and crises in life and, at some time, we all need a little assistance to help us cope. When one is experiencing physical illness and its resultant treatments, it usually produces emotional stresses ranging from indifference to crisis behaviors. With this thought in mind, every person becomes a mental health client in some way because an emotional reaction always follows a physical diagnosis, an uncomfortable procedure, or time spent as a patient. Nurses and other health care providers help provide the nurturing that all clients (not just those with mental illnesses) need; but they are now challenged to provide that care within ever-changing health care delivery environments.

CHANGES IN MENTAL HEALTH CARE

"According to a recent study by the World Health Organization, the World Bank, and Harvard University, mental disorders account for 4 out of the 10 leading causes of disability in established market economies worldwide . . . Other research has estimated that the cost of mental illnesses in the United States, including indirect costs such as days lost from work, was $148 billion in 1990, the last time the total bill was measured" (National Institute of Mental Health, 1999).

Health care is undergoing many changes today. Escalating costs in several countries are forcing officials to take a close look at where and how health care funds are spent. In the United States new patterns of providing health care services are emerging as preferred provider and health maintenance organizations. Social changes such as an aging population, an overburdened welfare system, and a cost-conscious U.S. Congress are exerting their influences on today's health care system.

The influence of many cultures and new technology is changing the way we look at health and illness. Today clients may not speak the same language. Technological advances are opening new areas of exploration, and discoveries about the biochemical nature of humans are challenging the foundations of our thinking.

The treatment and prevention of mental illness (and other health issues) are caught up in the web of change. As a result, nurses and all health care providers will be challenged to deliver effective, cost-accountable care, which will call for creativity and innovation. Change is a certainty, and adaptability is a key.

Change in Settings

Until recently, most psychiatric care was limited to the inpatient setting, either a unit at the local community hospital or a long-term care institution. Today, however, most institutions are closed, many inpatient psychiatric units are full, and emergency departments are becoming havens for those experiencing crisis. Some individuals with acute problems are denied care and told to return when "something happens" (Mentally ill, 1999).

When the large state mental health institutions began to discharge their clients, it was argued that most people could live in the community if they continued to receive medication and aftercare (Torrey, 1998). Many mentally ill persons were transferred to nursing homes and long-term care facilities. Changes in the system that once supported the mentally ill are now moving them into community health care systems, and the specialized "aftercare" that was promised is commonly not provided.

As a result of the unsupported release, many mentally troubled persons became sick again and eventually homeless. The seriously mentally ill now constitute more than one third of the homeless population (Torry and Zdanowicz, 1999). Jails and prisons have evolved into holding facilities for people with mental problems (Harrington, 1999). Many of the mentally ill are jailed just to get them off the streets. Others are found living at the fringes of society, sleeping in abandoned buildings, and depending on the generosity of others for food and clothing.

The treatment settings for people with mental illness have changed to follow the clients from the institution to the street, jail, neighborhood clinic, or local physician's office. Mental health care is an important component of overall health, and it must be addressed if we are to become capable, adaptable, and functional people. Health care providers must become skilled in assessing and working with clients suffering from mental or emotional disorders, no matter where the setting or what the situation.

Homelessness

Many families function just "one paycheck away from poverty." They can financially cope for the present; but add one stressor, and the whole situation becomes threatened. It is not uncommon to hear of the working-class family whose father was laid off his job. If work is not found soon, the family becomes unable to make the mortgage payments and is eventually forced out of their home onto the streets. Sad as it seems, this scenario has become a reality for many families.

Homelessness means to be without a permanent residence, a place to live. Homelessness means to have every possession you own stuffed into the back of the car (if you are lucky enough to own a car). Homelessness means your children cannot attend school because they have no permanent address, no phone number, and usually no immunization records.

Traditionally, homeless people were unmarried, intermittently employed, white male adults with an average age of 50. However, they seldom actually slept in the streets because of the availability of cheap hotels, missions, and SROs (sleeping room only). A study of Chicago's homeless population in the late 1950s revealed that 25% of the homeless people were on Social Security (and trying to live inexpensively), 25% were chronic alcoholics, 20% had a physical disability, 20% had a chronic mental illness, and 10% were maladjusted. These men are the "old homeless," the traditionally less fortunate members of society.

During the 1960s and 1970s, the number of homeless people declined in the United States; however, by the early 1980s a growing number of the "new homeless" began to appear, and that number has rapidly increased ever since. Today's homeless people are younger and much poorer than their counterparts of yesterday and have no actual shelter, much less a home. The numbers of women, children, and minorities have swelled the ranks of the homeless to significant numbers. Families without a home now make up 38% of the homeless population in a city (Myths and facts, 1999).

Loss of control over the daily events of their own lives leads homeless people toward a loss of self-worth, learned helplessness, and depression. Children who are homeless for any length of time experience serious threats to their current well-being and their future ability to succeed.

The health status of the homeless, both mental and physical, is poor, and the average age of death for a homeless person in the United States is about 50 (Farnam and others, 1999). About one third of today's homeless are mentally ill. Many of these people were relatively adjusted when they were discharged from an institution, but when the medications ran out and the aftercare was not provided, their psychiatric problems returned. Without adequate support, resources, and encouragement, many of the chronically mentally ill find it almost impossible to take steps to improve their lives.

Homelessness has become a national tragedy that in some way affects us all. When people cannot find health care for the smaller problems, they wait until immediate attention is required. This practice brings about a high incidence of severe disorders. The trauma of losing one's home, adjusting to life in a shelter or on the street, and struggling for a way out produces symptoms of psychological and emotional distress. Stress disorders are not uncommon among the homeless, even those with previously high levels of functioning.

The children of this subsociety endure hardships that most of us can only imagine. Low-birth-weight babies and infant illness are common. Studies of homeless women in New York City revealed that infant mortality is very high.

If the children survive infancy, they are at risk for double the incidence of respiratory infections and skin ailments, as well as the usual childhood diseases. Parasitic infestations, such as lice or scabies, occur in homeless children much more frequently than in the general population. Homeless children are also affected by poor educational opportunities, anxiety, depression, and behavioral difficulties.

Few homeless children are immunized, fewer are educated, and many live with hunger and chronic malnutrition. Developmental delays, including short attention spans; immature motor, speech, and interpersonal skills; and inappropriate social behaviors, are frequently encountered with homeless children. Poverty, inadequate shelter, lack of access to day care services, and the stresses of having no home all contribute to homeless children's lack of development. For homeless children, childhood is not the happy time of exploration and learning that it should be.

Adolescents are also found in greater numbers among the homeless than two decades ago. Estimates of homeless adolescents are as high as one-and-a-half million individuals. Many of these are the children of dysfunctional families who are frequently neglected, abused, and exploited. Homeless adolescents are at a much greater risk for hepatitis, AIDS, and other sexually transmitted diseases. In addition, life on the streets leads to high rates of substance abuse, depression, and frequent suicidal attempts. The future holds little promise for a teen without hopes, aspirations, or emotional support.

Adults with chronic mental illness constitute about one third of the homeless population. Because of their illness, the ability to function in daily life is severely limited. Self-care activities, interpersonal relationships, and abilities to work or attend school are compromised for mentally troubled individuals. Usually, financial resources are very limited, and many of the rooming houses that once provided inexpensive shelter have been converted to other uses or destroyed. Publicly financed housing, especially for the mentally ill, is difficult to obtain. Given the lack of community mental health services, one can understand why a large number of people with chronic mental illnesses are now wandering the streets of both large and small communities.

When research was conducted to compare the mentally ill homeless with non–mentally ill homeless, people with severe mental illnesses were similar to their counterparts in age, ethnicity, sex, and extent of substance abuse. However, the homeless mentally ill were in poorer health, homeless for longer periods of time, struggling with more barriers to employment, and had less contact with family or friends than the homeless without mental difficulties.

The actual number of homeless persons is difficult to determine, but estimates range from less than 1 million to more than 7 million. Homelessness is a national health problem that must be solved if we are to save a generation of fellow human beings from the despair of having no future. Health care problems for the homeless are monumental, but they can be addressed. As the providers of health care, we must consider new ways and means of working with this population if we are to protect and encourage the health of all people.

The Americans With Disabilities Act

The Americans With Disabilities Act (ADA) of 1990 is a federal statute designed to remove the barriers that prevented qualified people with disabilities from having the same employment opportunities that are available to persons without disabilities. The ADA requires employers to make "reasonable accommodation" for disabled individuals, thus allowing them to perform the essential functions of the job.

Under the ADA guidelines, a person is considered disabled when a physical or mental impairment "substantially limits one or more major life activities" (Equal Employment Opportunity Commission, 1992). A mental impairment is defined by the ADA as "any mental or psychological disorder, such as mental retardation, organic brain syndrome, emotional or mental illness, and specified learning abilities." If the condition substantially limits one's functioning, the person is covered by the ADA. Employers can no longer refuse to hire persons solely on the basis of disability and must make reasonable adjustments for the disabled employee. The implications of this legislation excite and challenge those who work with psychiatric clients.

The intent of the ADA is to tailor the needs of the job with the needs of the disabled individual. However, Congress cannot legislate social change. Only time and successful work experiences with mentally ill employees will remove the stigma of mental illness in the workplace.

This is our next challenge: to prepare our clients for gainful employment and, at the same time, convince employers that people with mental disorders can be reliable employees (see Think About box).

Cultural Influences

The world is shrinking. In the past a person would grow, live, procreate, and die within one community or geographical region. Today world travelers work in one part of the globe and commute to another area to raise their families. Waves of immigrants move from their homelands in search of a better life, and rapid forms of transportation move thousands of people around the world in a matter of hours instead of days. As more individuals become computer literate and users of the global computer networks, our world will shrink even more. Because of these changes, nurses and other health care providers will be encountering persons from various cultural backgrounds with greater frequency. Learning to interact effectively and respectfully is a challenge that faces all the world's citizens, but for health care workers this is especially important.

The mental problems of a culture can have a universal quality. There are some behaviors, such as those associated with depression, that all cultures define as mental health disorders. Other mental health problems may be specifically limited to the members of that group. These types of problems are called *culture-bound disorders* because they appear to be related to specific cultures. For example, the disorder the Hispanics call *susto* is an emotional anxiety that results from "soul loss."

Health, illness, and mental illness are defined differently throughout various cultures. The person who talks to himself may be considered "a nut" in one society and revered as a holy man in another. Their behaviors might be exactly the same, but the social setting in which they take place differs. The point is that mental illness is culturally defined to a large extent. To work effectively with clients from other cultures, health caregivers must discover how clients define mental illness.

As displaced individuals adapt to their new cultures, they combine elements of both the home and the host culture into their daily lives. The result is a unique blend of both worlds, a "third culture." Bicultural clients require a thorough cultural assessment to discover their individual frames of reference (how they view the world). Only then can therapeutic interventions be planned with the expectation of success. An effective therapy in one culture is not always successful when applied in another culture.

As more people emigrate throughout the world, health care providers will encounter many clients whose first language is not English. This presents many challenges, especially when a psychiatric component is involved. Even when the client speaks or understands some English, the stresses of illness (and the complexities of a modern health care system) increase anxiety, and clients often attempt to communicate by reverting back to their native language. Many times these communications can be misunderstood and result in poor treatment outcomes. The Cultural Aspects box offers an illustration of poor communication. If mental health care providers are to deliver effective care, we must be aware of the cultural backgrounds of our clients and develop our plans of care with each client's unique cultural heritage in mind. Caring for culturally diverse clients is another challenge, because our services

---

Think About

You are working in a community hospital. Today you find that one of your co-workers who told you that he has a history of mental illness has been assigned to your care team. You have never worked with this person before today.

◆ What is your initial reaction?
◆ How do you think this will affect the activities of the workplace?

Cultural Aspects

Sam was a Caucasian nurse working at a Native American reservation health center. He frequently monitored the physician's chronically ill clients, did his best to educate each of them about their conditions, and provided emotional support to help them cope with their conditions. Why then, he wondered, did he have such difficulty communicating with his clients?

On the suggestion of his physician, a long-term resident on the reservation, Sam began to look at how his behaviors affected his clients. After finding no real answer there, he consulted a tribal elder with his problem. All that he was told was that "the eyes are the window of the soul." This statement perplexed Sam until he realized that he was "staring down" his clients when he was interacting with them.

Sam was so intent on putting his client education messages across that he repeatedly missed an important nonverbal clue—each of his clients avoided direct eye contact and looked downward whenever Sam was instructing them. Once he realized that his problem was a culturally based miscommunication, he revised his method of teaching and changed his eye contact behaviors. His clients began to communicate with him. Sam had learned a valuable lesson: not all people communicate the same way.

How does Sam's experience affect your interactions with clients?

are only as effective as they are perceived to be by our clients.

THE MENTAL HEALTH CARE TEAM

Mental illness has a multifaceted nature that includes physical disorders, social factors, psychological issues, and spiritual concerns. To attempt to meet the many client needs and to provide care in both inpatient and community settings, interdisciplinary mental health care teams were introduced. A **mental health care team** is a group of professionally trained specialists who develop and implement comprehensive treatment plans for clients with mental and emotional problems.

Team Members

The ideal composition of an interdisciplinary (also called multidisciplinary) mental health care team is the client, a physician, a psychologist, a nurse, a dietitian, a social worker, a representative of the client's spiritual beliefs (e.g., minister or priest), an occupational therapist, and other specialists as needed. The main function of the team is to coordinate care as the client moves from inpatient to community settings and through the health care system. Refer to Table 2-2, Chapter 2, for a description of each team member's role in the health care team.

Interdisciplinary Interactions

Members of the mental health care team communicate frequently because scarce services must be allocated and clients need effective care. Some care teams meet often to monitor client progress, review the client's use of services, and establish treatment goals. Others may interact by phone or e-mail. All work with clients and each other to meet defined goals. To illustrate, nurses who care for hospitalized clients begin discharge planning upon admission and communicate with the care team. Discharge planners and social workers communicate with community members who provide services. When clients are ready for discharge, the care team is able to make a smooth transition back into the community for the client, because the interactions of each team member focused on the treatment goals.

The managed care system of health care delivery has the goal of delivering care that is clinically necessary, medically appropriate, and defined within benefit parameters.

Mental Health Care Delivery Settings

In the past, mental health care was obtained in the psychiatrist's office or the inpatient setting. Today mental health care is delivered in three general settings: the institution, the community, or the home. Mental health units in general hospitals and the mental health institutions are examples of institutional settings. Mental

health specialists are found in many community settings, ranging from prisons and jails to private clinics. Many work in neighborhood clinics or with social service agencies. Home care mental health is frequently delivered through psychiatric nurses and technicians who regularly visit clients in their home environments. Client care and support is the web that helps clients cope with their mental health problems within rapidly changing societies.

CHANGE AND MENTAL HEALTH CLIENTS

Throughout history mental illnesses have been labeled as being somehow "different" from physical maladies. People with mental illnesses were obviously not in this reality, so why should they care about how they are treated? This attitude prevailed for many centuries; consequently, persons with mental illnesses were neglected, abused, and confined without hope of improvement.

As new psychiatric theories arose, attitudes toward the mentally ill changed, but individuals were still viewed as culprits or victims who somehow caused their own problems. During this time, the role of the patient was to be a passive recipient of care. Therapies were designed and delivered without regard to appropriateness, and patients were expected to quietly cooperate. Relationships between clients and care providers ranged from patronizing to adversarial.

Today both the providers and consumers of mental health care are striving to change attitudes and practices. Involving clients in treatment means every party must assume an active role. This interaction involves the building of trust, mutual respect, and acceptance.

Competency

Are people with mental illness capable of making decisions about proper care and treatment of their problems? Society struggles to balance individual rights with the need to protect its citizens. Meanwhile, our legal system and those who work with the mentally ill are often challenged to provide the answer to this complex question.

To be considered **competent**, an individual must be able to (1) make a choice, (2) understand important information, (3) appreciate one's own situation, and (4) apply reasoning. Studies reveal that mental illness often coexists with competent decision making, but many individuals (up to 50%) show seriously impaired judgment. Many hospitalized clients with severe symptoms, such as paranoia or disorganized thought, are usually incompetent. Apply the four measures of competence described above when assessing a client's decision-making abilities. It may help solve the dilemma of discerning which clients are able to make reasonable treatment decisions.

The challenge of meeting the human needs of clients without violating their rights is especially true for clients with mental health problems. When people were discharged from institutions into their "least restrictive environments," their rights to freedom, autonomy, and self-determination were protected. However, the concept of the least restrictive setting begins to break down when clients are unable to provide the essentials of daily living for themselves and are in need of treatment.

Individuals are not exercising their rights to freedom when they wander the streets aimlessly, out of touch with reality. They are usually able to determine little for themselves and have virtually no ability to self-direct their lives (Wilk, 1994). In these cases, an institutional setting may prove to be a more beneficial environment.

To implement the concept of the least restrictive treatment environment, mental health care team members assess the available community resources and match their services to the unique needs and limitations of each client. In today's health care environment, the linking of mentally troubled clients with too few community resources is, and will likely remain, a challenge for us all.

Empowerment of Client

The traditional role of a client was passive. Clients were expected to accept the physician's diagnosis, therapies, and comments without question. They were also expected to be motivated, cooperative, and passive enough to get well. As a result, people became increasingly detached from the responsibility for their own health care and discontented with the system that delivered that care.

Today people are becoming more responsible and active consumers of health care, but many health care services remain tied to the old models of the passive client. Individuals entering the health care system are beginning to exercise the right of self-determination. They seek out information about their conditions, weigh the pros and cons of each treatment option, and select the ones that best suit them. Because the consumer's role has moved from a passive to an active one, the term *client* becomes more appropriate than the passively connoted term *patient.* Hopefully, the relationship between care providers and client develops into a dynamic interchange, with therapeutic goals that are mutually acceptable. This therapeutic partnership, however, involves responsibility.

Obligations of Client

To receive the most effective care, clients must fulfill certain obligations. These responsibilities are few, but they are important for success of treatment. First, clients must be *truthful.* Many times people are uncomfortable about sharing personal information. They may expect health care providers to pass judgment on their actions or refuse care. Nevertheless, honest, complete data are essential for planning care. Second, clients have an

obligation to be *responsible for their own behaviors.* Even people who periodically lose contact with reality are capable of assuming some responsibility. Third, clients have an obligation to *cooperate with treatment;* that is, assuming clients want to "get well." Consumers of mental health services who are willing to assume the obligations of truthfulness, responsibility, and cooperation can play an active role in successful diagnosis and treatment of their problems. Within the therapeutic relationship, care providers also have certain obligations.

Obligations of Care Providers

As clients assume certain obligations, so do the mental health care providers who work with them. From the psychiatrist to the technician, each assumes specific responsibilities when working with clients. However, all providers of mental health care have the obligation to perform the following four steps.

First and most important, *accept the client "as is."* Nurses do not have to like or approve of any behavior, but the *person* must be accepted as a worthy human being—capable of change. Do not pass judgment. We are here to help—not to conjure up emotionally based opinions.

Second, *demonstrate respect* for clients. Refer to clients by name. Ask permission before entering their living space, if necessary. Show approval for gains made in therapy. Express concern for their well-being, and remember to be polite. All these behaviors demonstrate respect for clients much more clearly than words. Even the most disturbed person responds to respectful care.

Third, *empower clients.* Much mental illness is associated with feelings of lack of control over their lives. Care providers who recognize this can provide small, but frequent, opportunities for decision making and success. As clients choose among various options, they are exercising some control over their environment. Hopefully, decisions gradually move from making choices to solving problems. During the process, each success provides encouragement for the next step and a sense of control.

Fourth, mental health professionals, especially nurses and therapists who work closely with clients, have the added obligation to provide educational opportunities—in short, to *educate.* Unless clients are comatose, they are capable of learning. New knowledge allows people to change. *Empowerment education* is an intervention that helps mentally troubled clients attain increased control of their lives (Schofield, 1998), and empowered clients are more willing to explore and change their behaviors. Table 33-1 summarizes the obligations of the therapeutic partnership.

Studies have demonstrated that clients who feel they have some control over their situation report fewer symptoms and less discomfort. They have speedier recoveries and are able to participate in the activities of

Table 33-1	Obligations of the Therapeutic Partnership
Clients	**Care providers**
To be truthful	To accept the client as a person capable of change
To be responsible for one's own behaviors	To demonstrate respect and acceptance of the person
To cooperate with treatment	To empower clients
	To educate clients

daily living earlier than clients who perceive little or no control. In short, clients need to be active participants in their own care.

Providers of Care

Membership in the health care profession is also changing. Once only doctors, nurses, and family members provided mental health care. Today assorted technicians, assistants, and aides provide many services that were once exclusively within the realm of psychiatry. Because each technician works within a narrow specialty, it becomes the nurse's responsibility to ensure that safe, coordinated health care is being delivered to clients. Nurses need to understand and exercise their roles in coordinating health care.

The services of nursing assistants and patient care technicians (PCTs) are just as important in the mental health setting as they are in the hospital setting. Certified nursing assistants (CNAs) have been employed in psychiatric institutions for many years, helping nurses with client care and treatments. Patient care technicians have advanced CNA training and are relatively new to the health care profession. Recently, however, both roles have expanded into the community, where they have met with success.

To illustrate, the Supportive Homemaker Program of Haverhill, Massachusetts (Holland, 1993) employs mental health supportive home care aides (HCAs) to provide emotional and social support for clients in their homes. The program is designed to serve several populations: children who are at risk for abuse or neglect, those people who lack family or social support, the depressed, the severely ill, and the senile elderly.

The program depends on the HCA's abilities. Those who demonstrate an acceptance of others, compassion, cultural awareness, patience, and a gentle sense of humor are selected. Once a modest training period is completed, each HCA is assigned a caseload and a psychiatric nurse coordinator, who provides support and guidance.

Through frequent visits, the HCA establishes a relationship with each client. Because they are nonthreatening, nonjudgmental, and represent no authority or power, supportive HCAs provide a reliable relationship, which helps to ease the anxiety and apprehension of being alone or unable to cope.

The main function of supportive HCAs is to act as helping individuals. These responsibilities include providing homemaker services, transportation, and instruction. Skills in the daily activities of living, home management, and even self-care are taught and reinforced on subsequent visits. The importance of good nutrition and medical care for children is stressed. If needed, clients are instructed on ways to obtain food, clothing, shelter, and education.

Supportive HCAs encourage clients to use the services of appropriate community resources. They act as advocates by instructing clients about how the services can help, assisting them in making contact with specific services, and even providing transportation for appointments. The success of these mental health care providers lies not with their academic or political prowess, but with one fundamental thought: they are there to care—to help, to make things better.

Other providers of care for mentally troubled people are the psychiatric technicians who are formally trained to provide mental health care in both inpatient and outpatient settings. "Psych techs" were once commonly employed in large state institutions, but as clients were discharged into the community, their numbers became smaller. Today psychiatric technicians can be found in practice settings ranging from community mental health centers to prisons. As mental health care moves into the community, larger numbers of care providers will be needed.

Expanded Roles for Nurses

The profession of nursing has undergone many changes in the past 20 years. The "handmaiden to the physician" model has been replaced by the role of a professional, with all its accompanying rights and obligations. Nurses of today are considered to be experts in the area of assisting people to cope with the impact of health problems on everyday living. They are guided by state nurse practice acts and the profession's standards of care. Appendix A offers a description of psychiatric nursing standards. Nurses participate fully as members of the treatment team. They also provide education for clients and their significant others, and coordinate the activities of various therapeutic interventions and support agencies. Nurses' roles are continuing to evolve, and the challenge every nurse must face is to grow with change.

As mental health care moves into the community, new roles are opening up for nurses. Hospitals no longer employ the majority of nurses because attempts to control costs have decreased the numbers of nurses per institution. Clients are being discharged from acute care facilities earlier and now require nursing services in their homes and communities. Because nurses help people to adjust to and cope with the changes in daily living that result from their illness or condition, they practice in a number of challenging new settings.

For example, nurses play a vital role in centers for the homeless where treatment teams (clinicians, social workers, a nurse, and a psychiatrist) assess each client for medical, psychiatric, and social service needs. The role of the nurse in these treatment centers is one of facilitator/advocate who assists clients in gaining access to services. Nurses commonly perform unconventional nursing tasks and must be flexible with treatment plans. Collaboration with the multidisciplinary treatment team and numerous community agencies assists them in referring clients to various resources. Other tasks performed by nurses in these settings include rescheduling missed appointments, assisting clients in filling out applications for services or employment interviews, clarifying instructions, and monitoring clients' physical and mental changes.

Preventive health care is another main responsibility of these nurses. Routine screening for weight, hypertension, and response to medications allows them many opportunities to instruct clients about more healthful living activities. Weekly lectures and discussions about proper nutrition, sexually transmitted diseases, and current health issues are planned and conducted by nurses. Realistic goals are set to encourage clients to commit to meeting their needs, and much support by all members of the staff helps clients to regain their self-esteem (see Case Study box). With the homeless mentally ill, successful outcomes are few, but the personal rewards and professional satisfactions are many.

Nurses also collaborate with physicians to plan and implement programs for people with serious mental illness. One such program employs only nurses as case managers because they value continuity of care and are knowledgeable and comfortable with medication management. **Nurse case managers** work with psychiatrists to develop treatment plans tailored to each client's special needs. Clients are encouraged to share their concerns with their nurse case manager, who evaluates the need for psychiatric consultation. Nurses and psychiatrists meet weekly for discussions and decisions about each client's medications, therapies, and referrals.

Nurses in this setting provide intake assessments and referral services, initial and ongoing medication services, supportive counseling by telephone or routine visits with clients, individual and group education, and advocacy for clients interacting with family, the legal system, or other parts of the health care system. Because of the nurse case manager's support and guidance, clients with severe mental illnesses are able to function more adequately

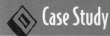

Case Study

A 30-year-old man presents to the treatment center complaining of overwhelming feelings of agitation and hostility. During the nurse's initial assessment, the client reveals that he has not been taking his psychotherapeutic medications because they make him too drowsy. "So, this is not an uncommon complaint," the nurse thinks; but on further questioning, the nurse discovers that the client becomes vulnerable to street predators when he sleeps after taking his medication. In fact, the client reveals that he has often been mugged and beaten while sleeping in subways.

On the nurse's request, the client's medications were adjusted. The client agreed to come to the center for daily administration and monitoring. After a few months, his behavior changes were so remarkable that he was able to become reunited with his family. He continues to visit the treatment center daily for support and evaluation.

◆ How can Maslow's hierarchy of needs be applied to this case?

◆ How did the nurse's assessment lead to changes in the client's life?

within their community, and costly and unnecessary psychiatric consultations are reduced. The nurse-physician collaborative practice model may prove to be one solution to the challenge of delivering mental health care to clients within their home environments.

Psychosocial rehabilitation is another area in which nurses are expanding their roles. Evolving as a social model of treatment rather than a medical model, psychosocial rehabilitation is a way of assisting people with mental health problems to readjust and adapt to life in the community. In these settings, nurses are able to use their full range of skills without the focus being placed on illness or disability. Wellness, wholeness, and the abilities of the individual are emphasized, whereas vocational, educational, residential, social, and personal adjustment services are offenders. Clients are encouraged to exercise freedom of choice and become consciously self-directed. Individual care plans, called personal service plans, are developed but controlled by clients who identify the goals that are important to them. Resources and support people are chosen by clients with guidance from the treatment team (referred to as a service delivery team).

Self-help is a fundamental concept of psychosocial rehabilitation. Care team members offer social and vocational coaching, but clients must act for themselves. The belief that all people have the inherent capacity for change and the focus on what the client can do have resulted in some remarkable successes. Nurses who practice within these settings truly work with persons in their environment to maximize wellness.

As health care moves into the community, the need for mental health clinical nurse specialists will continue to grow. Mental health home care nurses focus on prevention and wellness care, collaborate with other professionals, and serve as the client's advocate within the mental health delivery system. Clients who are facing the crises of illness are assisted by mental health home care nurses with both their physical and emotional difficulties. Because they are able to intervene during the early stages of dysfunction, the services of mental health home care nurses are proving to be successful as well as cost effective.

One of the most exciting expanded roles for nurses is that of **entrepreneur** or self-employed nurse. Today nurses are establishing their own clinics, acting as health care consultants, and working to provide a variety of health care services to business and industry. Mental health care nurses are involved in businesses that provide services for adults, children, employees, organizations, and public and government agencies. Nurses are accepting the challenge to seek out and create innovative models for the delivery of mental health care services to special populations.

MANAGING CHANGE

Because life is a dynamic process, all living things undergo change. Seasons, plants, people, and processes all change. Nurses and other health care providers must keep pace with continual changes in health care, new therapies, theories, medications, and more. Therefore it is important to understand the characteristics of change and how to successfully cope and adapt.

Change is defined as the process of making or becoming different. Change itself is neither inherently good nor bad. It is the reactions of the people involved in the process that tend to label or judge a change.

People resist change because it implies uncertainty, which brings about a disturbance in the status quo. We all resist change to some extent to maintain our equilibrium and keep things "the way they are." People resist change for several reasons. Although major problems may be present in the current situation, they are known and comfortable. Change brings about discomfort when the status quo is disrupted. Individuals may feel that their self-interests are threatened. They may have inaccurate perceptions about the nature or implications of the changes or become so threatened that they begin to use psychological defense mechanisms to defend their viewpoints. Some people offer resistance to change because they truly believe the changes will not be beneficial (Box 33-1). Dealing effectively with change requires a period of transition and psychological adaptation. Understanding the *change process* will help both care providers and clients adapt to the continuing process of change.

Box 33-1   Reasons People Resist Change

1. Problems are known and comfortable.
2. Change brings about discomfort.
3. Change disrupts the status quo.
4. Individuals feel their self-interests are threatened.
5. Individuals have inaccurate perceptions about the nature or implications of the change.
6. Individuals may believe the changes will not be beneficial.

The Change Process

There are two basic types of change: planned change and unplanned change (Morrison, 1993). Planned change is the deliberate effort to make things different within a system. Changes are carefully planned and implemented slowly and deliberately. When done appropriately, planned change meets with minimal hostility and resistance. Planned change is always the ideal, but seldom the reality.

Unplanned change is unexpected, not anticipated, and usually not desired. Change happens whether it is planned or unexpected. In health care settings, unplanned changes are daily occurrences. "Expect the unexpected" is a statement often made by managers and supervisors in the workplace to describe unplanned change.

Whether change is unanticipated or expected, intense reactions are provoked in some people. Although reactions to change are highly individual and can range from simple acceptance to outright hostility, most reactions can be generalized into three categories: anxiety, mistrust, and loss. All these reactions have effects on mental health clients.

When the comfort of a daily routine is lost, people (especially those with mental health problems) become anxious. Planned changes for these clients must be implemented slowly, in small steps, giving time for adjustment. Unexpected change, however, does not allow for this luxury, and anxiety levels increase.

Mistrust develops when people are unclear about what is happening. Once individuals feel threatened, resistance develops, and an "us versus them" attitude evolves. To keep mistrust at a minimum, maintain open communications with all those involved in the change. Listen to everyone's concerns and provide what information you can.

Change also involves loss when one gives up old, comfortable attitudes or behaviors. Phrases such as "in the old days" or "the way we used to do it" are expressions associated with loss. Replacing loss with hope by focusing on possible benefits helps people to cope with change, especially if it is unexpected. Hints for coping with unplanned changes are offered in Table 33-2.

Table 33-2 Coping With Unplanned Changes

Nursing action	Comments
Do not panic.	Remain calm no matter what happens.
	Keep your own reactions under control by staying in the "thinking" mode.
	Remember decisions made during high stress are more likely to be ineffective. Stay cool.
Analyze the situation.	Define the problems that are occurring as a result of the change.
	Assess why the change is happening now, and consider its possible effects.
	Assess resources and limitations.
Reset priorities.	Determine what needs to be done.
	List needs in order of importance and then communicate and act.
Match resources with priorities.	Match what needs to be done with the best available resource.
	Resources are always limited. Do the best you can with what you have.
Continuously evaluate.	This step is even more important when the change is unplanned.
	Monitor individuals and groups as they progress through the change process.
	Monitor the situation's dynamics.
	Be prepared for the possibility of other changes.

Mental health care providers must be especially adept at coping with unexpected changes. Change affects us all, but adaptability, healthy emotional responses, and a willingness to support ourselves and others go a long way toward meeting the challenge of coping successfully with changes in our busy world of today.

OTHER CHALLENGES

Life today is filled with a myriad of personal, professional, and social challenges. Personally, we are constantly challenged to move calmly through the struggles of everyday living. Professionally, we are charged with all the obligations and responsibilities of the helping professions, not to mention our duty to the people who become our clients. Socially, we are confronted with many complex and interrelated problems.

Challenges to Society

The social order of many countries is being disrupted by change. Third World countries must cope with the problems of providing the basic necessities of life (food, clothing, shelter) for their citizens. Health care and education are placed lower on the priority list when a country's people are going hungry or are without shelter. Add to this various political disputes, and one can see why so many challenges exist in countries throughout the world.

Modern industrial societies usually manage to feed and clothe the majority of their citizens, but numerous social problems remain. Family structures are changing in many societies; this one factor alone spins off new challenges related to child rearing, financial support, role changes, and group interactions. Homeless families are growing, and with homelessness comes the loss of opportunities for appropriate health care and a solid education. Violence is on the upswing because some persons cannot tolerate the stresses of the modern world.

Social problems affecting health care include challenges to immunize children; control the spread of sophisticated new communicable diseases; provide humane care for the ill, infirm, and aged; and educate the population about healthy living practices. Politically, nurses and all people interested in health are challenged to make health care more accessible, delivering primary care in convenient, familiar community settings.

Persons With AIDS

Individuals with HIV who progress to the next stage of the disease are known as "persons with AIDS," or PWAs. Because of the long incubation period, the changing nature of the virus, and the attitudes of many people, PWAs pose a special challenge for health care providers.

Early detection of HIV infections is important, especially for those who work with mental health clients because many individuals with HIV show signs of central nervous system damage that may present as a psychiatric illness. Many individuals with HIV demonstrate "mental symptoms" before the better known opportunistic infections develop. Clients may have a single complaint or multiple symptoms (Box 33-2). Many of these complaints can be mistaken for depression, so each must be carefully investigated.

Homeless youth and the chronically mentally ill are at an increased risk for contracting HIV. Lack of judgment, and high-risk sexual and substance abuse behaviors make these groups of people especially vulnerable. The incidence of HIV infection is increasing in the 15- to 25-year-old age group, which seems to be related to the lack of accurate information and the syndrome of "it can't happen to me" so common to many individuals of that age. Community mental and physical health care providers must meet the challenge to develop new comprehen-

Box 33-2 Mental Signs and Symptoms of HIV Infection

Agitation
Apathy
Confusion
Decreased memory function
Dementia
Poor appetite
Sleep disturbances
Slowed thinking
Tiredness, lethargy
Weight loss

sive knowledge and skills to serve an ever-increasing population of clients with HIV.

Information Overload

No single person can keep up with all the new knowledge constantly being generated. **Information overload** is a state of mind in which so many facts have been absorbed that they all become an unrelated jumble of stored information. It is easy to become overwhelmed with information today. More information has become available to the average citizen of today's world. In addition, megacommunications systems offer opportunities for an even greater availability of information. Clients are becoming more informed, and sometimes their information contains inaccuracies or half-truths. Health care providers have the responsibility to be accurately informed and knowledgeable about the health care information each client is receiving.

"But how do I cope with the bombardment of information?" you wonder. *Learn something new every day.* We cannot be expected to move through our daily activities and spend our remaining hours pondering over the latest facts or theories, but we can commit ourselves to making the effort to discover something we did not know this morning. Strive to learn at least one new piece of information a day. By the end of a year, you will have gained much new knowledge.

Be open to new information. Some things that sound silly in one time period become reality in another. People said in the 1950s that man would never walk on the moon. Now space travel is taken for granted. Do not discard data that does not fit into your way of thinking. Keep it tucked away; sooner or later it will prove itself to be accurate or false.

Learn to *think critically.* Use logical thinking and the problem-solving process to practice critical thinking skills. Maintain an open mind and a questioning attitude. Realize that knowing how to critically question and relate information is more important than having many facts at hand. This is one of our great challenges.

The Challenge to Care

People remember the health care workers who cared for them, who listened, who held their hand, and who supported them when times were rough. Caring is the essence of nursing and the power of the health care professions. Do not become so involved in the physical aspects that you forget to nurture the art of caring for people, because scientific evidence is lending new support for the actions that make up the art of caring.

As discussed in earlier chapters, studies in the field of psychoneuroimmunology (PNI) are demonstrating that connections between the mind and body are actually an intricate network that responds as a whole. Emotions are responses of a whole person, complete with physical and psychological reactions. Certain therapeutic actions, such as touch, have been found to reduce anxiety levels and may play a role in actually boosting the immune system by decreasing the immunosuppressive effects of stress. Other studies have demonstrated that therapeutic touch can decrease pain and promote wound healing. Currently, the U.S. government is funding research into the effects of therapeutic touch on the immune system's response to stress. Therapeutic emotional interventions are finally receiving scientific attention. We have known all along that caring is a powerful weapon in the search for health and wholeness.

A Look to the Future

As you have read throughout this text, all areas of human functioning are deeply interwoven. Physical illnesses are always accompanied by some level of emotional, intellectual, social, and spiritual distress, and the opposite is also true. Therefore "psychiatric" or "mental health" care is a critical component of every therapeutic situation. Caring for the physical body is not enough. For high levels of wellness and adaptation, the whole individual, every aspect of the dynamic being we call "the client," must be considered with every therapeutic action.

Health is defined by the client's criteria for wellness. Care providers emphasize clients' strengths and their abilities to adapt and to change. By working with clients' personal definitions of health, the focus is on their goals, and an understanding of the interactions between them and their complex and changing environments is gained.

Nurses help clients to adjust to the activities of daily living when clients are confronted by health problems. Because of this, nurses are in the position to shift the focus of health care from one that concentrates on "deficits and deficiencies" to one that considers the possibilities and positive achievements that are within the grasp of each client. This health-oriented point of view allows for successful interventions by concentrating on solutions that draw on clients' strengths and supportive resources.

The health care professions are undergoing change. Because mental distress or illness affects every aspect of a person's life, the care needs of individuals with acute and chronic mental health problems are many. Although several issues affecting mental health policies in the United States and elsewhere are being explored, too few resources are available for treating the numerous individuals who require therapeutic care. As a result, nurses and other health care providers must consider every interaction with their clients as an opportunity for encouraging high levels of mental health. If we are to make progress with the social problems of crime, violence, abuse, homelessness, and poverty, we must treat each mentally troubled person as our most important client because the mental health of a society depends on the mental health of each of its individual citizens.

It is an exciting time to be a health care provider. Maintain a positive attitude. Do your best, strive to learn, and you will turn most of your challenges into opportunities. Numerous challenges await us. Perhaps one of the greatest will be to bring caring into the community and ensure that health care services will be available to every individual. These are your challenges.

KEY CONCEPTS

◆ Health care is undergoing many changes relating to escalating costs, social changes, and technological advances.

◆ Treatment settings for people with mental illness have evolved from the institution to the street, jail, neighborhood clinic, community hospital, and local doctor's office.

◆ The growing number of homeless people challenges all health care providers to meet the many needs of this population.

◆ The Americans with Disabilities Act of 1990 states that people with mental health problems have the same opportunity for employment as other people.

◆ Learning to interact respectfully and effectively with people from different cultures is an important challenge for health care workers.

◆ The role of client has changed from passive participant to active consumer of health care services.

◆ To be considered competent, an individual must be able to make a choice, understand important information, appreciate one's own situation, and apply reasoning.

◆ Clients are obligated to be truthful, responsible, and cooperative with care.

◆ Care providers are obligated to accept the client "as is," demonstrate respect, empower clients, and educate.

◆ Today's mental health care providers include certified nursing assistants, home care aides, and psychiatric technicians.

◆ Expanded roles for nurses include positions in centers for the homeless, collaborating with physicians as case managers, working with psychosocial rehabilitation teams, and meeting the needs of special populations through nurse-owned businesses.

◆ Change, the process of making or becoming different, is inherently neither good nor bad.

◆ To cope with information overload, develop your critical thinking skills by using logical thinking and the problem-solving process.

◆ Early detection of HIV infections is especially important because many clients with HIV show signs of central nervous system damage that may present as a psychiatric illness.

◆ Actions such as therapeutic touch have been found to reduce anxiety levels, decrease pain, and promote wound healing, and these actions may play a role in actually boosting the immune system by decreasing the immunosuppressive effects of stress.

◆ Care providers are in the position to shift the focus of health care from one that concentrates on "deficits and deficiencies" to one that considers the possibilities and positive achievements that are within the grasp of each client.

Suggestions for Further Reading

In the article "Understanding the Seven Stages of Change" (*American Journal of Nursing* 95(4): 41, 1995), Jo Manion states that understanding the stages of change will help you survive and even grow from the change experience.

Internet addresses for general mental health information include the American Psychological Association PsychNet (www.apa.org), Help! A Consumer's Guide to Mental Health (www.iComm.ca/madmagic/help), and Psychlink (www.psychlink.com).

References

Equal Employment Opportunity Commission: *A technical assistance manual on the employee provisions (Title 1) of the Americans with Disabilities Act,* 1992, Washington, DC, U.S. Government Printing Office.

Farnam CR and others: Health status and risk factors of people with severe and persistent mental illness, *Journal of Psychosocial Nursing* 37(6):16, 1999.

Harrington SP: New bedlam: jails—not psychiatric hospitals—now care for the indigent mentally ill, *Humanist* 59(3):9, 1999.

Holland L: Mental health supportive home care aides, *Caring* (4):44, 1993.

Mentally ill denied care, *Chemist & Druggist,* p. 8, April 24, 1999.

Morrison M: *Professional skills for leadership: foundations of a successful career,* St. Louis, 1993, Mosby.

Myths and facts about homelessness, Washington, DC, 1999, National Law Center on Homelessness and Poverty.

National Institute of Mental Health: *The numbers count: mental illness in America,* National Institute of Mental Health Pub No. NIH 99-4584, Bethesda, Md, 1999, Department of Health & Human Services.

Schofield R: Empowerment education for individuals with serious mental illness, *Journal of Psychosocial Nursing* 36(11):35, 1998.

Torrey EF: *Out of the shadows: confronting America's mental illness crisis,* ed 2, New York, 1998, J Wiley.

Torrey EF, Zdanowicz MT: How freedom punishes the severely mentally ill, *USA Today,* July 7, 1999.

Wilk RJ: Are the rights of people with mental illness still important? *Social Work* 39(2):167, 1994.

Appendix A

Standards of Psychiatric–Mental Health Nursing Practice

Standard I. Assessment

The psychiatric–mental health nurse collects patient health data.

Standard II. Diagnosis

The psychiatric–mental health nurse analyzes the assessment data in determining diagnoses.

Standard III. Outcome Identification

The psychiatric–mental health nurse identifies expected outcomes individualized to the patient.

Standard IV. Planning

The psychiatric–mental health nurse develops a plan of care that is negotiated among the patient, nurse, family, and health care team and prescribes evidence-based interventions to attain expected outcomes.

Standard V. Implementation

The psychiatric–mental health nurse implements the interventions identified in the plan of care.

Standard Va. Counseling

The psychiatric–mental health nurse uses counseling interventions to assist patients in regaining or improving their previous coping abilities, fostering mental health, and preventing mental illness and disability.

Standard Vb. Milieu Therapy

The psychiatric–mental health nurse provides, structures, and maintains a therapeutic environment in collaboration with the patient and other health care providers.

Standard Vc. Self-Care Activities

The psychiatric–mental health nurse structures interventions around the patient's activities of daily living to foster self-care and mental and physical well-being.

Standard Vd. Psychobiological Interventions

The psychiatric–mental health nurse uses knowledge of psychobiological interventions and applies clinical skills to restore the patient's health and prevent further disability.

Standard Ve. Health Teaching

The psychiatric–mental health nurse, through health teaching, assists patients in achieving satisfying, productive, and healthy patterns of living.

Standard Vf. Case Management

The psychiatric–mental health nurse provides case management to coordinate comprehensive health services and ensure continuity of care.

Standard Vg. Health Promotion and Health Maintenance

The psychiatric–mental health nurse employs strategies and interventions to promote and maintain mental health and prevent mental illness.

Standard VI. Evaluation

The psychiatric–mental health nurse evaluates the patient's progress in attaining expected outcomes.

From American Nurses Association: *Scope and standards of psychiatric–mental health nursing practice*, Washington, DC, 2000, The Association.

Appendix B

DSM-IV–TR Classification of Adult Mental Disorders

Delirium, Dementia, Amnestic Disorders
Substance-Related Disorders
Schizophrenia and Other Psychotic Disorders
Mood Disorders
Anxiety Disorders
Somatoform Disorders
Factitious Disorders
Dissociative Disorders
Sexual and Gender Identity Disorders
Eating Disorders
Sleeping Disorders
Impulse-Control Disorder Not Elsewhere Classified
Adjustment Disorders
Personality Disorders
Other Conditions
    Psychological factors affecting the medical condition
    Noncompliance
    Relational problems
    Problems related to abuse or neglect
    Borderline intellectual functioning
    Identity problem
    Occupational problem
    Phase of life problem
    Medication-induced disorders
    Malingering
    Antisocial behavior
    Bereavement
    Age-related cognitive decline
    Academic problem
    Religious or spiritual problem

Modified from American Psychiatric Association: *Diagnostic and statistical manual of mental disorders*, ed 4, text revision, Washington, DC, 2000, The Association.

Appendix C

A Simple Method to Determine Tardive Dyskinesia Symptoms: AIMS Examination Procedure*

Patient Identification and Date

Observe the client unobtrusively at rest (e.g., in waiting room).

(The chair to be used in this examination should be a hard, firm one without arms).

After observing the patient, he or she may be rated on a scale according to the severity of symptoms:

0 = none
1 = minimal
2 = mild
3 = moderate
4 = severe

Ask the client whether there is anything in his or her mouth (i.e., gum, candy, etc.) and if there is, to remove it.

Ask client about the current condition of his or her teeth. Ask patient if he or she wears dentures. Do teeth or dentures bother client now?

Ask client whether he or she notices any movements in mouth, face, hands or feet. If yes, ask to describe and to what extent they currently bother patient or interfere with his/her activities.

| 0 | 1 | 2 | 3 | 4 |

Have client sit in chair with hands on knees, legs slightly apart, and feet flat on floor. (Look at entire body for movements while in this position.)

| 0 | 1 | 2 | 3 | 4 |

Ask client to sit with hands hanging unsupported. If male, between legs, if female and wearing a dress, hanging over knees. (Observe hands and other body areas.)

| 0 | 1 | 2 | 3 | 4 |

Ask patient to open mouth. (Observe tongue at rest within mouth.) Do this twice.

| 0 | 1 | 2 | 3 | 4 |

Ask client to protrude tongue. (Observe abnormalities of tongue movement.) Do this twice.

| 0 | 1 | 2 | 3 | 4 |

Ask client to tap thumb, with each finger, as rapidly as possible for 10 to 15 seconds; separately with right hand, then with left hand. (Observe facial and leg movements.)

| 0 | 1 | 2 | 3 | 4 |

From Sandoz Pharmaceuticals, East Hanover, NJ 07936.
*AIMS, Abnormal Involuntary Movement Scale.

Flex and extend client's left and right arms. (One at a time.)

0	1	2	3	4

Ask client to stand up. (Observe in profile. Observe all body areas again, hips included.)

0	1	2	3	4

Ask client to extend both arms outstretched in front with palms down. (Observe trunk, legs, and mouth.)

0	1	2	3	4

† Have client walk a few paces, turn, and walk back to chair. (Observe hands and gait.) Do this twice.

†Activated movements.

Appendix D

Mental Status Assessment at a Glance

1. **Appearance**
   _____ Manner of dress
   _____ Personal grooming
   _____ Facial expressions
   _____ Posture and gait

2. **Speech**
   _____ Manner of response (frank, evading)
   _____ Choice of words (to assess general intelligence, education, levels of function, thought)
   _____ Speech disorder

3. **Level of consciousness**
   _____ Level of alertness
   _____ Orientation (time, place, person)

4. **Attention span**
   _____ Ability to keep thoughts focused on one topic
   _____ Repeat a series of numbers
   _____ Serial 7s (ask client to subtract 7 from 100, 7 from 93, and so on)

5. **Memory**
   _____ Immediate memory (ask client to repeat words after 15 minutes)
   _____ Recent memory (ask client about yesterday's activities)
   _____ Remote memory (ask client about dates of birth, marriage, schooling)

6. **Understanding abstract relationships**
   _____ Understanding of proverbs (concrete or abstract)
   _____ Ability to understand similarities (e.g., "How are a bicycle and an automobile alike?")

7. **Arithmetic and reading ability**
   _____ Simple addition, subtraction, multiplication, and division (ask client to make change)
   _____ Ability to read newspaper, magazine

8. **General information knowledge**
   _____ Discuss newspaper or magazine article
   _____ General information questions (e.g., "How many days in a year? Where does the sun set?")

9. **Judgment**
   _____ Responses to family, work, financial problems
   _____ Responses to "What would you do if . . ." questions

10. **Emotional status**
    _____ Ask "How do you feel today?" or "How do you feel about . . ." questions
    _____ Affect
    _____ Current situation and coping behaviors

Modified from Jess LW: Investigating impaired mental status: an assessment guide you can use, *Nursing* 18(6):42, 1988.

Glossary

abstinence Nonuse of an addictive substance or behaviors.

abuse Process of causing an individual harm.

abused substances Chemicals that alter the individual's perception by affecting the central nervous system (CNS); also referred to as mind-altering substances.

acceptance Act of receiving or taking what is being offered or given.

acquired immunodeficiency syndrome (AIDS) A viral infection that prevents the body from warding off infectious diseases.

acting out Use of inappropriate, detrimental, or destructive behaviors to express current or past emotions.

acupuncture Insertion of fine needles into the skin at certain specific sites or meridians along the body to treat illness.

adaptation Change or response to stress of any kind; degree and nature of adaptation shown by a client, regularly evaluated by the nurse; in nursing, the effectiveness of nursing care, the course of the disease, and the ability of the client to cope with stress.

addiction Physical dependence on a drug that is taken or behavior that is performed despite the physical and psychosocial problems associated with its use.

addictive behaviors Obsessive-compulsive activities that take the form of certain repetitive behaviors, such as gambling, shopping, working, and engaging in excessive sexual activity.

adolescence Period of life between 11 and 21 years of age.

adolescent suicide Act of intentionally taking one's own life by a person between 11 and 21 years of age.

adulthood The period of life lasting from about 18 to approximately 65 years of age.

advocacy Process of providing a client with information, support, and feedback so that the client can make an informed decision.

affect Outward manifestation of a person's feelings or emotions.

affective Pertaining to emotion, mood, or feeling.

affective disorder Ineffective emotional state, ranging from deep depression to excited elation.

affective loss In dementia, the loss of mood, emotion, and personality.

ageism Practice of stereotyping older persons as feeble, dependent, and nonproductive.

aggression Forceful attitude or action that is expressed physically, symbolically, or verbally.

aging Process of growing older.

agitation Behavior that is verbally or physically offensive.

agnosia Inability to recognize familiar environmental objects or people (stimuli).

agoraphobia Anxiety about possible situations (especially open or public places) in which a panic attack may occur.

AIDS Acquired immunodeficiency syndrome, a viral infection that prevents the body from warding off infectious diseases.

akathisia Inability to sit still, commonly caused by antipsychotic drugs.

akinesia Absence of movement, physically and mentally.

alcohol Ethanol (ETOH), the results of the fermentation or distillation of yeast and grains, malts, or fruits.

alcoholism Chronic disease caused by prolonged or excessive alcohol use.

alexithymia Difficulty in identifying and describing emotions.

Alzheimer's disease Progressive, degenerative disorder that impedes the functioning of brain cells and synapses and results in impaired memory, thinking, and behavior.

ambivalence State in which an individual experiences conflicting feelings, attitudes, or drives.

amnesia Loss of memory that cannot be explained by normal forgetfulness.

amphetamines Class of drugs that act as central nervous system stimulants.

anergy Inability to start an activity.

anger Normal emotional response to a perceived threat, frustration, or distressing event; occurs in response to an individual's frustration level or feelings of being threatened or losing control.

anhedonia Loss of interest or pleasure from previously enjoyed activities.

anorexia nervosa Severe disturbance in eating behavior; can result in a body that is much lower than its ideal weight.

Antabuse Chemical disulfiram; when taken with alcohol, produces uncomfortable and possibly serious physical reactions.

anticholinergic Drug used to block the responses to parasympathetic stimulation, which results in dilated pupils, dry eyes and mouth, and rapid heart rate.

anticholinergic reaction Effect caused by drugs that block acetylcholine receptors and cause such symptoms as dry mouth, blurred vision, constipation, rapid heart beat, and urinary hesitancy.

anticipatory grief The process of grieving before an actual event occurs.

anticonvulsant Drug used to treat and prevent seizures.

antipsychotic Drug used to treat the symptoms of major mental disorders.

antisocial personality Pervasive pattern of disregard for and violation of the rights of others.

anxiety Vague, uneasy feeling experienced by individuals in response to real or imagined stress.

anxiety disorder Psychic tension that interferes with a person's ability to perform the activities of daily living.

anxiety state State that occurs when an individual's coping abilities are overwhelmed and emotional control is lost.

anxiety trait Learned component of the personality in which an individual reacts to relatively nonstressful situations with anxiety.

anxiolytics Group of drugs designed to reduce anxiety; the antianxiety medications.

apathy Lack of feelings, emotions, concern, or interests.

aphasia Disorder in which language function is defective or absent; inability to speak or understand verbal messages.

assault Any behavior that presents an immediate threat to another person.

assertiveness Ability to directly express one's feelings or needs in a way that respects the rights of other people and retains the individual's dignity.

assessment First step of the nursing process, which includes the gathering, clustering, and analysis of data relating to a client.

attention-deficit hyperactivity disorder Cluster of behaviors associated with inattention and impulsive actions.

attitudes Ideas that help make up our points of view; one's outlook.

autism Pervasive developmental disorder of the brain. Symptoms appear during the first 3 years of life and include disturbances in physical, social, and language skills; abnormal responses to sensations; and abnormal ways of relating to people, objects, and events.

autonomic nervous system System responsible for regulating the internal vital functions of the body, such as the cardiac and smooth muscles.

autonomic tone Ability of tissue to coordinate actions with other tissues. Neurotransmitters of both the sympathetic and the parasympathetic nervous systems affect the function of each organ or tissue, but one branch dominates and sets the tone of that tissue to coordinate with other tissues.

autonomy Ability to direct and control one's own activities, one's destiny.

avoidance behaviors Refusal to cope with anxiety-producing situations by ignoring them.

avoidant personality Extreme anxiety related to a fear of rejection and humiliation; to prevent possible rejection, individuals narrow their interests to a small range of activities with a very small, if any, support system.

battered wife Repeated abuse of someone, usually a woman.

battering Repeated abuse of someone, usually a woman, child, or elder.

battery Unlawful use of force on a person.

behavior Manner of conducting oneself; one's actions.

belief Conviction that is mentally accepted as true whether or not it is based in fact.

beneficence To actively do good.

bereavement Emotional and behavioral state of thoughts, feelings, and activities that follow a loss.

bereavement-related depression State of bereavement in which the griever feels the loss so intensely that despair, worthlessness, and depression overwhelm everything else in life.

bill of rights List of client's rights set forth by the American Hospital Association; offers some guidance and protection to clients by stating the responsibilities that a hospital and its staff have toward clients and their families during hospitalization; not a legally binding document.

binge eating Uncontrolled ingestion (in a certain period of time) of an amount of food that is definitely larger than most individuals would eat in similar circumstances.

biofeedback A process that provides visual or auditory information about autonomic body functions.

bipolar disorder Behavioral problems caused by sudden, dramatic shifts in emotional extremes.

bisexual Person who is attracted to and engages in sexual activities with members of both genders.

block grant Certain sum of money granted by the federal government to the states for health care.

body dysmorphic disorder Preoccupation with a physical difference or defect in one's body.

body image Person's subjective concept of his or her physical appearance.

borderline personality Instability in mood, thinking, behavior, personal relationships, and self-image.

bradykinesia Slowing down of body movements and mental state.

bulimia Uncontrolled ingestion of large amounts of food (called *binge eating*), followed by inappropriate methods to prevent weight gain (called *purging*).

caffeine Active ingredient of coffee, tea, and other beverages that stimulates the central nervous system.

calculation Ability to perform mathematical problems.

cannabis Leaves and flowers of the plant *Cannabis sativa;* also called marijuana.

career One's preparation for and advancements or achievements in a particular vocation.

caring Concern for the well-being of a person shown in ways such as attentive listening, comforting, honesty, acceptance, and sensitivity.

caregiver-client relationship A directed energy exchange between two people, a flow that moves clients toward more effective behaviors.

case management Assignment of a health care provider to assist a client in assessing health and social service systems and to ensure that all required services are obtained.

cataplexy Sudden episode of bilateral muscle weakness and loss of muscle tone that lasts for seconds to minutes.

catastrophic reaction Minor anxieties or frustrations that cascade into severe behavioral reactions in which the person becomes increasingly confused, agitated, and fearful and may wander, become noisy, act compulsively, or behave violently.

catatonia State or condition characterized by obvious motor disturbances, usually immobility with muscle rigidity, or (less commonly) excessive impulsive activity.

catchment area Delineated geographical region used for the planning of health care services.

central nervous system (CNS) Brain and spinal cord, which together control all the motor and sensory functions of the body.

cephalocaudal growth A pattern of growth and development in which the head of an organism develops first, followed by the extremities, then feet.

change process Series of steps that result in a difference.

chemical Substance, drug, or medication.

chemical dependency Psychophysiological state of being addicted to drugs or alcohol; also called *addiction*.

chemical restraint Antipsychotic medication; a medication that reduces or eliminates psychotic symptoms and quiets behavior.

child abuse Mistreatment of children through physical, sexual, or emotional abuse.

chronicity Long-term, persistent difficulties; in chronic mental disorders, periods of relative comfort and ease of functioning, alternating with relapses into acute psychiatric states.

chronic mental illness Recurrence of one or more psychiatric disorders, which results in significant functional disability.

clang associations Use of words that have rhythm.

closed system Set of interacting, related units with rigid, impermeable boundaries that close out information and energy and eventually shorten survival.

cocaine Processed extract of the coca plant, which causes central nervous stimulation and intense feelings of well-being.

code of ethics Statement encompassing the set of rules by which practitioners of a profession are expected to conform.

cognition Activities of the mind characterized by knowing, learning, judging, reasoning, and memory.

cognitive Pertaining to the mental processes of comprehension, judgment, memory, and reasoning.

cognitive loss Decline in cognitive abilities and intellect, including an inability to recall recent events and process new information, agnosia, apraxia, and aphasia.

commitment Personal bond to some course of action.

communication Reciprocal exchange of information, ideas, beliefs, feelings, and attitudes between two persons or among a group of persons.

communication disorder Problems with expressing and receiving messages, pronouncing words, and stuttering that interfere with a child's development.

communication style Rituals connected with greeting and departure, the lines of conversation, and the directness of communication.

community mental health centers Outpatient settings in which a comprehensive range of mental health services are made readily available to all members of a community.

community support system Organized network of caring and trained people committed to assisting the chronically mentally ill to meet their needs within the community.

comorbidity Two medical or psychiatric disorders present at the same time.

compassion Symptomatic consciousness of others' distress together with a desire to alleviate it.

competent State of being able to make a choice, understand important information, appreciate one's own situation, and apply reasoning.

compliance Act of following prescribed treatments.

complicated grief Persistent yearning for a deceased person and other related symptoms that often occur without the signs of depression but are associated with impaired psychological functioning and disturbances of mood, sleep, and self-esteem.

compulsion Distressing recurring behavior that must be performed to reduce anxiety.

compulsive overeating Pattern of eating to lessen emotional discomfort, anxiety, or distress.

conative loss Loss of the ability to make and carry out plans.

concrete thinking Inability to identify or describe feelings, experiences, and behavior abstractly.

conduct disorder Persistent pattern of unacceptable behaviors, which include defiance of authority, engaging in aggressive actions toward others, refusal to follow society's rules and norms, and violation of the rights of others.

confidence Belief in the nurse's ability to assist, to help clients cope with the difficulties and implications of their health problems; a trust or belief in one's own abilities.

confidentiality Sharing of client information only with those persons who are directly involved in the care of the client.

conscience Knowledge or feeling of what is right and wrong, often accompanied by a strong desire to do the "right thing."

consistency Behaviors that imply being steady and regular, dependable.

consultation Process in which the assistance of a specialist is sought to help identify ways in which to cope effectively with client management problems.

context Setting or environment in which an event occurs.

continuous mental health care team Group of specialists who assume full responsibility for the care of their clients during all stages of illness, in or out of the hospital.

contract law Division of private law that focuses on agreements between individuals or institutions.

controlled substance Certain drug classes manufactured, distributed, and dispensed according to the federal regulations of the 1970 Controlled Substances Act.

conversion disorder Somatoform disorder in which the individual presents with problems related to the sensory or motor functions.

coping mechanisms Any thought or action that is aimed at reducing stress.

coping resources Options, strategies, and methods for dealing with stress.

countertransference Barrier in the therapeutic relationship based in the nurse's emotional responses to the client.

courage Response that allows us to face and cope with those aspects of life that are dangerous, difficult, or painful.

covert modeling Act of mentally rehearsing a difficult performance or event before actually doing the activity.

crack Type of processed cocaine made by combining cocaine with ammonia or baking soda and heating the mixture to remove the hydrochloride molecule, resulting in chips or chunks of highly addicting cocaine, called *rocks*.

crime Actions or behaviors that break the laws of a society.

criminal law Division of public law designed to protect the members of a society.

crisis Period of severe emotional disorganization resulting from a lack of appropriate coping mechanisms or supports.

crisis intervention Short-term, active therapy that provides emotional first aid for victims of trauma with the goal of assisting individuals and families to manage the immediate crisis situation and return to precrisis levels of functioning.

crisis stabilization Goal of crisis intervention; process of assisting clients in coping with crisis situations by placing them in a 1 or 2-day treatment setting where equilibrium (homeostasis) can be reestablished.

cultural competence The process of continually learning about the cultures with which we work and developing cross-cultural therapeutic health care skills.

culture Set of learned values, beliefs, customs, and behaviors that is shared by a group of interacting individuals.

culture-bound disorder Mental problems that appear to be associated to members of a specific culture.

cyberspace Communications through the use of computers and their networks.

cyclothymic disorder Pattern of behaviors involving repeated mood swings, alternating between hypomania and depressive symptoms.

data collection Activities that elicit, retrieve, or discover information about a certain subject.

deceit Lying; act of representing as true something that is known to be false.

defamation Any false communication that results in harm.

defense mechanisms Unconscious, intrapsychic reaction that offers protection to the self from a stressful situation.

deinstitutionalization At the individual patient level, the transfer to a community setting of a patient who has been hospitalized for an extended period of time; at the mental health care system level, a shift in the focus of mental health care from the large, long-term institution to the community through the discharge of long-term patients and avoidance of unnecessary admissions.

delirium Change of consciousness that occurs over a short period of time.

delusions False beliefs that are resistant to reasoning or change.

dementia Loss of multiple abilities, including short- and long-term memory, language, and the ability to understand (conceptualize).

demonical exorcisms Religious ceremonies in which the patients were physically punished to drive away the possessing spirit.

denial Psychological defense mechanism in which one refuses to acknowledge painful facts.

dependent personality Anxiety associated with separation and abandonment with a deep fear of rejection that expresses itself as the need to be cared for.

depersonalization Feeling of unreality and alienation from self with ego and self-concept disorganization.

depression Emotional state characterized by feelings of sadness, disappointment, and despair.

derealization Loss of ego boundaries; inability to tell where one's body ends and the environment begins.

detoxification The process of withdrawing a substance under medical supervision.

development Increasing ability in skills or functions.

direct self-destructive behavior Any form of active suicidal behavior, such as threats, gestures, or attempts to intentionally end one's life.

disability Loss, absence, or impairment of physical or mental fitness.

discharge planning Process whereby nurses help clients cope with the hurdles of illness or surgery through early identification and intervention of potential problems following discharge from a health care facility.

discrimination Act of showing favor or disfavor to a person or group of people in a manner unacceptable to society.

disease Condition in which a physical dysfunction exists.

dissociation Disconnection from full awareness of self, time, or external circumstances.

dissociative disorder A disturbance in the normally interacting functions of consciousness: identity, memory, and perception.

dissociative identity disorder Repeated and persistent episodes in which one feels detached or unconnected to the self.

disturbed communications Interference in communication related to the sending or receiving of messages, inadequate mastery of the language, insufficient information, or no opportunity for feedback.

disulfiram (Antabuse) A chemical that produces uncomfortable and possibly serious physical reactions when taken with alcohol.

domestic violence Aggressive behaviors directed toward significant others.

drug-induced parkinsonism Group of symptoms that mimic Parkinson's disease, including tremors, muscle rigidity, and difficulty with voluntary movements.

dual diagnosis In mental health, the presence of two or more psychiatric disorders, one commonly being substance abuse.

duty to warn Duty to protect potential victims from possible harm by a psychiatric client.

dying process Experience of progressing through several psychological stages before the actual death occurs, which allows people to cope with the overwhelming emotional reactions associated with losing loved ones.

dynamics Interactions among the various forces operating in any system.

dyskinesia Inability to execute voluntary movements.

dyslexia Impaired ability to read, sometimes accompanied by a mixing of letters or syllables in a word when speaking.

dyspareunia Pain associated with sexual intercourse.

dyssomnia Sleep disorder characterized by abnormalities in the amount, quality, or timing of sleep.

dysthymia Daily moderate depression that lasts for longer than 2 years.

dystonia Impaired muscle tone.

eating disorder Ongoing disturbance in behaviors associated with the ingestion of food.

eccentric Odd, unconventional, irregular, out of the ordinary.

echolalia Purposeless imitation of another's speech, repetition of another's statement over and over.

echopraxia Purposeless imitation of another's movements.

ego In psychoanalysis, the part of the psyche that experiences and maintains conscious contact with reality; rational part of the personality; seat of such mental processes as perception and memory; develops defense mechanisms to cope with anxiety.

elder abuse Any action on the part of a caregiver to take advantage of an older adult, his or her emotional well-being, or property.

electroconvulsive therapy (ECT) Artificial induction of a grand mal seizure by passing a controlled electrical current through electrodes applied to one or both temples.

elopement Announced leaving or running away from an inpatient health care institution.

emotions Nonintellectual reactions to various stimuli, based on individual's perceptions.

empathy Ability to recognize and share the emotions and states of mind of another and to understand the meaning and significance of that person's behavior.

empowerment Active assumption of the rights, benefits, responsibilities, and obligations of a particular role.

encopresis Fecal incontinence in a child older than 4 years of age with no physical abnormalities; includes the repeated, usually voluntary, passage of feces in inappropriate places.

entrepreneur A self-employed person. In nursing, those who have established their own nurse-operated clinics, act as health care consultants, and provide a variety of health care services to business and industry.

enuresis Involuntary urinary incontinence of a child 5 years or older.

environmental control Ability of an individual to perceive and control his or her environment.

epilepsy Condition of abnormal electrical activity in the brain, characterized by recurrent episodes of seizure activity, abnormal behaviors, sensory disturbances, loss of or changes in consciousness, or a combination of these events.

equilibrium Attempt of a system or organism to maintain a steady state or balance within itself and among other systems.

erotic Inducing sexual feelings.

erratic Deviating from conventional or customary course; having no fixed purpose or direction.

ethical dilemma Uncertainty or disagreement about the moral principles that endorse different courses of action.

ethics Set of rules or values that govern right behavior.

ethnicity Broad term that refers to the socialization patterns, customs, and cultural habits of a particular group.

evaluation Process by which one compares data and makes a judgment.

exacerbation Periods marked by an increase in the signs and symptoms and seriousness of a problem or disorder.

exhibitionism Exposure of one's genitals to an unsuspecting person followed by sexual arousal.

expectations Behaviors that one assumes based on what the individual thinks another person expects or desires.

exploitation Use of another individual for selfish purposes, profit, or gain.

extended family Household group consisting of parents, children, grandparents, and other family members.

external loss Those losses outside the individual that relate to objects, possessions, the environment, loved ones, and support.

extrapyramidal side effects (EPSEs) Abnormal involuntary movement disorders caused by a drug-induced imbalance between two major neurotransmitters, dopamine and acetylcholine, in portions of the brain.

factitious disorder Signs and symptoms that are intentionally produced so that one may assume the sick role.

failure Lack of success; neglect or omission.

false imprisonment Detention of a competent person against his or her will.

family Group of people who are biologically or emotionally attached, interact regularly, and share concerns for the growth and development of each member.

fear Response to an appraisal of a dangerous stressor.

feedback Responses and intrapersonal communications of each person when messages are being sent and received.

felony Crime that is punishable by imprisonment or death.

fetishism Use of objects (e.g., panties, leather, rubber sheeting) for the purpose of sexual arousal.

flashback Vivid recollections of an event in which the individual relives a frightening, traumatic experience.

flight of ideas Abrupt change of topic in a rapid flow of speech.

flooding Method for treating phobias in which the client is rapidly and repeatedly exposed to the feared object or situation until anxiety levels diminish.

forensic evidence Objective information that is obtained from a victim and used in a court of law to determine guilt or innocence of an alleged perpetrator of violence.

fraud Act of giving of false information with the knowledge that it will be acted on.

frotteurism Practice of rubbing up against a nonconsenting person with the purpose of sexual arousal.

fugue Escape from reality; dissociative fugue: sudden, unexpected travel, with an inability to recall the past.

functional assessment Analysis of each client's abilities to perform the activities of daily living.

gang Group of people, generally adolescents, who act, look, and dress alike; share the same values; and follow similar codes of conduct.

gay Male or female homosexual.

gender The male or female sex; one's biological sex.

gender abuse Aggressive, violent, or exploitative behaviors that are directed toward members of one sex, usually female.

gender identity The personal identity of being male or female that one carries.

gender perception A view of one's maleness or femaleness.

gender role Expected cultural and social patterns of behavior based on one's sex.

generalized seizure Discharge of electrical activity within the brain that generally results in loss of consciousness.

genuineness Quality of being open, honest, sincere; actively involved.

gerontophobia Fear of aging and refusal to accept the elderly into the mainstream of society.

glycogenolysis The process of removing stored sugar from the liver and converting it to glucose for bodily energy.

gregarious Sociable, in need of the company of others.

grief Set of emotional reactions that accompany a loss.

grieving process The experience of coping with a significant loss.

growth Development from a lower or simpler to a higher or more complex form.

habituation Occurs when an individual depends on a substance to provide pleasure or relief from discomfort.

hallucination False sensory input with no external stimulus, usually in the form of smells, sounds, tastes, sight, or touch.

hallucinogen Chemical substance that alters one's reality.

health A state of physical, emotional, sociocultural, and spiritual well-being in which the psychological realms are in balance with the physical self in a state of homeostasis.

health-illness continuum Broad spectrum or scale by means of which a person's level of health can be described, ranging from high-level wellness to severe illness.

health maintenance organization Group of doctors, hospitals, and clinics who deliver health care to enrolled clients who pay a fixed, negotiated fee.

helping boundaries Professional limitations that define the needs of the nurse as distinctly different from the needs of the patient: what is too helpful and what is not and what fosters independence versus unhealthy dependence.

heroin A semisynthetic narcotic of opium.

heterosexual Person who expresses sexuality with members of the opposite sex.

histrionic personality Pattern of excessive emotional expression accompanied by attention-seeking behaviors.

HIV/AIDS Human immunodeficiency virus; a retrovirus that results in acquired immunodeficiency syndrome and its various resultant disorders.

hoarding Act of collecting and saving assorted, seemingly useless items.

holistic health care Philosophical concept designed to consider all aspects of human functioning and help clients achieve harmony within themselves and with others, nature, and the world.

homelessness Lack of a regular and adequate nighttime residence.

homeostasis Tendency of the body to achieve and maintain a steady internal state.

homicide The taking of anther's life: murder.

homosexual Person who expresses sexual desire or preference for members of one's own sex.

hope Multidimensional dynamic life force characterized by an anticipated and confident yet uncertain expectation of achieving a future good.

hospice Philosophy of care for people with terminal illnesses or conditions and their loved ones.

hospitalization Placing of an ill or injured person into an inpatient health care facility that provides continuous nursing care and an organized medical staff.

human dimensions Major facets or areas of being human, which include physical, emotional, intellectual, social, and spiritual functions.

humoral theory of disease Hippocrates's view that illness was the result of an imbalance of the body's humors of blood, phlegm, black bile, and yellow bile.

hypersomnia Sleep disorder characterized by excessive sleepiness.

hypertensive crisis Condition in which the blood pressure rises to extreme levels; commonly caused by an interaction between monoamine oxidase inhibitors and other substances.

hypochondriasis Somatoform disorder in which one has an intense fear or preoccupation of having a serious disease or medical condition based on a misinterpretation of body signs and symptoms.

hypomania Exaggerated sense of cheerfulness and well-being.

id In psychoanalysis the part of the psyche functioning in the unconscious that is the source of instinctive energy, impulses, and drives and is based on the pleasure principle and has strong tendencies toward self-preservation.

ideas of reference Incorrect perceptions of causal events as having great or significant meaning; finding special, personal messages in everyday events.

identity diffusion Failure to bring various childhood identifications into an effective adult personality.

illness State of social, emotional, intellectual, and physical dysfunction.

illusions False perceptions of actual stimuli.

imagery Formation of mental concepts, figures, or ideas.

impulse-control Ability to express one's emotions in appropriate or effective ways.

impulsivity Pattern of behavior in which actions are taken without forethought or regard to the consequences.

incest Inappropriate sexual activities with one or more members of one's family.

incongruent communications Interactions in which the verbal messages being sent do not match one's nonverbal communications.

indirect self-destructive behaviors Any behaviors that may result in harm to the individual's well-being or death in which people have no actual intention of ending their lives.

inferiority Feeling of being inadequate or less than others.

information overload Inability to process data because of their sheer volume.

informed consent Process of presenting clients with information about the benefits, risks, and side effects of specific treatments, thus enabling clients to make voluntary and competent decisions about their care.

inhalant Chemical substance that is introduced into the body by breathing in through the nose and mouth.

inpatient psychiatric care Health care facility that provides 24-hour-a-day care within a structured and protective setting.

insight The power or act of seeing into a situation; understanding the inner nature of things.

insomnia A disorder of falling asleep or maintaining a sound sleep.

institutionalization Result of adapting to an environment to the point at which one is unable or unwilling to live in a different environment.

integrity State of wholeness, of being complete.

intelligence Person's general knowledge, including orientation, memory, and ability to calculate and think abstractly.

internal loss Physical or emotional losses that involve some part of oneself.

interpersonal communications Interactions that occur between two or more persons consisting of the verbal and nonverbal messages that are sent and received during every interaction.

interview Purposeful, organized conversation with a client.

intoxication State of being under the influence of a chemical substance or drug.

intrapersonal communications Messages that are sent and received within oneself.

introspection Analysis of self, including one's feelings, reactions, attitudes, opinions, values, and behaviors.

invasion of privacy Violation of a person's space, body, belongings, or personal information.

involuntary commitment Request for mental health services that is initiated by someone other than the client.

involvement The process of actively interacting with the environment and those persons within it.

judgment Ability to evaluate choices and make appropriate decisions.

la belle indifference Lack of concern or indifference about the nature or the implications of the signs and symptoms of a somatoform disorder.

laryngeal-pharyngeal dystonia Life-threatening side effect of antipsychotic medications that occurs when the muscles of the throat become rigid and the client begins to gag, choke, and become cyanotic. Respiratory distress and asphyxia result if immediate intervention does not occur.

laws Controls by which a society governs itself.

learned helplessness Feeling of no control over self as a result of learning faulty attitudes and behaviors.

learning disorder Problems with learning to read, write, or calculate.

lesbian Woman who prefers homosexuality as a mode of sexual expression.

libel Written communication that results in harm.

libidinal energy Also called libido; psychic energy or instinctual drive associated with sexual desire, pleasure, or creativity.

life space Psychological field or space in which one moves, including oneself, other people, and objects.

limit setting Process of consistently reinforcing the established structure (rules, routine) of the therapeutic setting.

lithium Naturally occurring salt used to treat mania.

lobotomy Surgical procedure that disconnects the frontal lobes from the thalamus in the brain and results in a decrease in violent behaviors and mood swings.

locus of control Power an individual possesses to control his or her environment.

loose associations Thought disturbance in which the speaker rapidly shifts topics from one unrelated area to another.

loss Actual or potential state in which a valued object, person, or body part that was formerly present is lost or changed and can no longer be seen, felt, heard, known, or experienced.

lunacy Medieval term meaning a mental disorder caused by or relating to the moon.

machismo Compulsive masculinity evidenced by preoccupation with physical strength and athletic prowess, attempts to demonstrate daring, or violent and aggressive behaviors.

malingering Somatoform disorder in which one produces symptoms to meet a recognizable, external goal.

malpractice Failure to exercise an accepted degree of professional skill or learning, resulting in injury, loss, or damage.

mania Extreme emotional state characterized by excitement, great elation, overtalkativeness, increased motor activity, fleeting grandiose ideas, and agitated behaviors.

manic depression Behavioral problems caused by sudden, dramatic shifts in emotional extremes; older term for a bipolar disorder.

manipulation Controlling others for one's own purposes by influencing them in unfair or false ways.

marijuana Leaves and flowers of the plant *Cannabis sativa*.

marriage A legal state that bonds two people as a single family unit.

masochism Sexual arousal achieved by being the recipient of pain, humiliation, or suffering.

maturation Process of attaining complete physical and psychosocial development.

maturity The ability to accept responsibility for one's actions, delay gratification, and make priorities; the period in life from the end of adolescence until death.

memory Ability to recall past events, experience, and perceptions.

memory loss Natural part of the aging process relating to the inability to recall a certain detail or event.

mental health Relative state of mind in which a person who is healthy is able to cope with and adjust to the recurrent stresses of everyday living in an acceptable way.

mental health care team Group of professionally trained specialists who develop and implement comprehensive treatment plans for clients with mental/emotional problems.

mental illness Any disturbance of emotional equilibrium that results in maladaptive behaviors and impaired functioning.

mentally healthy adult A person who can cope with and adjust to the recurrent stresses of daily living in an acceptable way.

mental retardation Developmental disorder characterized by significantly below average intellectual level and limited abilities to function.

methadone Narcotic used to treat long-term heroin addiction.

middle adulthood Period of life from about 35 to around 65 years of age.

misdemeanor Crime that is punishable by fines or imprisonment of less than 1 year.

model Example or pattern that provides a matrix or framework for a theory.

monoamine oxidase inhibitors (MAOIs) Antidepressant drug that can produce serious drug and food interactions, such as cardiovascular and blood pressure reactions and CNS depression.

mood Subjective state of an individual's overall feelings.

mood disorder Prolonged emotional state that influences one's whole personality and life functioning.

morals Attitudes, beliefs, and values that define one's basis for right or wrong behavior.

mortality Condition of being subject to death.

mourning Process of working through or resolving one's grief.

mutism Refusal or inability to communicate.

mutuality Process through which the client assumes an appropriate level of autonomy without blocking the provision of necessary health care services.

narcissistic personality Pattern of behavior characterized by ideas of grandiosity and the need to be admired; belief that one is special, unique, or extra important.

narcolepsy Uncommon sleep disorder in which an individual has repeated attacks of sleep.

narcotic Natural, semisynthetic, or synthetic chemical substance that acts as a central nervous system depressant.

natural selection Theory that states that only the fittest organisms survive and evolve.

need Requirement; something that one cannot do without.

negative symptoms In schizophrenia, behaviors that indicate a lack of adaptive mechanisms, including flat affect, poor grooming, withdrawal, and poverty of speech.

neglect Lack of meeting a dependent person's (usually a child's) basic needs for food, clothing, shelter, love, and belonging.

negligence Omission or commission of an act that a reasonable and prudent person would or would not do.

neologism Invented or made-up word.

neuroleptic malignant syndrome (NMS) Serious and potentially fatal extrapyramidal side effect of antipsychotic or neuroleptic medications.

neuron The basic unit of the nervous system whose function is to transmit electrical information to other nerve cells.

neuropeptides Neurotransmitter composed of amino acid strings that interacts with the endocrine, immune, and nervous systems.

neurotransmitters Chemical found in the nervous system that facilitates the transmission of energy and acts as the body's chemical messenger system.

nicotine Addictive, active ingredient of tobacco.

noncompliance Informed decision made by a client not to follow a prescribed treatment program.

nonmaleficence The ethical principle that states do no harm.

nontherapeutic communications Messages that hinder effective communications.

nonverbal communications Messages that are sent and received without the use of words, which includes one's intrapersonal communications; the messages created through the body's motions and use of touch, space, and sight; unspoken interpersonal communications; and such behaviors as eye movement, gestures, movement of the body, expressions, posture, and eye contact.

norms Established rules of conduct that arise from a culture's behavioral standards.

nuclear family Household unit consisting of two parents and their offspring.

nurse case manager Professional nurses who work with psychiatrists to develop treatment plans tailored to each client's special needs.

nurse practice acts State regulations that define the limits and scope of nursing practice.

nursing (therapeutic) process Organizational framework for the practice of nursing that uses the steps of assessment, nursing diagnosis, planning, implementation, and evaluation for the delivery of client care.

nurture Act or process of promoting the development of persons or things.

obesity Abnormal increase in body fat; body weight that is more than 20% above one's ideal weight.

object constancy Awareness that a person or item still exists even though it cannot be perceived (seen, touched) at the time.

obsession Persistent, recurring, inappropriate, and distressing thoughts.

obsessive-compulsive personality Extreme anxiety about the uncertainty of the future; extremely orderly and overly preoccupied with details; devoted to work, has few leisure activities, and is consumed by the need for perfection.

obstructive sleep apnea Sleep disruptions caused by abnormalities of ventilation during sleep.

oculogyric crisis Dystonic reaction, usually a side-effect of psychotropic medication, in which the eyes involuntarily roll to the back of the head.

older adulthood Period of life from around 65 years of age to death.

open system Set of interacting, related units with permeable boundaries through which matter, energy, and information pass.

opiates Opioids; processed products of opium.

oppositional defiant disorder A pattern of negative, aggressive behaviors with authority figures in the child's life in which the child is constantly involved in power struggles, always fighting for control and attention.

outpatient mental health care Health care setting that provides comprehensive services for mentally ill clients within their home environments.

pain disorder Pain or discomfort that is the major focus of distress when no physical cause of the pain can be identified.

pain management Series of nursing interventions designed to assist clients in identifying, defining, and controlling pain.

panic attack Brief period of intense fear or discomfort accompanied by various physical and emotional reactions.

paranoia Suspicious system of thinking with delusions of persecution and grandeur; pattern of behaviors marked by suspiciousness and mistrust.

paraphilia Group of sexual variations that depart from society's traditional and acceptable modes of seeking sexual gratification.

parasomnias Sleep disorders characterized by abnormal behavioral or physical events during sleep.

parasuicidal behaviors Unsuccessful attempts and gestures of suicide that are associated with a low likelihood of success.

parasympathetic nervous system A branch of the autonomic nervous system that is designed to conserve energy and the sympathetic system's excitability. The main functions are to monitor and control the regulatory processes of the body, which it accomplishes by governing smooth muscle tone and glandular secretions.

partial seizure Discharge of electrical activity in the brain that results in a change in consciousness, sensory disturbances, or abnormal behaviors.

passive aggression Indirect expressions of anger through subtle, evasive, or manipulative behaviors.

passive suicide Act of taking of one's own life by refusing to eat, drink, or cooperate with care.

paternalism Attitude in which the care provider becomes the judge of what is best for clients, limiting clients' abilities to make decisions and increasing their dependency on others.

PCP (phencyclidine) Drug developed for use as an animal tranquilizer; in humans, produces mild depression with low doses and a schizophrenic-like reaction with higher amounts.

pedophilia Fondling or other types of sexual activity with a prepubescent child (usually younger than 13 years of age) initiated by an adult.

peer groups Group of people of similar age, interests, and developmental levels.

perception Use of the senses to gain information.

peripheral nervous system Thirty-one spinal nerves that originate in the spinal cord in addition to the 12 pairs of cranial nerves; further divided into a motor and an autonomic system.

perpetrator Person who executes, with or without planning, a crime or act of violence or aggression.

perseveration Repeating of the same idea in response to different questions or interactions.

personal identity Composite of behavioral traits and characteristics by which one is recognized as an individual.

personality Unique pattern of attitudes and behaviors each individual develops to adapt to a particular environment and its standards.

personality disorder Enduring pattern of inner experience and behavior that deviates markedly from the expectations of the individual's culture, is pervasive and inflexible, has an onset in adolescence or early adulthood, is stable over time, and leads to distress or impairment.

personifications According to Harry Stack Sullivan, distorted images of certain relationships that spill over or transfer into other relationships.

pervasive developmental disorder Problems severe enough to affect several areas of a child's functioning (including difficulty with social interaction skills, communication skills, and learning) and behavior that is different from other children of the same age and developmental level.

phobia Unnatural fear of people, animals, objects, situations, or occurrences.

phototherapy Exposure of clients to full-spectrum light for certain periods during the day for the relief of depressive symptoms that occur during the winter months.

physical properties In a therapeutic environment, temperature, lighting, sound, cleanliness, and aesthetics.

physiological stress response Mechanism that protects mammals during times of threat or illness; fight-or-flight response; a biochemical survival system designed to provide the body with the energy for fighting or fleeing.

pica Eating disorder characterized by ingestion of nonfood items, such as hair, string, or dirt for more than 1 month.

polysomnogram Device that monitors the client's electrophysical responses during sleep and includes such measurements as brain wave activity (electroencephalogram [EEG]), muscle movement (electromyogram [EMG]), and extraocular eye movements (electrooculogram [EOG]).

pornography Writings, pictures, or other messages that are intended to sexually arouse.

positive symptoms In schizophrenia, the signs related to maladaptive thoughts and behaviors, including hallucinations, speech problems, and bizarre behaviors.

postpartum depression A condition characterized by symptoms of tearfulness, irritability, hypochondria, sleeplessness, impairment of concentration, and headache in the days and weeks following childbirth.

posttraumatic stress disorder Problems that develop after a person experiences a psychologically distressing event; characterized by an oversensitivity or overinvolvement with stimuli that recall the traumatic event.

poverty Inability to secure the basic necessities of life, such as food, shelter, and clothing.

poverty of thought Lack of ability to produce new thoughts or follow a train of thought.

preferred provider organization Network of physicians, hospitals, and clinics that agree to provide medical care for the organization's members at a discount.

prejudice Displacement of unacceptable impulses and behaviors onto a culturally different group.

primary gain Physical signs and symptoms of an illness used to relieve an individual's anxieties by masking inner emotional turmoil.

principles Set of standards or code that guides actions.

private law Rules that define the relationships between individuals.

prostitution The selling of sexual favors.

proximal-distal growth The pattern of growth and development where growth occurs from near to far, midline to distal.

psyche Vital or spiritual aspect of the individual as opposed to the body or soma; total components of the id, ego, and superego, including all conscious and unconscious aspects.

psychiatric rehabilitation Multidisciplinary services that assist people with mental health problems to readjust and adapt to life in the community as actively and independently as possible; includes personal adjustment and social, residential, educational, and vocational services. Also called *psychosocial rehabilitation.*

psychoanalysis Branch of psychiatry founded by Sigmund Freud devoted to the study of the psychology of human behavior; also a type of therapy for certain emotional disorders that investigates the workings of the mind.

psychobiology Study of the biochemical foundations of thought, mood, emotion, affect, and behavior.

psychomotor agitation Increased motor behaviors, such as pacing, hand wringing, hair pulling, that are associated with emotional problems.

psychomotor depression Decreased motor activity, such as slowed body movements, stooping posture, and slumping.

psychopath Person with an antisocial personality disorder and a pervasive pattern of disregard for and violation of the rights of others, often using deceit and manipulation.

psychophysical disorders A disorder in which stress-related problems result in physical signs and symptoms.

psychosis Inability to recognize reality, relate to others, or cope with life's demands.

psychosocial rehabilitation Multidisciplinary services that assist people with mental health problems to readjust and adapt to life in the community as actively and independently as possible; includes personal adjustment and social, residential, educational, and vocational services. Also called *psychiatric rehabilitation.*

psychosomatic illness Popular term that describes emotionally (psycho) related physical (somatic) disorders.

psychotherapeutic drugs Chemicals that affect the mind and treat the symptoms of mental-emotional illness.

psychotherapy Any of a large number of related methods of treating mental-emotional disorders by psychological techniques rather than by physical means.

puberty Period in life at which the ability to reproduce is developed, beginning with a 24- to 36-month growth spurt and ending when the reproductive system is mature.

public law Rules that define the relationship between the government and its citizens.

purging Recurring inappropriate behaviors to prevent weight gain; usually associated with bulimia.

race Group of genetically related people who share certain physical characteristics.

rape Forced sexual assault.

rapport Dynamic process; an energy exchange between nurse and client that provides the background for all other nursing actions.

rational suicide Act of purposefully ending one's own life after conscious and rational deliberation.

reasonable and prudent care provider theory Principle by which the law judges a caregiver's actions by comparing what other caregivers would do in similar situations.

recidivism Relapse of a symptom, disease, or behavior pattern.

reformation Changes brought about by the division of the Catholic Church during the sixteenth century.

refugee A person who, because of war or persecution, flees from his or her home or country and seeks refuge elsewhere.

rehabilitation Process of assisting individuals with serious mental illness to effectively cope with their life situations.

relapse The recurrence of the substance-abusing behaviors after a significant period of abstinence.

religion Defined, organized, and practiced system of beliefs and practices usually involving a moral code.

religiosity Delusions of great spirituality; believing one has powers to communicate with God or become a spirit.

remission In chronic mental illness, times of partial or complete disappearance of symptoms.

resistance Client's attempts to avoid recognizing or exploring anxiety-provoking material.

resource linkage Process of matching client's needs with the most appropriate community services.

responding strategies Therapeutic techniques that relate to the nurse's actions or interventions while communicating.

responsibility State of being answerable for acts or decisions and able to fulfill obligations.

restraints Device or drug to aid the immobilization of a client.

rights Power, privilege, or existence to which one has a just claim.

risk factor Something that causes a person or group to be particularly vulnerable to an unwanted event.

risk taking Act of purposefully engaging oneself in unfamiliar activities, then observing one's responses.

role Expected pattern of behaviors associated with a certain position.

role performances Socially expected behavioral patterns.

rumination disorder Uncommon problem of childhood involving regurgitating and rechewing food.

sadism Sexual arousal achieved by inflicting physical or psychological pain or humiliation on another person.

schizoid personality Personalities that lack the desire or willingness to become involved in a close relationship, prefer solitary activities, are emotionally restricted, and communicate emotional detachment, coldness, and a lack of concern for others.

schizophrenia Condition associated with disturbing thought patterns, behaviors, and loss of contact with reality to the point where it impairs functioning.

schizotypal personality Interaction pattern of avoiding people with behaviors characterized by distortions and eccentricities (odd, strange, or peculiar actions).

seasonal affective disorder Levels of mild to moderate depression experienced during long winter days; symptoms begin to lift with the coming of spring.

seclusion Removal of a client to an area of decreased stimulation; isolation of one person from others.

secondary gain Situation in which the payoff for remaining ill outweighs the advantages of recovery and clients profit or avoid unpleasant situations by remaining ill.

seizure Convulsion that is the result of misfired electrical impulses within the brain.

self-actualization Need to achieve one's full potential.

self-awareness Consciousness of one's own individuality and personality.

self-concept All the attitudes, notions, beliefs, and convictions that make up an individual's self-knowledge, including perceptions of personal characteristics and abilities, interactions with other people and the environment, values associated with experiences and objects, and goals and ideals.

self-esteem Individual's judgment of his or her own worth.

self-ideal Personal standards of how one should behave.

self-injury Attempts to harm or hurt oneself.

self-protective responses Ways in which individuals behave to meet safety and security needs, ranging from adaptive to self-destructive.

sensorium Part of the consciousness that perceives, sorts, and integrates information.

sexual abuse Intentional engaging of children or others in inappropriate or illegal sexual activities.

sexual disorder Disturbances in sexual desire or functioning that cause marked distress and interpersonal difficulties.

sexual dysfunction A disturbance anywhere in the four stages (appetite, excitement, orgasm, and resolution) of the sexual response cycle.

sexuality Combination of physical, chemical, psychological, and functional characteristics that are expressed by one's gender identity and sexual behaviors.

sexual orientation Individual's sexual attraction to others. Also called *sexual preference.*

shaken baby syndrome Vigorous manual shaking of an infant who is being held by the extremities or shoulders, leading to whiplash-induced intracranial and intraocular bleeding and no external signs of head trauma.

sick role Actions and behaviors of a person who is ill and excused from everyday responsibilities.

signal anxiety Learned anxiety response to an anticipated event.

situational crisis Event or situation for which one is unprepared, resulting from environmental factors outside the individual.

situational depression Depressive responses tied to a specific event or situation that can be traced to a recognizable cause.

skill development Process of learning and applying more effective methods for coping with life and other people.

slander Verbal communications that result in harm.

sleep disorder Condition or problem that repeatedly disrupts an individual's pattern of sleep.

social isolation Removal of or withdrawal from the company and companionship of other people.

social relationship Relationship between two people based on sharing and enjoyment of each other's company.

soma The body, as distinguished from the mind or psyche.

somatic therapy Physical interventions that affect behavioral changes (e.g., electroconvulsive therapy).

somatization Act of focusing anxieties and emotional conflicts into physical symptoms.

somatoform disorder Disorder in which a child or adult has the signs and symptoms of illness or disease without a traceable physical cause.

space Area that surrounds a person.

speech cluttering Disorder of speech and language processing that results in unorganized, dysthymic, and frequently unintelligible speech.

spinal cord Long "relay station" of nerve tissue that extends from the base of the brain (foramen magnum) to the first or second lumbar vertebra in the lower back through the spinal canal of the spinal column.

spirituality A belief in a power greater than any human being.

splitting Emotionally dividing staff members or other people by complimenting one group and degrading another; performed by clients.

standards of care Written statement describing actions or conditions that direct client care; used to guide practice and evaluate performance; also called standards of practice.

stereotype Oversimplified mental picture of a cultural group.

stigma A sign or mark of shame, disapproval, or disgrace, of being shunned and/or rejected.

stress Any factor that requires a response or change in the functioning of an organism.

substance A drug of abuse, a medication, or a toxin.

substance (drug) abuse Inappropriate use of a drug, medication, or toxin whose use results in dependence, addiction, or withdrawal.

substance (chemical) dependency Occurs when a user must take his or her usual or an increasing dose of the drug to prevent the onset of withdrawal signs and symptoms.

substance use Act of taking a chemical substance.

suicidal attempt Serious self-directed action that is intended to do harm to or end one's own life.

suicidal gesture Suicidal actions that result in little or no injury to oneself but communicate a message.

suicidal ideation Thoughts or fantasies of suicide that are expressed but have no definite intent.

suicidal intention Level of seriousness about committing suicide.

suicidal threat Expressions of the intent to take one's life but without any action.

suicide Act of intentionally taking one's own life.

suicide precautions Standard interventions to prevent a suicide attempt from occurring.

suicidology Study of the nature of suicide.

sundown syndrome A group of behaviors characterized by confusion, agitation, and disruptive actions that occur in the late afternoon or evening. The cause is unknown but sundowning is associated with dementia, loss of cognitive functions, and physical or social stressors.

superego In psychoanalysis, that part of the psyche, functioning mostly in the unconscious, that develops when the standards of the parents and society are incorporated into the ego.

surgery Invasive procedure in which the body is entered through an artificially created opening, abnormal tissue or fluid is removed, and the opening is artificially closed.

surveillance Process of watching over adolescents to determine if they are safe, behaving within acceptable limits, making good decisions, or are in need of adult intervention.

sympathetic nervous system Division of the autonomic nervous system that prepares the body for immediate adaptation through the fight-or-flight mechanism.

synapse Small space or gap that separates nerve cells.

tardive dyskinesia Drug-induced condition that produces involuntary, repeated movements of the muscles of the face, trunk, arms, and legs; usually occurs following a long period of antipsychotic drug use.

temperament Genetically linked biological bases that underlie moods, energy levels, and attitudes.

terminal illness Illness or condition likely to result in death.

territoriality Need to gain control over an area of space and claim it for oneself.

theory Statement that predicts, explains, or describes a relationship between events, concepts, or ideas.

therapeutic communications Interactions that focus on the client, foster the therapeutic relationship, and are specifically designed to achieve client outcomes.

therapeutic environment (milieu) Inpatient psychiatric setting that provides safe, stable surroundings that are structured to enhance the client's response to treatment.

therapeutic relationship Series of interactions initiated by the nurse with the purpose of providing corrective interpersonal experiences.

therapeutic touch Facilitation of healing by the use of the hands to consciously direct energy.

third-party payments Payments for medical costs made by someone other than the client, usually through an insurance company or government program such as Medicare or Medicaid.

thought content What an individual is thinking.

thought processes How a person thinks, analyzes the world, and connects and organizes information.

torticollis Contraction of the cervical muscles that forces the neck into a twisted position.

tort law Division of private law that relates to compensation for a legal wrong committed against the person or property of another.

trance State resembling sleep in which consciousness remains but voluntary movement is lost, as in hypnosis.

transcultural nursing Part of nursing practice in which the nurse assesses, plans, and delivers culturally appropriate care.

transference Client's emotional response to the nurse based on earlier relationships with significant others.

transmission Conscious and unconscious response of the persons involved in the communication to the message received.

transsexualism Discomfort with his or her biological sex and a desire to surgically change sexual anatomy and live as a member of the other sex.

transvestism Practice of dressing in opposite-sex clothing for sexual gratification.

trauma Physical, emotional, or spiritual injury.

traumatic stress reaction A series of behavioral and emotional responses following an overwhelmingly stressful event.

trust Risk-taking process whereby an individual's situation depends on the future behavior of another person.

unconscious Part of the mental function in which thoughts, ideas, emotions, or memories are beyond awareness and not subject to ready recall.

unipolar disorder Classification of mood disorders that includes major depression and dysthymia.

vaginismus Persistent involuntary contractions of the perineal muscles around the outer third of the vagina whenever vaginal penetration is attempted.

value Dearly held belief about the worth of an idea, behavior, or item.

values clarification Method for discovering one's own values by assessing, exploring, and determining what those personal values are and how they affect personal decision making.

verbal communications Level of communication related to the spoken word, which includes the spoken and written word, use of language and symbols, and arrangement of words or phrases.

verbigeration The purposeless repetition of words or statements.

victim Person who has been caused harm through the actions of another.

victimization Process of causing harm; children suffer more victimizations than do adults, including more conventional crime, more family violence, and some forms unique to children, such as family abduction, neglect, and abuse.

violence Any behavior that threatens or harms another person or his or her property.

voluntary admission Request for mental health services that is originated by the client.

voyeurism Sexual arousal achieved by observing unsuspecting persons who are disrobing, naked, or engaging in sexual activity.

withdrawal Detoxification; process of allowing an addictive substance to leave the body; usually done under medical supervision.

word salad In schizophrenia, verbal communications in which a series of words is used that seem to be unrelated.

young adulthood Period of life that lasts from about 18 to 35 years of age.

Index

Chapter 1

The History of Mental Health Care

Review Worksheet

1. Write your definition of mental health and mental illness.

   _____

   _____

   _____

Match the following:

   a. Hippocrates   d. Dorthea Dix
   b. Plato   e. Benjamin Rush
   c. Philippe Pinel   f. Clifford Beers

2. _____ Surveyed conditions of mental hospitals in United States, Canada, and Scotland.

3. _____ Wrote a book that started the mental hygiene movement.

4. _____ Said life was a dynamic equilibrium maintained by the soul.

5. _____ Wrote the first American textbook on psychiatry.

6. _____ Viewed mental illness as the result of an imbalance of humors.

7. _____ Freed the mentally ill in France from their chains.

8. What made witch hunting so popular for 600 years (1200-1700)?

   _____

   _____

   _____

9. Which legislative act called for a neighborhood-based mental health care delivery system?
   a. Mental Health Systems Act of 1977
   b. National Mental Health Act of 1946
   c. Omnibus Budget Reform Act of 1987
   d. Community Mental Health Act of 1963

10. Which legislative act dramatically reduced federal funding for mental health and illness care?
   a. Mental Health Study Act of 1955
   b. Omnibus Budget Reconciliation Act of 1981
   c. Mental Health Systems Act of 1977
   d. Omnibus Budget Reform Act of 1987

Chapter 2
Current Mental Health Care Systems

Student's Name

_____

Date

_____

Review Worksheet

Define the following:

1. third-party payment _____

_____

2. preferred provider organization _____

_____

3. health maintenance organization _____

_____

4. diagnosis-related group _____

_____

5. What factor is considered when admitting a client to an inpatient psychiatric setting?

_____

6. List two outpatient psychiatric care settings.

   a. _____

   b. _____

7. Identify each health care team member to complete the puzzle.

ACROSS
2. PhD who does diagnostic testing
3. MD team leader
4. Member who assists clients with specialized needs
5. Member responsible for management of the environment

DOWN
1. Member who evaluates families and their interactions with environment

8. List four components of case management.

a. _____

b. _____

c. _____

d. _____

9. Define holistic health care.

_____

_____

_____

10. List two mental health problems associated with HIV/AIDS.

a. _____

b. _____

Chapter 3
Ethical and Legal Issues

Student's Name

_____

Date

_____

Review Worksheet

Match the following terms and their definitions.

    a. laws   d. nonmaleficence
    b. rights   e. ethics
    c. morals

1. _____ Serves as one's personal basis for right or wrong behaviors

2. _____ Power to which one has a just claim

3. _____ To do no harm

4. _____ Shared set of rules that govern right behavior

5. _____ Controls by which a society governs itself

6. Complete the crossword puzzle.

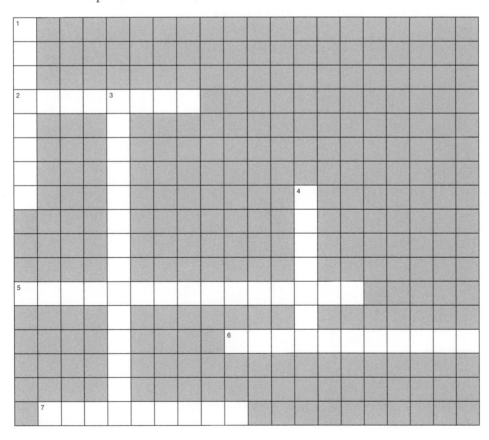

ACROSS
2. Right of people to act for themselves
5. Duty to respect private information
6. Duty to actively promote good
7. Duty to keep promises

DOWN
1. Duty to tell the truth
3. Duty to do no harm
4. Duty to treat all equally

7. Arrange the steps for resolving ethical dilemmas in order.

_____ Gather relevant information.

_____ Take action.

_____ Assume good will.

_____ List and rank values.

_____ Identify all elements of the situation.

8. List three areas of potential liability for nurses and other care providers.

a. _____

b. _____

c. _____

Match the following examples with the appropriate tort.
   a. "She's a nasty old lady who bites."
   b. "If you don't cooperate, I'll call the techs and we will lock you up."
   c. Leaving a suicidal client unattended and he harms himself.
   d. Searching a client's belongings without permission.
   e. Charting a medication that was not actually given.

9. _____ assault

10. _____ malpractice

11. _____ fraud

12. _____ slander

13. _____ invasion of privacy

Chapter 4
Sociocultural Issues

Student's Name

_____

Date

_____

Review Worksheet

Fill in the blanks.

1. _____ A group of people who share distinct physical characteristics.

2. _____ Learned behavior patterns with shared values system.

3. _____ Customs and cultural habits of a group.

4. _____ An oversimplified mental picture of a cultural group.

5. _____ An expected pattern of behavior associated with a certain position or rank.

6. List four characteristics of culture.

   a. _____

   b. _____

   c. _____

   d. _____

7. Complete the crossword puzzle.

ACROSS
1. Condition in which a physical dysfunction exists
3. Belief that illness is the result of an imbalance of energy forces
5. Belief that illness is the result of punishment
6. Results of living up to norms and role expectations

DOWN
2. A state of physical, social, and emotional dysfunction
4. A belief that is widespread in Haitian culture

8. List which area of the cultural assessment relates to each of the following statements.

   a. _____ "I practice Buddhism."

   b. _____ "Pleasing the ancestors is more important than today's problems."

   c. _____ He speaks Italian and Spanish.

   d. _____ She visits an herbalist monthly.

9. Describe how stereotyping can influence the care of mental health clients.

   _____

   _____

   _____

Chapter 5

Early Theories and Therapies

Student's Name

_____

Date

_____

From the list below, match the following people with the appropriate theory and fill in the blanks.

Hippocrates   Abraham Maslow   Carl Jung
Charles Darwin   Sigmund Freud   Carl Rogers
Jean Piaget   H.S. Sullivan   B.F. Skinner
Erik Erikson

1. _____ Introduced the theory that only the fittest survive through the process of natural selection.

2. _____ Used operant conditioning to change observable behavior through the use of positive and negative reinforcers.

3. _____ Developed client-centered therapy.

4. _____ Devised the psychoanalytic theory of human behavior.

5. _____ Constructed the theory of motivation based on human needs.

6. _____ Interpersonal psychology focused on the social nature of people and the role of anxiety in personality formation.

7. _____ Developed the eight stages of psychosocial development.

Fill in the blanks.

8. A _____ is defined as a statement that describes or explains a

_____ among ideas, concepts, or events.

9. A _____ is an example or pattern that provides a _____ for a theory.

Match the therapy with the statement that best describes it.
    a. actualizing therapy   e. gestalt therapy
    b. assertiveness training   f. interpersonal therapy
    c. behavior modification   g. logo therapy
    d. client-centered therapy   h. psychoanalysis

10. _____ Based on a person's need to search for meaning and values in life.

11. _____ Uses dream analysis and free association to uncover unconscious conflicts.

12. _____ Uses operant conditioning to change specific actions.

13. _____ Helps clients to uncover how their personifications (distorted images) affect their lives.

14. _____ The client directs the therapeutic relationship using the therapist as a guide to self-understanding.

15. _____ Teaches clients to express themselves in constructive, nonaggressive ways.

16. _____ Goal of therapy is self-actualization, not cure or relief of symptoms.

17. Describe how Maslow's theory is used in planning care for mentally ill clients.

_____

_____

_____

Chapter 6
Contemporary Theories and Therapies

Student's Name

_____

Date

_____

Review Worksheet

Briefly describe the following:

1. systems theory _____

2. life space _____

3. homeostasis _____

4. crisis _____

5. fight-or-flight response _____

Fill in the blanks.

6. The concept of equilibrium, devised by Lewin, states that each body system attempts to _____ _____ within itself and among other systems.

7. Thomas Szasz states that mental illness is a _____ , and every person is responsible for his or her own _____ .

Match the concept or therapy with the most appropriate selection.

    a. covert modeling   d. sociocultural theory
    b. social learning theory   e. individual therapy
    c. behavior modification   f. general adaptation theory

8. _____ Describes the physical responses of the body to stress and the processes by which they adapt.

9. _____ People learn by observing the outcomes of various events and then comparing themselves with others.

10. _____ Used by therapists to define positive behaviors and develop programs with specific reinforcements to change the specified behaviors.

11. _____ A process described as the act of mentally rehearsing an activity before actually engaging in the activity.

12. _____ The concept of self is developed through interactions with other people.

Chapter 7

Psychotherapeutic Drug Therapy

Student's Name

_____

Date

_____

Review Worksheet

1. Circle the correct parasympathetic nervous system action.
   a. The pupils of the eye dilate.
   b. Saliva, tears, and respiratory and gastrointestinal secretions decrease.
   c. The smooth muscles of the lungs constrict and restrict airways.
   d. The blood vessels in the heart and skeletal muscles dilate.

2. The _____ prepares the body for immediate adaptation through the fight-or-flight response.
   a. central nervous system
   b. peripheral nervous system
   c. sympathetic nervous system
   d. parasympathetic nervous system

3. List the four responsibilities (client care guidelines) for clients on psychotherapeutic drug therapy.
   a. _____
   b. _____
   c. _____
   d. _____

Match the following terms and their definitions.
   a. benzodiazepines   d. hypertensive crisis
   b. anticholinergic reaction e. tricyclic drugs
   c. EPSEs

4. _____ Treats depression

5. _____ Treats anxiety

6. _____ Dry mouth, blurred vision, sweating

7. _____ Akathisia, dyskinesia, akinesia

8. _____ Stiff neck, throbbing headache, tightness in the chest

9. What do you suspect is happening to the client who complains of feeling jittery, is unable to sit still, and has problems with eye movements?

   _____

   _____

   _____

10. An informed decision made by a client not to follow the prescribed treatment program is called

_____ .

Circle the correct answer.

11. Why must salt intake be monitored in clients who are receiving lithium?
   a. Salt and water compete for lithium in the tissues.
   b. Salt and lithium compete for excretion in the kidney.
   c. Salt competes with lithium for detoxification in the liver.
   d. People who take lithium crave large amounts of salt.

Chapter 8
Principles of Mental Health Care

Review Worksheet

Match the following terms and their definitions.

a. principle   d. responsibility
b. empathy   e. consistency
c. advocacy

1. _____ Capability of making and fulfilling obligations

2. _____ Reliability, stability

3. _____ The providing of information to make a decision

4. _____ Code that guides decisions and actions

5. _____ Ability to see the world as another person does

State which principle of mental health care is being used in the following situations.

6. All clients will be at breakfast by 0800.

   Principle: _____

7. Mr. J. is practicing anger control by counting to 10 before he speaks out.

   Principle: _____

8. Caregiver Jane sits with a mute client for 15 minutes every morning.

   Principle: _____

9. Nurse Dan is not intimidated by Mr. Jones's rough appearance and salty mannerisms.

   Principle: _____

10. Miss Sally is expected to arrive for her appointment at 1300 every other day.

    Principle: _____

11. Sam states he is being followed by the FBI. The caregiver responds with, "Would you like to talk about it?"

    Principle: _____

12. List the five steps of the therapeutic (nursing) process.

    a. _____

    b. _____

    c. _____

    d. _____

    e. _____

Chapter 9

The Therapeutic Environment

Student's Name

_____

Date

_____

Review Worksheet

1. John S. is a 30-year-old man who has overdosed on methamphetamine. He states that he feels unable to control his behavior. Do you think he should be admitted to an inpatient environment? _____ Explain your answer. _____

2. List three purposes of the inpatient therapeutic environment.

   a. _____

   b. _____

   c. _____

Describe one intervention for each of the following client needs.

3. nourishment _____

4. personal hygiene _____

5. sense of security _____

6. territory _____

7. communication _____

8. social relationships _____

9. acceptance _____

10. time _____

Fill in the blanks.

11. One of the greatest roadblocks for people with mental/emotional problems is the _____ attached to mental illness.

12. Repeated admissions to psychiatric inpatient facilities have become a way of life for many people with chronic mental illness. This situation is known as _____ .

13. Clients who do not follow their prescribed courses of treatment are called _____ .

Chapter 10

The Therapeutic Relationship

Student's Name

_____

Date

_____

Review Worksheet

Match the following terms and their definitions.

   a. trust   d. caring
   b. empathy   e. hope
   c. autonomy

1. _____ The ability to direct and control one's own activities

2. _____ Confident but uncertain view of the future

3. _____ Process in which one's situation depends on the future behavior of another person

4. _____ Energy that allows caregivers to accept and care for each client as a person

5. _____ Ability to share in the client's world

6. List steps to develop caring.

   a. _____

   b. _____

   c. _____

   d. _____

7. List four ways in which the caregiver instills hope in clients.

   a. _____

   b. _____

   c. _____

   d. _____

Identify the phase of the therapeutic relationship and fill in the blanks.

8. _____ Reviews progress toward meeting goal and prepares client for independence.

9. _____ Gathers data and explores feelings about client.

10. _____ Establishes a working agreement (caregiver-client contract) with client.

11. _____ Client and care provider work on meeting the mutually agreed-on goals.

Chapter 11

Therapeutic Communication

Student's Name

_____

Date

_____

Review Worksheet

1. Complete the crossword puzzle.

ACROSS

4. All persons have the right to live and have someone care for them
6. Desire to know both positive and negative sides of person
7. Ensures client's safety; anticipates problems and troubles
8. Consistent, open, and frank communications

DOWN

1. Nurse is present, available, and has tangible aid to offer
2. Communicates that it is acceptable to try new ways of thinking and behaving
3. Communications are clear, specific, and to the point
5. Belief in client's ability to solve problems and assume responsibility for his/her own life

List the communication as therapeutic (T) or nontherapeutic (NT).

2. _____ "Would you like to talk about it?"

3. _____ "Everything will be all right."

4. _____ "I'm glad you decided to do that."

5. _____ "You appear tense."

6. _____ "Dr. Dee is a very good psychiatrist. You should learn to trust him."

7. _____ "How did this make you feel?"

8. _____ "I'm not sure I understand."

Fill in the blanks.

9. A speech pattern that is associated with mentally ill clients in which the client shifts rapidly between unrelated ideas is called _____ .

10. A nontherapeutic communication technique in which the caregiver responds with cliches or trite expressions is called _____ .

Chapter 12

The Most Important Skill: Self-Awareness

Student's Name

_____

Date

_____

Review Worksheet

Match the following terms and their definitions.

- a. caring
- b. insight
- c. failure
- d. acceptance
- e. helping boundaries
- f. commitment
- g. nurturing

1. _____ Can provide opportunities for learning

2. _____ The recognition of and attendance to meeting needs

3. _____ A personal bond to a course of action

4. _____ The ability to understand the nature of things

5. _____ Helps to define the limits of the nurse's therapeutic behaviors

6. _____ The receiving of what is being offered

7. Her client committed suicide 3 days after he was discharged, and Rachel feels a great sense of failure. List three ways that she could grow from failure.

   a. _____

   b. _____

   c. _____

Fill in the blanks.

8. Peoples' values and belief systems have a strong impact on their _____ .

9. A caregiver's ability to care for clients depends on how well the caregiver _____ .

10. Introspection is the process of _____ .

11. Professional helping boundaries help define _____ .

12. The caregiver's most important commitment is to _____ .

Chapter 13

Mental Health Assessment Skills

Review Worksheet

Fill in the blanks.

1. The purpose of the assessment step of the nursing (therapeutic) process is _____

   _____ .

2. The holistic assessment focuses on five aspects or dimensions of a person. List these dimensions.

   a. _____

   b. _____

   c. _____

   d. _____

   e. _____

3. The purpose of the mental status examination is _____

   _____ .

4. The purpose of a physical assessment (examination) for mental health clients is _____

   _____ .

5. List 10 areas assessed with the mental status examination.

   a. _____

   b. _____

   c. _____

   d. _____

   e. _____

   f. _____

   g. _____

   h. _____

   i. _____

   j. _____

Chapter 14

Problems of Childhood

Review Worksheet

Circle the correct answer.

1. Temper tantrums are a common behavior in
   a. infants.
   b. 1- to 4-year-olds.
   c. 5- to 9-year-olds.
   d. children over 10 years old.

2. The effects of poverty on children
   a. are small and unimportant.
   b. have little impact on their mental health.
   c. can have a strong impact on children's growth and development.
   d. are not considered when making a diagnosis.

3. Mental health assistance should be sought for parent-child conflicts when the
   a. conflict worsens over a period of time.
   b. parents are tired of dealing with the conflict.
   c. child threatens to run away.
   d. child's behavior is out of control.

4. One of the most frequent anxieties of young children is a fear of
   a. strangers.
   b. new people and places.
   c. separation from their parents.
   d. separation from a favorite object.

5. Children with depression
   a. act out.
   b. giggle continually.
   c. lose interest in school and friends.
   d. often stop talking and stare into space.

Short answer

6. Somatoform disorders are thought to be caused by _____ .

7. Extremely traumatic events involving injury or threat to a child often result in the development of

   PTSD because _____ .

8. Children with enuresis can often be helped with _____

   _____ .

9. Autism is diagnosed when the child has serious problems with:

a. _____

b. _____

c. _____

10. Three general therapeutic interventions for children with mental health problems are:

a. _____

b. _____

c. _____

Chapter 15

Problems of Adolescence

Student's Name

_____

Date

_____

Review Worksheet

Short answer

1. Brian thinks through a problem by considering several options. He is learning to use and apply

_____ .

2. A teen's peer group has several important functions. The most important is _____

_____ .

3. When an adolescent's behaviors or problems impair performance (school, social, work) or threaten

   physical well-being, what is needed? _____ .

4. Describe the therapeutic intervention known as surveillance. _____

_____

Match the following terms and their definitions.
   a. behavioral disorder   f. sexual disorder
   b. emotional disorder   g. psychotic disorder
   c. eating disorder   h. suicidal problems
   d. chemical dependency   i. limit setting
   e. personality disorder   j. skill development

5. _____ Becomes preoccupied with ridding self of own characteristics and assuming those of the desired sex.

6. _____ Anorexia nervosa or bulimia.

7. _____ Symptoms include fighting, temper tantrums, running away from home, destroying property, and problems with authorities and school.

8. _____ Thoughts or actions to take one's own life.

9. _____ Problem solving, social interactions, working cooperatively in a group.

10. _____ Moods range from depression to hyperactivity, anxiety.

11. _____ Understanding the rules and consequences of breaking the rules.

12. _____ Moves from experimenting to burnout.

13. _____ Characterized by a loss of contact with reality.

14. _____ A major characteristic is impulsivity, the drive to engage in an act that is harmful to self or others.

Chapter 16

Problems of Adulthood

Student's Name

_____

Date

_____

Review Worksheet

1. Describe how a young adult's sense of personal identity affects his or her functioning.

   _____

   _____

2. How would you respond to a 20-year-old who wanted a baby so she would have someone to love her?

   _____

   _____

3. Describe three characteristics of a mentally healthy adult.

   a. _____

   b. _____

   c. _____

Short answer

4. When an individual's ability to problem solve in effective ways is limited, what commonly occurs?

   _____

5. A frequent source of problems for families with children is _____ .

6. Young adults are more vulnerable to contracting HIV/AIDS because _____

   _____ .

7. The most important therapeutic tool in the treatment of HIV/AIDS is _____ .

8. Beyond the diagnostic labels of mental illness lies _____ .

9. Middle-age adults are faced with accepting _____ .

10. Joe is a 23-year-old man with AIDS who has had sexual relationships with 12 women and 2 other men. How many women has Joe put at risk for contracting HIV? _____

    How many men? _____

Chapter 17

Problems of Late Adulthood

Review Worksheet

Define the following signs or symptoms.

1. hoarding _____

2. agnosia _____

3. apraxia _____

4. aphasia _____

5. conative loss _____

6. memory loss _____

7. delirium _____

8. Alzheimer's disease _____

9. List three general health care goals for the care of clients with Alzheimer's disease.

   a. _____

   b. _____

   c. _____

10. Explain the concept of respect and its importance to geriatric health care.

   _____

   _____

   _____

Chapter 18

Illness and Hospitalization

Review Worksheet

Circle the correct answer.

1. The experience of being hospitalized is a
   a. developmental crisis.
   b. personal crisis.
   c. situational crisis.
   d. maturational crisis.

2. An individual's state of health
   a. remains stable throughout life.
   b. is constantly changing.
   c. changes through childhood and then stabilizes as an adult.
   d. is in a state of disequilibrium.

3. The stage of illness in which a person experiences symptoms is called the
   a. first stage.
   b. second stage.
   c. third stage.
   d. fourth stage.

4. Nurses and other caregivers must always remember that _____ is just as important as good physical care.
   a. entertainment
   b. nutritional care
   c. financial arrangements
   d. psychosocial care

5. The way a person responds to the stresses of illness or hospitalization is based on
   a. how the person interprets the situation.
   b. how the person behaves when ill.
   c. how the person treats his or her physicians and nurses.
   d. his or her insurance coverage.

6. A refusal to acknowledge painful facts is called _____.

7. A feeling of having been mistreated, opposed, or injured is known as _____.

8. An overwhelming emotional state where one is unable to process information is known as

_____.

9. List the three stages of the hospitalization experience.

   a. _____

   b. _____

   c. _____

10. List three ways in which nurses can support family members and significant others.

   a. _____

   b. _____

   c. _____

Chapter 19

Loss and Grief

Student's Name

_____

Date

_____

Review Worksheet

Define the following terms.

1. external losses _____

2. internal losses _____

3. grief _____

4. the grieving process _____

5. mourning _____

6. List two types of dysfunctional (unresolved) grief.

   a. _____

   b. _____

7. List the five stages of dying, as defined by Elizabeth Kübler-Ross.

   a. _____

   b. _____

   c. _____

   d. _____

   e. _____

Circle the correct answer.

8. Mary was widowed about 10 months ago. Although she seems to be adjusting well to the loss of her husband, lately she has been refusing invitations to social events. When she is visited by friends, she continually reminisces about her past. During her last visit, she told a friend that she was not really interested in her activities and would prefer to be left alone. Mary is suffering from
   a. denial.
   b. normal grief.
   c. complicated grief.
   d. complex grief.

9. Health care providers should share in the grief experience with the loved ones of a deceased person, but they should remember that their primary goal is
   a. to work through their own grief.
   b. to provide support for the grievers.
   c. to provide care for the body.
   d. to complete the documentation of the death.

10. Mr. Clark is a 26-year-old man who was recently diagnosed with a fatal illness. During one of his visits to the clinic, he tells the medical assistant that he has decided to refuse further treatment for his condition. How will this decision change the goals of care for this client?
   a. The goal will change to providing support for his choice.
   b. The goal will change to persuade him to reconsider his choice.
   c. The goal to keep him alive as long as possible will remain the same.
   d. The goal to cure the illness will remain the same.

Chapter 20
Anxiety Disorders

Student's Name
_____

Date
_____

Review Worksheet

Identify the level of anxiety (mild, moderate, severe, panic) for the following behaviors.

1. _____ After the news of her father's accident, Maria feels "overloaded." She begins to wring her hands, pace, and wander around the room moaning.

2. _____ Sam is awaiting the results of his examination. He appears to be calm and relaxed.

3. _____ Rose has just learned that she is being evicted from her home. She reacts by sitting immobilized. When questioned, she is unable to think or speak logically.

4. _____ Marian is preparing to free-climb a challenging mountain. She feels energized and concentrates on reaching her destination.

5. Describe maladaptive anxiety and list two examples. _____

   _____

   a. _____

   b. _____

6. List three behavioral addictions (compulsions).

   a. _____

   b. _____

   c. _____

7. Identify two useful purposes of anxiety.

   a. _____

   b. _____

Indicate if the following interventions are therapeutic (TI) or nontherapeutic (NI).

8. _____ Telling the client that everything will be all right as soon as the medication takes effect.

9. _____ Teaching the client to problem solve.

10. _____ Assessing every child for the presence of anxiety and stress.

Chapter 21

Depression and Other Mood Disorders

Review Worksheet

Student's Name

_____

Date

_____

Identify the level of depression and circle the correct answer.

1. Linda is a 22-year-old woman who has recently developed feelings of sadness and loss following a breakup with her boyfriend. She has noticed no appetite or sleep changes.
   a. mild depression
   b. moderate depression
   c. severe depression

2. Harold has become unable to concentrate or follow through with tasks. Lately even his appearance has begun to suffer. Today he spent the day staring at a blank television screen.
   a. mild depression
   b. moderate depression
   c. severe depression

3. Rosie has to drag herself from chore to chore throughout the day. She feels helpless and ineffective when she has to care for her children and believes there is no escape from her unhappy situation.
   a. mild depression
   b. moderate depression
   c. severe depression

Short answer

4. What dietary restrictions should be taught to clients taking MAOIs? _____

   _____

5. Toxicity should be suspected when lithium levels are above _____ .

6. Describe the behaviors associated with hypomania. _____

   _____

7. The main characteristic of _____ is sudden or dramatic shifts in moods.

8. The drug classes most frequently used to treat mood disorders are _____

   _____ and _____ .

List one therapeutic intervention for the following complaints.

9. Feelings of wanting to commit suicide _____

   _____

10. Excessive sweating after taking a tricyclic antidepressant _____

_____

11. Client began antidepressant drug therapy 5 days ago. Today she has suddenly developed confusion and delirium. _____

_____

12. Rex has been taking lithium for about 3 months. Yesterday he urinated more than 4 quarts in less than 24 hours. List two interventions. _____

_____

13. Conchita tells you that she cannot talk to other people because they will find out how stupid she really is. _____

_____

Chapter 22

Physical Problems, Psychological Sources

Student's Name

_____

Date

_____

Review Worksheet

Match the following terms and their definitions.

- a. primary gain
- b. secondary gain
- c. hypochondriasis
- d. conversion disorder
- e. malingering
- f. physiological stress response
- g. body dysmorphic disorder

1. _____ Intense fear of having a disease.

2. _____ Often presents as seizure disorder in children under 10 years of age.

3. _____ Relieves anxiety by masking inner emotional turmoil.

4. _____ Produces symptoms to meet a recognizable goal.

5. _____ Being relieved of responsibilities, having dependency needs met.

6. _____ A preoccupation with a physical difference or defect in one's body.

7. _____ The fight-or-flight response.

8. The purpose of the physiological stress response is to
   a. decrease stress.
   b. keep hormone levels functional.
   c. protect the individual from anxiety.
   d. protect the individual from threat or illness.

9. When the body is under continual or repeated stress, it responds by activating the fight-or-flight mechanism, which can result in
   a. an energized feeling.
   b. an emotional discharge.
   c. anger that is directed outward.
   d. physical signs and symptoms of an illness, disease, or disability.

10. The _____ theory states that individuals are biochemically patterned to react to stress in childhood.

11. In somatoform disorders, the development of physical symptoms is the result of attempts to

_____ .

12. Because of the chronic nature of the disorder and the fact that they are "doctor shoppers," clients with _____ are difficult to treat.

13. List three therapeutic interventions for clients with somatoform disorders.

a. _____

b. _____

c. _____

Chapter 23
Eating and Sleeping Disorders

Review Worksheet

Match the following terms and their definitions.

a. anorexia nervosa	f. narcolepsy
b. bulimia	g. parasomnia
c. obesity	h. dyssomnia
d. insomnia	i. polysomnogram
e. hypersomnia	j. sleep apnea

1. _____ An abnormality in the amount, quality, or timing of sleep.

2. _____ A disorder of binge eating and the use of inappropriate methods to prevent weight gain.

3. _____ A disorder of falling or staying asleep.

4. _____ Monitors the body's electrophysical responses during sleep.

5. _____ A condition in which an individual refuses to maintain a normal body weight because of an intense fear of becoming fat.

6. _____ Repeated attacks of sleep.

7. _____ Excessive sleepiness.

8. _____ Excessive body weight.

9. _____ Abnormal behavior or physical events that happen during sleep.

10. _____ Sleep problems that are caused by abnormal ventilation during sleep.

11. The main goal for nurses and other health care providers in treating clients with eating disorders is

_____ .

12. List three nursing diagnoses for clients with eating disorders.

a. _____

b. _____

c. _____

Chapter 24
Dissociative Disorders

Student's Name

_____

Date

_____

Review Worksheet

1. Complete the crossword puzzle.

ACROSS

3. Disconnection from full awareness of self, time, and/or external circumstances
4. To escape or run away from reality
7. Failure to bring various childhood identifications into adult personality (two words)
8. Persons are able to struggle with life's problems while feeling good about living if this is healthy

DOWN

1. Loss of memory
2. A state resembling sleep in which consciousness remains but voluntary movement is lost
3. During an episode, one feels detached or unconnected to the self
5. One of the main causes of dissociative disorders
6. Often expressed through various levels of anxiety and involves feelings of being weak, inadequate, and helpless (more than one word)

2. Bruce has been admitted with a diagnosis of depersonalization disorder. Develop three therapeutic interventions for him.

a. _____

b. _____

c. _____

3. Develop the primary treatment goal for Bruce. _____

_____

4. Explain identity diffusion. _____

_____

Chapter 25

Anger and Aggression

Student's Name

_____

Date

_____

Review Worksheet

Short answer

1. A forceful behaviors that results in injury, abuse, or harm to another is called _____ .

2. Children and adolescents often _____ in an attempt to establish and test the limits of appropriate behavior.

3. _____ is the abuse of members of one sex by members of another.

4. Models of anger and aggression that focus on the interactions of individuals within their social environment and locate the source of violence in interpersonal frustrations are based in the _____ group of theories.

5. Categorize four factors that contribute to the use of aggressive behaviors.

   a. _____

   b. _____

   c. _____

   d. _____

Identify the stage in the assault cycle that most closely matches the listed behaviors.

6. _____ Cries, apologizes, tries to atone (make up) for behaviors.

7. _____ Becomes restless, irritable, argues, paces.

8. _____ Loses control, fights, kicks, bites, screams.

9. _____ Loses ability to reason; becomes flushed or pale.

Indicate if the following statements are true (T) or false (F).

10. _____ The most important intervention is to rapidly assess a potentially violent client.

11. _____ The use of restraints or seclusion is the last level of intervention for an aggressive client.

12. _____ The most therapeutic and experienced care providers never experience feelings of anger or aggression.

Circle the correct answer.

13. The client confides in a friend that she would like to punch her therapist in the face, then smiles sweetly when interacting with the therapist. The client is demonstrating
   a. assertive behaviors.
   b. active-aggressive behaviors.
   c. passive-aggressive behaviors.
   d. impulse-control behaviors.

Chapter 26
Violence

Student's Name
_____

Date
_____

Review Worksheet

Short answer

1. Harm that is caused through a failure to provide for basic needs or by placing an individual's health or welfare at unreasonable risk is called _____ .

2. A term used to describe repeated physical abuse of someone, usually a woman, child, or elder, is _____ .

3. _____ is the intentional misuse of someone or something that results in harm, injury, or trauma.

4. Information that is gathered for legal purposes and helps the law find and convict the perpetrator of a violent act or crime is called _____ .

5. _____ is any behavior that threatens, harms, or injures a person or property.

6. _____ theories state that boys are socialized throughout their childhood to behave more aggressively and violently than girls.

7. A major care goal for victims of violence is _____ .

8. The essential feature of _____ is the development of characteristic symptoms following exposure to extreme traumatic stressors.

9. Every nurse needs to be alert for the possibility of _____ whenever there is a history of unexplained lethargy, fussiness, or irritability in an infant.

10. The most frequent abusers of the elderly are _____ .

Case Scenario: Bonnie R., a 19-year-old mother of two, arrives in the emergency room with her 18-month-old son, Billy. She gives you a vague history of Billy being pushed off the bed by his older brother about 3 or 4 days ago. Since then Billy has been irritable and fussy. He refuses to eat and cries "all the time." Whenever Billy tries to walk, his left leg crumples and he falls. Because of his constant fussing, Bonnie admits to having "smacked him" yesterday so he would "stop screaming."

11. What information in Billy's history provides you with a clue to the possibility of child abuse?

_____

12. What information should your physical assessment include?

_____

13. What is the first priority of care for Billy at this time?

_____

As you assist the physician in placing Billy in traction, you become angry at the thought of Billy having to endure so much unnecessary pain. By the time Billy is finally settled, you are absolutely furious with Billy's mother.

14. How do you cope with these emotions and still remain therapeutic with Billy and his mother?

_____

_____

_____

Chapter 27

Suicide

Review Worksheet

Identify the terms that best describe the behaviors characterized in the following statements.

1. _____ Jerry smokes cigarettes, drives his motorcycle too fast, and likes to feel the thrill of being chased by the police.

2. _____ Heather repeatedly scratches herself until she bleeds because the pain "lets me know I'm still here."

3. _____ Sam states that he will attempt suicide again, but he has not acted so far.

4. _____ Mary overdosed with sleeping medications because she "is tired of fighting."

5. _____ Yesterday John gave his cherished car to his best friend. Last night he died from a gunshot wound to the head.

Indicate if the following statements are true (T) or false (F).

6. _____ Suicidal thoughts or intentions can exist in clients with any medical or mental health disorder.

7. _____ Suicide rates are lower in people who use drugs or alcohol.

8. _____ All suicidal persons are depressed.

9. _____ People who talk about suicide will not attempt to do it.

10. _____ It is harmful to discuss suicide with clients.

Case Scenario: David has recently lost his job, custody of his children, and his car because he was unable to make the monthly payments. He is being admitted following a week-long drunk. He has repeatedly stated that he would be better off dead.

11. The first priority for this client is _____

_____ .

12. It has been assessed that David is a high suicide risk. The type of observation that he requires is

called _____ .

13. Staff members attempt to make a "no self-harm contract" with David. Explain a no self-harm contract. _____

14. David's nurse helps him to explore coping mechanisms that were successful in the past. The purpose of this is to _____ .

Chapter 28

Substance-Related Disorders

Review Worksheet

1. Physical dependence on a drug that is taken despite the problems associated with its use is called

   _____ .

2. _____ occurs when an individual who was previously drug free has re-turned to substance-abusing behaviors.

3. When a person is not using an addictive substance, he or she is practicing _____ .

4. _____ occurs when increasingly larger amounts of a substance are required to produce the desired effect.

5. The incidence of _____ rises when women drink alcohol during pregnancy.

6. Older adults frequently abuse _____ .

Identify the type of substance abuse and circle the correct answer.

7. Jerry has "chugged" large amounts of the substance and now is beginning to show signs of respiratory failure.
   a. antibiotics
   b. amphetamines
   c. alcohol
   d. inhalants

8. The physical assessment of Maria reveals constricted pupils, euphoria, and drowsiness.
   a. PCP
   b. heroin
   c. cocaine
   d. marijuana

9. After injecting or inhaling it, Jamie experiences intense feelings of well-being that last for less than an hour.
   a. alcohol
   b. acid
   c. caffeine
   d. cocaine

10. Stan had a flashback 2 weeks after taking:
    a. alcohol
    b. acid
    c. caffeine
    d. cocaine

11. Amber is unable to sit still, her pulse rate is over 120, and she is constantly talking and fidgeting.
    a. alcohol
    b. acid
    c. amphetamines
    d. alfalfa

12. List four ways that nurses and other care providers act as therapeutic agents when caring for individuals with substance abuse problems.

    a. _____

    b. _____

    c. _____

    d. _____

Chapter 29

Sexual Disorders

Review Worksheet

Identify the terms that most closely describe the behaviors characterized in the following statements.

1. _____ Prefers sexual relationships with persons of the opposite sex.

2. _____ The practice of seeking sexual excitement from wearing the clothing of the opposite sex.

3. _____ An inconsistency between the child's biological sex and his/her identity as a boy or girl.

4. _____ A sexual behavior that departs from society's acceptable modes of seeking sexual gratification.

5. _____ The process of establishing an integrated or complete identity as a homosexual.

6. List four types of homosexual relationships.

a. _____

b. _____

c. _____

d. _____

7. List three theories that attempt to explain why an individual prefers a certain mode of sexual expression.

a. _____

b. _____

c. _____

8. To effectively care for clients with sexual problems, care providers must first examine their own

_____ and _____ .

Chapter 30
Personality Disorders

Student's Name
_____

Date
_____

Review Worksheet

Match the following terms and their definitions.

a. personality
b. temperament
c. dual diagnosis
d. manipulation
e. paranoia
f. psychopath
g. impulsivity
h. deceit

1. _____ A suspicious system of thinking with delusions of persecution and grandeur

2. _____ Controlling others for one's own purposes by influencing them in unfair or false ways

3. _____ Traits and attitudes that identify one as an individual

4. _____ The act of representing as true something that is actually known to be false

5. _____ The biological basis that underlies moods, energy levels, and attitudes

6. _____ Acting without forethought or regard to the consequences

7. _____ Suffering from two or more mental health problems or conditions

8. _____ A pattern of disregard for and violation of the rights of others

9. List three main characteristics of a personality disorder.

a. _____

b. _____

c. _____

10. Paul is unable to control his anger, acts impulsively, and abuses drugs. He has no friends but refuses to seek help. Why do clients like Paul with maladaptive social responses not always benefit from psychotherapy?

_____

_____

11. Identify three classes of medications used to treat clients who have been diagnosed with personality disorders.

a. _____

b. _____

c. _____

Chapter 31

Schizophrenia and Other Psychoses

Student's Name

_____

Date

_____

Review Worksheet

Identify the terms that most closely describe the behaviors characterized in the following statements.

1. _____ Disorders marked by a loss of contact with reality.

2. _____ Lack of energy or motivation.

3. _____ Abnormal involuntary movement disorders caused by a drug-induced imbalance between two major neurotransmitters in the brain.

4. _____ False sensory inputs with no external stimulus.

5. _____ The idea that people or the media are talking about oneself.

6. _____ Inability to recognize familiar environmental objects or people.

7. _____ False perceptions of real objects or persons.

8. _____ Inability to tell where one's body ends and the environment begins.

9. _____ Lack of ability to produce new thoughts or follow a train of thought.

10. Sam is delusional. Describe his behavior. _____

    _____

    _____

11. Lisa is sitting in the corner with her hand covering her mouth. She is whispering, giggling, and appears to be deeply involved in a conversation, but no one is around. This misperception is called

    _____ .

12. Jeremy tells you that Jesus is talking to him because he is the only one left who can save the world.

    This misperception is called _____ .

13. The major responsibilities when caring for clients who are receiving antipsychotic drug therapy are:

    _____

    _____

    _____

Chapter 32

Chronic Mental Health Disorders

Review Worksheet

Short answer

1. Most chronic mental health problems are characterized by periods of
   _____ and _____ .

2. Psychiatric diagnoses serve only to _____ or _____
   certain behaviors because each person's experiences with mental illness is unique.

3. Explain two goals of care for chronically mentally ill individuals.

   a. _____

   b. _____

4. Individuals with _____ are suffering from two psychiatric disorders, one of
   which is usually substance related.

5. List four psychological characteristics of chronic mental illness.

   a. _____

   b. _____

   c. _____

   d. _____

Indicate if the following statements are true (T) or false (F).

6. _____ People with chronic mental illness are unable to care for themselves.

7. _____ The sexual practices of chronically mentally troubled persons place them at an increased risk for
   contracting and transmitting HIV/AIDS.

8. _____ Psychiatric rehabilitation programs teach severely mentally ill clients about the skills needed to
   effectively perform the activities of daily living, including proper nutrition, activity, and rest
   habits.

9. _____ It is inappropriate to ask a client to describe the meaning of his or her hallucinations.

10. _____ Mental health nursing is a critical component of every situation no matter what the diagnosis.

Chapter 33

Challenges for the Future

Student's Name

_____

Date

_____

Review Worksheet

1. List three treatment settings for clients with mental health problems.

   a. _____

   b. _____

   c. _____

Short answer

2. Children who are _____ experience serious threats to their current and future well-being.

3. The "old homeless" tended to be adult, unmarried _____ with an average age of _____ years old.

4. People with _____ make up about one third of the homeless population.

5. The _____ is a federal law that removes the employment barriers for people with mental or physical disabilities.

6. Mental problems that are limited to a specific cultural group of people are called

   _____ .

Indicate if the following statements are true (T) or false (F).

7. _____ Nurses can choose to be self-employed and establish their own practices.

8. _____ Supportive HCAs plan nursing care for the clients in their caseload.

9. _____ A basic concept of psychosocial rehabilitation is self-help.

10. _____ Under certain circumstances changes can be bad for people or organizations.

11. _____ Many people with HIV will demonstrate mental signs and symptoms before physical signs and symptoms.

12. _____ Change involves loss and discomfort.

13. _____ The first step in coping with unplanned change is to reset priorities.